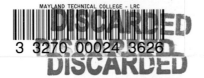

D0095825

ADVANCED AND CRITICAL CARE ONCOLOGY NURSING

Managing Primary Complications

Cynthia C. Chernecky, PhD, RN, CNS, AOCN
Associate Professor, Nursing
Department of Adult Health Nursing
School of Nursing
Medical College of Georgia
Augusta, Georgia

Barbara J. Berger, MSN, RN, CCRN
Clinical Nurse Specialist/Intensive Care Unit and Education Coordinator
University Hospitals
Bedford Medical Center
Bedford, Ohio

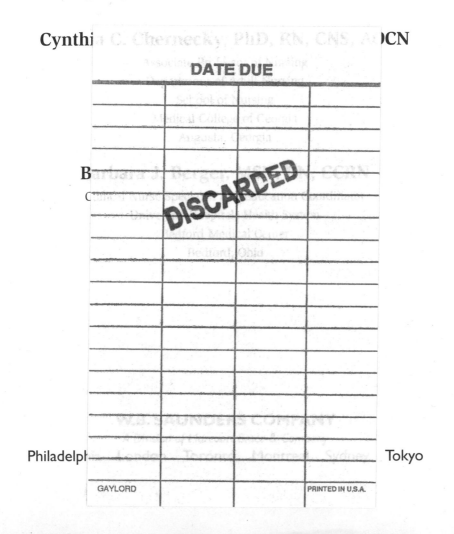

W.B. SAUNDERS COMPANY
A Harcourt Health Sciences Company

Philadelphia   London   Toronto   Montreal   Sydney   Tokyo

W.B. SAUNDERS COMPANY
A Division of Harcourt Brace & Company

The Curtis Center
Independence Square West
Philadelphia, Pennsylvania 19106

Library of Congress Cataloging-in-Publication Data

Chernecky, Cynthia C.
    Advanced and critical care oncology nursing : managing primary
complications / Cynthia C. Chernecky, Barbara J. Berger.
        p.   cm.
    ISBN 0-7216-6860-7
    1. Cancer—Complications. 2. Medical emergencies. 3. Cancer—Nursing.
I. Berger, Barbara J. II. Title.
    [DNLM: 1. Neoplasms—complications—nurses' instruction.
2. Critical Care—nurses' instruction.   WY 156 C521a 1998]
RC262.C436   1998
616.99'2025—DC21
DNLM/DLC
                                                                        97-7109

ADVANCED AND CRITICAL CARE ONCOLOGY NURSING   ISBN 0-7216-6860-7

Printed in the United States of America.

Last digit is the print number: 9   8   7   6   5   4   3   2   1

NOTICE

Medical-surgical nursing is an ever-changing field. Standard safety precautions must be followed, but as new research and clinical experience broaden our knowledge, changes in treatment and drug therapy become necessary or appropriate. The editors of this work have carefully checked the generic and trade drug names and verified drug dosages to ensure that the dosage information in this work is accurate and in accord with the standards accepted at the time of publication. Readers are advised, however, to check the product information currently provided by the manufacturer of each drug to be administered to be certain that changes have not been made in the recommended dose or in the contraindications for administration. This is of particular importance in regard to new or infrequently used drugs. It is the responsibility of the treating physician, relying on experience and knowledge of the patient, to determine dosages and the best treatment for the patient. The editors cannot be responsible for misuse or misapplication of the material in this work.

THE PUBLISHER

CONTRIBUTORS

Barbara J. Berger, MSN, RN, CCRN
Clinical Nurse Specialist and
   Education Coordinator
University Hospitals Health System
Bedford Medical Center
Bedford, Ohio
Hepatic Encephalopathy,
   Hyponatremia

Michelle Budzinski-Braunscheidel,
   BSN, RN, C
Staff Nurse
Cleveland Clinic Foundation
Cleveland, Ohio
Lactic Acidosis—Type B

Karen E. Byrd, RN, MSN, AOCN
Clinical Nurse Specialist, Adult
   Oncology
North Carolina Baptist
   Hospital/Bowman-Grey School of
   Medicine of
   Wake Forest University
Winston-Salem, North Carolina
Bronchiolitis Obliterans

Roger Carpenter, RN, MSN
Professional Education Coordinator
University Hospitals of Cleveland
Cleveland, Ohio
Fever

Cynthia C. Chernecky, PhD, RN,
   CNS, AOCN
Associate Professor of Nursing
Department of Adult Nursing
School of Nursing
Medical College of Georgia
Augusta, Georgia
Hyperkalemia, Hyponatremia

Patricia Manda Collins, MSN, RN,
   OCN
Adjunct Assistant Professor
University of Miami
Miami, Florida
Malignant Pleural Effusions

Wendy Cooper, RN, BSN, OCN
Ambulatory Oncology
   Clinician/Educator
South Fulton Medical Center
East Point, Georgia
Hyperkalemia

Colleen L. Corish, RN, MN, OCN
Bone Marrow Transplant Coordinator
Medical University of South Carolina
Charleston, South Carolina
Bronchiolitis Obliterans

Barbara Daly, PhD, RN, FAAN
Associate Professor
School of Nursing and School of
   Medicine
Case Western Reserve University
Cleveland, Ohio
   and
Co-Director, Clinical Ethics Service
University Hospitals of Cleveland
Cleveland, Ohio
Ethics Case Study

Gail Wych Davidson, RN, BSN
Patient Care Resource Manager
Division of Surgical Oncology
Arthur G. James Cancer Hospital and
   Research Institute
Columbus, Ohio
Malignant Ascites

Peggy Dragonette, MS, RN, CCRN
Clinical Nurse Specialist
University Hospitals of Cleveland
    and
Clinical Instructor
Frances Payne Bolton School of
    Nursing
Case Western Reserve University
Cleveland, Ohio
*Malignant Pericardial Effusion and
    Cardiac Tamponade*

Jean Ellsworth-Wolk, RN, MS, OCN
Oncology Clinical Nurse Specialist
Lakewood Hospital
Lakewood, Ohio
Acute Pancreatitis

Helen Foley, MSN, RN
Clinical Faculty Member
Frances Payne Bolton School of
    Nursing
Case Western Reserve University
Cleveland, Ohio
Hepatic Veno-Occlusive Disease

**Denise Ann Forster, MSN, RN,
    CRRN, CETN, LSW, CANP**
Spinal Cord Injury Program Nurse
    Practitioner, Program Manager
MetroHealth at Home, Home Care
    Agency
MetroHealth Medical Center
Cleveland, Ohio
Spinal Cord Compression

**Eileen M. Glynn-Tucker, RN, MS,
    AOCN**
Oncology Clinical Nurse Specialist
Outpatient Oncology Team Leader
Lake Forest Hospital
Lake Forest, Illinois
*Hypomagnesemia,
    Malnutrition/Cachexia*

Beth Griebel, MSN, RN
Nursing Staff Development Specialist
Arthur G. James Cancer Hospital and
    Research Institute
Columbus, Ohio
Malignant Ascites

Madeline Heffner, RN, BSN, CPNP
Hemophilia Nurse Coordinator
University of Cincinnati Medical
    Center
Cincinnati, Ohio
Hyperuricemia

Janice L. Hickman, MSN, RN, CS
Clinical Nurse Specialist
Neuroscience Intensive Care Unit
University Hospitals of Cleveland
Cleveland, Ohio
    and
Clinical Faculty
Frances Payne Bolton School of
    Nursing
Case Western Reserve University
Cleveland, Ohio
Increased Intracranial Pressure

Wendy Holmes, MSN, RN
Associate Professor
Yale University School of Nursing
New Haven, Connecticut
    and
Clinical Nurse Specialist
Bone Marrow Transplantation
Yale-New Haven Hospital
New Haven, Connecticut
*Hyperleukocytosis in Childhood
    Leukemia*

Bette K. Idemoto, MSN, RN, CS, CCRN
Vascular Clinical Nurse Specialist
University Hospitals of Cleveland
Cleveland, Ohio
and
Clinical Faculty
Frances Payne Bolton School of
Nursing
Case Western Reserve University
Cleveland, Ohio
Hypokalemia

Molly A. Johantgen, MSN, RN, CCRN
Clinical Nurse Specialist, Critical Care
The Christ Hospital
Cincinnati, Ohio
Carotid Artery Rupture

Annemarie Marwitz Kallenbach, RN, BSN, MS, CCRN, TNS
Surgical Intensive Care Unit Patient
Coordinator
Lutheran General Hospital Advocate
Park Ridge, Illinois
Acute Respiratory Distress Syndrome

Catherine Ann Kernich, RN, MSN
Clinical Nurse Specialist
Department of Neurology
University Hospitals of Cleveland
Cleveland, Ohio
and
Clinical Faculty
Frances Payne Bolton School of
Nursing
Case Western Reserve University
Cleveland, Ohio
Seizures

J. Christopher Ladaika, BSN, RN, CCRN
Clinical Nurse
Medical Intensive Care Unit
University Hospitals of Cleveland
Cleveland, Ohio
Hepatic Encephalopathy

Deborah A. Liedtke, MSN, RN, OCN
Head Nurse, Manager
Bone Marrow Transplant and Solid
Tumor Services
University Hospitals of Cleveland
Cleveland, Ohio
Perirectal Infection

Molly Loney, RN, MSN, OCN
Oncology Clinical Nurse Specialist
Columbia St. Luke's Medical Center
A Ministry of the Sisters of Charity of
St. Augustine
Cleveland, Ohio
and
Clinical Faculty
Frances Payne Bolton School of
Nursing
Case Western Reserve University
Cleveland, Ohio
and
Clinical Faculty
Kent State University School of
Nursing
Kent, Ohio
Superior Vena Cava Syndrome

Melissa Manojlovich, MS, RN, CCRN
Nursing Instructor
Henry Ford Community College
5101 Evergreen Road
Dearborn, Michigan
and
Staff Nurse, Medical Intensive Care
Unit
Detroit Receiving Hospital
Dearborn, Michigan
Esophageal Varices

Vicki D. Marsee, RN, BSN, MBA, CNAA
President
Healthcare Leadership Consultants
Tampa, Florida
and
Guest Lecturer
University of South Florida
Tampa, Florida
Ethical Perspectives

Jan L. Hawthorne Maxson, MSN, RN, AOCN
Care Manager
Women's Surgical Oncology
University Hospitals of Cleveland
Cleveland, Ohio
and
Clinical Faculty
Frances Payne Bolton School of Nursing
Case Western Reserve University
Cleveland, Ohio
Syndrome of Inappropriate Antidiuretic Hormone Secretion

Deborah Kryspin Meriney, RN, MN, OCN
Instructor
University of Pittsburgh School of Nursing
Pittsburgh, Pennsylvania
Hypercalcemia

Wendy Rowehl Miano, MSN, RN, AOCN
Associate Director, Ireland Cancer Center
University Hospitals of Cleveland
Cleveland, Ohio
and

Clinical Faculty Member
Frances Payne Bolton School of Nursing
Case Western Reserve University
Cleveland, Ohio
Hepatic Veno-Occlusive Disease

Christine Miaskowski, PhD, RN, FAAN
Professor and Chair
Department of Physiological Nursing
University of California
San Francisco, California
Pain Management: Somatic, Visceral, and Neuropathic

Lisa M. Moles, RN, MSN
Pediatric Nurse Practitioner
Cardiothoracic Surgery
Children's Hospital Medical Center
Cincinnati, Ohio
Typhlitis in Pediatrics

Kathleen Murphy-Ende, RN, PhD, FNP, OCN
Nurse Practitioner
Department of Clinical Oncology
Meriter-Physicians Plus
Madison, Wisconsin
Disseminated Intravascular Coagulation

Patricia Novak-Smith, MS, RN, OCN
Clinical Case Manager, Gynecologic Oncology
University Hospital
Denver, Colorado
Hemorrhage Secondary to Cervical Cancer

Phyllis G. Peterson, RN, MN,AOCN
Assistant Professor, Division of
    Nursing
Our Lady of Holy Cross College
New Orleans, Louisiana
Sepsis and Septic Shock

Anna M. Pignanelli, BSN, RN, C
Clinical Instructor
Cleveland Clinic Foundation
Cleveland, Ohio
Lactic Acidosis—Type B

Linda S. Polman, RN, BSN,
    CPON
Clinical Nurse III, Hematology-
    Oncology Stem Cell Transplant Unit
Children's Hospital Medical Center
Cincinnati, Ohio
Hyperuricemia

Carol S. Potter, RN, MS, AOCN
Oncology Clinical Nurse Specialist
Glenbrook Hospital
Glenview, Illinois
Lambert-Eaton Myasthenic Syndrome

Rosanne M. Radziewicz, MSN, RN,
    CS
Psychiatric Clinical Nurse
    Specialist
MetroHealth Medical Center
Cleveland, Ohio
Suicidal Ideation

Sara J. Reeder, PhD, RN
Assistant Professor
University of Pittsburgh School of
    Nursing
Pittsburgh, Pennsylvania
Hypercalcemia

Marti Reiser, RN, MSN, CCRN
Instructor and Skills Lab Coordinator
Frances Payne Bolton School of
    Nursing
Case Western Reserve University
Cleveland, Ohio
                    and
Staff Nurse (PRN)
University Hospitals of Cleveland
Cleveland, Ohio
Airway Obstruction

Jeanene (Gigi) Robison, MSN, RN,
    OCN
Oncology Clinical Nurse
    Specialist
The Christ Hospital
Cincinnati, Ohio
Tumor Lysis Syndrome

Margaret Quinn Rosenzweig, CRNP-
    C, MSN, AOCN
Clinical Instructor
University of Pittsburgh School of
    Nursing
Pittsburgh, Pennsylvania
Graft vs. Host Disease

Karen Schulz, RN, MSN
Clinical Nurse Specialist
Department of Surgery
Columbia-St. Luke's Medical Center
A Ministry of the Sisters of Charity of
    St. Augustine
Cleveland, Ohio
                    and
Clinical Faculty
Frances Payne Bolton School of
    Nursing
Case Western Reserve University
Cleveland, Ohio
Hypernatremia

Jennifer Simpson, MSN, CRNP
University of Pittsburgh Cancer
   Institute
Pittsburgh, Pennsylvania
Graft vs. Host Disease

Jane Stearns, RN, MSN
Director of Clinical Services
Visiting Nurses Association of
   Cleveland
Cleveland, Ohio
Hemorrhagic Cystitis

Roberta Anne Strohl, RN, MN, AOCN
Clinical Associate Professor
Department of Radiation Oncology
University of Maryland at Baltimore
Baltimore, Maryland
Pathologic Fracture

Paula Timmerman, RN, MSN, AOCN
Oncology Clinical Nurse Specialist
Good Samaritan Hospital
Downers Grove, Illinois
Pulmonary Fibrosis

Gretchen A. Vaughn, RN, MSN
Clinical Nurse Specialist,
   Hematology/Oncology
Children's Hospital Medical Center
Cincinnati, Ohio
      and
Clinical Faculty
University of Cincinnati College of
   Nursing and Health
Cincinnati, Ohio
Typhlitis in Pediatrics

Susanne Vendlinski, BSN, MSN, RN,
  OCN
Instructor
The University of Akron College of
   Nursing
Akron, Ohio
      and
Staff Nurse (per diem)
Akron General Medical and Hospice
   Care Center of the Visiting Nurse
   Service
Akron, Ohio
Diabetes Insipidus

Constance G. Visovsky, MS, RN,
  ACNP
Instructor
Frances Payne Bolton School of
   Nursing
Case Western Reserve University
Cleveland, Ohio
Airway Obstruction

Cynthia L. von Hohenleiten, MN,
  RN, OCN
Nurse Practitioner, Medical Oncology
The Emory Clinic
Atlanta, Georgia
Anaphylaxis from Chemotherapy

Jennifer S. Webster, MN, MPH, RN,
  OCN
Clinical Nurse Specialist, Bone
   Marrow Transplant
Emory University Hospital
Atlanta, Georgia
Anaphylaxis from Chemotherapy

Michael Wrigley, RN, MA
Clinical Nurse, Medical Intensive Care
   Unit
University Hospitals of Cleveland
Cleveland, Ohio
Hepatic Encephalopathy

REVIEWERS

Individual chapters have been reviewed by the following people:

Connie Barden, RN, MSN, CCRN
Clinical Specialist/Case Manager
Mt. Sinai Medical Center
Miami Beach, Florida

Bonnie J. Beach, RN, BSN
Mariner Health Care
Sun City Center, Florida

Catherine M. Bender, PhD, RN
Assistant Professor
Health and Community System
       and
University of Pittsburgh Cancer
    Institute
Pittsburgh, Pennsylvania

Bennie Berry, RN, MSN, CCRN
Staff Nurse, Critical Care
South Fulton Medical Center
East Point, Georgia

Margaret L. Burns, RN, MSN
Staff Nurse
Alton Ochsner Medical Foundation
New Orleans, Louisiana

Dorothy A. Calabrese, MSN, RN,
   CURN, OCN
Cleveland Clinic Foundation
Cleveland, Ohio

Roger Carpenter, RN, MSN
Professional Education Coordinator
University Hospitals of Cleveland
Cleveland, Ohio

Danielle M. Gale, RN, MS, AOCN
Oncology/Biotherapy Care Manager
Lutheran General Hospital
Park Ridge, Illinois

Kathleen M. Hill, RN, MSN, CCRN
Summa St. Thomas School of Nursing
Akron, Ohio

Rosalyn Jordan, RN, ADN
Staff Nurse, Hematology/Oncology
    Unit
Pitt County Memorial Hospital
Greenville, North Carolina

Deborah G. Klein, RN, MSN, CCRN,
   CS
Clinical Nurse Specialist
Trauma/Critical Care Nursing
MetroHealth Medical Center
Cleveland, Ohio

Michele Konnick, MS, RN, CCRN,
   CEN
Indiana University Northwest
Gary, Indiana

Mary Ann Lamont Krall, BS, MS, MSN, RN
Quality Management Nurse, Medicine and Intensive Care
Department of Veterans Affairs Medical Center
Cleveland, Ohio
and
Clinical Faculty
Frances Payne Bolton School of Nursing
Case Western Reserve University
Cleveland, Ohio

Beatrice C. Lampkin, M.D.
Professor of Pediatrics
University of Cincinnati College of Medicine
Cincinnati, Ohio

Deborah A. Liedtke, MSN, RN, OCN
Head Nurse Manager
Bone Marrow Transplant and Solid Tumor Services
University Hospitals of Cleveland
Cleveland, Ohio

Aline T. Mierzejewski, RN, MS, CCRN
Manager, Oncology Critical Care
H. Lee Moffitt Cancer Center and Research Institute
Tampa, Florida

Donna Moses, RN, C, MSN
Educational Nurse Specialist—Trauma
Pitt County Memorial Hospital
Greenville, South Carolina

Kathleen Murphy-Ende, RN, PhD, FNP, OCN
Nurse Practitioner
Department of Clinical Oncology
Meriter-Physicians Plus
Madison, Wisconsin

Becky M. Overcasher, RN, BSN
Neurosurgical Nurse Coordinator
University Hospitals of Cleveland
Cleveland, Ohio

Julie S. Piorkowski, BSPh
Ohio State Board of Pharmacy License
Children's Hospital Medical Center
Cincinnati, Ohio

Penny J. Reiss, RN, MS, CS
Medical-Surgical Clinical Specialist
Good Samaritan Hospital
Downers Grove, Illinois

Karen Ridgeway, RN, MSN
Board of Directors
Children's Cancer Center
Tampa, Florida

Sandra L. Siedlecki, RN, MSN, CEN
University of Akron
Akron, Ohio

Jose I. Suarez, M.D.
Department of Neurology
The Johns Hopkins Medical Institutions
Baltimore, Maryland

Lisa Maree Troesch, RN, BSN, OCN
Arthur G. James Cancer Hospital and Research Institute
Columbus, Ohio

Rachel K. Vanek, RN, C, MSN
Acute Care Nurse Practitioner
Medical Intensive Care Unit
University Hospitals of Cleveland
Cleveland, Ohio

Dave G. Watson, Sr., BA
Cancer Help in Progress
Tampa, Florida

David W. Woodruff, MSN, RN, CCRN
University of Akron
Akron, Ohio

PREFACE

As nurses we care, hope, struggle, and succeed. As a profession we know that our effectiveness increases when we work together for the good of the client. This book is an example of collaboration between oncology and critical care practitioners and the strength that comes from multispecialty professional accountability, the outcome of which is seamless care for the client and family, regardless of the setting. This book extends the example of collaboration between critical care and oncology nurses to other professional health care specialists and includes expertise from authors, contributors, and reviewers. In addition, this text demonstrates a collaborative, in-depth understanding of survival; quality of life; ethics; physical, psychosocial, and emotional demands; and prognosis for oncology clients in crisis and their families. Comprehensive teaching and client/family preparation is included for each primary oncologic complication to assist the nurse working with oncology clients in any setting. Each chapter of this book was either co-authored or written and reviewed, at minimum, by an oncology and a critical care nurse. The knowledge and expertise of both specialties were combined with the most current literature and survival statistics for different types of cancers. The pathophysiology of oncologic complications, risk, treatment approaches, prognosis, assessment findings, and nursing and medical interventions are followed by anticipated outcomes and discharge needs, client education in lay terminology, and likely client/family questions and possible answers. Chapters on ethics related to the oncology client in crisis and his or her family are included to foster further comprehensive care and to provide a logical framework to guide ethical decision-making. Each chapter concludes with test questions designed to help the reader reinforce content and study for certification examinations. The quality of the "need-to-know" information is excellent. When a client experiences an oncologic emergency or primary complication, the book's clarity and format will help the reader quickly find what is needed without wading through extremely long, detailed chapters. The result is a reference that provides, for caregivers in all settings, needed information when working with oncology clients actually or potentially experiencing primary complications of their disease or treatment. We believe we have succeeded in collaborating for the good of the client, family, significant others, community, and nursing profession.

ACKNOWLEDGMENTS

Dedication, caring, trust, and integrity are not just words to me. I have experienced all of these in this project. The professional nurses, oncology and critical care alike, saw the need for a text that would improve care and worked collaboratively and endlessly to meet this goal. I thank each of you personally and all the endless colleagues we consulted for information, who are too numerous to mention. I am thankful to the Medical College of Georgia, in particular, to Dean Vickie Lambert, the School of Nursing faculty, and Jenny Whitlock for their support and enthusiasm; and the Augusta Chapter of the Oncology Nursing Society and my nursing colleagues at the Medical College of Georgia Hospitals and Clinics oncology units and critical care units for their full support and expertise. I also thank my colleague and friend Barbara Berger, who exemplifies professionalism, collaboration, trust, hard work, and an inexhaustible belief in the discipline of nursing. Once again we have made a great team and have had some laughs along the way! I would also like to acknowledge the community of the Orthodox Church of America that supported my spiritual strength, which was necessary to fulfill this project. In particular, I want to thank my mother, Olga Chernecky; my godmother and aunt, Helen Prohorik; my cousins Paula, Karyn, Jonathan and Philip; my nieces Ellie and Annie and nephew Michael; and priests John Townsend, Kirrill Gvosdev, Michael Zaparyniuk, Gregory Koo, Peter Smith, and their Matushkas, and all the deacons, subdeacons, readers, and altar boys. I would also like to thank those who continue to show by example the meaning of the Orthodox faith—namely, Vera Gargano, Barbara and Paul Connelly, Julie Powell, Elaine Calugar, Matushka Joanna Sandiford, Tatiana Koletchko, Pavel Koletchko, Sasha Lisnichuk, Micah Spence, Vincent Hunter, Ray Graves, Liubow Liagin, Rostislav Liagin, choir directors Phyllis Skiba and Dr. Jeff Zdrale, Bonita Zdrale, Clair and Phyllis Gindlesperger, Dr. Leon and Barbara Sheean, Dr. Maria King, Marge Barriusso, Anna Waluchnewicz (who is 105 years young!), Lynn Bennett, Monk Makarios of the Monastery of the Glorious Ascension, and fellow Orthodox Christians at St. Vladimir's Orthodox Theological Seminary and St. Tikon's Orthodox Theological Seminary. Oh, what teamwork can accomplish is truly amazing! So what have I learned throughout my years that I may share with others? It is this; Truth is eternal and knowledge is changeable; I no longer mix these up!

Cynthia C. Chernecky, PhD, RN, CNS, AOCN

This book is designed to help improve the continuity of care for oncology clients in all settings. In particular, I thank my nursing peers from the Medical Intensive Care Unit and the Bone Marrow Transplant/Solid Tumor Unit at University Hospitals of Cleveland for the inspiration to expand our plan for chapter authorship or authorship/review as a collaboration between the two specialties. The staff nurses and managers from these two units work together with bioethicist and nurse Barbara Daly, PhD, RN, FAAN, to learn why and how their approaches to oncology care might differ. In the process, they gain a greater understanding of the needs of oncology clients and their families over the entire continuum of the illness. This leads to a more seamless plan for clients who receive care in both settings.

With extreme gratitude and respect for their dedication to making this text fulfill its promise, I thank my critical care, oncology, and other acute care colleagues in readily and meticulously preparing a resource designed to complement the rest of the oncology and critical care literature. I also thank my patient-focused colleague, mentor, teacher, and supervisor, Martha Allen, MSN, RN, Chief Operating Officer; and the incredibly visionary Arlene Rak, President and Chief Executive Officer, both of UHHS Bedford Medical Center, for their vocal support and positive anticipation of this book as a resource that will help enhance our own oncology nursing care. For their professional recommendations that led us to many of our qualified chapter authors, I acknowledge and thank both Molly Loney, RN, MSN, OCN (chapter author), and Charlene Phelps, MSN, RN, FAAN, Senior Vice President of Nursing, University Hospitals of Cleveland. I thank my husband, Stephan Berger, and my parents, Alice and Arlington Adams, for their patience and support during the time this manuscript was being prepared. Finally, I thank my co-editor and co-author, Cynthia Chernecky, the most optimistic person I have ever known, for the invitation to join her once again in the compilation of a text of which I am extremely proud and of which I am convinced will help make oncology client care more focused and comprehensive in any setting.

Barbara J. Berger, MSN, RN, CCRN

CONTENTS

BODY SYSTEM CROSS-REFERENCE

The following list is a list of body systems and which primary oncologic complications affect each body system. Each primary oncologic complication listed corresponds to a chapter title, where the reader can find necessary information helpful in caring for a client experiencing the complication or body system alteration. The reader is advised that two chapters, "Ethical Perspectives" (1) and "Ethics Case Study" (2), provide valuable assistance when working with clients experiencing any type or location of cancer.

CARDIOVASCULAR
Anaphylaxis from chemotherapy
Carotid artery rupture
Disseminated Intravascular Coagulation
Hemorrhage secondary to cervical cancer
Hypercalcemia
Hyperkalemia
Hypernatremia
Hypokalemia
Malignant ascites
Malignant pericardial effusion and cardiac tamponade
Pulmonary fibrosis
Sepsis and septic shock
Syndrome of inappropriate antidiuretic hormone secretion
Spinal cord compression
Superior vena cava syndrome
Tumor lysis syndrome

ENDOCRINE
Diabetes Insipidus
Fever
Syndrome of inappropriate antidiuretic hormone secretion

FLUID AND ELEC-TROLYTE BALANCE/ HEMODYNAMICS
Acute respiratory distress syndrome
Anaphylaxis from chemotherapy
Bronchiolitis obliterans
Carotid artery rupture
Diabetes insipidus
Disseminated intravascular coagulation
Esophageal varicies
Fever
Graft vs. Host Disease
Hemorrhage secondary to cervical cancer
Hemorrhagic cystitis
Hepatic veno-occlusive disease
Hypercalcemia

Hyperkalemia
Hypernatremia
Hypokalemia
Hypomagnesemia
Hyponatremia
Lactic acidosis type B
Malignant ascites
Malignant pericardial effusion and cardiac tamponade
Malnutrition/cachexia
Pain Management: Somatic, Visceral, and Neuropathic
Perirectal infection
Pulmonary fibrosis
Seizures
Sepsis and septic shock
Syndrome of inappropriate antidiuretic hormone secretion
Spinal cord compression
Superior vena cava syndrome
Tumor lysis syndrome
Typhlitis

GASTROINTESTINAL
Acute pancreatitis
Acute respiratory distress syndrome
Airway obstruction
Bronchiolitis obliterans
Disseminated Intravascular Coagulation
Graft vs. Host Disease
Hypercalcemia
Hyperkalemia
Hyperleukocytosis in childhood leukemia
Hypokalemia
Hypomagnesemia
Increased intracranial pressure
Lambert-Eaton myasthenic syndrome
Malignant ascites
Malnutrition/cachexia
Perirectal infection
Sepsis and septic shock
Syndrome of inappropriate antidiuretic hormone secretion
Spinal cord compression

Suicidal ideation
Tumor lysis syndrome
Typhlitis

HEPATIC
Bronchiolitis obliterans
Disseminated Intravascular Coagulation
Graft vs. Host Disease
Hepatic veno-occlusive disease
Malignant ascites
Pain Management: Somatic, Visceral, and Neuropathic
Seizures
Syndrome of inappropriate antidiuretic hormone secretion

IMMUNE
Acute respiratory distress syndrome
Anaphylaxis from chemotherapy
Bronchiolitis obliterans
Fever
Graft vs. Host Disease
Hemorrhage secondary to cervical cancer
Hyperleukocytosis in childhood leukemia
Lambert-Eaton myasthenic syndrome
Malnutrition/cachexia
Seizures
Sepsis and septic shock

INTEGUMENTARY
Anaphylaxis from chemotherapy
Bronchiolitis obliterans
Carotid artery rupture
Graft vs. Host Disease
Pain Management: Somatic, Visceral, and Neuropathic
Perirectal infection
Seizures
Sepsis and septic shock
Spinal cord compression

MENTAL HEALTH
Bronchiolitis obliterans
Diabetse insipidus
Hypercalcemia

Increased intracranial pressure
Malnutrition/cachexia
Pain Management: Somatic, Visceral, and Neuropathic
Sepsis and septic shock
Spinal cord compression
Suicidal ideation
Superior vena cava syndrome

MUSCULOSKELETAL
Bronchiolitis obliterans
Diabetes insipidus
Hypercalcemia
Hyperkalemia
Hypokalemia
Lambert-Eaton myasthenic syndrome
Pain Management: Somatic, Visceral, and Neuropathic
Pathologic fracture
Spinal cord compression
Tumor lysis syndrome

NEUROLOGIC
Bronchiolitis obliterans
Carotid artery rupture
Cerebral metastasis
Diabetes insipidus
Hepatic encephalopathy
Hypercalcemia
Hyperleukocytosis in childhood leukemia
Hypernatremia
Hypokalemia
Hypomagnesemia
Increased intracranial pressure
Lactic acidosis type B
Lambert-Eaton myasthenic syndrome
Pain Management: Somatic, Visceral, and Neuropathic
Seizures
Sepsis and septic shock
Syndrome of inappropriate antidiuretic hormone secretion
Spinal cord compression
Suicidal ideation
Superior vena cava syndrome
Tumor lysis syndrome

NUTRITIONAL/ METABOLIC

Acute respiratory distress syndrome
Bronchiolitis obliterans
Diabetes insipidus
Graft vs. Host Disease
Hypercalcemia
Hyperkalemia
Hypernatremia
Hypomagnesemia
Hypokalemia
Malnutrition/cachexia
Seizures
Sepsis and septic shock
Syndrome of inappropriate antidiuretic hormone secretion
Spinal cord compression
Suicidal ideation
Typhlitis
Tumor lysis syndrome

PULMONARY

Acute respiratory distress syndrome
Airway obstruction
Anaphylaxis from chemotherapy
Bronchiolitis obliterans
Diabetes insipidus
Disseminated Intravascular Coagulation
Hepatic veno-occlusive disease
Hyperleukocytosis in childhood leukemia
Hypernatremia
Lactic acidosis type B
Lambert-Eaton myasthenic syndrome
Malignant ascites
Malignant pericardial effusion and cardiac tamponade
Malignant pleural effusion
Pain Management: Somatic, Visceral, and Neuropathic

Pulmonary fibrosis
Syndrome of inappropriate antidiuretic hormone secretion
Spinal cord compression
Suicidal ideation
Superior vena cava syndrome

REPRODUCTIVE

Bronchiolitis obliterans
Disseminated Intravascular Coagulation
Hemorrhage secondary to cervical cancer
Lambert-Eaton myasthenic syndrome
Malignant ascites
Pain Management: Somatic, Visceral, and Neuropathic
Syndrome of inappropriate antidiuretic hormone secretion

Spinal cord compression
Suicidal ideation

URINARY/RENAL

Bronchiolitis obliterans
Diabetes insipidus
Hemorrhagic cystitis
Hepatic veno-occlusive disease
Hypercalcemia
Hyperkalemia
Hypernatremia
Hyperuricemia
Hypokalemia
Hypomagnesemia
Malnutrition/cachexia
Pain Management: Somatic, Visceral, and Neuropathic
Syndrome of inappropriate antidiuretic hormone secretion
Spinal cord compression
Tumor lysis syndrome

DISEASE SITE CROSS-REFERENCE

The following is a list of locations in the body that may be involved in cancer. Under each disease site are listed primary complications that may be caused by cancer in that area of the body. Each primary complication corresponds to a chapter title, where the reader can find necessary information helpful in caring for a client experiencing the complication. The reader is advised that two chapters, "Ethical Perspectives" (1), and "Ethics Case Study" (2), provide valuable assistance when working with clients experiencing any type or location of cancer.

ADRENAL GLAND
Hypernatremia
Hyponatremia

BLADDER/KIDNEY
Hepatic veno-occlusive
  disease
Hemorrhagic cystitis
Hypercalcemia
Hyperkalemia
Hypernatremia
Hypokalemia
Lambert-Eaton
  myasthenic syndrome
Malnutrition/cachexia
Pain Management:
  Somatic, Visceral, and
  Neuropathic
Pathologic fracture
Syndrome of
  inappropriate
  antidiuretic hormone
  secretion
Spinal cord compression

BREAST
Acute respiratory distress
  syndrome
Anaphylaxis from
  chemotherapy
Diabetes insipidus
Disseminated
  Intravascular
  Coagulation
Hepatic encephalopathy
Hepatic veno-occlusive
  disease
Hypercalcemia
Lactic acidosis type B
Lambert-Eaton
  myasthenic syndrome
Malignant ascites
Malignant pericardial
  effusion and cardiac
  tamponade
Malignant pleural
  effusion
Pain Management:
  Somatic, Visceral, and
  Neuropathic
Pathologic fracture
Seizures
Spinal cord compression
Suicidal ideation
Superior vena cava
  syndrome
Tumor lysis syndrome
Typhlitis

CENTRAL NERVOUS SYSTEM
Diabetes insipidus
Hyponatremia
Increased intracranial
  pressure
Pain Management:
  Somatic, Visceral, and
  Neuropathic
Pulmonary fibrosis
Seizures
Syndrome of
  inappropriate
  antidiuretic hormone
  secretion
Spinal cord compression
Suicidal ideation
Superior vena cava
  syndrome

CERVIX/UTERINE
Hemorrhagic cystitis
Hemorrhage secondary to
  cervical cancer
Malignant ascites
Pain Management:
  Somatic, Visceral, and
  Neuropathic
Syndrome of
  inappropriate
  antidiuretic hormone
  secretion
Suicidal ideation

COLON/RECTAL
Disseminated
  Intravascular
  Coagulation
Graft vs. Host Disease
Hemorrhagic cystitis
Hepatic encephalopathy
Hypercalcemia
Hypokalemia
Hypomagnesemia
Hyponatremia
Lactic acidosis type B
Lambert-Eaton
  myasthenic syndrome
Malignant ascites
Malnutrition/cachexia
Pain Management:
  Somatic, Visceral, and
  Neuropathic
Perirectal infection
Sepsis and septic shock
Syndrome of
  inappropriate
  antidiuretic hormone

secretion
Spinal cord compression
Superior vena cava
  syndrome
Tumor lysis syndrome

GALLBLADDER
Disseminated
  Intravascular
  Coagulation
Hepatic encephalopathy

GASTRIC/SMALL INTESTINE
Hepatic encephalopathy

HEAD AND NECK
Airway obstruction
Anaphylaxis from
  chemotherapy
Carotid artery rupture
Diabetes insipidus
Hypercalcemia
Hypomagnesemia
Hypernatremia
Hyponatremia
Lambert-Eaton
  myasthenic syndrome
Malnutrition/cachexia
Pain Management:
  Somatic, Visceral, and
  Neuropathic
Seizures
Sepsis and septic shock
Syndrome of
  inappropriate
  antidiuretic hormone
  secretion
Suicidal ideation
Superior vena cava
  syndrome

HODGKIN'S DISEASE
Airway obstruction
Anaphylaxis from
  chemotherapy
Fever
Hyperkalemia
Hyponatremia
Lactic acidosis type B
Malnutrition/cachexia
Pain Management:
  Somatic, Visceral, and
  Neuropathic
Pulmonary fibrosis
Sepsis and septic shock
Syndrome of
  inappropriate
  antidiuretic hormone

secretion
Superior vena cava
  syndrome
Tumor lysis syndrome

KIDNEY (SEE BLADDER/KIDNEY)

LARYNX (SEE HEAD AND NECK)

LEUKEMIA
Acute respiratory distress
  syndrome
Anaphylaxis from
  chemotherapy
Bronchiolitis obliterans
Diabetes insipidus
Disseminated
  Intravascular
  Coagulation
Fever
Graft vs. Host Disease
Hepatic veno-occlusive
  disease
Hypercalcemia
Hyperkalemia
Hyperleukocytosis in
  childhood leukemia
Hypokalemia
Hyponatremia
Lactic acidosis type B
Malignant pericardial
  effusion and cardiac
  tamponade
Malnutrition/cachexia
Pain Management:
  Somatic, Visceral, and
  Neuropathic
Perirectal infection
Pulmonary fibrosis
Seizures
Sepsis and septic shock
Syndrome of
  inappropriate
  antidiuretic hormone
  secretion
Typhlitis
Tumor lysis syndrome

LIVER
Hepatic encephalopathy
Tumor lysis syndrome

LUNG
Acute respiratory distress
  syndrome
Airway obstruction
Diabetes insipidus

Disseminated
  Intravascular
  Coagulation
Hepatic encephalopathy
Hypercalcemia
Hyperkalemia
Hypomagnesemia
Hyponatremia
Lactic acidosis type B
Lambert-Eaton
  myasthenic syndrome
Malignant pericardial
  effusion and cardiac
  tamponade
Malignant pleural
  effusion
Malnutrition/cachexia
Pain Management:
  Somatic, Visceral, and
  Neuropathic
Pathologic fracture
Perirectal infection
Pulmonary fibrosis
Seizures
Sepsis and septic shock
Syndrome of
  inappropriate
  antidiuretic hormone
  secretion
Spinal cord compression
Suicidal ideation
Superior vena cava
  syndrome
Tumor lysis syndrome

LYMPHOMA
Acute respiratory distress
  syndrome
Airway obstruction
Anaphylaxis from
  chemotherapy
Bronchiolitis obliterans
Diabetes insipidus
Disseminated
  Intravascular
  Coagulation
Fever
Graft vs. Host Disease
Hepatic encephalopathy
Hepatic veno-occlusive
  disease
Hypercalcemia
Hyperkalemia
Lactic acidosis type B
Lambert-Eaton
  myasthenic syndrome
Malignant ascites
Malignant pericardial
  effusion and cardiac
  tamponade

Malignant pleural
  effusion
Malnutrition/cachexia
Pain Management:
  Somatic, Visceral, and
  Neuropathic
Pathologic fracture
Perirectal infection
Sepsis and septic shock
Syndrome of
  inappropriate
  antidiuretic hormone
  secretion
Spinal cord compression
Suicidal ideation
Superior vena cava
  syndrome
Tumor lysis syndrome
Typhlitis

MEDULLOBLASTOMA
Tumor lysis syndrome

MELANOMA
Bronchiolitis obliterans
Disseminated
  Intravascular
  Coagulation
Malignant pericardial
  effusion and cardiac
  tamponade
Malnutrition/cachexia
Pain Management:
  Somatic, Visceral, and
  Neuropathic
Seizures
Sepsis and septic shock
Spinal cord compression

MERKEL CARCINOMA
Tumor lysis syndrome

MULTIPLE MYELOMA
Bronchiolitis obliterans
Graft vs. Host Disease
Hypercalcemia
Hypernatremia
Hyponatremia
Lactic acidosis type B
Malnutrition/cachexia
Pain Management:
  Somatic, Visceral, and
  Neuropathic
Pathologic fracture
Pulmonary fibrosis
Sepsis and septic shock
Spinal cord compression
Tumor lysis syndrome
Typhlitis

NEUROBLASTOMA
Tumor lysis syndrome

OVARY
Anaphylaxis from
  chemotherapy
Disseminated
  Intravascular
  Coagulation
Hypercalcemia
Hyponatremia
Lambert-Eaton
  myasthenic syndrome
Malignant ascites
Malnutrition/cachexia
Pain Management:
  Somatic, Visceral, and
  Neuropathic
Sepsis and septic shock
Syndrome of
  inappropriate
  antidiuretic hormone
  secretion
Suicidal ideation
Tumor lysis syndrome

PANCREAS
Diabetes insipidus
Disseminated
  Intravascular
  Coagulation
Hepatic encephalopathy
Hypokalemia
Hyponatremia
Malnutrition/cachexia
Pain Management:
  Somatic, Visceral, and
  Neuropathic
Syndrome of
  inappropriate
  antidiuretic hormone
  secretion
Suicidal ideation

PROSTATE
Disseminated
  Intravascular
  Coagulation
Hemorrhagic cystitis
Hypercalcemia
Hyponatremia
Lambert-Eaton
  myasthenic syndrome
Malnutrition/cachexia
Pain Management:
  Somatic, Visceral, and
  Neuropathic
Pathologic fracture
Syndrome of
  inappropriate
  antidiuretic hormone
  secretion
Spinal cord compression

**RECTUM (SEE
COLON/RECTAL)**

**RHABDOMYO-
SARCOMA**
Tumor lysis syndrome

SARCOMA
Anaphylaxis from
  chemotherapy
Fever
Hypercalcemia
Hyperkalemia
Hyponatremia
Lactic acidosis type B
Malignant pericardial
  effusion and cardiac
  tamponade
Pain Management:
  Somatic, Visceral, and
  Neuropathic
Perirectal infection
Syndrome of
  inappropriate
  antidiuretic hormone
  secretion
Spinal cord compression
Superior vena cava
  syndrome
Tumor lysis syndrome

SEMINOMA
Tumor lysis syndrome

TESTICULAR
Anaphylaxis from
  chemotherapy
Hepatic encephalopathy
Hypomagnesemia
Pain Management:
  Somatic, Visceral, and
  Neuropathic
Pulmonary fibrosis
Superior vena cava
  syndrome

THYROID
Hypercalcemia
Pain Management:
  Somatic, Visceral, and
  Neuropathic
Pathologic fracture
Suicidal ideation
Superior vena cava
  syndrome

VULVA
Tumor lysis syndrome

WILM'S TUMOR
Pulmonary fibrosis

CHAPTER 1

ETHICAL PERSPECTIVES

Vicki D. Marsee, RN, BSN, MBA, CNAA

CHAPTER OBJECTIVES

At the completion of this chapter, the reader will be able to:

Describe the discipline and subdisciplines of ethics.

Discuss ethical theories, principles, and values.

Describe an ethical conflict resolution model.

Differentiate three types of advance directives.

OVERVIEW

ETHICS has many meanings to many people. There are ethical viewpoints on topics ranging from business to family life to politics, but one of the most profound arenas for ethical discussion is in emergency oncologic health care. It is in this arena that decisions must be made about life prolongation, where decisions must be tailored to individual circumstances, needs, and desires, while balancing the benefits against the risks. It is an arena that many times offers several right answers to the same question, even though each answer would lead to a different outcome, and it is an arena in which those whose duty it is to administer the decisions may or may not be in agreement with the final choices.

Nurses, clients, families, and other health care providers share an interest in maximizing positive outcomes by making the best decisions for the welfare of the client. Given this common goal, how then does ethical conflict occur? When it does occur, who has the authority to make a final decision? Furthermore, how can the nurse facilitate conflict resolution and effectively support clients and their families with quite possibly the most important decisions of their lives?

The nurse is in an excellent position to be of assistance in situations of ethical disagreement. As an expert in information gathering, analysis, and interpretation, the nurse possesses most of the tools necessary for effective intervention. All that is needed is a working knowledge of values clarification and the ability to apply ethical principles systematically within the appropriate theoretical framework.

THE DISCIPLINE OF ETHICS

Ethics as a discipline attempts to (1) study moral actions, behaviors, and attitudes descriptively and analytically, and to (2) prescribe what actions, behaviors, and attitudes *ought* to be (Young, 1989, p. 38). Therefore, ethics can be described as a discipline that studies what we do, why we do it, and what ought to be done.

Descriptive ethics is a scientific study of morality. It seeks to provide information on current moral thinking through data collection on moral decision making and to describe and explain which moral views are, in fact, accepted within certain social frameworks. Since morality arises, in part, from the social nature of the community, it provides us with general rules of conduct and standards of evaluation (Fowler, 1987, p. 25). Of course, morality differs among cultures and generations, and it influences lawmaking. Descriptive ethics is generally not considered a subdiscipline of ethics, although it is closely associated with it.

Metaethics, also called analytic ethics, is a subdiscipline of the broader field of ethics. It attempts to analyze and justify moral reasoning and moral concepts such as "a right" or "a duty." Although important from a philosophical standpoint, it is not necessarily of assistance to the nurse in decision-making situations with oncology clients. Normative ethics is also a subdiscipline of ethics. It deals with norms or standards of behavior and with actions that *ought* to be done. It is comprised of judgments of value, rights, duties, and responsibilities. It equates obligations of duty with "oughts."

Branching from normative ethics is the category of applied ethics, which is comprised of many different fields (Fowler, 1987). For example, business has its own ethics concerns, as do law, medicine, and nursing. Applied ethics is more useful to the nurse because it encompasses the principles and values of biomedical ethics, also known as bioethics (Fig. 1–1).

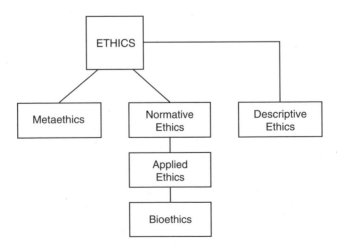

Figure 1–1 Ethics subdisciplines and subcategories.

Table 1–1	
Theories	
Consequentialism (utilitarianism)	Acts are right as long as they produce good consequences.
Nonconsequentialism (deontologism)	Acts are right based on the inherent rightness or wrongness of the act itself.

ETHICAL DECISION MAKING

Oncology clients experiencing emergency situations need assistance to make decisions in their own best interests. Nurses are in an ideal position to provide this service because of their familiarity with the client's history, present state of health, and simply because they *know* the client. To provide maximal assistance, nurses must possess an understanding of the theories, principles, and values upon which the language and substance of ethics are based. (See Tables 1–1 to 1–3.)

Furthermore, nurses must be well informed about their professional codes of ethics (see ANA, *Code for Nurses with Interpretative Statements,* 1985; ANA, *The Nonnegotiable Nature of the ANA Code for Nurses with Interpretative Statements,* 1994b), as well as about current professional-association position statements regarding ethical controversies (see Oncology Nursing Society, *Support of Oncology Nurses in Confronting Ethical Dimensions of Nursing Practice,* 1995; ANA, Position Statement on Ethics and Human

Table 1–2	
Principles	
Autonomy	An obligation exists to respect the decision-making capacities of autonomous clients.
	The client has a right to self-determination, including the ability to choose among medically indicated treatments and the ability to refuse any unwanted treatments.
Beneficence	An obligation exists to provide for the good of the client, to provide benefits and to balance the benefits against the risks.
Nonmaleficence	An obligation exists to avoid the causation of harm to the client.
Justice	An obligation exists to promote fairness in the distribution of benefits and risks.

Table 1–3
Values

Confidentiality	Respect for the client's privacy of information.
Fidelity	The keeping of one's promises and commitments, to others and to oneself.
Integrity	Adherence to a moral code of values; honesty.
Veracity	Truthfulness.

Rights, 1991; ANA, *Mechanisms through Which State Nurses Associations Consider Ethical and Human Rights Issues,* 1994a), and about the scope of their practice according to their state nurse practice act. Being thus informed greatly enhances the ability to effectively assist clients and families to make decisions.

PERSONAL VALUES CLARIFICATION

Values clarification attempts to answer questions about *who* we are, *what* we believe in, and *why* we behave the way we do. Such understanding of one's own values is essential to the ethical decision-making process.

Nurses are obligated to support their client's autonomy as well as to adhere to the values of beneficence, nonmaleficence, and justice. Sometimes these values are in conflict with one another, and one value may need to be prioritized higher than another. It is important for the nurse to be able to recognize and differentiate his or her own values from those of the client's. If there exists an insurmountable conflict between the two persons' value systems, the client's care must be assigned to another nurse.

ETHICS AND HUMAN VALUES COMMITTEES

Ethics and human values committees are interdisciplinary groups that offer advice about ethical problems that arise in clinical care. They generally provide consultations or a forum for discussion; however, not all will issue formal recommendations nor will all initiate policy. Most are viewed as intermediaries in the negotiation of legal-ethical concerns, particularly in the case of those clients who are incompetent or when significant disagreement exists among health care professionals, clients, and families.

Ethics committees also have a responsibility to educate the staff of a facility, the clients, and the community at large on ethical issues related to health care (Savage, 1994). Oncology and critical care nurses should be active participants in such education because of their valuable clinical experiences. Knowledge of oncology topics can indeed be vital in an emergency situation. Since nurses work closely with clients, families, and other members of the health care team, they are in a pivotal position to articulate educational issues needing to be addressed.

Access to ethics and human values committees is beneficial to nursing practice involving oncology clients in that it promotes interdisciplinary interaction and understanding of differing ethical perspectives. Such forums also provide opportunity for heightened awareness of ethnic and cultural factors influencing client choices. This, in turn, enhances support for autonomous decision making.

RESOLVING ETHICAL DILEMMAS

Not every issue requires an ethics and human values committee meeting. Nurses can initiate the resolution process with the client and members of the provider team. Each situation should be approached systematically, although the process may require modification of the different phases, and some of the phases may overlap (Fig. 1-2).

Phase 1   *Recognize* the need for intervention. In this phase the nurse must be aware of the actual or potential development of a conflict. In many cases timely intervention during this phase will prove to be preventive.

Phase 2   *Identify* the key players. Certainly the client and physician are always considered key players. Are there significant others? Which nurse is considered the primary nurse, or is there a nurse with whom the client has developed a trusting rapport?

Phase 3   *Define and clarify* the issues as the key players see them. Is there a knowledge or information deficit? Many times one or more of the parties simply does not have enough information or understanding about the situation, so decisions are delayed.

Phase 4   *Relate* the issues to ethical principles, values, or concepts that will have meaning for the key players. Use lay terms where appropriate. For example, when you are discussing the client with the health care team, it may be appropriate to say, "In order to respect the client's autonomy . . ."; but when you are talking directly with the client, it may be more appropriate to say, "In order to preserve your right to make your health care decisions, we'd like to . . . 'get your permission' or 'inform you.'"

Phase 5   *Analyze* alternative choices and consequences. Weigh the risks and benefits and discuss them with the health care team. Subjective judgments about the pros and cons of each

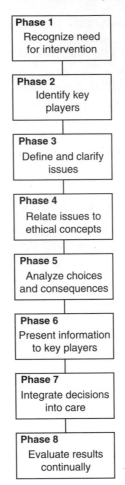

Figure 1-2 Phases of ethical dilemma resolution.

choice are a natural occurrence and do not diminish the value of the analysis.

Phase 6   *Present* the information to the key players. Share the analysis with the client and key significant others as the client desires. Many ethics committees include the client in the analysis phase during a committee consultation and, if so, phases 5 and 6 will occur simultaneously.

Phase 7   *Implement* the decisions and integrate them into the client's plan of care. This phase is complicated, because as new issues arise, previous phases may need to be repeated.

Phase 8   *Evaluate* the results of each decision in an ongoing manner.

No decision is irrevocable, nor is one decision applicable to all situations. The decision to maintain the current course of action or to choose an alternative must be made. Continue the evaluation phase throughout the intervention. Document the work of each phase in the client's record in accordance with your facility's policies.

FUTILITY

Promoting the well-being of the client complies with the ethical principle of *beneficence,* or doing good for the client. However, it is not uncommon for nurses to experience frustration when medical interventions are perceived to be useless. The ethical values of beneficence and *nonmaleficence* often conflict as oncology nurses assist with emergency procedures in futile situations.

Futility is an elusive concept because of its relativity. An intervention may be effective for one physiologic system but not effective for the client holistically. Furthermore, because the effectiveness of interventions among clients as individuals varies, futility is a subjective decision in each case.

Schneiderman, Jecker, and Jonsen (1990) propose defining futility as "any effort to achieve a result that is possible but that reasoning or experience suggests is highly improbable and that cannot be systematically reproduced" (p. 951). This definition attributes respect and credibility to the physician's experience and judgment in deciding whether or not to provide specific interventions.

Although physicians have no obligation to provide treatment that clearly will have no physiologic benefit to the client (Hastings Center, 1987, p. 32), many times the benefit is not, or cannot be, accurately projected in advance of treatment. When contemplating whether an intervention will be futile or not, improvement of the client's prognosis, comfort, or overall state of well-being should be the primary factors considered.

For example, if vasoactive and antidysrhythmic infusions produce acceptable blood pressure and cardiac rate and rhythm, but the client is ventilatory dependent and obtunded, should not the goal of treatment intervention shift from single-system maintenance to holistic functionality? Furthermore, the use of scarce resources for futile care, with resultant costs to the client and family as well as to society at large, causes conflict in balancing the values of beneficence and justice.

The value of *justice* refers to a proper balance between access to an adequate level of care and appropriate distribution of resources. Applying justice may limit a client's liberty to demand scarce health care resources to the detriment of other clients who would more likely benefit (Hastings Center, 1987, p. 8).

Futility should be distinguished from hopelessness. "Futility refers to the objective quality of an action whereas hope describes a subjective attitude"

(Schneiderman, Jecker, and Jonsen, 1990). A person can believe an intervention to be futile but still hope it will work. In oncologic emergency situations, in which hope is still possible for the client and family but for which progression of the course of illness renders interventions in all likelihood futile, consideration must to be given to continue the provision of aggressive care until the client and family can accept the reality of the situation.

WITHHOLDING AND WITHDRAWING

When a client has been determined to be near the end of his or her life, decisions will be made to withhold additional therapies and to discontinue current life-prolonging interventions. Some of the decisions will be dictated by client preference (e.g., the client has signed an advance directive prohibiting mechanical ventilation), but many will be implemented based on the physician's judgment (e.g., perhaps intravenous vasoactive medications are no longer warranted).

Membership in ethics networks or organizations can provide information about current ethical issues relevant to the care of clients experiencing oncologic emergencies. According to the Hastings Center (1987), four factors must guide decision making in the care of the terminally ill:

1. The utmost regard for the client's well-being.
2. The value of autonomy.
3. The integrity of health care professionals.
4. The value of justice.

None of the values should be ranked higher than another, and each should play an integral role in the decision-making process.

Nurses can rely on their professional organizations to provide ethical guidance for withholding or withdrawing interventions in the terminally ill (AACN, 1990; AACN, 1989; AACN, 1985; ANA, 1992a; ANA, 1992b). Nurses must be well acquainted with the ethical and legal scope of their professional practice to provide end-of-life care to their clients. They must make choices in their clinical practice that are in accord with their own moral belief system. "The integrity of health care professionals is relevant not only to their obligations to the client but also to their own conscientious moral and religious beliefs" (Hastings Center, 1987, p. 8).

CLIENT DECISION MAKING

In Western society high priority is given to individual autonomy. Oncology clients are encouraged to decide the course of their health care for themselves. Nurses respect the client's decisions and encourage autonomy by providing information about and support for treatment options chosen by the client. Many ethical questions arise as a practical matter in delivering emergency oncologic bedside care as a result of the value placed on autonomy.

INFORMED CONSENT

The principle of autonomy is the moral basis for obtaining informed consent as well as accepting informed refusal. It respects the oncology client's right to make decisions. The nurse is in an ideal position to assist the client in obtaining information about various treatment options in order to make informed decisions and give consent.

Informed consent is a process (Berry, Dodd, Hinds, and Ferrell, 1996), not an episodic event or a document. It is a continuous exchange of information among all the parties involved with the client, who has the right to withdraw consent as desired.

ADVANCE DIRECTIVES

The Patient Self-Determination Act of 1991 is a federal law requiring health care agencies to inform clients about the availability of advance directives. The concept of *directing* decisions about one's care in *advance* of the need for care supports autonomous decision making. Clients may choose to make decisions for themselves by means of a living will document, or they may choose to appoint someone else, through a health care surrogate document, to make health care decisions if a future need occurs.

Advance directives make clear to health care providers the desires and decisions of the client in the event decision-making capacity is lost. A *living will* is a written document prepared while a client is fully competent. Its contents describe the client's decision preferences about types of life-prolonging procedures and whether to use, withhold, or withdraw them in a situation of terminal illness. Another type of advance directive entails the appointment of a *health care surrogate*. The client appoints another individual to make health care decisions in the event the client becomes incapacitated. A *durable power of attorney* is a third type of advance directive, which confers to an individual appointed by the client the authority to handle the latter's business affairs, such as banking or property transfer, and who in forty-eight states (Fade, 1994) can additionally function as a health care surrogate.

Three criteria recommended by the Hastings Center (1987) upon which the surrogate should base decisions are:

1. The client's previously indicated explicit directions, or in the absence of any directions,
2. Knowledge of the client's preferences and values, or in the absence of such knowledge,
3. Presumption of how a reasonable person in the client's circumstances would choose.

It is important for every nurse to be familiar with the advance directive laws in his or her state of practice. Clients have the right to rescind or revise advance directives at any time, and advance directives never override the capable, competent client's current decision.

HOPE

The *hope experience* (Nowotny, 1989) describes the formation on the part of the client of new goals, new strategies, and feelings of safety and comfort. Oncology clients have hope that they will overcome their cancer, adjust to new lifestyles, and get on with their lives. Hope allows them to envision the future after the current crisis has passed. Fostering hope during an oncologic emergency is reassuring to the client, but nurses must be careful to avoid giving "false" hope. Since hope can play a therapeutic role in the coping process (Owen, 1989; Herth, 1989) for clients with cancer, the values of veracity and integrity can provide guidance to nurses as they nurture their clients' hopes. This can be a realistic endeavor if nurses help their clients set short-term, attainable goals and reinforce all positive or successful outcomes regardless of how small.

RESEARCH/CLINICAL TRIALS

The most pressing ethical issue for the oncology nurse in clinical trial research is that of informed consent. Oncology clients willingly consent to participation in clinical research trials when they think it is in their best interest. The many unknowns surrounding the variables and potential outcomes of the study result in questions without definite answers. Yet, clients consent because they hope to achieve greater benefit than would be obtained with standard therapy.

It is helpful for the nurse to understand the underlying theoretical basis for research. Prestifilippo et al. (1993) describe research as a class of activities designed to contribute to the expansion of generalized knowledge (utilitarianism), whereas standard clinical practice is a class of activities designed to contribute to the well-being of an individual client (deontology). It is well known that the objective of a randomized clinical trial is to determine which of two treatments is superior for a specific disease in a specific population. The nurse can facilitate education of the client about the overall concept of cancer therapy research. The client may fear randomization into a "no treatment" category and needs to understand there is no placebo experimentation.

Oncology clients want the therapy that is most likely to result in a cure or a remission and least likely to bring about serious adverse consequences. Although standard therapy has already been tested and outcomes are known, Lantos (1993) says oncology clients choose clinical trials because research is conducted with therapies that are *potentially* better. Although cancer clients are provided with as much information as possible to encourage autonomy and truly informed consent about clinical trial research therapy, they may still defer the decision to their physician. Tabak (1995) explains that clients facing experimental therapy are confronted with physical, mental, and emotional barriers that degrade their decision-making ability to a much greater extent than is found in clients who are not in life-threatening situations.

ALTERNATIVE THERAPY

Oncology clients have a right to freedom of choice in selecting their modes of cancer intervention. When an alternative to traditional therapy is chosen by the client, nurses may experience ethical conflict because the duty to support the client's autonomy somehow contradicts the value of beneficence. For example, the nurse is obligated to provide safe and effective care but is prohibited from administering unconventional drug or medical therapies not approved by the FDA (Fletcher, 1992).

To provide information to oncology clients, nurses must become knowledgeable about alternative therapies. Although it is not within the scope of their practice to recommend therapy, it is their obligation to support the client's right to information about particular therapies.

The nurse should solicit information from the client with the goal of ascertaining the adequacy of the information. Montbriand (1993) suggests establishing a rapport with the client by asking open-ended questions, listening with sensitivity, and carefully probing for information. This protocol, when used with a nonbiased attitude, will assure the client that his or her views are respected. Fletcher (1992) suggests inquiring whether or not the risks, benefits, and costs of the treatment have been fully disclosed. The goal of the nurse is not to persuade the client in one direction or the other, but to clarify the rationale for the decision in an effort to promote fully informed consent.

PALLIATIVE CARE

The goal of all cancer interventions, including palliative care, should be to advance the client's interests as defined by the client. Clients choosing to forego further aggressive therapies continue to have advanced nursing needs. Ethical issues arise in palliative care when a perceived conflict of values occurs.

Given the goals of promoting comfort, respecting dignity, and supporting autonomy, the nurse is challenged to balance ethical values in managing the client's care. Of immense importance is the issue of pain control. According to Lisson (1989), pain is an ethical issue from the client's point of view because the more severe the pain, the more it overshadows the client's self-defining human qualities of intelligence, autonomy, and self-esteem.

Providing effective pain relief is of the highest priority if the client so desires. However, enough medication to relieve the pain may have the effect of shortening the client's life by causing hypotension and/or severe respiratory depression. Nurses are well within ethical and legal boundaries in providing such pain relief as long as the intent of the intervention is to *relieve pain* and not to *shorten life*. The Council on Ethical and Judicial Affairs (1992, p. 2231) states that "the administration of a drug necessary to ease the pain of a client who is terminally ill and suffering excruciating pain may be appropriate medical treatment even though the effect of the drug may shorten life." The reader is referred to Chapter 33 of this volume for further discussion on pain management.

EUTHANASIA AND PHYSICIAN-ASSISTED SUICIDE

Euthanasia is commonly defined as the act of bringing about the death of a hopelessly ill and suffering person in a relatively quick and painless way for reasons of mercy (Council on Ethical and Judicial Affairs, 1992, p. 2229). Physician-assisted suicide, on the other hand, entails making a means of suicide available for the client, who then carries out the act. The difference is whether the physician serves as the agent of administration of the service.

Thinking varies about the appropriateness of euthanasia and physician-assisted suicide from an ethical point of view. Although euthanasia is illegal throughout the United States, there is support both for and against it. Those who favor it do so on the basis of support for autonomy. Those who do not favor it fear that the concepts would ultimately extend euthanasia and physician-assisted suicide to populations unable to exercise autonomy, such as the incapable and the incompetent.

Professional nurses' associations have taken a definitive stance against euthanasia and physician-assisted suicide (ANA, 1985; ANA, 1994c; ANA, 1994d; ONS, 1995). Although nurses are prohibited from assisting with euthanasia or suicide, misinterpretations and misperceptions appear to abound as to what constitutes euthanasia or physician-assisted suicide.

Neither withholding interventions at the request of the client or health care surrogate nor withdrawing life-prolonging interventions in futile situations at the request of the physician constitutes euthanasia or assisted suicide. Some nurses equate the actions of withholding and/or withdrawing with the concepts of euthanasia and assisted suicide and perceive them to be one and the same. It is important for nurses to conduct their own personal values clarification analysis and come to terms with their thinking on ethics topics. Only then can they rationally choose challenging professional assignments without incurring internal personal moral conflict.

Whether withdrawing, withholding, maintaining, or accelerating interventions, nurses are obligated to improve the care of those who are dying by tending to their physical and psychosocial needs. The need for expert balancing of beneficence and autonomy in nursing practice becomes evident during the care of oncology clients.

CHAPTER SUMMARY

Ethical decision making and dilemma resolution are processes that continue to be developed and practiced by health care professionals at all levels. Oncology nurses are intimately involved in the process because of their key role in oncologic emergencies and because of their unique nurse–client relationship.

Nurses frequently encounter ethical dilemmas when caring for their oncology clients, especially during emergency situations. Through clarification of their own value systems, facilitation of multidisciplinary client care conferences, and practice with dilemma resolution models, nurses can provide sound rationality to the process of ethical decision making.

TEST QUESTIONS

1. The subdiscipline of ethics dealing with health care issues is:
   A. Metaethics
   B. Bioethics
   C. Descriptive
   D. Normative

1. Answer: B
Bioethics is also known as biomedical ethics.

2. The ethical theory that defines the right thing to do based on the outcome of the act is:
   A. Consequentialism
   B. Nonconsequentialism
   C. Beneficence
   D. Nonmaleficence

2. Answer: A
Consequentialism, also called utilitarianism, takes the position that acts are right if the total net outcome is good.

3. The ethical theory that defines an act as right or wrong based on the rightness or wrongness of the act itself, independent of the outcome, is:
   A. Consequentialism
   B. Nonconsequentialism
   C. Beneficence
   D. Nonmaleficence

3. Answer: B
Nonconsequentialism, also known as deontologism, regards the rightness or wrongness of an act as independent of its total outcome, such quality being inherent in the rightness or wrongness of the act itself.

4. The ethical value obligating one to tell the truth is:
   A. Confidentiality
   B. Integrity
   C. Veracity
   D. Fidelity

4. Answer: C
Veracity is the value obligating one to tell the truth.

5. The ethical principle that refers to a client's right to self-determination is:
   A. Beneficence
   B. Justice
   C. Autonomy
   D. Nonmaleficence

5. Answer: C
Autonomy is the obligation to respect the client's capacity to choose among medically indicated treatments and to refuse any unwanted treatments.

6. The ability of a client to make decisions now, while mentally capable, in the event of incapacitation in future health care crises is called:
   A. Utilitarianism
   B. Confidentiality
   C. Morality
   D. Advance directive

6. Answer: D
Advance directives—in the form of living wills, health care surrogates, and durable powers of attorney—allow decision making by the capable client for future events.

7. Informed consent is:
   A. Permission to perform a procedure
   B. A document with the client's signature
   C. A process of fully informing the client
   D. Release of information

7. Answer: C
Informed consent is a process ensuring that the client is fully informed when making choices about therapy, including potential outcomes, side effects, and alternatives.

8. Alternative therapy can be an ethical issue because:
   A. The client may not be aware of the risks, benefits, and costs.
   B. It is illegal.
   C. It is nonprofessional
   D. It is not approved by the FDA.

8. Answer: A
The client has a right to make his or her own decisions about therapy based on his or her being fully informed about the risks, benefits, and costs.

9. The client's condition has deteriorated to the point that further aggressive treatment is deemed futile. The physician has prescribed discontinuance of antidysrhythmics, vasoactive medications, and ventilatory support. In the *presence* of advance directives, which ethical principle has guided the decision to remove therapy?

9. Answer: A
Competent, capable clients may choose interventions for future medical crises in which they would no longer be able to make their own decisions. Withdrawal of life-prolonging interventions would comply with the client's decision and therefore support the concept of autonomy.

A. Autonomy
B. Beneficence
C. Justice
D. Nonmaleficence

10. The same client's condition has deteriorated to the point that further aggressive treatment is deemed futile. The physician has prescribed discontinuance of antidysrhythmics, vasoactive medications, and ventilatory support. In the *absence* of advance directives, which ethical principle has guided the decision to remove therapy?
   A. Autonomy
   B. Beneficence
   C. Justice
   D. Nonmaleficence

10. Answer: B
It is not in the best interests of the client to continue futile interventions. Discontinuing life-prolonging mechanisms in the presence of futility supports the concept of beneficence.

REFERENCES

AACN: Position Statement: AACN Clarification of Resuscitation Status in Critical Care Settings. Newport Beach, CA: AACN, 1985, p. 1.

AACN; Position Statement: AACN Role of the Critical Care Nurse as Patient Advocate. Newport Beach, CA: AACN, 1989, p. 1.

AACN: Postion Statement: AACN Withholding and/or Withdrawing Life-Sustaining Treatment. Newport Beach, CA: AACN, 1990, pp. 1–2.

ANA: Code for Nurse with Interpretive Statements. Kansas City, MO: ANA, 1985.

ANA: Position Statement on Ethics and Human Rights. Washington, DC: ANA, 1991.

ANA: Position Statement: Foregoing Artificial Nutrition and Hydration. Washington,DC: ANA, 1992a, pp 1–3.

ANA: Position Statement: Nursing Care and Do-Not-Resuscitate Decisions. Washington, DC: ANA, 1992b, pp. 1–3.

ANA: Mechanisms Through Which State Nurses Associations Consider Ethical and Human Rights Issues. Washington, DC: ANA, 1994a.

ANA: The Nonnegotiable Nature of the ANA Code for Nurses with Interpretive Statements. Washington, DC: ANA, 1994b.

ANA: Position Statement: Active Euthanasia. Washington, DC: ANA, 1994c.

ANA: Position Statement: Assisted Suicide. Washington, DC: ANA, 1994d.

Beauchamp TL: The "Four-Principles" Approach. *In* Gillon R (ed): Principles of Health Care Ethics. New York: John Wiley, 1994.

Berry D, Dodd M, Hinds P, Ferrell B: Informed consent: Process and clinical issues. Oncol Nurs Forum 23(3):507–512, 1996.

Calman K: The ethics of allocation of scarce health care resources: A view from the centre. J Med Ethics 20(2):71–74, 1994.

Council on Ethical and Judicial Affairs, American Medical Association, Report D: Guidelines for the Appropriate Use of Do-Not-Resuscitate Orders. Reprinted in JAMA 265(14), 1991.

Council on Ethical and Judicial Affairs, American Medical Association, Report B: Decisions
    Near the End of Life. Reprinted in JAMA 267:2229–2233, 1992.
Council on Ethical and Judicial Affairs: Code of Medical Ethics Reports. Vol. 5, No. 2, Report
    59, 1994, pp. 269–275.
Emanual E: Euthanasia: Historical, ethical, and empiric perspectives. Arch Intern Med 154(17):
    1890–1901, 1994.
Fade A: Advance directives: Keeping up with changing legislation. Nursing Dynamics 3(1):13–15, 1994.
Fletcher D: Unconventional cancer treatments: Professional, legal and ethical issues. Oncol
    Nurs Forum 19(9):1351–1354, 1992.
Fowler M: Introduction to ethics and ethical theory. In Cleary, PL (sponsoring ed): Ethics at the
    Bedside. Philadelphia: JB Lippincott, 1987.
Hastings Center: Guidelines on the Termination of Life-Sustaining Treatment and the Care of
    the Dying. Bloomington: Indiana University Press, 1987.
Herth, K: The relationship between level of hope and level of coping response and other vari-
    ables in patients with cancer. Oncol Nurs Forum 16(1):7–72, 1989.
Jassak P, Ryan M: Ethical issues in clinical research. Semin Oncol Nurs 5(2):102–108, 1989.
Johns J: Advance directives and opportunities for nurses. Image: J Nurs Sch 28(2):149–153, 1996.
Lantos J: Informed consent. Cancer (Suppl 72)(9):2811–2815, 1993.
Levine R: Ethics of clinical trials: Do they help the patient? Cancer (Suppl 72)(9):2805–2810, 1993.
Lisson E: Ethical issues in pain management. Semin Oncol Nurs 5(2):114–119, 1989.
Lynn J: Choices of curative and palliative care for cancer patients. CA-A Cancer Journal for
    Clinicians 36(2):100–104, 1986.
Montbriand M: Freedom of choice: An issue concerning alternate therapies chosen by patients
    with cancer. Oncol Nurs Forum 20(8):1195–1201, 1993.
Nowotny M: Assessment of hope in patients with cancer: Development of an instrument. Oncol
    Nurs Forum 16(1):57–61, 1989.
ONS: Oncology Nursing Society's Support of Oncology Nurses in Confronting Ethical Dimen-
    sions of Nursing Practice. Oncol Nurs Forum 22(2):255, 1995.
Otte D, Allen K: Ethical principles in the nursing care of the terminally ill adult. Oncol Nurs
    Forum 14(5):87–91, 1987.
Owen D: Nurses' perspectives on the meaning of hope in patients with cancer: A qualitative
    study. Oncol Nurs Forum 16(1):75–79, 1989.
Pillar B, Jacox A, Redman B: Technology, its assessment, and nursing. Nurs Outlook
    38(1):16–19, 1990.
Prestifilippo J, Antman K, Berkman B, Kaufman D, Lantos J, Lawrence W, Levine R, McKenna
    R: The ethical treatment of cancer. Cancer (Suppl 72)(9):2816–2819, 1993.
Savage T: The nurses' role on ethics committees and as an ethics consultant. Semin Nurs
    Manag 2(1):41–47, 1994.
Schneiderman L, Jecker N, Jonsen A: Medical futility: Its meaning and ethical implications.
    Ann Intern Med 112(12):949–954, 1990.
Seroka A: Values clarification and ethical decision making. Semin Nurs Manag 2(1):8–15, 1994.
Tabak N: Decision making in consenting to experimental cancer therapy. Cancer Nurs
    18(2):89–96, 1995.
Taylor C: Medical futility and nurses. Image: J Nurs Sch 27(4):301–306, 1995.
Veatch RM, Fry ST: Case studies in nursing ethics. Philadelphia: JB Lippincott, 1987.
Young E: Life and death in the ICU: Ethical considerations. In Civetta J, Taylor R, Kirby R (eds):
    Introduction to Critical Care. Philadelphia: JB Lippincott, 1989, pp. 37–58.

Chapter 2

Ethics Case Study

Barbara Daly, PhD, RN, FAAN

CHAPTER OBJECTIVES

At the completion of this chapter, the reader will be able to:

Identify frequently encountered ethical issues arising in the care of critically ill oncology clients.

Describe nursing interventions that are ethically appropriate in caring for the dying client and his or her family.

Evaluate the application of selected ethical principles in a hypothetical case.

OVERVIEW

THE FOLLOWING case study illustrates the moral complexities often involved in caring for critically ill oncology clients. It is presented in two parts in order to illustrate the dynamic nature of ethical dilemmas and the need to frequently re-evaluate responses in light of new information, new events, and changes in the nurse–client relationship. Each part of the case is followed by a discussion of the client's situation and the ethical problems it poses. Interventions that utilize the problem-solving approach described in Chapter 1 are described, and reference is made to the particular ethical principles or values these interventions draw into question.

CASE STUDY: PART 1

Mrs. T is a 54-year-old woman with non-small cell carcinoma of the lung. She has been divorced for 22 years. She has a 34-year-old daughter and a 29-year-old son, both of whom live in the same city with her, as does her mother, two sisters, and a brother. Her father is deceased.

Mrs. T was originally diagnosed with cancer a year ago. She underwent a right upper lobectomy at that time, followed by radiation therapy. She had metastasis to the hilar nodes at the time of surgery, and she has completed a course of chemotherapy. Her hospitalization at the time of surgery was prolonged because of respiratory insufficiency, probably related to chronic obstructive pulmonary disease (COPD). Prior to her surgery, Mrs. T was a heavy smoker; she has no other concurrent health problems.

Since her diagnosis and original surgery, Mrs. T was scrupulous in following medical advice. She stopped smoking, began an exercise program, and was eager to participate in an experimental protocol of combination therapy for her cancer. She was relatively symptom-free until she developed a community-acquired pneumonia. She was hospitalized by her oncologist for this 48 hours ago, and IV antibiotics were administered. She then became septic and was transferred to the intensive care unit (ICU).

On arrival in the ICU, Mrs. T was acutely short of breath. Her blood pressure was 78/54, her pulse was 118, and a pulse oximeter demonstrated her oxygen saturation to be 88%. She was immediately intubated, and a dopamine infusion was begun. Despite positive pressure ventilation and an FiO_2 of 80%, Mrs. T's arterial pO_2 remained at 68 mmHg. Pulmonary artery pressures were consistent with relative hypovolemia, peripheral vasodilation, and depressed cardiac output, typical of septic shock. Atracurium was administered to induce paralysis, with morphine used for deep sedation. With the addition of dobutamine and positive end expiratory pressure (PEEP) on the ventilator, Mrs. T's pO_2 was raised to 84 mmHg, and her blood pressure stabilized.

Mrs. T's daughter and sister were with her when the deterioration in her condition necessitated transfer to the ICU. They called other family members and remained in the waiting room outside of the ICU. Upon seeing Mrs. T, they were tearful and quite anxious. They seemed overwhelmed when the unit physician explained Mrs. T's condition to them and told them that her prognosis was quite poor, given the presence of sepsis in the context of metastatic cancer and diminished pulmonary reserve. At the bedside, Mrs. T's nurse explained the equipment and answered their questions about her condition.

Mrs. T's condition remained critical. Although her oxygenation remained adequate, she continued to require increasing amounts of dobutamine to maintain an adequate blood pressure. When Mrs. T's daughter and son visited, the nurse raised the subject of resuscitation by asking if Mrs. T had ever talked about her wishes should she become critically ill. Mrs. T's daughter, Linda, became quite angry, demanding to know why the nurse was asking this. The nurse explained that this was routine practice when clients were as sick as Mrs. T and that the nurses and doctors needed to know what her wishes were. Linda responded that Mrs. T would want everything done, that she was "a fighter." She asked if there was something the nurse was not telling her or if something had changed since the last visit. When the nurse again tried to reassure Linda that she was only trying to be sure that this treatment was in accord with Mrs. T's wishes, since she could not speak for herself, Linda seemed to relax. She and her brother stayed with their mother for the next hour, frequently talking to her and encouraging her to keep fighting, assuring her that she could "beat this."

Discussion

The situation described above is quite typical of that encountered by critical care professionals, faced with caring for a client in an acute crisis. In such situations, physicians and nurses are hampered by lack of detailed knowledge of the client's history and a lack of understanding of the client's value system, while faced with the need to make decisions quickly and maintain the standards of care necessary to preserve life. In addition to initiating interventions designed to address the client's physiologic problems, the nurse is also obligated to adhere to ethical standards.

As discussed in Chapter 1, the preeminent principle directing medical decisions in the United States is autonomy. The commitment to fostering the right of individuals to make their own decisions about medical care underlies both the negative duty to refrain from controlling client decisions and the positive duty to ensure that clients are well informed prior to decisions. When clients are unable to speak for themselves, in the absence of a durable power of attorney, decision-making rights pass to their families. The moral justification for this tradition lies in the assumption that the individual's family is most likely to have that person's best interest in mind—that the family is most likely to know either what the person's wishes would be or at least what the person might want, given his or her values and experiences. Even in the absence of clear knowledge of client preference, the "substituted-judgment standard" asserts that a family member with similar cultural, social, and religious background is in a better position to judge what is in the client's best interest than are professionals with no prior contact with the person.

In addition to the obligation to honor autonomy, health professionals have special duties of beneficence. Doing good, or benefiting the individual, is central to the meaning of both nursing and medicine. As long as professionals and clients share a common understanding of what constitutes "good," professionals are able to honor autonomous choices of clients and also fulfill their duty to benefit the client. When the professionals' judgment of what would be in the client's best interest differs from the choices made by the client, potential for conflict exists.

In the case study presented thus far, the nurse caring for Mrs. T attempted to support the client's autonomy by gathering more data about her previous wishes. This is not only an appropriate objective but an essential one, given the situation of grave illness and likelihood of further deterioration in the client's condition. However, the challenge to practitioners in addressing ethical issues stems not only from the demands posed by ethical principles but also from the inherent difficulties of communicating effectively in situations marked by enormous stress and ambiguities.

From the perspective of Mrs. T's family, their mother had suffered a life-threatening complication. The ICU probably represented, as it does to many, a place of rescue, staffed by specialists whose purpose is to help her in successfully fighting off this new threat to her life. In this context, to abruptly raise of the possibility of withholding care and "giving up" may be seen as threatening and incomprehensible. As such, the nurse's actions may contribute to suspicion and a lack of trust between the family and ICU staff, who perceive themselves as fulfilling an important obligation to their client.

While the practice of having critical care specialists assume responsibility for managing care in the ICU is preferred in most large, academic health centers, it does present added problems in communication. In the case study described, the physicians and nurses were hampered by inadequate knowledge of this client and her family. Although it was essential that they determine her wishes regarding aggressive interventions, in order to do this effectively, they had to learn more about what conversations had been held previously, discover whether others had ever addressed the issue, and try to assess the family's overall goals and coping abilities. This information could best be obtained through collaboration with the medical and nursing staff who knew Mrs. T before her recent admission to the ICU.

It is certainly encumbent upon the nurse to talk with clients and their families about treatment goals and preferences, but fulfilling this responsibility without generating mistrust entails having an adequate database from which to work. Occasionally there is not enough time to gather information before decisions are called for, such as when an arrest is imminent, but in most cases nurses and physicians should delay initiating conversations about treatment goals until learning about discussions and decisions that have preceded a client's transfer to the ICU.

CASE STUDY: PART 2

By the third day in the ICU, Mrs. T's condition had stabilized, although she demonstrated significant pulmonary shunting, which required an FiO_2 of 60% to maintain adequate oxygenation, and she continued to require dobutamine for support of her cardiac output. Mrs. T was sedated with a propofol infusion and remained somnolent. On day 4, her blood pressure dropped precipitously, and she began to have ventricular dysrhythmias. By day 5, ECG changes and positive cardiac enzymes confirmed that she had suffered a myocardial infarction.

The ICU team now had two concerns. First, the occurrence of an acute cardiac event presented an additional immediate threat to survival. Second, even if Mrs. T could be supported through the first few days following infarction, when the risk of death is highest, impairment in ventricular function would further hamper her already poor chance of being weaned from the ventilator, given her diminished pulmonary reserve. With this change in her condition, it was essential to re-evaluate treatment goals.

Since her admission, Mrs. T's family had remained in close attendance. One family member was always present, sleeping in the waiting room at night. They asked many questions of the staff, often focusing on minute details of care, such as insisting that Mrs. T's hands be elevated at all times to reduce the peripheral edema often accompanying sepsis. Mrs. T's daughter, Linda, seemed to take the role of decision maker, although all family members were involved to some extent. Linda had taken a leave of absence from her job as an executive assistant at a local manufacturing firm and spent most of every day at the hospital.

During the week Mrs. T had now been in the ICU, her primary nurse established a beginning relationship with Linda and learned more about Mrs. T's life. Linda described her mother as a "tough woman" who had raised her children to be like herself, "strong and independent." She had always worked, supporting the family even before her divorce. She had coped with her diagnosis of cancer, according to Linda, in her usual fashion of "taking charge," insisting on remaining in her own home alone rather than recuperating in the home of one of her children. She did not have strong ties to any church or religious group.

As she got to know Linda, Mrs. T's primary nurse also became concerned about the impact of the illness on Linda herself. Linda conveyed a strong sense of duty, trying to act as her mother's surrogate and cope with the crisis of her mother's illness as her mother would—with strength, assertiveness, and optimism. However, she appeared increasingly fatigued and anxious as the days went on. As Mrs. T's condition worsened, the nurse was faced with the challenge of how to support Linda through the re-evaluation of treatment goals while also acting as an advocate for Mrs. T.

Discussion

With significant changes in the condition of the client, it is imperative that the critical care staff make a formal plan to address decisions about treatment goals, just as they would make specific plans to address physiologic changes. As suggested in Chapter 1, an organized approach to problem solving is most helpful when initiated before problems escalate and adversarial relationships develop. In Mrs. T's case, such an approach will reduce the likelihood of either avoiding discussion with her family members because of reluctance to confront assumed differences in opinion about treatment goals, or of approaching the family on the spur of the moment without adequate planning.

The eight-phase resolution process can be applied to both actual and potential ethical problems. The worsening of Mrs. T's condition, the increasing stress and fatigue exhibited by her daughter, and the potential for conflicting opinions about treatment goals are factors that lead to the recognition of the need for intervention (phase 1).

A number of individuals should be involved to some extent in discussions about Mrs. T's treatment (phase 2). Of course, it is preferable to be able to talk directly with the client about treatment choices. In the case of clients, such as Mrs. T, who are receiving continuous sedation to improve ventilation, it may be appropriate to stop the sedative infusion for a few hours to determine if the client can regain decision-making capacity. If this is not possible, in the absence of a designated durable power of attorney for health care, the client's family members must assume primary decision-making authority for the client.

All caregivers who have significant involvement in the client's care should be invited to participate in discussions in some way. This will obviously include the client's primary nurse and ICU physician, but nurses and physicians who cared for the client prior to ICU transfer should also be included. Ancillary staff who have cared for the client, such as respiratory therapists or social workers, may also have important information that should be considered. Although in Mrs. T's case she did not have a close religious adviser, clergy who have known the client and/or family can also be of great assistance in reaching decisions.

In the third and fourth phases of the resolution process issues are defined and clarified, and then they are examined in the light of ethical principles. The actual issue confronting the staff at this point (part 2 of the case study) is the need to re-evaluate treatment goals because of changes in the client's physical condition. A potential issue is the possibility that Mrs. T's family may identify a goal that the ICU staff believe is unattainable or that the family may identify a goal that the ICU staff believe is neither a valid substitute for Mrs. T's own wishes nor in her best interest.

Several potential goals could be adopted in Mrs. T's case, each representing an alternative choice with attendant consequences (phase 5). In the great majority of situations of critical illness, the consensus among members of the health team and family members is that the goal of treatment is to preserve and extend life at all costs, with the consequence that every available therapy that has any chance of success is used, including resuscitation in the event of cardiac arrest. The ultimate consequences of implementing a plan to achieve this goal are always uncertain, but they may include survival with a significantly diminished quality of life. Another treatment goal would be to extend and preserve life without adding to the client's burden of suffering. The decision might then be made to maintain therapy at the current level but refrain from additional interventions, such as cardiopulmonary resuscitation (CPR). In other situations, the primary treatment goal might be to maintain comfort and reduce the suffering caused by continued interventions. A treatment withdrawal plan would then be appropriate, with the understanding that death would follow.

The focus of deliberations about treatment must be twofold, including identification of the goal of therapy and specification of the medical and prognostic facts of the client's condition. Identifying the goal of therapy is a process primarily governed by the ethical mandates of promoting individual autonomy and fulfilling the professional duties of beneficence and nonmaleficence. The goal chosen is also essentially influenced by the medical and prognostic facts, including the availability of various interventions and the likely outcomes of each. A common mistake in discussing treatment plans with clients and families is to ask them to make choices about specific interventions, such as whether or not to start dialysis or whether or not to institute a "Do Not Resuscitate" order, without first clarifying the goal of treatment. The clinicians, or clinical experts, should decide which therapies are appropriate, once the client or family has identified the goal of treatment, having been informed of the relevant facts by the clinical team.

Because the potential for ethical conflict exists in Mrs. T's case, the way in which the discussion of goals and options is carried out (phase 6) is of utmost importance Following certain guidelines ensures the proper handling of such discussions. First, meetings should be scheduled so that all involved individuals can attend; thus, each person must be notified at least several hours, if not a day, in advance. Timely notification is particularly important in the event of numerous family members, some of whom may need to make arrangements to be absent from work. If the client is not able to participate, it is best to hold the discussion away from the bedside so that everyone can be seated comfortably and discussion is thereby facilitated. Family members are always anxious in such situations, and it can be helpful to begin the meeting by simply explaining how the discussion will proceed. For example, the nurse or physician might make necessary introductions of everyone present, then say something like: "We appreciate your arranging to come here so we can talk about Mrs. T's condition and make decisions together about her care. As you know, she has recently had some additional problems with her heart, and we would like to first review what we know about her condition today and answer any questions you may have. Then we need to talk together about where to go from here. Since Mrs. T cannot tell us directly what her wishes are, we need everyone's input in deciding what our goals should be at this point, given what you know about her and what her current condition is." This statement should be followed by a brief summary of Mrs. T's condition, with an explanation of the significance of cardiac involvement.

After everyone's questions have been answered, it is sometimes helpful to also review the client's previous treatment goals and choices and the group's understanding of the values that led to those goals and choices. In Mrs. T's case, the ICU team could either ask the family to describe once more how she felt about her medical care, or they could say something like, "From our discussion with you, we understand that your mother was very committed to fighting her cancer, and that this is consistent with how she faced many challenges in her life. You've described her to us as a very strong woman who was quite independent."

These first two parts of the discussion—defining the course of discussion and reviewing treatment goals and options—serve to establish a common understanding among all those present. Now the issues should be identified precisely. It is imperative at this point that the ICU team be clear about their views and express them directly. For example, if the team believes that there is virtually no chance for survival, this should be stated. If there is some chance that Mrs. T will survive, but with a very low probability of ever being weaned from the ventilator, this should be stated. The next question for the group to address is what goal would best represent Mrs. T's own views and preferences, given these facts.

By focusing the discussion on what decision the client would make, were she able, several things are accomplished. This approach minimizes the likelihood that the family feels the full burden of decision-making responsibility and enables them, rather, to feel they are sharing in the decision making with the physicians and nurses. It is the duty of health professionals to support the preferences of the client, despite possible disagreement by some family members. Reference to the values, preferences, and life history of the client forms a basis for substituted judgment, and establishes a context for implementing what would be closest to the client's own decision, instead of deferring simply to the desires and preferences of those present or making the family members feel they are being asked to allow their loved one to die. Finally, focusing the discussion on goals clearly communicates that decisions to restrict life-support treatment in any way, even by withdrawing interventions, do not constitute "giving up" or abandoning the client. Whether the goal becomes continuing the current interventions, maximizing comfort, or avoiding additional treatment burdens, further development of the plan of care (phase 7), based on the discussion, will be necessary, and the results of the decisions must be evaluated (phase 8).

Obviously, such discussions require careful planning and coordination among the caregivers. It is often helpful for the ICU staff to have a care conference before meeting with the family to ensure that every member has the opportunity to think through his or her own beliefs about treatment goals and to reach consensus before approaching the family. This is also an appropriate time to consider how to respond if no agreement can be reached between the family and ICU team.

In situations such as Mrs. T's, family members often delay making decisions to change treatment goals and limit treatment. This can be a result of many factors, such as denial of the impending death of their loved one; persistent distrust of the medical or nursing staff; disagreement among family members; reluctance to participate in the decision making; hope that events will obviate the need for a choice; and most often, simple uncertainty about the best course of action. Whatever the reason for the family's delay, the critical care staff should be prepared to allow the family members time to think about the decision at hand, to talk among themselves, and to achieve some degree of comfort within themselves with their decision. Even if the family initially insists on treatment goals that are unrealistic or objectionable to critical care staff, it is usually best to allow some time before approaching them again. In the unusual case in which critical care staff feel that acting in accord with family wishes would require them to harm the client or violate their own ethical duties of beneficence and nonmaleficence, hospital ethics committees and possibly the hospital's legal office should be consulted.

CHAPTER SUMMARY

The case of Mrs. T illustrates a dilemma seen in oncologic critical care with increasing frequency. The tremendous range in treatment options available today, the complexity of modern tertiary care centers, and the variability in values among members of a culturally diverse society all contribute to the likelihood of ethical dilemmas. Mrs. T's situation presents the common challenges of identifying appropriate treatment goals and plans for the client, fulfilling ethical responsibilities to the client, while also addressing the emotional needs of the client's family. Although the occurrence of conflict and dilemmas may not be entirely avoidable, the use of a thoughtful, carefully planned approach can do much to alleviate both the moral and emotional distress associated with such situations.

CHAPTER 3

ACUTE PANCREATITIS

Jean Ellsworth-Wolk, RN, MS, OCN

CHAPTER OBJECTIVES

At the completion of this chapter, the reader will be able to:

Define acute pancreatitis.

State risk factors associated with acute pancreatitis in the oncology client.

Describe nursing care as it relates to oncology clients with acute pancreatitis.

Anticipate and prepare the client and family for a possible poor outcome.

OVERVIEW

ACUTE pancreatitis is an inflammatory process of the pancreas that is caused by the premature activation of pancreatic enzymes. This process results in autodigestion of the pancreatic gland and can lead to systemic complications. Precipitating factors are many and may include drugs, viruses, and metabolic conditions. The severity of this disease can range from mild and self-limiting to severe and fatal. Acute pancreatitis is a rare, yet serious complication in the oncology population and is seen most frequently in the bone marrow transplant population (Soergel, 1993). Once diagnosed, the elderly population can expect a poorer disease outcome (Marshall, 1993).

DESCRIPTION

Acute pancreatitis is characterized by an inflammatory process within the pancreas precipitated by the premature activation of pancreatic enzymes. These enzymes are normally secreted in an inactive form for the digestion of fats, carbohydrates, and proteins. The etiology of this premature activation can be multifactorial, and the theories of causation are still unclear but may include obstruction of the ampulla of Vater or common bile duct. Depending on the degree and extent of pancreatic inflammatory involvement and/or necrosis, the intensity of the disease ranges from mild to severe. Two types of acute pancreatitis can be distinguished morphologically—edematous, or interstitial, pancreatitis and necrotizing pancreatitis.

Edematous acute pancreatitis is characterized by interstitial edema, engorgement of capillaries, and dilation of lymphatic vessels. Necrotizing pancreatitis is characterized by pancreatic cell death and may initiate an inflammatory response that extends beyond the pancreas. Surrounding blood vessels may rupture, or the exudation of peritoneal fluid may sequester and become infected, leading to tissue necrosis, peritonitis, shock, and death. Distinction between the two morphologic types is essential to predict the severity of the course of the disease, as well as the outcome. The factors responsible for the transformation of edematous pancreatitis to the necrotizing form are largely unknown.

The pathophysiology of severe pancreatitis can be traced to the extravasation of the pancreatic enzymes. These toxic proteolytic enzymes cause widespread chemical inflammation of tissue. As a result, there is considerable loss and sequestration of protein-rich fluid from the vascular space, leading to hypovolemia and hypotension. Some of these enzymes also enter the systemic circulation and produce vasodilation and increased vascular permeability with a resultant loss of circulating fluid volume, contributing to hypovolemia, hypotension, and systemic hypoperfusion.

Multisystem complications of acute pancreatitis include almost every organ system and impact significantly on the morbidity and mortality of this disease. These complications can occur early in the course of the disease or as late as two weeks following the resolution of the acute phase. The etiologies of these complications range from enzyme impairment of the pancreatic function to pancreatic tissue necrosis (Table 3–1).

Differential diagnosis can be difficult, so it is necessary to look at the total picture of physical symptoms, laboratory data, and radiologic tests. The primary goals of medical treatment are to rest the pancreas, relieve the pain, and maintain intravascular fluid volume. Management of secondary complications are related to the organ system involved.

RISK PROFILE

Cancers: Pancreatic cancer, islet cell tumors, metastatic carcinoma to the pancreas.

Conditions: Alcoholism, biliary disease, immunosuppression, hypercalcemia, Zollinger-Ellison syndrome, long-term steroid therapy, radiation therapy, hyperparathyroidism, graft vs. host disease (GVHD), post endoscopic retrograde cholangiopancreatography (ERCP), hyperlipidemia.

Pediatrics: Post bone marrow transplant.

Environment: Viral; adenoviruses, mumps, *coxsackie, Staphylococcus,* scarlet fever, hepatitis B, *Campylobacter, Mycoplasma.*

Foods: Long-term hyperalimentation (biliary sludge), high-fat diets.

Table 3–1
Complications of Acute Pancreatitis

Complications	Physiologic Mechanism

Pulmonary
  Atelectasis
  Pleural effusion
  Acute respiratory distress syndrome
	Enzyme activity

Cardiovascular Hypotension	Enzyme activity Increased vascular permeability

Metabolic
  Hyperglycemia
  Metabolic acidosis
  Hypocalcemia
  Hypokalemia
	Pancreatic malfunction

Renal
  Prerenal failure
  Acute tubular necrosis
	Enzyme activity

Hematologic
  Thrombosis
  Disseminated intravascular coagulation
  Gastrointestinal/pancreatic bleed
	Enzyme activity
	Vascular stasis

Septic
  Pancreatic abscess
  Infected pseudocyst
  Peritonitis	

Central nervous system Pancreatic encephalopathy	

Drugs: Prednisone, 6-mercaptopurine, L-asparaginase, estrogens, Azothioprine, interleukin 2, cyclosporine, and combination chemotherapy (see Table 3–2 for other medications).

PROGNOSIS

The severity of symptoms of acute pancreatitis is dependent on the morphologic involvement, which is either edematous interstitial pancreatitis or necrotizing, fulminant pancreatitis. It is unclear what mechanism of action detemines which form will predominate. The edematous interstitial form is usually a mild cause that is self-limiting. In 5 to 15% of the cases the disease takes the fulminant course. The prognosis can be predicted by the morphologic type and the presence of the following systemic complications:

Table 3–2
Drugs Associated with Acute Pancreatitis

Acetaminophen	Hydrochlorothiazide	Procainamide
Amphetamines	Indomethacin	Propoxyphene
Calcium	Lipids	Rifampin
Chlorthalidone	Manganese	Salicylates
Cholestyramine	Mefenamic acid	Sulfa antibiotics
Cimetidine	Methyldopa	Sulindac
Clonidine	Nitrofurantoin	Tetracycline
Diazoxide	Opiates	Thiazides
Ethacrynic acid	Pentamidine	Valproic acid
Furosemide	Phenformin	Vitamin D
Histamine	Phenolphthalein	

1. *Cardiovascular* (systolic blood pressure [BP] < 80 mmHg for at least 15 minutes).
2. *Respiratory* (PO_2 < 60 mmHg, requiring O_2 > 24 hours).
3. *Renal* (serum creatinine > 1.4 mg% during hospitalization).
4. *Sepsis-like picture* (temperature > 39°C, white blood cells [WBC] > 20,000/mm³).

Category of Pancreatitis	Mortality
Interstitial with complications	Low
Necrotizing without complications	Low
Necrotizing with complications	High

Additionally, a very reliable determinant of prognosis is measurement of criteria on Ranson's Scale (Marshall, 1993). Three or more of the following criteria predict a severe course of the disease:

1. Age over 55 years.
2. WBC > 16,000/mm³.
3. Blood glucose > 200 mg/dl.
4. Base deficit over 4 mEq/L.
5. Serum lactate-dehydrogenase (LD) over 350 IU/L.
6. Aspartate aminotransferase (AST) over 250 IU/L.

Development of the following criteria in the first 48 hours indicates a worsening prognosis:

7. Hematocrit drop of > 10 percentage points.
8. Blood urea nitrogen (BUN) increase > 5 mg/dl.
9. Arterial pO_2 of < 60 mmHg.
10. Serum calcium of < 8 mg/dl.
11. Estimated fluid sequestration in abdomen of $> 6L$.

When 5 or 6 of the 11 Ranson criteria are present, the mortality rate is about 40%, and it increases if more criteria are present.

TREATMENT

Surgery: Severe/necrotizing fulminant—surgical debridement of necrotic pancreatic tissue; surgical incision and drainage (I and D) of pancreatic abscess, pseudocyst, or hemorrhage.

Chemotherapy: Not indicated.

Radiation: Not indicated.

Medications

Intravenous normal saline (NS), Ringer's lactate for intravascular volume replacement.
Antiemetic medications for nausea control.
Meperidine (Demerol) for pain management. Morphine is contraindicated, as it causes contraction of the sphincter of Oddi.
Insulin for management of hyperglycemia.
H_2 receptor blocker to reduce gastric secretions.
Intravenous antibiotics if fever $> 39°$ C.
Intravenous calcium gluconate for calcium replacement.

Procedures

Place nasogastric (NG) tube to intermittent suction to remove gastric secretions.
Arterial blood gas (ABG) monitoring for metabolic acidosis.
Oxygen therapy for oxygenation of tissues.
Dialysis for renal failure.
Peritoneal lavage to remove vasoactive substances from the peritoneum.

Other

Nothing by mouth (NPO).
Bed rest.
For severe/necrotizing fulminant pancreatitis:
- Placement of pulmonary artery catheter for monitoring of intravascular pressures.
- Intravenous hyperalimentation (HAL) for prolonged NPO status.

ASSESSMENT CRITERIA: ACUTE PANCREATITIS

	Mild/Edematous	Severe/Necrotizing
Vital signs		
Temperature	<39° C	>39° C
Pulse	Rapid	Rapid
Respirations	Tachypneic	Tachypneic
Blood pressure	Hypotensive	Systolic BP <80 mmHg
Central venous pressure	Normal	Below normal
History		
Conditions	Bone marrow transplant Alcoholic binge Highly fatty meal—recent Long-term hyperalimentation	
Hallmark physical signs and symptoms	Severe upper abdominal pain that is described as knifelike, twisting, relentless. May radiate to either costal margin or be referred to the lower back.	
Additional physical signs and symptoms	Mental aberrations, vomiting, nausea, low-grade fever, abdominal distension, abdominal guarding, abdominal tympany, hypoactive/absent bowel sounds, jaundice. **Severe/necrotizing pancreatitis:** Weakness, sweating, abdominal rigidity, ascites, rebound tenderness, palpable abdominal mass, Grey Turner's sign (a bluish discoloration of the lower abdominal flanks), Cullen's sign (a bluish discoloration of the umbilical area).	
Psychosocial signs	Anxiety	
Lab values		
Amylase, serum	Initially high but may normalize	
Amylase, urine	High	
Lipase, serum	High	
Triglycerides, serum	High	
Glucose	High	
Calcium	Low	
Magnesium	Low	
Potassium	Low or high	
Albumin	Low	
WBC	High	
Bilirubin	May be high	
Liver enzymes	May be high	
Prothrombin time	Prolonged	
ABGs	Hypoxemia, metabolic acidosis	
Creatinine	May be >1.5 mg%	

(continued)

ASSESSMENT CRITERIA: ACUTE PANCREATITIS (continued)

Diagnostic tests

Abdominal films	Assess potential areas of ileus.
Chest films	Assess atelectasis, pleural effusion, pneumonia.
ERCP	Assess abnormalities of the pancreatic duct.
Abdominal CT/ Ultrasonography/Magnetic resonance imaging (MRI)	Assess size of pancreas. Identify fluid collections, abscesses, or mass lesions. Identify if interstitial or necrotizing pancreatitis.

NURSING DIAGNOSIS

Pain related to:
- Anxiety and fear.
- Tissue damage.
- Inflammation, necrosis.
- Immobility.
- Peritoneal irritation from activated pancreatic exocrine enzymes.

Fluid volume deficit related to:
- Hemorrhage.
- Diaphoresis.
- Anorexia.
- Vomiting.
- Presence of NG tube.
- NPO regimen.
- Vascular fluid leak caused by pancreatic enzyme release.

Ineffective breathing patterns related to:
- Severe abdominal pain and distension.
- Need to maintain knee-chest position to alleviate pain.

Impaired gas exchange related to:
- Atelectasis.
- Pleural effusions.
- Acute respiratory distress syndrome (ARDS).
- Fluid overload during fluid administration.
- Splinting from pain.

Altered nutrition: **less than body requirements** related to:
- Anorexia, NPO status.
- Nausea and vomiting.
- Altered production of digestive enzymes.

Anxiety related to:
- Lack of knowledge regarding illness and cause of pain.
- Severity of illness.

Impairment of tissue integrity: oral mucous membranes related to dehydration.

Knowledge deficit: related to unfamiliarity with sequelae and treatment for pancreatitis.

NURSING INTERVENTIONS

Immediate nursing interventions

Assess pulse, respirations, blood pressure, and temperature q1h and PRN until stable.

Send serum electrolytes (Ca^{++}, glucose, Mg^{++}) panel, serum amylase, urine amylase, complete blood count (CBC) with differential.

Establish patent IV access and obtain volumetric infusion pump.

Measure hourly intake and output.

NPO status.

Position client for comfort, in sitting position or with knees on chest.

Anticipated physician orders and interventions

NG tube to low intermittent suction.

Demerol 100 to 150 mg IM q3–4h PRN for abdominal pain (other narcotics may cause contraction of the sphincter of Oddi).

IV fluid replacement according to severity of circulatory volume deficit (NS, Ringer's lactate, colloids).

Chest x-ray.

Ultrasound of abdomen.

CT (computed tomography) scan of pancreas.

Plain films of abdomen.

Anticholinergic drug therapy (to suppress gastrointestinal secretions).

IV electrolyte replacement according to deficits (hypocalcemia, hypokalemia, hypomagnesemia).

Severe acute pancreatitis: Additional anticipated physician orders and interventions

Pulmonary artery catheterization.

IV fluid replacement, including fresh frozen plasma, colloids, crystalloids, and blood products.

Vasopressor therapy: dopamine 2–5 µg/kg/minute or more to maintain systolic BP.

Peritoneal lavage.

Surgical intervention.

Antibiotic therapy.

Insulin therapy.

Nutritional support–total parenteral nutrition.

Ongoing nursing assessment, monitoring, and interventions

Assess:
- Breath sounds q1h and PRN.
- Level of comfort q3–4h and PRN and medicate accordingly.

- Nasal and oral mucous membranes q1h and provide mouth care PRN.
- Restlessness/anxiety and provide reassurance and antianxiety agents accordingly.

Measure:
- I and O q1h and PRN (urine output should be > 30 ml/hour).
- Nasogastric drainage.
- Pulmonary capillary wedge pressure if pulmonary artery catheter is present.
- Weight qd.
- Bedside blood glucose monitoring.

Send:
- Repeat serum electrolyte panel q24h and PRN.
- ABGs PRN.

Implement:
- Bed rest.
- NPO.
- Oral care.

TEACHING/EDUCATION

Select items, based on client's pathophysiology.

Nasogastric tube/NPO status: *Rationale:* The pain you are having now is because your pancreas is irritated. Eating and drinking would make it more irritated. So until it rests for a while you won't be allowed to eat or drink anything. We will make sure your mouth won't get dry. We also need to suction all the fluids out of your stomach, so we need to put in a tube through your nose into your stomach.

Intravenous blood samples: *Rationale:* Several blood and urine samples will be taken over the next few days. They are needed to check the condition of your pancreas.

Pain medication: *Rationale:* There is no reason for you to be in pain. You need to let us know when you are having pain, and we will give you an injection to take away the pain.

Intravenous fluid therapy: *Rationale:* You will need fluids while you can't eat anything, so you'll be getting them through your vein. You will also be getting other medications through your IV.

Diagnostic tests: *Rationale:* You will need to have some x-rays to help us know the condition of your pancreas.

Intensive care monitoring: *Rationale:* You need to be monitored more closely to see that your blood pressure and lungs are okay. You will have more IV lines and be connected to monitors.

EVALUATION/DESIRED OUTCOMES

1. Serum and urine amylase will return to normal within 72 hours.
2. Blood pressure will be within normal limits (WNL) within 48 hours.
3. Renal perfusion will be maintained as evidenced by urine output > 30 ml/hour.
4. Lungs are clear to auscultation within 48 hours.
5. Pain is relieved within 8 hours.
6. NG tube is discontinued within 72 hours.
7. Client is free of signs and symptoms of acute pancreatitis within 7 days.
8. Serum electrolytes are WNL within 72 hours.
9. Pancreatic abscess and signs and symptoms of long-term complications are understood by the client and the family.

DISCHARGE PLANNING

Client, post acute pancreatitis, may need: Training of the client and significant others in signs and symptoms of pancreatic abscess.

FOLLOW-UP CARE

Anticipated care: Physician office visit within 1 month.

Anticipated client/family questions and possible answers

What is pancreatitis?

"Your pancreas is an important organ; it helps your body digest the food you eat and helps your body use the food for energy. Sometimes a drug or a virus can irritate the pancreas so that it's not working right. It can cause a lot of problems when it's not working right, like pain, make you sick to your stomach, make your blood pressure drop. The only way to make it better is to let it rest by not having any food to digest."

What caused this problem with my pancreas?

"It might have been a combination of things, but most likely it was caused by a drug you were taking or by an infection."

Will this problem with my pancreas happen again?

"It is possible that this may happen again, and you need to know that if the abdominal pain starts again, or if you have a fever, call your doctor right away."

"It may happen again, and there are some things you can do to help prevent it. Avoid drinking alcohol and eating meals with a lot of fat, like fried foods, and avoid using lots of butter."

CHAPTER SUMMARY

Acute pancreatitis is an inflammatory process of the pancreas that is a rare but a potentially fatal complication in the oncology population. It occurs most frequently in the bone marrow transplant population. The disease ranges in severity from a mild self-limiting form to a fulminant state. Causes may include various drugs, viruses, long-term hyperalimentation, biliary disease, or immunosuppressive states. Nursing interventions and treatment are related to the severity of the disease and the occurrence of systemic complications. The occurrence of any of the systemic complications may constitute an acute oncologic emergency.

TEST QUESTIONS

1. The most useful laboratory test for the early diagnosis of acute pancreatitis is serum:
   A. Lipase
   B. Amylase
   C. Aspartate aminotransferase
   D. Bilirubin

1. Answer: B
The serum amylase will be elevated in the early stages of the onset of acute pancreatitis.

2. The primary cause of acute pancreatitis in the oncology population is:
   A. Malignant transformation of the pancreas
   B. Treatment-induced immunosuppressive state
   C. Toxic drug effects
   D. Radiation toxicity

2. Answer: B
The individuals at greatest risk in the oncology population are bone marrow recipients who experience GVHD. These clients are in a severely immunosuppressed state.

3. Initial treatment of acute pancreatitis includes:
   A. TPN, oxygen, and surgical exploration
   B. Analgesia, inhibition of pancreatic enzyme secretion, and fluid replacement
   C. Invasive monitoring, IV antibiotics, rest
   D. Needle aspiration pancreatic enzymes, ventilatory support, and enteral feeding

3. Answer: B
The three primary goals in initial management of acute pancreatitis are to treat the cardinal sign of abdominal pain, maintain blood pressure by fluid replacement, and halt secretion of pancreatic enzymes.

4. The hallmark symptom of acute pancreatitis is:
   A. Abdominal pain
   B. Hypotension
   C. Nausea and vomiting
   D. Abdominal distension

4. Answer: A
The hallmark symptom of acute pancreatitis is upper abdominal pain described as "knifelike, twisting, relentless" and may be referred to the lower back.

5. A frequent electrolyte imbalance associated with acute pancreatitis is:
   A. Hypercalcemia
   B. Hypermagnesemia
   C. Hyponatremia
   D. Hypokalemia

5. Answer: D
Hypokalemia may be present with prolonged vomiting, but serum potassium may be elevated if acute renal failure develops as a systemic complication.

6. The most important common complication of acute pancreatitis is:
   A. Immobility
   B. Paralytic ileus
   C. Fluid volume deficit
   D. Pneumonia

6. Answer: C
Fluid volume deficit may have multiple causes and may lead to hypovolemic shock or ARDS.

7. What is the pathobiologic mechanism that transforms the edematous form of acute pancreatitis into the necrotizing form?
   A. Hypotension
   B. Unknown mechanism
   C. Hypoxemia
   D. Pancreatic enzyme activity

7. Answer: B
To date, the underlying mechanism that causes the transformation from edematous pancreatitis to the necrotizing form is unknown.

8. The underlying pathophysiologic mechanism of acute pancreatitis is:
   A. Stimulation of the gallbladder
   B. Blockage of the pancreatic duct
   C. Premature activation of pancreatic enzymes
   D. Increased permeability of intestinal vasculature

8. Answer: C
The inflammation of acute pancreatitis is caused by the premature activation of pancreatic enzymes. This activation can be precipitated by drugs, viruses, disease conditions, or other miscellaneous etiologies.

9. Complications of acute pancreatitis amenable to surgical intervention include:
   A. Abscess
   B. Pseudocyst
   C. Hemorrhage
   D. All of the above

9. Answer: D
In order to prevent a fatal outcome, surgical intervention is absolutely essential in each of these three situations.

10. Essential nursing interventions for acute pancreatitis must focus on:
    A. Volume replacement
    B. Nutritional replacement
    C. Promoting comfort, monitoring vital signs judiciously, and assessing for potential complications
    D. Respiratory support

10. Answer: C
Besides providing comfort, nursing interventions must focus on meticulous assessment of the client's physical status in order to intervene in a timely manner.

REFERENCES

Banks P: Medical management of acute pancreatitis and complications. *In* Go V, Lebenthal E, et al (eds): The Pancreas: Biology, Pathobiology and Disease, 2nd ed. New York: Raven Press, 1993, pp. 593–610.

Chabner B: Miscellaneous agents. *In* Devita V, Hellman S, et al (eds): Cancer: Principles and Practice of Oncology, 4th ed. Philadelphia: JB Lippincott, 1993, p. 387.

Ko CW, Schoch HG, Lee SP, et al: Acute pancreatitis in marrow transplant: Prevalence at autopsy and risk factor analysis (Abstract). Proceedings of Annual Digestive Disease Conference, San Diego, California, May, 1995.

Everson G: Gallbladder function in gallstone disease. Gastroenterol Clin North Am 20(1):85–110, 1991.

Krumberger J: Acute pancreatitis. Crit Care Nurs Clin North Am 51:185–202, 1993.

Lin A, Feller ER: Pancreatic carcinoma as a cause of unexplained pancreatitis: Report of ten cases. Ann Intern Med 113(2):166–167, 1990.

Marshall JB: Acute pancreatitis: A review with an emphasis on new developments. Arch Intern Med 153(10):1185–1198, 1993.

McDonald G, Tirumali N: Intestinal and liver toxicity of antineoplastic drugs. West J Med 140(2):250–259, 1984.

Niemann T, Trigg M, Winick N, et al: Disseminated adenoviral infection presenting as acute pancreatitis. Hum Pathol 24(10):1145–1149, 1993.

Noone J: Acute pancreatitis: An Orem approach to nursing assessment and care. Crit Care Nurs 15(4):27–37, 1995.

Roubein L, Levin B: Gastrointestinal complications. *In* Holland J, Frei E, et al. (eds): Cancer Medicine, 3rd ed. Philadelphia: Lea and Febiger, 1993, pp. 2370–2381.

Soergel K: Acute pancreatitis. *In* Scharschmidt B, Feldman M (eds): Gastrointestinal Disease: Pathophysiology/Diagnosis/Management, 5th ed. Philadelphia: WB Saunders, 1993, pp. 1628–1653.

Yeung KY, Haidak DJ, Brown JA, et al: Metastasis induced acute pancreatitis in small cell bronchogenic carcinoma. Arch Intern Med 139:552–554, 1979.

CHAPTER 4

ACUTE RESPIRATORY DISTRESS SYNDROME

Annemarie Marwitz Kallenbach, RN, BSN, MS, CCRN, TNS

CHAPTER OBJECTIVES

At the completion of this chapter, the reader will be able to:

Define acute respiratory distress syndrome (ARDS).

Describe the pathophysiology of ARDS.

Describe clinical findings in the client with ARDS.

State risk factors associated with ARDS in the oncology client.

Describe nursing care as it relates to ARDS in the oncology client.

Anticipate and prepare the client with ARDS for future care needs.

OVERVIEW

ARDS is a profound form of respiratory failure. It is characterized by refractory hypoxemia and bilateral fluffy infiltrates on chest x-ray with a normal pulmonary capillary wedge (no evidence of left ventricular dysfunction). ARDS occurs in oncology clients who develop sepsis, pneumonia, or diffuse pulmonary infection. Neutropenic clients are at greatest risk of developing infection leading to sepsis. ARDS is differentiated from pulmonary fibrosis and interstitial pneumonitis by pulmonary biopsy. There is no direct treatment for ARDS. Instead, treatment is directed at reversal of the underlying cause and avoidance of complications and further deterioration.

DESCRIPTION

Incidence

In the United States, the incidence of ARDS is estimated to be 200,000 cases per year from all causes (Atkins, 1994). Although the syndrome was first described by Asbaugh in 1967 (Kollef and Schuster, 1995), its true incidence unknown, as consensus to its description was made only recently (Bernard et al., 1994). Forty to 60% of bone marrow transplant (BMT) clients develop adverse pulmonary sequelae, including ARDS, with 30 to 40% of BMT clients requiring intensive care unit (ICU) care. Mortality of BMT clients with respiratory compromise and mechanical ventilation ranges from 75 to 98% (Affessa et al., 1992).

Definition

ARDS is a syndrome of inflammation and increased lung capillary permeability. Originally called acute respiratory distress syndrome, the syndrome was subsequently labeled adult respiratory distress syndrome to differentiate it from the syndrome seen in premature infants. In the American-European Consensus conference on ARDS in 1994, it was decided to return to the original name, because the syndrome is not limited to adults. ARDS is associated with a grouping of physiologic, radiographic, and clinical findings that cannot be explained by increased left heart or pulmonary capillary pressures. Hallmark criteria are acute onset, refractory arterial hypoxemia, and diffuse radiologic infiltrates. In the oncology population ARDS is associated most with sepsis syndrome, aspiration, primary pneumonia, and diffuse pulmonary infection. Neutropenic clients are at high risk.

Pathophysiology

Because ARDS is associated with sepsis syndrome, aspiration, primary pneumonia, and diffuse pulmonary infection, these pathophysiologic processes initiate concurrent mechanisms. In sepsis, mediators and inflammation operate to contain, suppress, and eliminate infecting organisms and to clear damaged tissue of cellular debris and foreign material. This system may escape regulatory control. Mediators (Table 4–1) fall into numerous classes: *protein systems (humoral)*—complement, kinins, plasmins, and coagulation factors; *actual cells (cellular)*—lymphocytes, polymorphonuclear granulocytes, macrophages, and platelets; and *biochemical mediators*—histamine, tumor necrosis factor, interleukin 1 (IL-1), prostaglandins, and oxygen-free radicals (McFadden and Sartorius, 1992).

Alveolar epithelial disruption occurs from decreased blood flow in hypoperfusion states, damage from aspirates, direct vasoactive mediator damage due to the endotoxins and exotoxins released from bacterial, viral, and fungal pathogens and to inflammation. As the alveolar epithelium is disrupted, the alveoli are flooded with fluid and protein. This flooding destroys surfactant. Type I pneumocytes are damaged and result in degeneration and swelling of the alveoli. The normally thin membrane of the alveolar and capillary walls necessary for gas diffusion thickens, which results in the decreased diffusion of gas (oxygen). Type II pneumocyte damage and resulting decreased surfactant production lead to an increase in surface tension

Table 4–1
Mediators

Mediators	Action
Arachidonic acid metabolites (leukotrienes, prostaglandins, thromboxanes)	Affect vasomotor tone. Stimulate platelet aggregation. Affect macrophage/T-cell interaction. Affect temperature regulation. Influence cellular activation and mediator release. Provide bronchial smooth muscle tone.
Complement—amplifies inflammatory and immune responses.	Induces inflammation. Directs target cell lysis. Activates phagocytes. Causes opsonization.
Interleukins—stimulate neuroendocrine activity and provide a link between immune, nervous, and endocrine systems.	Stimulate leukocytosis. Enhance B-cell and T-cell activity. Diminish endothelium anticoagulation. Trigger vasodilator mediators. Stimulate acute phase reactants. Increase amino acid flux. Decrease vascular responsiveness to catecholamines. Stimulate neuroendocrine activation.
Kinins—regulate microvascular perfusion and enhance immune response.	Vasodilate. Increase capillary permeability. Stimulate WBC chemotaxis. Stimulate neutrophils. Contract smooth muscle.
Nitric oxide	Vasodilates.
Oxygen-free radicals—are locally produced during oxidative metabolism.	Alter cell membrane fluidity, secretory function, and ionic gradient. Alter cell receptor function. Cause denaturation of protein.
Platelet-activating factor—is a lipid mediator to activate platelets.	Causes platelet aggregation. Causes neutrophil adhesion. Causes neutrophil degranulation. Increases vascular permeability. Increases vasomotor changes.
Proteases—digest proteins.	Digest bacteria.
Tumor necrosis factor—mediates toxic effects of endotoxin.	Causes release of IL-1, PAF, and eicosanaoids. Increases collagenase for tissues remodeling. Causes increased WBC/endothelial interaction. Decreases vascular responsiveness to catecholamines.

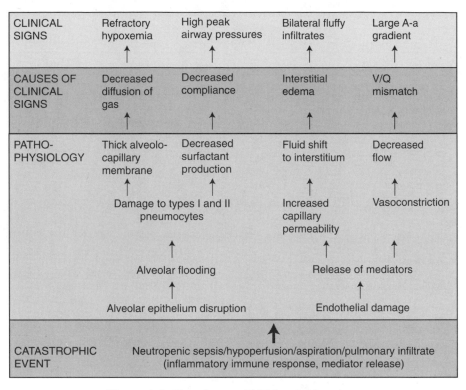

Figure 4–1 Clinical signs of ARDS pathophysiology.

within the alveoli. Another factor increasing the alveolar surface tension is the incorporation of surfactant into fibrin to form a hyaline membrane. The lungs, therefore, have decreased compliance or become stiff.

Endothelial damage also causes the release of mediators, with a twofold effect. First, there is increased capillary permeability, which results in fluid and protein movement into the interstitium of the lung and interstitial pulmonary edema. The release of mediators secondarily causes pulmonary vasoconstriction, which causes decreased blood flow to portions of the lung, resulting in ventilation perfusion (V/Q) mismatching (Fig. 4–1).

In summary, the decreased gas diffusion, increased lung compliance, interstitial edema, and V/Q mismatching result in progressive alveolar collapse and intrapulmonary shunting. These processes are evident in the refractory hypoxemia, high airway pressures, and bilateral fluffy infiltrates on chest x-ray.

Clinical findings

Clients in the early phase of developing ARDS present with tachypnea and anxiety. Wheezing and fine rales may be found upon auscultation of the lungs. Initial chest radiographs remain clear. Initial arterial blood gases (ABGs) will

Table 4–2
Oxygenation

	Normal Lungs	Acute Lung Injury (ALI)	Acute Respiratory Distress Syndrome (ARDS)
FiO_2	0.21 (room air)		> 0.50
PaO_2	80–100 mmHg		
FiO_2/PaO_2 ratio	400–500	< 300	< 200

demonstrate a respiratory alkalosis (increased pH due to decreased $PaCO_2$) as a result of hyperventilation caused by hypoxemia. Serial ABGs will demonstrate decreasing PaO_2 with the same or increasing supplemental oxygen (Table 4–2). Pulse oximetry changes will occur slowly and late.

RISK PROFILE

Cancers: Leukemias, hematologic malignancy, other cancers treated with high-dose chemotherapy and/or bone marrow transplant due to long neutropenic nadir (Bricksel and Whedon, 1995; Forman, 1994; McFadden and Sartorius, 1992; Whedon, 1991).

Pediatrics: Leukemia.

Conditions: Septic shock, hypotension, low perfusion states, profound neutropenia (Heyll et al., 1991), long nadir, sepsis syndrome (Bricksel and Whedon, 1995; Forman, 1994; McFadden and Sartorius, 1992; Whedon, 1991), infection, streptococcal infection (Elting, Bodey, and Keefe, 1992), aspiration, pneumonia, diffuse pulmonary infection, mucositis, and gastritis. Concomitant mucositis with its high oral bacterial load and risk of aspiration due to dysphagia also increases risk. Use of H_2 agonist and antacids increases the pH of the gastric environment and may predispose clients to higher levels of bacteria in the gut and to translocation outside of the GI tract.

Pediatrics: Stomatococcus mucilaginous in neutropenia (Henwick, Koehler, and Patrick, 1993).

Environment: Bacteria sources: fresh flowers, standing water, plants.

Table 4–3
Experimental Drugs

Note: Studies have not shown improvement in morbidity or mortality; therefore, no recommendation for use of these drugs has been made.

Drugs	Proposed Action
Antioxidants	Act as scavenger of oxygen-free radicals.
Nitrous oxide	Provides selective pulmonary vasodilation (no systemic effect) and therefore reduces pulmonary artery pressures and intrapulmonary shunting, with an increase in PaO_2/FiO_2 ratio, and no change in mean arterial pressure (MAP) or cardiac output.
Exogenous surfactant	Improves air-space stability and has antibacterial and immunologic properties. Therefore, results in reduced airway pressures, improved ventilation, and reduced incidence of nosocomial pneumonia.
Prostaglandins	Block platelet aggregation, modulate inflammation, cause vasodilation, and therefore improve oxygenation ratios.
Nonsteroid anti-inflammatory drugs	Inhibit endotoxin-induced increases in circulating tumor necrosis factor.
Ketoconazole	Inhibits thromboxane synthesis and inhibits the biosynthesis of the leukotrienes.
Pentoxifylline	Phosphodiesterase inhibitor (inhibits the chemotaxis and activation of neutrophils).
Antiendotoxin and anticytokines	Inhibit endotoxin and cytokines.

Source: Data from Kollef M, Schuster DP: The acute respiratory distress syndrome. N Eng J Med 332(1):27–37, 1995.

Foods: Fresh food containing live bacteria.

Drugs: Chemotherapy and total body irradiation that cause neutropenia (especially with longer nadir); conditioning for bone marrow transplant; chemotherapy that denudes or ulcerates oral and gastrointestinal mucosa. Concomitant mucositis with its high oral bacterial load and risk of aspiration due to dysphagia also increases risk. Use of H_2 agonist and antacids increase the pH of the gastric environment and may predispose clients to higher levels of bacteria in the gut.

PROGNOSIS

ARDS mortality rates vary from 16 to 78% depending on the source and definition. In the neutropenic septic client with ARDS, mortality approaches 72 to 96% (Paz, Crilley, Weinar, and Brodsky, 1993). If there is multiple organ failure with sepsis, mortality approaches 100%.

TREATMENT

Treatment is supportive, with the use of supplemental oxygen and mechanical ventilation when necessary. Intake and output (I and O) must remain even, as increased lung water worsens condition and prognosis. Nutrition, infection protection, and antibiotic therapy are important components of supportive therapy. Many experimental therapies are being used to try to improve morbidity and mortality (Table 4–3).

Surgery: None.

Chemotherapy: None.

Radiation: None.

Medications

Antibiotics: early empirical administration, late administration based on culture result.

For administration of experimental drugs, see Table 4–3.

Combinations of analgesics and sedation are used to reduce oxygen demands. Anesthetic adjuncts such as propofol and neuromuscular blockade are added when oxygenation cannot be maintained.

Procedures

Mechanical ventilation. Use of positive end expiratory pressure (PEEP) is advocated to keep FiO_2 at the lowest possible level. FiO_2 of greater than 0.50 is considered to carry a risk for oxygen toxicity and causes further damage to the lungs.

Pulmonary artery catheters may be inserted to rule out contributing cardiac conditions (e.g., decreased cardiac output, left heart failure) and to closely evaluate and maximize fluid, vasoactive drug, and PEEP utilization (Haupt, Kaufman, and Carlson, 1992).

Experimental: permissive hypercapnia ventilation (Atkins, Egloff, and Willms, 1994).

Experimental: inverse ratio ventilation (Manthous and Schmidt, 1993).

Other

Care in an ICU.

Experimental: extracorporeal membrane oxygenation (Dirkes, Dickinson, and Valentine, 1992).

Experimental in adults: exogenous surfactant (Jacobson, Park, Psych, and Holcroft, 1993).

ASSESSMENT CRITERIA:
ACUTE RESPIRATORY DISTRESS SYNDROME

Vital signs	Tachypnea, tachycardia, decreased SaO_2
History	Neutropenia, infection, mucositis
Hallmark physical signs and symptoms	Dyspnea
Additional physical signs and symptoms	Diminished breath sounds
Psychosocial signs	Anxiety
Lab values	(Early) respiratory alkalosis (pH > 7.4, $PaCO_2$ < 40)
	PaO_2: FiO_2 <200 on ABG
	A-a (Alveolar-arterial) gradient
	Shunt (Q_s/Q_t) >10%
	ANC <500 neutrophils/mm³
Diagnostic tests	Bilateral fluffy infiltrates on chest x-ray
	Pulmonary artery catheterization
	Pulmonary artery wedge pressure (PAWP) <18 mm Hg
	Cardiac output—normal (4–8 L/minute)
Other	Increased peak inspiratory pressure
	Increased static effective compliance
	$$= \frac{\text{Tidal volume}}{\text{Plateau pressure} - \text{PEEP}}$$
	(Normal >50 ml/cm H_2O)
	Increased dynamic compliance
	$$= \frac{\text{Tidal volume}}{\text{Peak inspiratory pressure} - \text{PEEP}}$$
	(Normal 40–50 ml/cm H_2O)

NURSING DIAGNOSIS

Impaired gas exchange related to ARDS process.
Ineffective breathing pattern related to increased lung compliance and high oxygen demands.
Anxiety related to dyspnea.

Impaired verbal communication due to mechanical ventilation.

Altered nutrition, less than body requirements related to NPO status due to mechanical ventilation, high metabolic demands.

High risk for impaired skin integrity related to mucositis and endotracheal (ET) tube placement.

NURSING INTERVENTIONS

Immediate nursing interventions

Respiratory monitoring.

Oxygen therapy.

Mechanical ventilation.

Hemodynamic monitoring (McCloskey and Bulechek, 1994).

Maintain a patent airway.

Auscultate breath sounds.

Monitor respiratory and oxygenation status.

Remove secretions by encouraging coughing.

Administer/monitor respiratory treatments (e.g., bronchodilators, nebulizer treatments) as appropriate.

Perform/monitor chest physical therapy as appropriate.

Assist with incentive spirometer as appropriate.

Assist with ET intubation as necessary.

Gather necessary intubation and emergency equipment and position client, administering medications as ordered and monitoring for complication during intubation procedure.

Verify ET placement with a chest radiograph, ensuring cannulation of the trachea 1 to 4 cm above the level of the carina.

Apply suction as needed.

Institute measures to prevent self-extubation.

Monitor effects of ventilator changes on oxygenation: ABGs, SaO_2, SvO_2, and end tidal CO_2, shunt, $A\text{-}aDO_2$, client's subjective response.

Administer oxygen and monitor its effectiveness.

Maintain SpO_2 >90%.

Optimize heart rate, preload, afterload, and contractility.

Administer positive inotropic/contractility medications.

Evaluate side effects of negative inotropic medications.

Administer vasodilator and/or vasoconstrictor medications as appropriate.

Anticipated physician orders and interventions

Ventilation perfusion scan.

Mechanical ventilation: Increase/decrease FiO_2 to maintain SaO_2 >90%.

Pulmonary artery catheter insertion.

Pan culture with fever spike.

Sputum culture when change in color of sputum.

Total parenteral nutrition or gastric feeding.

Treatment of infection source or highly suspicious source.

Ongoing nursing assessment, monitoring, and interventions

Infection protection.

Nutrition therapy.

Anxiety reduction.

Circulatory care.

Pain management.

Skin monitoring. (McCloskey and Bulechek, 1994)

Assess:

- Lung sounds q4h and PRN.
- Respiratory rate q1h.
- SpO_2 continuously.
- SvO_2 continuously.
- PaO_2 q4h during acute desaturation period or while titrating FiO_2 up to maintain SaO_2 > 90%, then qd.
- Peak airway pressure q1h with ventilator setting and respiratory rate monitoring. Notify MD for trend upward.
- Exhaled tidal volume by continuous alarm settings.
- Effects of ventilator changes on oxygenation: ABG, SaO_2, SvO_2 and end tidal CO_2, A-aDO_2, client's subjective response.
- Blood pressure, heart rate (continuously), and cardiac output q8h and PRN with increasing levels of PEEP.
- Side effects of negative inotropic medications.
- Oxygen delivery/oxygen consumption parameters with changes in hemoglobin, cardiac output, and SaO_2.
- Degree of shunt, vital capacity, dead space, maximal ventilator volume (MVV), inspiratory force, and forced expiratory volume in one second (FEV1) for readiness to wean from mechanical ventilation daily.
- Respiratory secretions with suctioning.
- Electrolytes (especially potassium, magnesium, and phosphorus) qd.
- Nutrition needs within first 3 days.
- Tube feeding residual q8h.
- Bowel sounds q4h.
- Elimination pattern qd.

Measure:

- Vital signs q1h and PRN.

- Pulmonary artery pressures q1h verify correlation with pulmonary capillary wedge pressure q shift.
- Cardiac output/index, systemic vascular resistance (SVR) q shift and PRN, especially with changes in PEEP.
- Central venous pressure (CVP) q1h.
- I and O q1h.
- Weights qd at time of I and O total.

Send:
- Cultures q 3 days.
- ABGs as above.
- Complete blood count with differential qd until absolute neutrophil count (ANC) > 500.
- Electrolytes qd.

Implement:
- Neutropenic precautions.
- Ventilator care protocols.
- Maintain safe/stable artificial airway.
- Maintain ET tube at correct centimeter marking at lip.
- Change ET placement position q24h, inspecting for skin integrity.
- Check ET cuff for minimal cuff pressure, using minimal leak technique.
- Institute measures to prevent self-extubation.
- Minimize leverage and traction of artificial airway.
- Pulmonary hygiene routines (e.g., respiratory treatments; chest physical therapy; incentive spirometer; deep breathing and coughing; suctioning).
- FiO_2 weaning to maintain adequate PaO_2.
- Gastric feeding protocols.
- Skin care protocols.
- Communication plan with health care team, client, and family.

TEACHING/EDUCATION

Intensive care regimen: *Rationale:* Because you/your family member need close monitoring, a breathing machine and electronic equipment to monitor heart rate and rhythm, blood pressure, and heart pressures are used. A catheter is placed into the heart to measure and regulate body fluid levels.

Equipment/alarm use: *Rationale:* There are many pieces of equipment, noises, and alarms that help the health care team do its work to closely monitor your/your family member's care. If you see anything you do not understand, please ask the health care team.

Mechanical ventilator: *Rationale:* Because the work and effort of breathing is difficult, you/your family member is attached to a breathing machine. This machine provides high levels of oxygen and also supports the work of breathing.

Arterial catheter/ABGs: *Rationale:* A small tube has been inserted into the wrist to directly obtain blood to measure how well oxygen is getting to the lung tissue.

Pulse oximeter: *Rationale:* The red light attached to your/your family member's finger or ear gives us constant information about how the oxygen is getting to the tissues of the body.

Daily chest x-ray: *Rationale:* We take an x-ray every day to measure the progress of your/your family member's lung function.

Wrist restraints: *Rationale:* Because of the risk of accidental removal of any of the important equipment in place, your arms have been gently tied down as a reminder not to pull at the equipment.

EVALUATION/DESIRED OUTCOMES

The client will demonstrate the following:

1. Adequate airway patency and gas exchange as evidenced by SaO_2 > 90% on lowest possible FiO_2.
2. Improving circulation and perfusion as evidenced by cardiac output within normal limits, urine output > 30 ml/hour.
3. Improving homeostatic electrolyte, acid-base balance—i.e., pH and electrolytes (e.g., calcium, magnesium, phosphorus) within normal range, output greater than or equal to intake.
4. Adequate nutritional support, as evidenced by intake of calories to meet metabolic needs.
5. Comprehensive antibiotic coverage for organisms that have been cultured or are highly suspect; no evidence of secondary respiratory complications (e.g., pneumothorax, atelectasis, aspiration, or accidental extubation).
6. Restoration of comfort.
7. Knowledge of health problem to sustain health as evidenced by appropriate questions and verbalized understanding of intensive care routine, equipment and procedures, prognosis, and treatment plan.
8. Tolerance of identified physical activities without fatigue and excess energy expenditure as evidenced by maintenance of functional level.

DISCHARGE PLANNING

ARDS client may need:

Long-term ventilation.
Help in end-of-life or quality-of-life ethical decision making.

FOLLOW-UP CARE

Anticipated care

Follow-up with pulmonologist for 3 to 6 months.
Periodic chest x-ray follow-up.
Avoidance and early detection of respiratory tract infection.
Client to keep a copy of the chest x-ray as a baseline.

Anticipated client/family questions and possible answers

How long will it take before my chest x-ray returns to normal?

"The chest x-ray can take up to a year, if ever, to return to normal."

Will I ever get off the ventilator?

"With ARDS the person can have a short stay in the ICU (3 days) or a very long stay. Many times a person may reach a plateau where he or she does not get better or worse. Long-term or chronic use of a breathing machine may be needed. Sometimes this care is provided outside the ICU a subacute setting."

How can I prepare for the future?

"Sometimes when a person is ill enough to be in intensive care for a long time (longer than a week), their condition worsens because of complications or failure of other body parts. If either occurs, it would be important to know how you want to live. If we need to make decisions with you, we will gather the whole health care team together (including a person from the hospital ethics department when necessary) to discuss what is the best treatment plan for you/your family member."

CHAPTER SUMMARY

Care of the oncology client with ARDS requires a thorough understanding of the clinical findings and related pathophysiology. The client presents with dyspnea and anxiety. Initial ABG findings include respiratory alkalosis due to hyperventilation and a decrease in PaO_2. As the client worsens, the hypoxemia worsens and becomes refractory to oxygen therapy without mechanical ventilation. Chest radiographic exam shows diffuse bilateral infiltrates without evidence of left ventricular failure. High airway pressures are found due to the decreased compliance of the lungs.

Intensive nursing care has been found to decrease mortality. Oncology clients with ARDS need mechanical ventilation with PEEP. Respiratory monitoring includes client assessment, ventilator–client interface assessment, serial ABGs, and continuous pulse oximetry to ensure adequate oxygenation. Close fluid monitoring with the aid of a pulmonary artery catheter is done to maximize hemodynamic status and minimize fluid administration.

Keeping the client in zero balance is critical to reduction in morbidity and mortality.

Because there is no direct treatment for ARDS, care is directed at treating the underlying cause, which, in the oncology client, is usually neutropenic sepsis and hypotension. Treatment for the oncology client with ARDS is also supportive in nature: It includes protection from secondary infection, monitoring and reduction of risk of respiratory barotrauma, and maintenance of nutritional and functional status. Prevention of complications and of a worsening of condition is a critical component to survival.

The needs of the client and family require constant education and support to reduce anxiety. Anxiety is induced from the cancer diagnosis, the critical nature of ARDS, the intensive care environment, and the overwhelming amount of information about the disease and its care that must be assimilated.

Survival from ARDS is possible, but it requires a comprehensive collaborative team approach between the many members of the health care team, the client, and the client's family. Collaboration must occur between the oncology and intensive care teams. Referral, resources, and education before the client comes to the ICU must be provided proactively in institutions where high-level chemotherapy, total body irradiation, and bone marrow transplantation occur.

TEST QUESTIONS

1. ARDS is an acronym for:
   A. Adult respiratory distress syndrome
   B. Acute respiratory distress syndrome
   C. Acute lung injury respiratory distress syndrome
   D. Aspiration respiratory distress syndrome

1. Answer: B
ARDS occurs in both adults and children. It is more severe then acute lung injury but shares common features with it. The syndrome was renamed in 1992 at the American-European Consensus conference.

2. ARDS is characterized by the following pulmonary artery reading:
   A. Elevated PAD
   B. Elevated PAWP
   C. Normal PAWP
   D. Normal CVP

2. Answer: C
ARDS is differentiated from cardiogenic pulmonary edema by a normal left heart pressure as demonstrated by a normal left ventricular end diastolic pressure (LVEDP) or pulmonary artery wedge pressure (PAWP).

3. ARDS etiology in the oncology client is *not* due to:
   A. Neutropenia
   B. Infection
   C. Direct result of chemotherapy agents
   D. Pulmonary capillary leak

3. Answer: C
ARDS in the oncology client is seen as a result of sepsis syndrome, which is more frequent in the neutropenic client or the client with infection. Pathophysiology includes pulmonary capillary leak.

4. Peak inspiratory pressures in ARDS:
   A. Increase
   B. Decrease
   C. Do not change
   D. Range from 25 to 30 cm H_2O

4. Answer: A
Increased stiffness (decreased compliance) is seen in ARDS. Normal compliance is < 50 ml/cm H_2O.

5. Chest x-ray appearance in ARDS is:
   A. Unilateral infiltrate
   B. Pneumothorax
   C. Flattened diaphragm
   D. Bilateral fluffy infiltrates

5. Answer: D
Classic chest x-ray pattern is bilateral fluffy infiltrates due to interstitial edema.

6. Refractory hypoxemia refers to:
   A. Low PaO_2 despite $FiO_2 > 50\%$
   B. Saturation $< 90\%$
   C. PaO_2 of 80
   D. SvO_2 below normal

6. Answer: A
In ARDS there is a large shunt that does not allow oxygen to reach the arterial blood; *it does not improve* without a large amount of inspired oxygen. SvO_2 (mixed venous saturation) is not usually affected in ARDS for unknown reasons.

7. The ratio of PaO_2 to FiO_2 in ARDS is:
   A. 500
   B. 400
   C. < 300
   D. < 200

7. Answer: D
Normal ratio is 500 (on room air 21% PaO_2 equals 100 $= 0.21 \times 500$). ARDS is defined by the ratio's being less than 200.

8. Pulmonary vasoconstriction in ARDS is *not* due to:
   A. Mediator release
   B. Neutrophil degradation
   C. Shunt
   D. Increased $PaCO_2$

8. Answer: D
Shunt is due to mediator and neutrophil factors; it is worsened by the need of the lung to shunt oxygen away from unventilated areas. Decreased $PaCO_2$ causes vasoconstriction.

9. Serial arterial blood gases (ABGs) are necessary to detect changes in:
   A. SvO_2
   B. SpO_2
   C. PaO_2
   D. $PaCO_2$

9. Answer: C
ABGs are necessary to trend the PaO_2 to FiO_2 ratio and is the best indicator of ARDS progression and regression. SpO_2 trends oxygen saturation without the need to draw ABGs. SvO_2 must be drawn from the distal port of a pulmonary artery catheter or read from a fiberoptic sensor on a pulmonary catheter. $PaCO_2$ can be drawn and trended from venous blood.

10. Complications from mechanical ventilation do *not* include:
    A. Pneumothorax
    B. Accidental extubation
    C. Pneumonia
    D. Oxygen desaturation

10. Answer: D
Mechanical ventilation is not without risk. Vigilant nursing care can decrease the rate of complications.

REFERENCES

Affessa B, Tefferi A, Hoagland HC, Letendre L, Peters S: Outcomes of recipients of bone marrow transplants who require intensive care unit support. Mayo Clin Proc 67:117–122, 1992.

Atkins P, Egloff M, Willms D: Respiratory consequences of multisystem crisis: The adult respiratory distress syndrome. Crit Care Nurs Q 16(4):27–38, 1994.

Bernard G, Artigas A, Brigham K, Carlet J, Falke K, Hudson L, Lamy M, Legall J, Morris A, Spragg R, and the Consensus Committee: The American-European Consensus conference on ARDS: Definitions, mechanisms, relevant outcomes and clinical trial coordination. Am J Respir Crit Care Med 149:818–824, 1994.

Bricksel PC, Whedon MB: Bone Marrow Transplantation: Administrative and Clinical Strategies. Boston: Jones and Bartlett, 1995.

Dirkes S, Dickinson S, Valentine J: Acute respiratory failure and ECMO. Crit Care Nurs Q 12(7):39–47, 1992.

Elting L, Bodey G, Keefe B: Septicemia and shock syndrome to viridans streptococci: A case-control study of predisposing factors. Clin Infect Dis 14(6):1201–1207, 1992.

Forman SJ (ed): Bone Marrow Transplantation. Boston: Blackwell Scientific Publications, 1994, p. 517.

Haupt MT, Kaufman BS, Carlson RW: Fluid resuscitation in patients with increased vascular permeability. Crit Care Clin 8(2):341–353, 1992.

Henwick S, Koehler M, Patrick C: Complications of bacteremia due to Stomatococcus mucilaginosus in neutropenic children. Clin Infect Dis 17(4):667–671, 1993.

Heyll A, Aul C, Gogolin F, Thomas M, Arning M, Gehrt A, Hadding U: Granulocyte colony-stimulating factor (G-CSF) treatment in neutropenic leukemia client with diffuse interstitial pulmonary infiltrates. Ann Hematol 63(6):328–332, 1991.

Jacobson W, Park G, Psych T, Holcroft J: Surfactant and adult respiratory distress syndrome. Br J Anesth 70:522–526, 1993.

Kollef M, Schuster DP: The acute respiratory distress syndrome. N Engl J Med 332(1):27–37, 1995.

Manthous C, Schmidt G: Inverse ratio ventilation in ARDS: Improved oxygenation with autoPEEP. Chest 103(3):953–954, 1993.

McCloskey J, Bulechek G (eds): Nursing Interventions Classification. St. Louis, MO: Mosby Year Book, 1992.

McFadden ME, Sartorius SE: Multiple systems organ failure in the patient with cancer. Oncol Nurs Forum 19(5):719–724, 1992.

Paz HL, Crilley P, Weinar M, Brodsky I: Outcomes of patients requiring medical ICU admission following bone marrow transplantation. Chest 104(2):527–531, 1993.

Schilero GJ, Oropello J, Benjamin E: Impairment in gas exchanged after granulocyte colony stimulating factor (G-CSF) in a client with the adult respiratory distress syndrome. Chest 107(1):276–278, 1995.

Secor VH: Multisystem organ failure: A pathophysiologic approach. Lewisville, TX: Barbara Clark Mims Associates, 1994, pp. 15–43.

Whedon MB: Bone Marrow Transplantation: Principles, Practice and Nursing Insights. Boston: Jones and Bartlett, 1991.

CHAPTER 5

AIRWAY OBSTRUCTION

Marti Reiser, RN, MSN, CCRN

AND

Constance Visovsky, MS, RN, ACNP

CHAPTER OBJECTIVES

At the completion of this chapter, the reader will be able to:

Define airway obstruction.

Discuss early recognition of airway obstruction.

Describe the cancers that place the client most at risk of airway obstruction.

Formulate an appropriate plan of care for a client experiencing airway obstruction.

Prioritize and initiate emergency nursing interventions designed to relieve airway obstruction.

OVERVIEW

CERTAINLY one of the most frightening and life-threatening acute complications of the oncologic client is airway obstruction. Rapid assessment and intervention of this oncologic emergency is mandatory. The causes of airway obstruction in the client with cancer are multifactorial. Primary disease, metastatic disease, treatment factors, and co-morbidities all can potentiate airway obstruction requiring acute care interventions.

DESCRIPTION

Upper airway obstruction occurs when air flow from the nose, mouth, and throat into the lower airway is impaired. Rapid recognition of this occurrence by the nurse is required to prevent respiratory arrest. Airway obstruction in the client with cancer is most often associated with tumors that occlude the upper airway. Cancers of the head, neck, thyroid, esophagus, lung, and superior mediastinal tumors, as well as metastatic disease, are most commonly associated with airway obstruction (Woodlock, 1993). Tumors that arise in or metastasize to the chest are directly related to pulmonary and cardiac complications. For example, a lung tumor may cause compression of vital structures, resulting in respiratory failure (Shelton, 1996).

Conditions such as malignant pericardial and pleural effusions, superior vena cava syndrome, pneumonia, pulmonary embolism, as well as mechanical obstruction of the airway via direct tumor invasion can require immediate acute care interventions (Shuey, 1994). Many individuals with cancer have some associated co-morbidity that may predispose them to airway obstruction. Emphysema, secondary to cigarette smoking, is frequently associated with lung cancer and may require the client to be mechanically ventilated at some point in the disease course.

Toxicities to the lung are a potential complication of high-dose chemotherapy and radiation treatments. Radiation-induced pneumonitis occurs in approximately 20% of clients and can persist for up to 12 months after the completion of treatment. Five percent of clients experience pulmonary fibrosis due to chemotherapy treatments with bleomycin, which results in a decrease in both diffusion of gases and total lung capacity (Bakemier and Qazi, 1993; McCoy-Adabody and Borger, 1996). The percentage of pulmonary toxicity from bleomycin increases to 17% when cumulative doses exceed 550 IU (international units). Other chemotherapeutic agents implicated in pulmonary toxicity include cyclophosphamide, carmustine, busulfan, mitomycin, methotrexate, and chlorambucil (Polomano, Weintraub, and Wurster, 1994). Both primary and metastatic lesions to the chest have the capability to cause significant pulmonary and cardiac compromise requiring acute care interventions. Lung and mediastinal tumors potentiate such complications as superior vena cava syndrome, syndrome of inappropriate antidiuretic hormone, pulmonary embolism, and malignant pleural effusion. Multimodal cancer treatment involving both high-dose chemotherapy and radiation treatments can lead to further airway compromise due to toxicities associated with treatment.

RISK PROFILE

Cancers: Head and neck cancer, specifically, cancer of the larynx, tongue, and thyroid; lung cancer (commonly bronchogenic carcinoma); malignant mesothelioma; superior mediastinal tumors (commonly lymphomas and lung cancer); hematologic malignancies; and esophageal cancer.

Conditions: Pneumonia, superior vena cava syndrome, malignant pleural effusion, radiation-induced pulmonary toxicity, chemotherapy-induced pulmonary toxicity, chronic obstructive pulmonary disease (COPD), pre-existing or concurrent cardiac compromise, chronic graft vs. host disease.

Environment: Allergens, which may be responsible for airway edema; smoking; asbestos exposure.

Foods: None.

Drugs: Bleomycin, cyclophosphamide, busulfan, chlorambucil, melphalan, carmustine (BCNU), lomustine, semustine, chlorozotocin, and methotrexate.

PROGNOSIS

Cancer clients most likely to survive a critical event, such as mechanical ventilation, are those with solid tumors who have been intubated for airway obstruction or those with newly diagnosed cancer, presenting as an oncologic emergency (Shelton, 1996). Early, rapid recognition and intervention is associated with a decline in mortality and morbidity resulting from airway obstruction. Clients at high risk for the development of airway obstruction will require intensive and vigilant monitoring and intervention by both medical and nursing professionals. Prognosis is directly related to the underlying etiology, functional status, nutritional state, and age of the client. Additionally, simultaneous treatment with radiation and chemotherapy may predispose clients to difficult weaning and prolonged ventilatory support (Polomano et al., 1994).

The treatment plan should clearly address such issues as co-morbidities, stage of disease, cancer prognosis, the wishes of both client and significant others regarding critical care interventions, and treatment options (Shelton, 1996).

TREATMENT

Procedures: Secure and maintain a patent airway by hyperextending the neck and/or by the use of an oral or nasal airway. Anticipate the need to suction the client if necessary and to manually ventilate the apneic client. Nasal or oral intubation using an endotracheal tube may follow.

Surgery: An emergency cricothyrotomy or tracheostomy may be performed in cases where intubation is contraindicated, or impossible due to large tumor burden. Surgery may also consist of debulking a large, obstructive tumor. Bronchoscopic laser treatment to relieve malignant airway obstruction has recently shown promising results. Laser bronchoscopy is performed as a palliative measure aimed at decreasing the feeling of "smothering" (asphyxia) present when large central airways are obstructed. Stent placement may be considered if the underlying etiology of the obstruction is due to superior vena cava syndrome. The reader is referred to the Chapter 41 for further information on this particular pathologic cause of airway obstruction.

Such surgical treatments are often followed by either radiation or chemotherapy. The course of critically ill oncology clients is often complicated by infection, bleeding tendencies, metabolic abnormalities, and compromised organ function. The practitioner should anticipate that the need for intensive care following surgery will be greater in this population (Polomano et al., 1994).

Chemotherapy: After emergency procedures and surgery, chemotherapy may be used to reduce the tumor in size or to sensitize the tumor for radiation therapy.

Radiation: Radiation is the treatment of choice for a large, obstructive tumor, especially in cases where the potential of respiratory obstruction is high. Tumor histology determines the radiation dosage. Lymphomas require a relatively small dose of radiation (2000 to 4000 cGys), but a larger treatment field, such as the mantle field. Solid tumors require a higher dose (5000 to 6000 cGys over 5 to 7 weeks) and are irradiated directly (Shuey, 1994). Tumors within the bronchi can be treated with laser therapy or focused-beam radiotherapy via the endotracheal tube (Nally, 1996).

Medications: Theophylline to reduce bronchospasm; epinephrine, isoetharine (Bronkosol), metaproterenol (Alupent), isoproterenol (Isuprel) aerosols to reduce bronchospasm; corticosteroids to reduce inflammation and edema and to possibly ameliorate lung toxicities associated with radiation or chemotherapy (Harwood, 1996); morphine for pain relief and reduction in oxygen demands; racemic epinephrine to reduce laryngeal edema.

Other: Fibrinolytic therapy may be considered in superior vena cava syndrome complicated by thrombosis (Shuey, 1994). Long- or short-term mechanical ventilation may be indicated. Palliative thoracentesis may be used for symptom management of intractable dyspnea.

ASSESSMENT CRITERIA: AIRWAY OBSTRUCTION

Vital signs	Heart rate and blood pressure elevated or within normal limits; respiratory rate increased or decreased. Tachycardia; tachypnea with wheezing and stridor.
History	See Risk Profile.
Hallmark physical signs and symptoms	Air hunger with labored breathing, acute anxiety with feeling of "smothering" (asphyxia), dyspnea, shortness of breath, stridor, wheezing, restlessness. "Crowing" respirations in pediatric patients with upper airway obstruction.
Additional physical signs and symptoms	Use of respiratory accessory muscles, sternal and intercostal muscle retractions, cough, orthopnea. Diminished or absent breath sounds distal to lesion, crackles or rhonchi or combination.
Psychosocial signs	Restlessness, feeling of suffocation, and eventually confusion.

(continued)

ASSESSMENT CRITERIA: AIRWAY OBSTRUCTION *(continued)*

Lab values	
ABGs	PaO$_2$: low
	PaCO$_2$: low if hyperventilating, high if hypoventilating.
	pH and NaHCO$_3$: vary depending on underlying cause.
	O$_2$ saturation <90%.
Diagnostic tests	CT scan of the chest, MRI, chest x-ray, bronchoscopy, esophageal radiography to identify cause and degree of obstruction.
Other	Assess hydration and institute fluid replacement or diuretics.

NURSING DIAGNOSIS

Ineffective airway clearance related to mechanical obstruction.

Anxiety related to dyspnea and hypoxia.

Acute confusion related to hypoxia.

Impaired gas exchange related to V/Q mismatch, tumor obstruction, infiltration, and edema.

Altered tissue perfusion related to V/Q mismatch.

Impaired physical mobility related to hypoxia and dyspnea.

Fear related to severe breathlessness and risk for death.

Ineffective family coping related to fear and anxiety.

NURSING INTERVENTIONS

Immediate nursing interventions

Open airway by tilting the head and inserting an oral airway.

Apply O$_2$ by nasal cannula or mask.

Prepare for oral or nasal intubation; prepare for possible emergency cricothyrotomy or tracheostomy.

Assess vital signs q5min.

Perform respiratory assessment immediately following opening of airway and q5min until respiratory distress subsides.

Monitor oxygen saturation via pulse oximetry.

Use suctioning as needed.

Send arterial blood sample for STAT arterial blood gas (ABG).

Establish IV access.

Prepare for arterial line.

Notify primary care provider, family, and chaplain.

Anticipated physician orders and interventions

Intubation and/or tracheostomy.

Arterial line.

Possible pulmonary artery catheter insertion.

Stat and serial ABGs.

Stat electrolytes, blood urea nitrogen (BUN), creatinine, blood glucose.

Stat chest x-ray (portable) to check endotracheal tube/tracheostomy (ETT/trach) placement and identify cause of airway obstruction.

MRI or CAT scan.

Positive pressure ventilation.

Continuous pulse oximetry.

Intake and output (I and O).

Daily weights.

Ongoing nursing assessment, monitoring, and interventions

Assess:
- Level of consciousness q1h and PRN.
- Patency of artificial airway and be alert for complications.
- Respiratory status q1h and PRN: breath sounds, oxygen saturation, mechanical ventilation settings and client tolerance, evidence of mediastinal shift.
- For signs and symptoms of infection related to neutropenia.

Measure:
- Vital signs q1h.
- I and O q1h for 24 hours, daily weights.

Send:
- Serial ABGs and electrolytes PRN until values normalize or return to baseline.

Implement:
- Continuous pulse oximetry.
- Ventilator changes (at the lowest FIO_2 to maintain a $PaO_2 > 60$ mmHg in order to avoid oxygen toxicity).
- Suctioning PRN.
- IV replacement therapy.
- Tube feedings.
- Sedation PRN to adequately ventilate client.
- Position changes q2h and PRN.
- Chest physical therapy q2h and PRN (unless client is thrombocytopenic).
- Bronchodilators as prescribed.
- Pain medications as needed.

- Comfort measures.
- Mouth care q4h and PRN.

TEACHING/EDUCATION

Artificial airway: *Rationale:* An artificial airway is needed to supply oxygen to you. The airway prevents you from talking, but this is only temporary. You will be able to talk when the airway is removed. A breathing machine may be necessary until the cause of airway obstruction is identified and treated.

IV fluids and arterial line: *Rationale:* You will need an IV line in your vein to give you fluids because you will be unable to eat or drink while the artificial airway is in place. Another special IV line will be placed in your artery to take many blood samples painlessly.

Purpose of suctioning: *Rationale:* A tube will be put in your airway to remove phlegm and allow you to breathe more easily.

Purpose of pulse oximetry: *Rationale:* A clip will be placed on your finger that tells the nurse the amount of oxygen in your blood.

Purpose of sedation: *Rationale:* The nurse will give you medication that allows you to relax and let the breathing machine breathe for you.

Purpose of NPO/tube feeding: *Rationale:* With a breathing tube in place, it would be dangerous to let you swallow food, because it could easily enter your lungs. A tube will be put in your nose to feed you with liquid tube feeding that is a much safer for you to get your nutrition.

EVALUATION/DESIRED OUTCOMES

1. Clear breath sounds bilaterally.
2. ABGs within normal limits for the client.
3. SaO_2 (pulse oximetry) greater than 90%.
4. Return of vital signs within normal limits for the client.
5. Absence of hypoxia-related confusion.
6. Improved pulmonary status.
7. Return of pulmonary function tests to previous norm for the client.
8. Relief of anxiety by client and family.
9. The cause and related signs and symptoms of airway obstruction will be understood by the client and/or family.
10. Radiation treatment and/or chemotherapy regimen will be instituted.

DISCHARGE PLANNING

The client with airway obstruction may need:

Discharge planning is highly dependent on the etiology of the airway obstruction. For some clients, prolonged acute care in the home may be necessary, as the client may need to be discharged with a permanent tracheostomy, requiring suction equipment and visiting nurse services. Family and/or caregivers will need instruction in tracheostomy care, suctioning, coughing, and deep-breathing strategies, postural drainage, and enteral feeding. For those clients for whom survival is extremely limited, in-home or inpatient hospice care will be needed.

FOLLOW-UP CARE

Anticipated care

Home care or visiting nurse support services, or both, to assist with airway management.
Feeding tube management.
Pain and symptom management.
Management of radiation-induced and/or chemotherapy-induced side effects.
Frequent follow-up visits with the primary care provider.

Anticipated client/family questions and possible answers

Can an obstruction of the airway happen again?
"This is possible if the underlying cause (tumor growth, edema, etc.) continues or recurs. It is important for you to know and recognize the signs of impending airway obstruction and what to do if it does happen."

If this were to happen to me again, do I have to go through all of this treatment?
"Considering your options, and conveying your wishes to both your family and health care professionals can ensure that you receive the care and treatment you desire. Your desires can be carried out with a power of attorney for health care or with a living will. If your airway were to become obstructed again, some of the same treatments could be used."

CHAPTER SUMMARY

Airway obstruction is an acute and possibly fatal complication of both primary and metastatic disease. The multifactorial nature of this complication requires treatment regimens to be highly individualized. Likewise, prognostic factors vary, as they are highly correlated with the underlying etiology of the airway obstruction. Consideration must be given to the disease course, as well as to any past or present cancer treatment. Such treatments may increase the risk of post surgical problems (Polomano et al., 1994).

Critical care and oncology nurses have a pivotal role in the assessment and collaborative care of individuals with cancer who have experienced airway obstruction. Such collaborative efforts can result in improved client outcomes, as many factors must be considered in treatment planning and intervention. Since untreated airway obstruction can result in both increased morbidity and mortality, prompt recognition and treatment of this oncologic emergency is imperative.

TEST QUESTIONS

1. Hallmark signs of airway obstruction include:
   A. Air hunger
   B. Cheyne-Stokes respirations
   C. Blood glucose over 80 mg/dl
   D. Tongue pain

1. Answer: A
Air hunger is an early sign of upper airway obstruction.

2. The primary nursing diagnosis for airway obstruction is:
   A. Anxiety
   B. Ineffective coping
   C. Ineffective breathing pattern
   D. Ineffective airway clearance

2. Answer: D
Ineffective airway clearance due to the obstruction is the primary nursing diagnosis.

3. What is the *first* nursing intervention for airway obstruction?
   A. Call 911.
   B. Open the airway.
   C. Call the physician.
   D. Administer bronkosol aerosol treatment.

3. Answer: B
Opening the airway with a head tilt is the *first* intervention performed.

4. An important consideration in the treatment of airway obstruction is:
   A. Allaying the client's fear and anxiety
   B. Documenting the event
   C. Suctioning q2h
   D. Starting an IV line

4. Answer: A
Fear and anxiety accompany air hunger and, if not relieved, can contribute to airway compromise.

5. Pediatric clients with airway obstruction classically present with:
   A. Crowing respirations
   B. Cough
   C. Crackles
   D. Rhonchi

5. Answer: A
Pediatric clients develop "crowing" respirations with upper airway obstruction.

6. The primary goal of treatment for a client with airway obstruction is:
   A. Return of the client's ABGs to their normal levels
   B. Chest x-ray within normal limits
   C. Oxygen saturation 96%
   D. Blood glucose ≤112 mg/dl

6. Answer: A
Returning the client to his or her normal ABG levels is a primary goal of treatment.

7. Surgical treatment of airway obstruction may include all *except:*
   A. Laser bronchoscopy
   B. Tracheostomy
   C. Cricothyrotomy
   D. Pneumonectomy

7. Answer: D
A pneumonectomy (complete removal of a lung) is not indicated in airway obstruction. Tracheostomy and cricothyrotomy provide a patent airway. Laser bronchoscopy can help decrease the client's feeling of smothering.

8. Airway obstruction is frequently associated with which type of cancer?
   A. Cervical
   B. Ovarian
   C. Head and neck
   D. Breast

8. Answer: C
Head and neck cancers, specifically, cancer of the larynx, tongue, thyroid, and esophagus, are most frequently associated with airway obstruction.

9. Medications used to treat airway obstruction include all but:
   A. Aspirin
   B. Epinephrine
   C. Bronkosol
   D. Corticosteroids

9. Answer: A
Aspirin has antiplatelet, anti-inflammatory, and antipyretic properties, but plays no role in the treatment of airway obstruction.

10. This chemotherapeutic agent has been implicated in leading to pulmonary fibrosis:
    A. Vincristine
    B. Cytoxan
    C. Bleomycin
    D. Prednisone

10. Answer: C
Bleomycin has been implicated in 17% of pulmonary toxicities when cumulative doses exceed 550 IU.

REFERENCES

Bakemeir R, Qazi R: Basic concepts of cancer chemotherapy and principles of medical oncology. *In* Rubin P (ed): Clinical Oncology: A Multidisciplinary Approach for Physicians and Students, 7th ed. Philadelphia: WB Saunders Co, 1993.

Boggs RL, Wooldridge-King M: AACN Procedure Manual for Critical Care, 3rd ed. Philadelphia: WB Saunders Co, 1993.

Carpenito L: Nursing Diagnosis: Application to Clinical Practice, 6th ed. Philadelphia: JB Lippincott, 1995.

Clochesy JM, Breu C, Cardin S, Rudy EB, Whittaker A: Critical Care Nursing. Philadelphia: WB Saunders Co, 1993.

de Souza A, Keal R, Hudson N, Leverment J, Spyt T: Use of expandable wire stents for malignant airway obstruction. Ann Thorac Surg 57(6):1573–1577, 1994.

Elpern E: Lung cancer. *In* Groenwald S, Frogge M, Goodman M, Yarbro C (eds): Cancer Nursing: Principles and Practice, 3rd ed., Boston: Jones and Bartlett, 1993, pp. 1175–1198.

Harwood K: Dyspnea. *In* Groenwald S, Frogge M, Goodman M, Yarbro C (eds): Cancer Symptom Management. Boston: Jones and Bartlett, 1996, pp. 31–39.

Kersten LD: Comprehensive Respiratory Nursing. Philadelphia: WB Saunders Co, 1989.

Kovac A: Upper airway trauma and obstruction: A review of causes, evaluation and management. Respir Care 38(4):351–359, 1993.

McCoy-Adabody A, Borger D: Selected critical care complications of cancer therapy. AACN Clinical Issues in Critical Care Nursing 7(1):26–36, 1996.

Nally A: Critical care of the patient with lung cancer. AACN Clinical Issues in Critical Care Nursing 7(1):79–94, 1996.

Polomano R, Weintraub F, Wurster A: Surgical critical care for cancer patients. Semin Oncol Nurs 10(3):165–176, 1994.

Shelton B: Issues and trends in critical care of patients with cancer. AACN Clinical Issues in Critical Care Nursing 7(1):9–25, 1996.

Shelton B, Baker L, Stecker S: Critical care of the patient with hematologic malignancy. AACN Clinical Issues in Critical Care Nursing 7(1):65–78, 1996.

Shuey K: Heart, lung and endocrine complications of solid tumors. Semin Oncol Nurs 10(3):177–188, 1994.

Wilkes G, Ingwersen K, Burke M: Oncology Nursing Drug Reference. Philadelphia: WB Saunders Co, 1994.

Woodlock T: Oncologic emergencies. *In* Rosenthal S, Carignan JR, Smith BD (eds): Medical Care of the Cancer Patient, 2nd ed. Philadelphia: WB Saunders Co, 1993.

CHAPTER 6

ANAPHYLAXIS FROM CHEMOTHERAPY

Cynthia von Hohenleiten, MN, RN, OCN

AND

Jennifer S. Webster, MN, MPH, RN, OCN

CHAPTER OBJECTIVES

At the completion of this chapter, the reader will be able to:

Define chemotherapy-related anaphylaxis.

Identify chemotherapeutic agents that put clients at risk for anaphylaxis.

State medical and pharmaceutical interventions for the oncology client experiencing anaphylaxis from chemotherapy.

Describe nursing care of the oncology client experiencing anaphylaxis from chemotherapy.

Anticipate education and discharge needs of the client who has experienced anaphylaxis from chemotherapy.

OVERVIEW

HYPERSENSITIVITY reactions to chemotherapeutic agents, ranging from mild to severe, have been described in the oncology medical literature. No definitive measurements of the incidence of chemotherapeutic hypersensitivity in the oncology population are available, but Weiss (1992) reports that hypersensitivity reactions have been recorded for every chemotherapeutic agent except dactinomycin and the nitrosoureas. Weiss estimates that certain agents may cause hypersensitivity reactions in 5 to 15% of oncology clients. This chapter discusses the life-endangering hypersensitivities, or anaphylaxis. Anaphylaxis is defined as an acute, systemic, potentially life-threatening reaction to an antigen in which mast cell mediator release causes respiratory and/or cardiovascular system dysfunction (Sullivan, 1988), usually within seconds or minutes of exposure to the antigen. The focus of this chapter is the nursing care of the oncology client experiencing anaphylaxis from chemotherapy.

DESCRIPTION

Mast cells are the primary cells involved in anaphylaxis. They are present throughout the tissues of the human body but are in highest concentrations in connective tissue, the lungs, the lining of the gastrointestinal (GI) tract, and the blood vessels (Church and Caulfield, 1993). Each mast cell contains tens of thousands of immunoglobulin E (IgE) receptors on the cell surface and stores of chemicals such as histamine, heparin, and serotonin (Sheffer and Horan, 1993). IgE, produced by the B-lymphocytes in response to exposure to an antigen, is the primary antibody involved in the commencement of an immediate allergic response (Gould, 1993). Antigen-specific IgE binds to mast cells and sensitizes them to the antigen. As a sensitized mast cell is subsequently exposed to the antigen, a series of reactions occur that result in degranulation of the mast cell and release of the chemical mediators. These primary chemical mediators are responsible for the multiple and often varied clinical manifestations of anaphylaxis by producing three major physiologic effects: vasodilation, increased permeability of capillary membranes, and contraction of vascular smooth muscle (Sheffer and Horan, 1993). Edema, reduced circulating blood volume, hypotension, and bronchoconstriction are the result. Without intervention, respiratory insufficiency, decreased cardiac output, shock, and death may occur.

Clinical presentation

The onset of anaphylaxis is usually precipitous, generally following within a few minutes of exposure to the antigen. Symptoms may range from mild to severe. The client may initially experience cutaneous warmth and/or tingling and a sensation of anxiety or impending doom. As the reaction progresses a wide variety of symptoms may appear. The signs and symptoms are presented in detail in the Assessment Criteria section of this chapter.

RISK PROFILE

Cancers: Anaphylaxis can occur during drug therapy for all types of cancers. Certain cancer diagnoses have been reported to be associated with more severe and more frequent hypersensitivity reactions than others: acute lymphocytic leukemia treated with L-asparaginase, craniospinal tumors treated with teniposide (O'Dwyer, King, Fortner, and Leyland-Jones, 1986), and lymphomas treated with bleomycin.

Conditions: A history of allergy to drugs of the same chemical class may increase risk; however, cross-reactivity is variable and unpredictable. Clients with chronic obstructive pulmonary disease (COPD) or asthma may be less sensitive to initial treatment with epinephrine and may require higher doses or alternate drugs for anaphylaxis management. Clients with cardiac disease may experience more severe or more protracted symptoms of anaphylaxis, such as hypotension and dysrhythmia.

Environment: None.

Foods: None.

Drugs: Previous exposure to the chemotherapeutic agent, infrequent administration (weekly vs. daily), intravenous (IV) route of administration, bolus injection, drugs that are proteins or heavy metals, and the use of Cremophor EL or benzyl alcohol as diluents (Weiss and Baker, 1987). Clients receiving beta-adrenergic blocking drugs will be resistant to the effects of epinephrine and albuterol used to treat anaphylaxis. Angiotensin-converting enzyme inhibitors can augment mast cell mediator release, thus prolonging the reaction (Sullivan, 1988).

Since very few antineoplastic agents have not had at least one reported case of hypersensitivity reaction, all clients receiving chemotherapy should be instructed to report any unusual symptoms. Antianaphylaxis medication should be near at hand, and clients should be observed closely during the first few minutes of each infusion. By definition, a true IgE-mediated Type I anaphylactic reaction requires at least one previous exposure to the drug and is therefore most common with repeated administration; however, anaphylactoid symptoms have occurred on initial exposure to a drug. Anaphylactoid reactions are mediated by drugs that directly trigger the release of histamine by mast cells, creating symptoms that mimic anaphylaxis (O'Brien and Souberbielle, 1992). The names of drugs, the relative frequency of reactions, and pertinent observations are listed in Table 6–1.

PROGNOSIS

Anaphylaxis can result in acute cardiopulmonary failure and death within minutes. Respiratory complications cause 70% of deaths, and cardiovascular complications account for 24% of deaths following anaphylaxis (Corren and Schocket, 1990). The drug of choice for the initial management of anaphylaxis is epinephrine, and failure to use this drug early in the course of anaphylaxis increases the likelihood of a fatal outcome (Sullivan, 1988). Positive outcomes are directly related to the early recognition of symptoms, discontinuation of the drug, prompt treatment, and supportive therapy.

TREATMENT

Surgery: Cricothyrotomy if endotracheal intubation is unsuccessful in the management of severe airway obstruction.

Table 6–1
Drugs with a Documented Incidence of Anaphylaxis

Drug	Incidence	Comments
L-asparaginase	6–43% (Weiss, 1984)	Higher incidence with IV versus IM route. Risk increases with cumulative doses and longer intervals between doses. A skin test is recommended prior to each dose; however, reactions may occur in the absence of a positive skin test.
Cisplatin	5% (Weiss and Baker, 1987)	Higher incidence when given in combination with other chemotherapeutic agents and as an intravesical treatment (Weiss and Bruno, 1981). May be possible to continue therapy despite hypersensitivity by pre-medicating and prolonging infusion > 6 hours.
Taxol	10% (Weiss et al. 1990)	Premedication and prolongation of infusion over 24 hours has reduced the incidence of hypersensitivity reactions to < 10%. Reactions usually occur with the first or second drug doses.
Teniposide and Etoposide	3.6–6.5% (O'Dwyer et al., 1986) 1–3% (Weiss and Baker, 1987)	More common with high cumulative doses, but reactions can occur during first exposure. No reported reactions to oral formulation.
Melphalan	3.9% (Cornwell, Pajak, and McIntyre, 1979)	IV route more allergenic than oral melphalan.
Carboplatin	2.5–10% (Weiss and Baker, 1987)	Cross-reactivity possible if client is hypersensitive to cisplatin.
Cytarabine	Few case reports (Weiss, 1992)	Uncommon. Initiated by moderate to high doses of drug.
Methotrexate	Occasional	No relation to dose or treatment duration. May cause acute onset of interstitial pneumonitis.
Cyclophosphamide	Rare case reports (Kim, Kesarwala, and Colvin, 1985)	Variable cross-reactivity with other alkylating agents.
Bleomycin	Febrile reactions occur 1–4 hours after adminis-tration in 20–25% of clients treated. Anaphylactoid symptoms may occur in rare cases.	Severe anaphylactoid reactions more prevalent in persons with lymphoma. Febrile reactions may progress to respiratory distress and hypotension. Give test dose before therapy.
Doxorubicin, Daunorubicin, and Mitoxantrone	Occasional severe reactions	Prior urticaria or "flare" at injection site warrants close monitoring with future doses (Craig and Capizzi, 1985).
Diaziquone (AZQ)	1–2% (Castleberry, Ragab, and Steuber, 1990)	Reactions occurred after at least three doses.
5-Fluorouracil	Rare	Angioedema and hypotension.

Chemotherapy

Discontinue the drug immediately.

In clients sensitized to cisplatin, Taxol, etoposide, and the anthracyclines, measures such as prolonging the infusion time, premedicating with diphenhydramine, and administering decadron and H_2 antagonists 12 and 6 hours before treatment have effectively prevented recurrent hypersensitivity reactions (Weiss, 1992).

If anaphylaxis occurs with L-asparaginase derived from *E. coli*, therapy may be continued by substituting chrysanthemia-derived L-asparaginase.

Radiation: Not indicated.

Medications

Subcutaneous epinephrine 300 to 500 µg.

Avoid IV bolus injections because they may cause potentially fatal cardiac dysrhythmia (Corren and Schocket, 1990).

Rapid IV fluid replacement with crystalloids or colloids.

Diphenhydramine 1 mg/kg IV and cimetidine 4 mg/kg IV for urticaria and hypotension.

Bronchodilator inhalation for lower airway symptoms.

Aminophylline IV infusion for persistent bronchospasm.

Hydrocortisone sodium succinate 100 to 500 mg IV initially, then repeated in 6 hours for possible late-phase reactions (Sheffer and Pennoyer, 1984).

For hypotension or airway obstruction *resistant* to initial treatment: epinephrine by continuous IV infusion (Sullivan, 1988) (see p. 75 for dose).

Norepinephrine infusion for profound or refractory hypotension.

Antidysrhythmic medications for dysrhythmia.

Clients who are being treated with beta-adrenergic blocking agents at the time of anaphylaxis are unlikely to respond to epinephrine therapy. Alternate measures to sustain blood pressure such as isoproterenol (Isuprel) in conjunction with H_1 and H_2 antagonists may be required. Aerosolized atropine sulfate may be given in place of beta agonists to treat bronchospasm in clients who are receiving beta-blockers (Corren and Schocket, 1990).

Procedures

Supplemental inspired oxygen.

Oropharyngeal airway followed by endotracheal intubation and assisted ventilation for airway obstruction unresponsive to epinephrine.

Continuous cardiac monitoring.

Placement of pulmonary artery catheter in clients requiring IV vasopressor support.

Intra-aortic balloon pump for resistant hypotension.

ASSESSMENT CRITERIA:
ANAPHYLAXIS FROM CHEMOTHERAPY

Signs and symptoms of anaphylaxis can occur within an hour of drug administration, but usually appear during the first few minutes of IV infusion. The response may be protracted despite aggressive therapy or can be recurrent. Recurrent anaphylactic reactions may appear up to 8 hours after initial remission of symptoms in approximately one-fourth of severe cases (Sullivan, 1988). This so-called biphasic reaction mimics the symptoms experienced in the first phase of anaphylaxis and can occur despite corticosteroid therapy. Due to the unpredictable and life-threatening nature of this response, clients should be closely monitored for at least 8 hours after initial stabilization.

Vital signs	
Temperature	At baseline. May be elevated with cytarabine and bleomycin.
Pulse	Rapid and weak due to H_1 and H_2 receptor activation. Supraventricular and ventricular rhythm disturbances possible.
Respirations	Tachypneic, dyspneic. Upper airway symptoms: hoarseness, stridor, "lump" in throat. Lower airway symptoms: wheezing, intercostal and suprasternal muscle retractions.
Systolic blood pressure	<90 mmHg
Central venous pressure (CVP)	<2 mmHg
Mean arterial pressure (MAP)	<60–70 mmHg
History	Previous hypersensitivity to prescribed drug. History of allergies, especially prior sensitivity to antineoplastic agents of the same class, e.g., alkylating agents, heavy metals. Use of beta-adrenergic blocking drugs or angiotensin-converting enzyme inhibitors. Pre-existing asthma, COPD, cardiac disease. Recent exposure to food, drugs, insect stings, blood products with the potential to cause anaphylaxis.
Hallmark physical signs and symptoms	Chest tightness, dizziness, flushed appearance, hypotension, inspiratory stridor, pruritis, tachycardia, urticaria, wheezing.
Additional signs and symptoms	Abdominal pain, diarrhea, nausea, rhinoconjunctivitis, uterine cramping, vomiting. Late manifestations: seizures, dysrhythmia, metabolic acidosis.
Psychosocial signs	Anxiety, sense of impending doom, restlessness.

ASSESSMENT CRITERIA:
ANAPHYLAXIX FROM CHEMOTHERAPY (continued)

Lab values	Normal values at onset of anaphylaxis.
	Hypoxemia, hypercarbia, and acidosis may ensue if reaction is severe and protracted.
pO_2	Low
pCO_2	High
pH	Low
Anion gap	High
Urine specific gravity	High. (Vasodilation may cause hypotension and a relative fluid volume deficit.)
Diagnostic tests	Serum mast cell tryptase level: peaks within 1 hour after the onset of anaphylaxis and remains elevated for several hours after acute episode.
	Intradermal skin test or intravenous test dose may be used prior to drug administration to identify clients at risk for hypersensitivity.

NURSING DIAGNOSIS

Ineffective airway clearance related to airway edema and secretions associated with anaphylaxis.

Impaired gas exchange related to bronchospasm associated with anaphylaxis.

Decreased cardiac output related to vasodilation and increased vasopermeability associated with histamine release.

Fluid volume deficit related to vasodilation.

Inability to sustain spontaneous ventilation related to cardiopulmonary arrest due to respiratory tract obstruction and/or shock.

Potential for injury due to falls related to orthostatic hypotension.

Risk for impaired skin integrity related to urticaria and pruritis.

Abdominal *pain* and cramping related to smooth muscle contraction in the gastrointestinal tract.

Anxiety related to the acute symptoms of anaphylaxis.

Knowledge deficit regarding subjective symptoms to report that are associated with anaphylaxis.

NURSING INTERVENTIONS

Interventions prior to drug administration

Review allergy history and current medications. Note if the client is currently taking beta blockers or has a history of asthma or COPD.

Record baseline blood pressure, pulse, respirations, and mental status.

Ensure that emergency medication and equipment (oxygen, ambu bag, airway, intubation tray) are readily available.

Establish a patent IV line.

Premedicate with prophylactic medications (e.g., antihistamines, corticosteroids), if prescribed.

Educate the client about the potential risks associated with each drug and the early subjective signs of anaphylaxis to report to the nurse.

Immediate nursing interventions

Discontinue drug infusion and keep the vein open.

Stay with the client and have another staff member notify the physician.

Assess pulse, respirations, breath sounds, blood pressure, and oxygen saturation q5min until stable, then q15min × 4, q1h × 4, then q4h.

Reassure the client and family.

If the airway is compromised:
- Extend neck and insert oropharyngeal airway if severe airway edema is not already present.
- Administer high-flow oxygen.
- Call for respiratory therapy assistance.
- Place suction equipment and intubation tray at bedside.
- Send STAT arterial blood gas (ABG).
- Prepare to assist with intubation if required.

If the client is hypotensive:
- Place the client in a supine position with the feet elevated if tolerated.
- Ensure patent IV access for rapid IV infusions.
- Measure hourly intake and output (I and O). Insert indwelling urinary catheter, if necessary.
- Initiate fall precautions to prevent injury from orthostasis.
- Initiate continuous ECG monitoring.
- Prepare for pulmonary artery catheter placement if vasopressor therapy is required.
- Apply shock trousers for lower-extremity compression, if necessary (Sullivan, 1988).

Anticipated physician orders and interventions

STAT epinephrine 300 to 500 µg. SQ (0.3–0.5 ml of 1:1000 solution). Repeat every 10 minutes until symptoms subside.

Pediatrics: Epinephrine 0.01 ml/kg of 1:1000 solution up to 0.3 ml every 10 minutes (Corren and Schocket, 1990).

Diphenhydramine 50 mg IV + famotidine 20 mg (or cimetidine 300 mg) IV push over 5 minutes.

Pediatrics: Diphenhydramine 1 mg/kg up to 50 mg; cimetidine 4 mg/kg up to 300 mg (Corren and Schocket, 1990).

Oxygen at 5 L/minute nasal cannula.

STAT ABGs and serum electrolyte panel.

Methylprednisolone 125 mg IV push. Repeat 6 hours after onset of reaction to prevent recurrent symptoms.

If the client is hypotensive:
- 0.9% NaCl rapid IV infusion up to 3 L.

If hypotension continues despite above measures:
- IV epinephrine infusion at 2 to 4 µg/minute (1 mg epinephrine in 500 ml solution at a rate of 1 to 2 ml/minute) (Sullivan, 1988).
- Norepinephrine IV infusion to maintain systolic blood pressure > 90–100 mmHg. Substitute isoproterenol if the client is taking a beta-blocking drug (Corren and Schocket, 1990).
- Intra-aortic balloon pump if blood pressure fails to respond to volume expansion and vasopressors.
- Antidysrhythmic drugs PRN dysrhythmia.

If severe upper airway obstruction:
- Endotracheal intubation.
- Crycothyrotomy if edema prevents intubation.

If severe lower airway obstruction:
- 2% racemic epinephrine inhalation (0.5 ml), *or* aerosolized albuterol inhalation.
- Aerosolized atropine sulfate for clients receiving beta-blocking drugs (Corren and Schocket, 1990).
- Aminophylline IV infusion.

Ongoing nursing assessment, monitoring, and interventions

Assess:
- Breath sounds q4h and PRN.
- Oxygen saturation continuously × 8 hours after onset of symptoms.
- For signs of congestive heart failure (jugular vein distention [JVD], S_3, tachypnea, crackles, peripheral edema) related to rapid volume replacement q4h × 24 hours.
- Skin color, temperature, turgor q8h.
- Level of consciousness q8h and PRN.
- For dysrhythmia continuously × 8 hours after onset of symptoms.
- For GI symptoms: nausea, vomiting, abdominal pain q8h.
- Anxiety level PRN.

Measure:
- Blood pressure, pulse, and respirations q5min until stable, then q15min × 4, then q1h × 4, then q4h.

- Cardiac output q2h during vasopressor support and hourly with titration.
- I and O q4h × 24 hours.
- Weight qd.

Send:
- ABG PRN for desaturation.
- Electrolyte panel 12 hours following start of IV fluid support.

Implement:
- Notify attending physician, pharmacist, and protocol nurse (if applicable) of adverse drug reaction. Document in medical record.
- Precautions against falls due to vasodilation and potential orthostasis.

TEACHING/EDUCATION

Signs and symptoms of anaphylaxis: *Rationale:* Certain chemotherapy drugs may cause an allergic reaction. If signs of an allergic reaction appear while you are taking chemotherapy drugs, tell your nurse immediately. The signs to look for are (1) itching or tingling of the skin; (2) any redness or blotching of the skin; (3) tightness in the chest, feeling flushed or warm; (4) feeling dizzy; (5) difficulty breathing; (6) nausea, vomiting, or diarrhea; (7) a sudden feeling of anxiety or that death is near.

Decrease/discontinue chemotherapy: *Rationale:* Certain chemotherapy drugs may cause an allergic reaction. If signs of an allergic reaction appear while you are taking chemotherapy drugs, some of your drugs may be stopped. You may receive medicine to lessen the chances of an allergic reaction. There may be a delay in your chemotherapy treatment.

Use of adrenaline or epinephrine: *Rationale:* Adrenaline (or epinephrine) is a medicine that can reduce or reverse the release of the substances that are provoking the allergic reaction. Adrenaline may be given by injection directly into a vein, or it may be injected under the skin by means of a small thin needle.

Use of Benadryl/diphenhydramine: *Rationale:* Benadryl (or diphenhydramine) is a medicine that can reduce or stop the skin from itching and stops the release of one of the substances (histamine) that causes the allergic response. Benadryl is injected directly into the vein.

Use of aminophylline: *Rationale:* Aminophylline dilates the tubes in your lungs that carry air, making it easier for you to breathe. Aminophylline is administered as a bag of medicine that drips through a needle directly into your vein.

Use of oxygen: *Rationale:* If you are having difficulty breathing, you may receive oxygen through a mask that covers your nose and mouth or through tubing that has prongs which rest at the openings of your nose. The oxygen will be at a higher concentration than what is in the air, so if you aren't breathing in as much air, you are still getting enough oxygen.

Use of hydrocortisone/methylprednisolone: *Rationale:* Hydrocortisone is a medicine that can reduce late or delayed allergic reactions. Hydrocortisone is injected directly into the vein.

Use of IV fluids or blood products: *Rationale:* If you have a low blood pressure, you may receive fluid or blood products (such as packed red blood cells or albumin) to boost the amount of fluid you have circulating in your bloodstream, which raises your blood pressure.

Use of nebulized albuterol: *Rationale:* If you continue to have trouble breathing, a special "breathing treatment" may be ordered. A respiratory therapist will help you to inhale a vapor or mist containing the medicine albuterol. This medicine should relax the tubes in your lungs that carry air, making it easier for you to breathe.

ABGs: *Rationale:* The oxygen level in your blood may need to be checked. This test is done by inserting a thin needle into a blood vessel in your wrist and collecting blood.

Use of an oropharyngeal airway and intubation: *Rationale:* If you are having a great deal of difficulty breathing, the doctor may insert a tube through your mouth down into your lungs, which can then be attached to a machine that will help you breathe. This is done only in extreme emergencies, and you will be asleep for this procedure.

EVALUATION/DESIRED OUTCOMES

1. Signs of anaphylaxis are recognized and treatments initiated within 5 minutes of the first appearance of symptoms.
2. Acute respiratory distress (wheezing, inspiratory stridor, chest tightness) subsides within 10 minutes of treatment.
3. Oxygen therapy is discontinued within 8 hours of onset of symptoms.
4. Blood pressure stabilizes within 1 hour of treatment.
5. IV fluids/blood products are discontinued within 12 hours of onset.
6. Pruritis and skin flushing resolve within 30 minutes of treatment.
7. Plans for continued chemotherapy regimen *or* alternative chemotherapy treatment will be in place within 24 hours. If the same chemotherapeutic agent is to be used, medication orders for anaphylaxis prophylaxis will be in place.
8. The client and family understand the cause of anaphylaxis and the signs and symptoms of recurrence.

DISCHARGE PLANNING

The client who has experienced chemotherapy anaphylaxis will need:

Short-term IV fluids and oxygen until fully recovered.

Close monitoring for at least 8 hours after initial stabilization to identify a possible recurrent anaphylactic reaction.

Extensive documentation of the reaction, signs and symptoms, and treatments.

A record that clearly indicates the name of the agent that precipitated the anaphylaxis.

Education of the client and family to notify all future health care workers of the anaphylaxis, the name of the chemotherapeutic agent that precipitated the incident, and the specific symptoms that accompanied the reaction.

If the client is to be discharged immediately after the adverse event, advise the client to avoid situations that may contribute to hypotension (e.g., hot tubs, exercise, saunas, hot sunshine) for a minimum of 12 hours.

FOLLOW-UP CARE

Anticipated care

A plan for resumption of scheduled chemotherapy or an alternative chemotherapy course within 24 hours of the anaphylaxis.

Upon resumption of chemotherapy, orders for premedications such as diphenhydramine or hydrocortisone as prophylaxis against a repeat episode of anaphylaxis. Possibly a course of chemotherapy desensitization, in which the client is exposed to very small amounts of the drug in order to develop a tolerance that will allow administration of the full chemotherapy dose. Desensitization may occur over days or weeks.

A physician office visit within 1 week.

Anticipated client/family questions and possible answers

Will I be able to continue with my chemotherapy?

"Your doctor will decide whether to continue with the same chemotherapy drugs or switch you to different chemotherapy agents. Many times there are other drugs that can be used to treat your disease; however, if the physician thinks that this particular agent is the best one for you, there are medicines we can give you to prevent this reaction from happening again."

Could this reaction happen again?

"It is possible that you could have the same reaction again. However, we will try to prevent that from happening by giving medicines such as hydrocortisone or diphenhydramine, which lessen the body's ability to react so strongly to the chemotherapy."

Is there anything I can do to prevent this reaction from happening again?

"The best way to prevent this from happening again is to make sure that everyone providing health care to you knows about your reaction to this drug. Please write down the name of the drug. If anyone asks you if you have any allergies, you must mention this agent. Your medical records will have extensive documentation of the reaction, but there may be a time when you don't have the records with you. Alerting health care workers about your allergy will allow them to plan to give you medications that may prevent a recurrence of the reaction if you should require this chemotherapy drug again. Wearing an arm bracelet with the chemotherapy drug name will also serve as a reminder and alert to health care professionals."

CHAPTER SUMMARY

Anaphylaxis may occur in any client receiving chemotherapy. Certain chemotherapeutic agents are more likely to cause anaphylaxis, and the oncology nurse should become familiar with them. Symptoms of anaphylaxis usually occur precipitously, can be life-threatening, and require immediate action. Early recognition and management of these symptoms greatly reduce morbidity and mortality. Nurses should know the hallmark signs of anaphylaxis and the initial interventions. Teaching the client how to prevent future anaphylaxis and to recognize symptoms if they do occur is also a critical component of the nurse's role.

TEST QUESTIONS

1. Anaphylaxis is:
   A. Rare in clients receiving chemotherapy.
   B. An acute, systemic, potentially life-threatening reaction to an antigen.
   C. Always preventable with the appropriate premedications.
   D. Easily recognized by trained health care personnel.

1. Answer: B
Anaphylaxis is a well-documented side effect of certain chemotherapeutic agents. It is not always preventable and may not be easily recognizable to health care personnel.

2. The risk of anaphylaxis increases if:
   A. The client is elderly.
   B. The client has a history of reactions to narcotics.
   C. The chemotherapeutic agent is administered by IV bolus injection.
   D. The client has a history of food allergies.

2. Answer: C
A higher risk of anaphylaxis from chemotherapy is associated with the IV route of administration and bolus injection. Age and food allergies do not increase risk. A history of allergy to drugs of the same chemical class may increase risk. However, there is no association between narcotic allergy and chemotherapy anaphylaxis.

3. A chemotherapeutic agent commonly associated with anaphylaxis is:
   A. Mitoxantrone
   B. Dacarbazine
   C. L-asparaginase
   D. Doxorubicin

3. Answer: C
L-asparaginase is the chemotherapeutic agent most commonly associated with anaphylaxis, with a documented incidence rate of 6 to 43%. The other agents listed have occasional case reports of severe reactions.

4. The potential for an anaphylactic reaction to L-asparaginase may be identified by:
   A. Administering a small amount of the agent by IV bolus.
   B. Administering a small amount of the agent as a skin test.
   C. Identifying the client with a history of asthma.
   D. Identifying the client with a history of blood product reactions.

4. Answer: B
Clients who are about to receive L-asparaginase usually receive an initial test dose under the skin. However, the absence of a positive skin test is not a complete guarantee that the client will not experience anaphylaxis to the full chemotherapy dose.

5. Hallmark signs and symptoms of anaphylaxis include:
   A. Hypertension, drowsiness, coughing
   B. Seizures, metabolic acidosis
   C. Chest tightness, wheezing, pruritis
   D. Bradycardia, coma

5. Answer: C
Chest tightness, dizziness, flushed appearance, hypotension, inspiratory stridor, pruritis, tachycardia, and wheezing are the classic signs of anaphylaxis.

6. Upon recognizing the symptoms of anaphylaxis, the *first* action the nurse should take is to:
   A. Discontinue the drug infusion and keep the vein open.
   B. Notify the physician of the suspected anaphylaxis.
   C. Raise the head of the bed to assist client respirations.
   D. If the client is hypotensive, place the client in a supine position with the feet elevated.

6. Answer: A
All of the described answers are appropriate. However, the first priority should be to reduce client exposure to the agent by discontinuing the infusion.

7. Upon notifying the physician of the anaphylaxis, which medications should the nurse be prepared to administer first?
   A. Epinephrine, diphenhydramine
   B. Oxygen therapy
   C. IV fluids or albumin
   D. Methylprednisolone

7. Answer: A
Epinephrine and diphenhydramine are the first-line drugs of choice during an anaphylactic reaction. The other treatments would all be administered based on the symptoms of the client.

8. Ongoing nursing assessment and monitoring should occur:
   A. Until the client is stabilized.
   B. For at least 1 hour after the client is stabilized.
   C. For at least 8 hours after the client is stabilized.
   D. For at least 24 hours after the client is stabilized.

8. Answer: C.
Recurrent anaphylactic reactions may occur up to 8 hours after the initial transmission of symptoms. Therefore, clients need to be closely monitored for at least 8 hours.

9. A client who has experienced anaphylaxis from chemotherapy will need to know:
   A. What foods he or she may eat.
   B. What activities may contribute to hypertension.
   C. If others in the family have a history of drug reactions.
   D. The cause of the anaphylaxis and the signs and symptoms of recurrence.

9. Answer: D
The client is often the first to recognize signs of recurrence and can summon help more quickly if he or she readily identifies the symptoms.

10. Discharge planning should include:
    A. A plan for desensitization to the chemotherapeutic agent.
    B. A resumption of normal activity levels.
    C. Education of the client and family to notify all future health care workers of the anaphylaxis and the name of the agent.
    D. Oxygen therapy at home.

10. Answer: C
Education of the client to prevent future anaphylactic reactions is crucial. Desensitization is not a common occurrence after anaphylaxis, although it is an option. The client may need to reduce normal activity level for a day following discharge. Due to the short-lived nature of anaphylactic reactions, clients should not require oxygen at home.

REFERENCES

Castleberry RP, Ragab AH, Steuber CP: AZQ in the treatment of recurrent pediatric brain and other malignant solid tumors. A Pediatric Oncology Group phase II study. Invest New Drugs 8:401–406, 1990.

Church M, Caulfield J: Mast cell and basophil functions. In Holgate ST, Church MK (eds): Allergy. London: Gower Medical Publishing, 1993, pp. 5.1–5.12.

Cornwell GG, Pajak TF, McIntyre OR: Hypersensitivity reactions to I.V. melphalan during treatment of multiple myeloma: Cancer and Leukemia Group B experience. Cancer Treat Rep 63:399–403, 1979.

Corren J, Schocket AL: Anaphylaxis: A preventable emergency. Postgrad Med 87(5):167–178, 1990.

Craig JB, Capizzi RL: The prevention and treatment of immediate hypersensitivity reactions from cancer chemotherapy. Semin Oncol Nurs 1(4):285–291, 1985.

Gould HJ: IgE structure, synthesis and interaction with receptors. In Holgate ST, Church MK (eds): Allergy. London: Gower Medical Publishing, 1993, pp. 2.1–2.13.

Hammond E: Anaphylactic reactions to chemotherapeutic agents. J Assoc Pediatr Oncol Nurs 5(3):16–19, 1988.

Kim HC, Kesarwala HH, Colvin M: Hypersensitivity reaction to a metabolite of cyclophosphamide. J Allergy Clin Immunol 76:591–594, 1985.

Kreamer KM: Anaphylaxis resulting from chemotherapy. Oncol Nurs Forum 8(4):13–16, 1981.

Lascari AD, Strano AJ, Johnson WW: Methotrexate-induced sudden fatal pulmonary reaction. Cancer 40:1393–1397, 1977.

O'Brien MER, Souberbielle BE: Allergic reactions to cytotoxic drugs—an update. Ann Oncol 3(8):605–610, 1992.

O'Dwyer PJ, King SA, Fortner CL, Leyland-Jones B: Hypersensitivity reactions to teniposide (VM-26): An analysis. J Clin Oncol 4:1262–1269, 1986.

Saunders MP, Denton CP, O'Brien MER, Blake P, Gore M, Wiltshaw E: Hypersensitivity reactions to cisplatin and carboplatin—a report on six cases. Ann Oncol 3:574–576, 1992.

Schneider SM, Distelhorst CW: Chemotherapy-induced emergencies. Semin Oncol 16(6):572–578, 1989.

Sheffer AL, Horan RG: Anaphylaxis. In Holgate ST, Church MK (eds): Allergy. London: Gower Medical Publishing, 1993, pp. 27.1–27.10.

Sheffer AL, Pennoyer DS: Management of adverse drug reactions. J Allergy Clin Immunol 10:580–588, 1984.

Sullivan TJ: Systemic anaphylaxis. In Lichtenstein LM, Fauci AS (eds): Current Therapy in Allergy, Immunology and Rheumatology. Toronto: BC Decker, 1988, pp. 91–98.

Weiss RB: Hypersensitivity reactions. Semin Oncol 19(5):458–477, 1992.

Weiss RB: Hypersensitivity reactions to cancer chemotherapy. *In* Perry MC, Yarbro JW (eds): Toxicity of Chemotherapy. Orlando, FL: Grune and Stratton, 1984, pp. 101–123.

Weiss RB, Baker JR: Hypersensitivity reactions from antineoplastic agents. Cancer Metastasis Rev 6:413–432, 1987.

Weiss RB, Bruno S: Hypersensitivity reactions to cancer chemotherapeutic agents. Ann Intern Med 94:66–72, 1981.

Weiss RB, Donehower RC, Wiernik PH, Ohnuma T, Gralla RJ, Trump DL, Baker JR Jr, Van Echo DA, Von Hoff, DD, Leyland-Jones B: Hypersensitivity reactions from taxol. J Clin Oncol 8:1263–1268, 1990.

CHAPTER 7

BRONCHIOLITIS OBLITERANS

Colleen L. Corish, RN, MN, OCN

AND

Karen E. Byrd, RN, MSN, OCN

CHAPTER OBJECTIVES

At the completion of this chapter, the reader will be able to:

Define bronchiolitis obliterans.

State risk factors associated with bronchiolitis obliterans in the oncology client.

Describe nursing care as it relates to oncology clients with bronchiolitis obliterans.

Anticipate and prepare the client with bronchiolitis obliterans for future care needs.

OVERVIEW

BRONCHIOLITIS obliterans is a phenomenon that has been studied and documented in the literature since 1901 (Holland, Wingard, Beschorner, Saral, and Santos, 1988, p. 621). As stated by Ezri et al. (1994), "Bronchiolitis Obliterans . . . is a relatively rare disease whose precise prevalence is unknown" (p. 1). This disease entity mainly damages the small conducting airways with physiologic and radiologic findings that are very similar to chronic obstructive pulmonary disease (COPD) (King, 1989, p. 69). King also notes that some of the processes may appear restrictive or both restrictive and obstructive, resulting in confusing bronchiolitis obliterans with other diffuse infiltrative ventilatory lung disorders (p. 69). The etiologies implicated include viral, toxic fume exposure, connective tissue disease, drugs, or organ transplantation ("immune" bronchiolitis obliterans), and idiopathic (Ezri et al., 1994, pp. 3–4). For the purpose of this chapter, bronchiolitis obliterans will be discussed as it applies to the oncology population; specifically, individuals who have undergone an allogeneic bone marrow transplant (BMT). It has been documented that the incidence of bronchiolitis obliterans is approximately 2 to 10% in clients who have undergone allogeneic BMT (Paz et al., 1993, p. 109).

While the incidence is rare, a few cases have been documented as occurring in the autologous transplant population.

DESCRIPTION

Bronchiolitis obliterans is a pulmonary disease that primarily affects the conductive bronchioles with partial or complete obliteration of the bronchiolar lumen either by plugs of granulation tissue or by fibrosis and scarring (Ezri et al., 1994, and King, 1989). Bronchiolitis obliterans as a result of granulation tissue deposition is sometimes referred to as "proliferative" bronchiolitis obliterans. Conversely, bronchiolitis obliterans caused by scarring is referred to as "constrictive" or "obstructive."

Proliferative bronchiolitis obliterans is most often characterized by an inflammatory process involving the respiratory bronchioles and alveoli. The resulting defect is restrictive. The significance of understanding the exact defect is in establishing prognosis and response to treatment. The restrictive, inflammatory defect is potentially reversible. On the other hand, obstructive bronchiolitis obliterans is irreversible owing to established fibrosis affecting the proximal bronchioles (Ezri et al., 1994). In the hematology/oncology literature, bronchiolitis obliterans has been described in clients experiencing irradiation pneumonitis (Kaufman and Komorowski, 1990), amphotericin B toxicity (Roncoroni, Corrado, Besuschio, Pavlovsky, and Narvaiz, 1990), autologous BMT (Paz, Crilley, Patchefsky, Schiffman, and Brodsky, 1992), and allogeneic BMT (King, 1989).

Bronchiolitis obliterans in the BMT patient

The exact pathogenesis of bronchiolitis obliterans in the allogeneic BMT patient has not been determined. However, Ezri et al. (1994), King (1989), and Crawford and Clark (1993) all agree that the presence of chronic graft vs. host disease (GVHD) probably has an impact on the development of this pulmonary complication.

Ezri et al. (1994) described an "enhanced expression of major histocompatibility (MHC) class II antigens on bronchiolar epithelium . . . associated with cytotoxic T lymphocyte infiltration" (p. 4). The assumption is that this is the initiating factor of a vicious cycle of inflammation and fibrosis. Similarly, King (1989) discusses a "lymphocytic bronchitis, characterized by lymphocyte-associated necrosis of the bronchial mucosa and submucosal glands" (p. 82). In this case lymphocytic bronchitis is thought to be pulmonary manifestation of GVHD (King, 1989). King (1989) also discusses two additional theories to explain the pathogenesis. Many BMT patients with suspected bronchiolitis obliterans who have undergone lung biopsy have shown marked lymphocyte or plasma cell infiltration of the terminal respiratory bronchioles and obliteration of the bronchiolar lumina with interstitial fibrosis. Since chronic GVHD is associated with a fibrosing mechanism in other organs, it would seem possible that bronchiolar fibrosis would be an additional manifestation of chronic GVHD. Additionally, chronic GVHD often contributes to esophageal and sinus disease that may result in recurrent esophageal aspiration, which could contribute and further complicate the lung injury.

Crawford and Clark (1993) describe a review of 21 BMT clients with pulmonary symptoms. Sixteen of the 21 patients demonstrated small airway involvement with bronchiolitis, only occasionally with fibrinous obliteration of the bronchiolar lumen. The other five clients who were described only showed evidence of bronchitis or interstitial pneumonia. This study illustrates the fact that bronchiolitis obliterans is not always the causative factor in BMT clients with respiratory symptoms.

Paz et al. (1992) described the first reported cases of bronchiolitis obliterans in clients who had undergone autologous BMT without demonstrating chronic GVHD. Preparative regimens, the possibility of underlying infection, underlying connective tissue disorder, or autoimmune response were postulated as possible initiators; however, no clear causative factor was identified in these clients. The important point is to consider the possibility of bronchiolitis obliterans in clients who present after autologous BMT with clinical signs and symptoms consistent with the disorder. For further information on GVHD, the reader is referred to Chapter 13.

Clients usually present with respiratory complaints such as dry, nonproductive cough, dyspnea on exertion, bibasilar rales, and scattered wheezes, and hypoxemia (King, 1989). The chest x-ray may be read as normal or hyperinflated. Most sources report that physical examination is not particularly helpful in the early diagnosis. Clients will need to undergo further evaluation with pulmonary function tests and most likely lung biopsy to confirm the diagnosis.

RISK PROFILE

The risk factors below have been documented in both adult and pediatric clients.

Cancers: Any malignancy or hematologic disorder in which allogeneic BMT is a treatment option (rare incidence in autologous BMT).

Conditions: Chronic GVHD; the interaction of chronic GVHD and methotrexate; possibly low serum immunoglobulin level; irradiation pneumonitis; older age (in adults).

Environment: None.

Foods: None.

Drugs: Methotrexate (for immunosuppression of GVHD) and amphotericin B (single case report).

PROGNOSIS

Clients undergoing a BMT are at risk for multiple pulmonary side effects. An accurate differential diagnosis is necessary when establishing the prognosis of the individual. Once bronchiolitis obliterans has been established, the prognosis is usually poor. Epler (1988) reported that bronchiolitis obliterans in association with BMT has a poor prognosis and does not respond well to steroids (p. 555). Fort and Graham-Pole (1990) stated that bronchiolitis obliterans is both irreversible and unresponsive to treatment; bronchiolitis obliterans progresses to recurrent pneumothoraxes and hypoxia, which result in death (pp. 407–408). In one study, it was established that 29 of the clients (20%) had developed late-onset pulmonary syndrome (LOPS) that had no identifying infectious component (Schwarer, Hughes, Trotman-Dickenson, Krausz, and Goldman, 1992, p. 1003). Six patients (21%) died, making LOPS the most frequent cause of nonrelapse death in clients 6 months post-BMT (p. 1005). This study used the term LOPS to include airflow obstruction associated with bronchiolitis obliterans and/or interstitial lung disease. Paz et al. (1993) studied 104 clients who underwent allogeneic BMT, 3.9% of whom developed bronchiolitis obliterans (p. 109). Two (50%) of these clients died from the complication (p. 109). Crawford and Clark (1993) observed, "The clinical course is variable, but the process usually is fatal in cases with rapidly progressive or severe obstruction" (p. 748).

TREATMENT

Surgery: No known surgical treatment.

Chemotherapy: Cyclophosphamide—not yet established (Crawford and Clark, 1993, p. 747).

Radiation: No known radiation treatment.

Medications

> Corticosteroids, sometimes in conjunction with cyclosporine.
> Investigation of the immunologic mechanism of GVHD (Epler, 1988, pp. 555–556).
> Azathioprine.
> FK 506 and thalidomide—not yet established (Crawford and Clark, 1993, p. 747).
> Adjunct therapy.
> Trimethoprim-sulfamethoxazole.
> Penicillin.
> Immunoglobulin G (IgG) (if serum levels low).
> Bronchodilator (small percentage of users respond).
> Inhaled corticosteroids (not yet established).

Procedures: No known procedural treatment.

ASSESSMENT CRITERIA: BRONCHIOLITIS OBLITERANS

Vital signs

Temperature	Normal or elevated
Pulse	Rapid
Respiratory rate	Rapid, dyspneic
Blood pressure	Normal, elevated, or decreased

History

Symptoms, conditions	Dry, nonproductive cough, wheezing, and dyspnea on exertion (DOE); chronic GVHD; infection (pneumonia, sinusitis, etc.).

Hallmark physical signs and symptoms — Cough, wheeze, DOE with a normal chest x-ray.

Additional physical signs and symptoms — Cachexia

Psychosocial signs — Anxiety, fear, confusion, exhaustion

Lab values

CBC with differential and platelet count	Elevated WBC (if counts were previously normal) or decreased WBC, with decreased neutrophils and thrombocytopenia. (Results will vary depending on the patient situation: presence of infection, previous bone marrow recovery, or the presence of GVHD.)
BUN	Increased
Creatinine	Increased
Total bilirubin	Moderately elevated (GVHD)
Transaminases	Elevated (three to six times higher than normal in GVHD)
Alkaline phosphatase	Elevated (five to ten times higher than normal in GVHD)
Immunoglobulins	Decreased IgG levels (controversial)

Cultures

Blood	Positive (if underlying infection present) or negative
Urine	Positive (if underlying infection present) or negative
Sputum	Positive (if underlying infection present) or negative

Diagnostic tests

Chest x-ray (posteroanterior and lateral)	Normal, hyperinflated, or diffuse interstitial infiltrates

Pulmonary function tests

Spirometry	Forced expiratory volume (FEV_1) and flow rates are decreased.
Lung volumes	Functional residual capacity (FRC) is increased, and total lung capacity (TLC) is normal.

ASSESSMENT CRITERIA: BRONCHIOLITIS OBLITERANS *(continued)*

Diffusing capacity	Decreased
ABG	Hypoxemia, hypocarbia
Bronchoscopy	Variable findings (dependent on underlying infection)
Transbronchial or open lung biopsy	Positive
Computerized tomography (CT) of the lung	Usually not beneficial.
Other	Assess activity tolerance.
	Assess nutritional status.

NURSING DIAGNOSIS

The nursing diagnoses will vary depending on specific client situations. Some of the common diagnoses and etiologies are listed below.

Activity intolerance related to dyspnea on exertion secondary to bronchiolitis obliterans.

Anxiety related to acute onset of disease and uncertain outcome.

Impaired gas exchange related to restrictive and/or obstructive respiratory dysfunction secondary to bronchiolitis obliterans.

Risk for infection related to suppressed immune system secondary to treatment (e.g., preparative chemotherapy regimen and immunosuppressive agents); also related to injured respiratory system secondary bronchiolitis obliterans.

Powerlessness related to inability to have control over situation secondary to acute onset of bronchiolitis obliterans.

NURSING INTERVENTIONS

Immediate nursing interventions

Assess respirations, pulse, blood pressure, and temperature initially; then follow up with assessment of respiratory status q2h. Apply pulse oximeter.

Place oxygen and suction equipment at the bedside.

Maintain client safety.

Reassure client that his or her needs will be met.

Ensure patent IV access.

Anticipated physician orders and interventions

Arterial blood gases (ABGs).

Oxygen therapy.

STAT chest x-ray.

STAT labs, including complete blood count (CBC) with platelet count, chemistry panel, coagulation panel.

Antibiotics.

Pulse oximeter.

Bronchoscopy.

Transbronchial or open lung biopsy.

Immunosuppressive therapy initiated for chronic GVHD (corticosteroids, cyclosporine, etc.).

Bronchodilator therapy.

IV replacement of IgG.

Ongoing nursing assessment, monitoring, and interventions

Assess:
- Level of consciousness q4h and PRN.
- Signs of chronic GVHD (skin, gastrointestinal tract, and liver).
- Signs of infection (bacterial, fungal, or viral).
- Activity tolerance.
- Emotional response.
- IV site for redness, edema, or pain q4h and PRN.

Measure:
- Pulse oximetry q2h and PRN.
- Blood pressure, pulse, respiration, and temperature q4h and PRN.
- Weight qd.

Initiate:
- Oxygen therapy as ordered.
- Drug therapy as ordered.
- Activity restrictions PRN, as ordered.
- Ethical discussions and planning with the client, family or significant other, and health care team, as appropriate.

TEACHING/EDUCATION

Chest x-ray: *Rationale:* An x-ray of the lungs is made to assess or evaluate complaints of shortness of breath.

Vital signs: *Rationale:* The nurse will be taking your blood pressure, pulse, respiratory rate, and temperature frequently to make sure they are not too high or too low.

ABGs: *Rationale:* A blood sample is drawn from the artery in the wrist to assess if there is enough oxygen in the bloodstream.

Pulse oximeter placement: *Rationale:* A plastic clip or sticky tape is placed on a finger to tell us if there is enough oxygen in the bloodstream. The machine beeps because it is monitoring the heart beat; if an alarm sounds, call the nurse.

Oxygen: *Rationale:* Oxygen is given either through the nostrils or over the nose and mouth to help relieve shortness of breath.

Activity restriction: *Rationale:* It may be necessary to limit your activity level because of your shortness of breath; your condition may cause you to tire easily; the nurses will help you with your meals, your bath, and walking to the bathroom.

IV blood samples: *Rationale:* Samples are needed to check the amount of oxygen and other parts of the blood such as sugar and kidney function; it may be necessary to take several samples; if you have a central line, the blood will be drawn from this line.

Drug therapy—steroids: *Rationale:* You may be started on a drug called a steroid to decrease the congestion in your lungs in order to help you breathe better; the drugs may make you feel anxious or cause swelling; please tell your doctor or nurse if you notice any of these changes.

Other drugs: *Rationale:* The doctor may start you on other drugs during your treatment; the nurse will explain any new drugs to you; please ask for explanations of anything you do not understand.

Pulmonary function tests (PFTs): *Rationale:* It may be necessary to test how well your lungs are working; you will be asked to breathe into a machine that puts the results on a graph for your doctor to read.

Bronchoscopy: *Rationale:* A tube may need to be placed through your nose and down into your lungs; the tube has a tiny camera on the end so the doctor can look at your lungs; the doctor may also take a sample of lung tissue to look at under a microscope; the doctor will give you medicine so the procedure will not be uncomfortable.

Intensive care unit: *Rationale:* It may be necessary to transfer you to an intensive care unit so you can be watched more closely by the critical care nurses.

EVALUATION/DESIRED OUTCOMES

1. Shortness of breath is relieved within 4 hours.
2. Differential diagnoses are established within 48 hours.
3. Drug therapy is initiated within 2 hours; the need for concomitant antibiotic therapy will be evaluated.
4. Blood and platelet transfusion needs are established within 4 hours and blood products are initiated within 6 hours.
5. The unstable client is transferred to intensive care unit within 4 hours, if assessment establishes need.
6. Bronchoscopy and PFTs performed within 24 hours.

DISCHARGE PLANNING

The prognosis for clients diagnosed with bronchiolitis obliterans after BMT is usually poor (Crawford and Clark, 1993; Ezri et al., 1994). Although few clients leave the hospital, we have outlined potential discharge planning needs.

Bronchiolitis obliterans client may need:

Oxygen therapy.
Enteral or parenteral nutrition to meet the increasing nutritional needs.
Home nursing visits, hospice (if bronchiolitis obliterans is progressive), or significant other to manage enteral and parenteral nutritional needs.
Short-term intermediate care facility, daily home nursing visits, or trained significant other to administer IV antibiotics or IV IgG, if needed.
Custodial caregiver for assistance with activities of daily living.
Chaplain or social worker to assist psychosocial adjustment to diagnosis.

FOLLOW-UP CARE

Anticipated care

Physician office visit within 1 to 2 weeks.
Pulmonary function tests, chest x-ray, and bronchoscopy monthly if condition continues to deteriorate.
Outpatient lab testing for CBC and platelet count weekly.
Other lab testing as appropriate (liver functions, blood urea nitrogen [BUN]/creatinine, immunoglobulins, etc.).
Evaluation of any signs of infection (cultures).
Home nursing visits (frequency will depend on the needs of the client).

Anticipated client/family questions and possible answers

Will I get better?
"It is hard to know at this point. We will be watching you closely to see how your body accepts this treatment."
"It depends on how you respond to the treatments. Each person responds differently."

How have other people done who have had this same problem?
"Each person responds differently. Some do well, while others have more problems. We will have to evaluate your progress as we go along."
"Everyone is different. Let's concentrate on what we can do to make you better."

Is there anything I can do to make this better?
"The disease will get better if and when your body accepts the treatment. You can help yourself by (1) not doing things that make you breathe harder,

such as exercise not approved by your doctor; (2) avoiding people who have a cold or the flu so you won't get an infection; (3) eating a healthful diet so your body can help fight these problems; (4) not returning to work unless your doctor says it is okay; (5) letting your doctor know if you are upset; have trouble sleeping; are unable to eat; feel helpless, out of control, or just really angry at everyone and everything."

Why do I need to keep repeating these tests?

"To see if you are accepting the treatment or if changes need to be made that might help things get better."

Why did I get a bone marrow transplant if this was going to happen?

"There are risks with treatment for any disease or medical problem. If you did not get the bone marrow transplant, your cancer would have come back, and there may have been no way to control it."

"When you were making the decision to have the bone marrow transplant, we discussed that it was your best option for survival despite possible side effects or problems."

"This is a rare complication of a bone marrow transplant. The transplant was necessary for treatment of your type of cancer. We need to work together to see what we can do to best treat your problems."

CHAPTER SUMMARY

Bronchiolitis obliterans is a disease that occurs infrequently in the BMT population. It affects approximately 10% of patients suffering from chronic graft vs. host disease. But, it has also been identified in the autologous population. The disease can present as a mixed restrictive and obstructive process that makes definitive diagnosis difficult. The nurse must have strong assessment skills when caring for a client suspected of having bronchiolitis obliterans because of the insidious onset of the disease. Treatment is usually supportive, with a high mortality in affected clients. Since the nursing care of these clients is supportive and the prognosis is poor, a major role of the nurse is to be a psychosocial resource for the client and significant others.

TEST QUESTIONS

1. The development of bronchiolitis obliterans is associated with:
   A. Pneumocystis carinii
   B. Graft vs. host disease (GVHD)
   C. Tuberculosis
   D. Fungal sepsis

1. Answer: B
Bronchiolitis obliterans has been associated with the presence of GVHD in allogeneic and autologous BMT clients.

2. The diagnostic testing for bron-
   chiolitis obliterans includes all of
   the following *except:*
   A. Pulmonary function tests
      (PFTs)
   B. Arterial blood gases (ABGs)
   C. Echocardiogram (ECHO)
   D. Bronchoscopy

2. Answer: C
An ECHO is done to assess the cardiac output, which is not part of the
diagnostic testing for bronchiolitis
obliterans.

3. Etiologies implicated in the
   development of bronchiolitis
   obliterans include all of those
   listed below *except:*
   A. Toxic fume exposure
   B. Bone marrow transplant
   C. Viral exposure
   D. Electrical shock.

3. Answer: D
Electrical shock has not been implicated in the development of bronchiolitis obliterans.

4. Bronchiolitis obliterans results
   primarily in:
   A. Restrictive and constrictive
      lung disease
   B. Only restrictive lung disease
   C. Only constrictive lung disease
   D. Neither restrictive nor con-
      strictive lung disease

4. Answer: A
It has been established that during
the disease process, both restrictive
and constrictive lung disease develops.

5. Investigational drug therapies for
   treatment of bronchiolitis obliter-
   ans includes the following
   chemotherapy agent:
   A. Methotrexate
   B. Mitoxantrone
   C. Cisplatin
   D. Cyclophosphamide

5. Answer: D
Cyclophosphamide has been evaluated as part of the treatment regimen, but definitive results have not
been established.

6. One nursing diagnosis not appro-
   priate for the client diagnosed
   with bronchiolitis obliterans is:
   A. Risk for infection
   B. Impaired gas exchange
   C. Alteration in cardiac output
   D. Anxiety

6. Answer: C
Cardiac output is not usually affected by bronchiolitis obliterans.

7. Signs of bronchiolitis obliterans include:
   A. Cough and dyspnea on exertion
   B. Edema
   C. Decreased transaminases and increased immunoglobulins
   D. Negative lung biopsy

7. Answer: A
Cough and dyspnea on exertion are usually the presenting signs of a client diagnosed with bronchiolitis obliterans.

8. A common risk factor for developing bronchiolitis obliterans is:
   A. Allogeneic BMT
   B. High serum IgG levels
   C. Veno-occlusive disease
   D. Lung cancer

8. Answer: A
Allogeneic BMT has been identified as a risk factor because of the high incidence of GVHD in this population. GVHD has been implicated in the development of bronchiolitis obliterans.

9. A client being evaluated for bronchiolitis obliterans would most likely be taught about which of the following diagnostic procedures:
   A. Endoscopy
   B. Bone marrow biopsy
   C. Thoracentesis
   D. Bronchoscopy

9. Answer: D
Bronchoscopy is usually one of the first diagnostic procedures to be done to rule out infection in the population with new onset respiratory difficulty.

10. An expected outcome for a client diagnosed with bronchiolitis obliterans is:
    A. Foley catheter will be discontinued within 48 hours.
    B. Chest tube will be inserted within 24 hours.
    C. Differential diagnosis will be established within 48 hours.
    D. Ambulating in room three times a day (TID)

10. Answer: C
Differential diagnosis is important in determining the course of treatment and prognosis for the client.

REFERENCES

Crawford S, Clark J: Bronchiolitis associated with bone marrow transplantation. Clin Chest
    Med 14(4):741–749, 1993.

Epler G: Bronchiolitis obliterans and airways obstruction associated with graft-versus-host dis-
    ease. Clin Chest Med 9(4):551–556, 1988.

Ezri T, Kunichezky S, Eliraz A, Soroker D, Halperin D, Schattner A: Bronchiotitis oblierans:
    Current concepts. Q J Med 87:1–10, 1994.

Fort J, Graham-Pole J: Pulmonary complications of bone marrow transplants. *In* Johnson FL,
    Pochedly C (eds): Bone Marrow Transplants in Children. New York: Raven Press, 1990,
    pp. 397–411.

Holland K, Wingard J, Beschorner W, Saral R, Santos G: Bronchiolitis obliterans in bone mar-
    row transplantation and its relationship to chronic graft-v-host disease and low serum
    IgG. Blood 72(2):621–627, 1988.

Kaufman J, Komorowski R: Bronchiolitis obliterans: A new clinical-pathologic complication of
    irradiation pneumonitis. Chest 97(5):1243–1244, 1990.

King T: Bronchiolitis obliterans. Lung 167:69–93, 1989.

Paz H, Crilley P, Patchefsky A, Schiffman R, Brodsky I: Bronchiolitis obliterans after autologous
    bone marrow transplantation. Chest 101(3):775–778, 1992.

Paz H, Crilley P, Topolsky D, Coll W, Patchefsky A, Brodsky I: Bronchiolitis obliterans after
    bone marrow transplantation: The effect of preconditioning. Respiration 60:109–114, 1993.

Roncoroni A, Corrado C, Besuschio S, Pavlovsky S, Narvaiz M: Bronchiolitis obliterans possibly
    associated with amphotericin B. J Infect Dis 161:589, 1990.

Schwarer A, Hughes JM, Trotman-Dickenson G, Krausz T, Goldman J: A chronic pulmonary
    syndrome associated with graft-versus-host disease after allogenic marrow transplanta-
    tion. Transplantation 54(6):1002–1008, 1992.

CHAPTER 8

CAROTID ARTERY RUPTURE

Molly A. Johantgen, MSN, RN, CCRN

CHAPTER OBJECTIVES

At the completion of this chapter, the reader will be able to:

Describe the conditions that may lead to carotid artery rupture.

Describe the nursing care as it relates to the oncology client with carotid artery rupture.

Prepare the client and significant others regarding the care associated with the client who is at high risk for rupture of the carotid artery.

OVERVIEW

THE RUPTURE of a carotid artery is a life-threatening and very likely death-producing event. The development of carotid artery rupture occurs in 3.5% of clients who have undergone radical surgery of the head and neck. The incidence of rupture of the artery is further increased with radiation therapy, which diminishes the healing of the suture line and enhances the formation of fistula (Cutright, 1992). Control of the potentially massive bleeding, and therefore the ability to save a life, is based on the extent of the erosion of the artery and speed of transport of the client to an operating room.

DESCRIPTION

The carotid artery is exposed to potential damage or weakness following extensive surgery associated with the removal of tumors in the head and neck regions. The tumor that is excised may itself invade the artery to cause weakness of the artery wall. The surgery poses multiple factors that decrease healing of the area, such as edema, removal of lymph tissue, and increased venous drainage. Further, if the client undergoes radiation therapy postoperatively, the therapies will increase tissue destruction and limit wound healing. These factors therefore increase the risk of infection, the development of a fistula, and the development of necrotic tissue. Infection, large amounts of drainage, and a necrotic process may cause the wall of the artery to weaken.

Once the artery wall is damaged, it may rupture, with erosion from any of the causative factors or increased pressure from within the artery itself, such as that caused by coughing (Belcher, 1992).

RISK PROFILE

All risk factors below are greater risks when occurring in the elderly client.

Cancers: Head and neck, specifically tumors that affect the neck region near the carotid artery.

Conditions: Local neck infection, sepsis (causing destruction of surrounding tissue), diabetes mellitus, immune deficiencies, and malnutrition (causing slow healing); clients receiving therapy to the neck, such as radiation (causing destruction of healthy tissue and reduced wound healing).

Environment: Radical neck surgery.

Foods: None.

Drugs: Full-strength skin cleansers and antiseptic agents that are cytotoxic to normal tissue, such as povidone iodine, iodophor, sodium hypochlorite solution (Dakin's), hydrogen peroxide, and acetic acid. Most wound cleansers need to be diluted to maintain cell viability. Normal saline provides a nontoxic cleansing solution for wound care (Bergstrom, Bennett, Carlson, et al., 1994; Burkey, Weinberg, and Brenden, 1993; Foresman, Payne, Becker, Lewis, and Rodeheaver, 1993).

PROGNOSIS

The prognosis of clients who rupture a carotid artery is extremely poor, but no mortality statistics are known. Hemorrhage from the carotid artery is usually extensive, and the ability to control the bleeding is difficult at best. Ligation of the artery is the only method that effectively stops the bleeding, but the ability to provide immediate surgical intervention can be improbable.

TREATMENT

Surgery: Ligation of the carotid artery above and below the area of rupture.

Chemotherapy: Not indicated.

Radiation: Not indicated.

Medications

IV normal saline, volume expanders, and/or blood products to treat hypovolemic shock and cerebral ischemia.

Antianxiety medications or analgesics for comfort if the client is alert.

Procedures

Placement of large-bore peripheral catheter for administration of fluids.
Suction airway to maintain patency.
Inflate cuff on tracheostomy if in place.
Provide digital external compression to carotid artery, using a gloved hand and one 4 × 4 gauze sponge.

Other: Type and crossmatch for multiple units of blood as a precaution in clients who are at risk for carotid artery rupture.

ASSESSMENT CRITERIA: CAROTID ARTERY RUPTURE

Vital signs

Pulse	Rapid and weak
Respirations	Tachypneic, dyspneic
Blood pressure	Systolic blood pressure <90 mmHg or 20 mmHg below baseline
Central venous pressure (CVP)	<2 mmHg

History

Symptoms, conditions	Wound infection; wound dehiscence; fistula.

Hallmark physical signs and symptoms	Bleeding from surgical wound; initially bleeding may be a trickle but quickly progresses to rapid, pulsating flow.

Additional physical signs and symptoms	May be preceded by coughing or straining.

Psychosocial signs	Anxiety

Lab values

Hemoglobin/hematocrit	Low

Diagnostic tests

Oxygen saturation	Diminished

NURSING DIAGNOSIS

Nursing diagnoses and etiologies that may affect the client with carotid artery rupture are as follows.

Tissue perfusion, altered cerebral and cardiopulmonary related to hemorrhage of the carotid artery.

(Potential for) ineffective airway clearance related to bleeding into

oropharynx or compression of the trachea secondary to hemorrhage of the carotid artery.

Anxiety related to the emergency procedures being performed and high risk of death.

NURSING INTERVENTIONS

Immediate nursing interventions

For clients at high risk of carotid artery rupture:

- Have emergency equipment and body substance isolation equipment (gloves, gown, goggles) available for use in the event hemorrhage should occur. See Table 8–1.
- Place venous access device to enable rapid infusion of IV fluids.
- Send blood sample for type and crossmatch or type and screen if the client's religious beliefs allow the use of blood products in the event hemorrhage should occur.

For client with actual carotid artery rupture:

- Assess wound for extent of bleeding, level of consciousness, respirations, pulse, and blood pressure.
- Apply digital pressure, using gloved hands and other personal protective equipment if required.
- Suction oral airway and inflate tracheostomy cuff if applicable.
- Provide emotional support by explaining the activities occurring and by speaking in a calm, reassuring manner.

Anticipated physician orders and interventions

Administration of normal saline, blood, or volume expanders based on the client's condition.

Intubation of the trachea to maintain the airway.

Antianxiety medication or analgesic as required.

TABLE 8–1
Emergency Equipment for Carotid Artery Rupture

Suction equipment	1 box of gloves
1 Yankauer catheter	4 packages of sterile 4 × 4 gauze
1 cuffed tracheostomy tube with 12 ml syringe if indicated	2 liters of normal saline
4 fluid-resistant gowns	4 sterile towels
4 face shields	4 bath towels

Source: Adapted from Schwartz SS, Yuska CM: Common patient care issues following surgery for head and neck cancer. *Semin Oncol Nurs* 15(3):191–194, 1989.

Transport to an operating room for ligation of the carotid artery.
Transfer to an intensive care unit postoperatively.

Ongoing nursing assessment, monitoring, and interventions

Assess:
- Level of consciousness q1h and PRN.
- Motor or sensory deficits q1h and PRN.
- Suture line for bleeding q5min × 6, then q30min × 4, then q1h.
- IV site for patency and signs of infiltration (redness, edema, pain).

Measure:
- Blood pressure, pulse, and respiration q1h and PRN.
- Intake and output (I and O) q1h until client stable.
- Oxygen saturation via pulse oximetry continuously × 24 hours, then PRN.

Send:
- Hemoglobin/hematocrit q6h × 24 hours.
- Serum electrolytes, creatinine, and blood urea nitrogen (BUN) q6h × 24 hours.
- Serum calcium and complete blood count (CBC) with differential in 24 hours.
- Arterial blood gases in 24 hours and PRN.

Implement:
- Suctioning of the airway PRN.

TEACHING/EDUCATION

The extent of teaching is based on the client's desire for emergency procedures to be implemented. In the terminally ill client, surgery may not be indicated.

Risk for hemorrhage: *Rationale:* Since you had surgery (and radiation treatments) to remove the cancer in your neck, one of the major blood vessels in your neck, called the carotid artery, may become weakened. If the artery wall becomes too weak, a hole may open up, and blood will be pumped out of your body very rapidly. Unless the bleeding can be quickly stopped, you could bleed to death.

Digital pressure/ligation of the artery: *Rationale:* If bleeding should occur, pressure is applied with the fingertips directly over the hole in the artery. Pressure will continue until you can be taken to the operating room, where a doctor can tie off the artery to stop the bleeding completely.

IV access placement: *Rationale:* You may lose a lot of blood if the blood vessel opens up. To replace the blood, we need a way to get it to you. The IV line allows us to give you blood and fluid very quickly. Medications can be given painlessly and quickly with the IV as well.

Maintaining the airway: *Rationale:* When pressure is held over the bleeding area in the artery, the pressure may cause you to have trouble breathing. If you can't breathe because of the pressure on your neck, the doctors may put a breathing tube down your throat so that we can help you breathe with a machine. More oxygen can be given to you through this tube. Blood may also get into your throat. To get the blood out of your throat, we may put a large tube into your throat and suction the blood out so you can breathe more easily.

EVALUATION/DESIRED OUTCOMES

1. Hemorrhage will be controlled so that the client does not die of exsanguination.
2. Client is able to have normal movement and sensation and normal level of consciousness postoperatively.
3. Hemoglobin/hematocrit increases to low-normal to normal values within 48 hours.
4. If the client and significant others have decided against resuscitation measures, the client will be calm and peaceful in dying with dignity.

DISCHARGE PLANNING

High-risk client may need:

Frank and open discussion describing the extremely poor prognosis if rupture should occur, since immediate surgical intervention cannot be ensured.

Training of client and significant others of the signs of carotid artery rupture and how to initiate emergency procedures, including digital pressure, if desired.

Training of client and significant others about how to assist client in having a peaceful death if emergency procedures are not desired.

Intermediate care facility, hospice, daily home nursing visits, or family caregivers to manage wound care.

Postoperative client may need:

Intermediate care facility, hospice, daily home nursing visits, or family caregivers to manage wound care.

FOLLOW-UP CARE

Anticipated care

Physician office visit within 2 weeks.
Outpatient lab testing for CBC within 1 week for the postoperative client.

Daily home nursing visit for wound care management for clients discharged.

Anticipated client/family questions and possible answers

Could the carotid artery rupture again?

"It is possible that until the area around your surgery heals, another place in the blood vessel may weaken and bleed. We will help you take care of your neck until it heals. Once the wound is healed, the likelihood of the blood vessel bleeding is very low."

Why will a nurse be coming to my home?

"The nurse will come to look at your neck and make sure that it is healing properly. The nurse may also clean the wound and teach your family how to take care of it. He or she will teach your family how to prepare your home for the possibility that you could have bleeding from the blood vessel and what to do if bleeding should occur."

CHAPTER SUMMARY

Carotid artery rupture is a medical emergency that occurs in 3.5% of people with radical neck surgery from tumors of the head and neck. The prognosis is poor, since hemorrhage is rapid and difficult to control. Weakening of the artery wall may be due to invasion of tumor into the wall, infection, drainage, and/or tissue destruction from irradiation. A realistic portrayal of the event, if it should occur, is important to discuss with the high-risk client and significant others. Prevention of rupture of the artery by limiting wound infections and promoting healing may be the only positive intervention for carotid artery rupture. If hemorrhage should occur, digital pressure with fluid resuscitation and maintenance of oxygenation are provided. When possible, the carotid artery is ligated above and below the region of rupture. Emotional support of the client and significant others during this tragic situation is paramount in the terminally ill client (Bildstein, 1993).

TEST QUESTIONS

1. The carotid artery is most vulnerable to rupture if the client has:
   A. A history of hypotension
   B. Been receiving chemotherapy
   C. Undergone radical neck surgery and radiation therapy to the head and neck
   D. Brain metastasis

1. Answer: C
Radical neck surgery and irradiation increase the risk of carotid artery wall weakness.

2. Following surgery, all of the following factors may weaken the carotid artery further, *except:*
   A. Wound infection
   B. Fistula formation
   C. Invasion of the tumor into the artery wall
   D. Chemotherapy

2. Answer: D
All of these factors increase exposure of the artery wall to destructive forces, except the use of chemotherapy.

3. The incidence of carotid artery rupture in clients who have head and neck cancer is:
   A. Less than 1%
   B. 3.5%
   C. 25%
   D. 50%

3. Answer: B
The incidence of carotid artery rupture is 3.5% of those who have been diagnosed with cancer of the head and neck.

4. The initial intervention for rupture of the carotid artery is to:
   A. Apply pressure to the area with gloved fingertips and 1 to 2 gauze sponges
   B. Insert gauze sponges into the client's mouth
   C. Place the client in the Trendelenberg position
   D. Make the client NPO

4. Answer: A
Because the client is in danger of exsanguination, direct pressure must be applied to the vessel itself. Using fingertips and limited sponges enhances control of the bleeding. Inserting sponges into the mouth or placing the client in the Trendelenberg position obstructs the airway.

5. The initial goal of therapy for clients with carotid artery rupture is to:
   A. Limit expansion of the cancer
   B. Maintain nutrition
   C. Prevent infection
   D. Control hemorrhage

5. Answer: D
The client will exsanguinate if bleeding is not controlled immediately. The other goals help prevent weakening of the wall of the artery.

6. In treating carotid artery rupture, a primary intervention should be to:
   A. Administer antianxiety therapy and chemotherapy
   B. Maintain the airway and cerebral perfusion
   C. Administer fluids and nutrition
   D. Maintain a calming atmosphere and limit surgical interventions

6. Answer: B
Maintaining the airway and cerebral perfusion is the primary intervention. Appropriate additional interventions include administering antianxiety therapy, administering fluids, and maintaining a calm atmosphere.

7. The only effective medical therapy for carotid artery rupture is:
   A. Bypass of the carotid artery
   B. Ligation of the carotid artery
   C. Placement of a gortex graft into the artery wall
   D. Excision of the carotid artery

7. Answer: B
Ligation of the artery both above and below the area that has ruptured will control the bleeding. Use of the other techniques is not technically possible or required.

8. Client education concerning the potential for carotid artery rupture should include:
   A. Factors that may increase fatigue
   B. Mouth care
   C. Poor prognosis if rupture should occur
   D. Activity restrictions

8. Answer: C
The client and significant other(s) must have a knowledge base to make an informed decision for care and effective training to respond to the potential crisis.

9. The terminal client who experiences carotid artery rupture should:
   A. Receive emergency surgery
   B. Be provided nutritional support
   C. Be allowed to die with dignity and comfort
   D. Receive fluid resuscitation

9. Answer: C
The terminal client should be allowed dignity in dying, since the prognosis with carotid artery rupture is very poor in the best of situations. Emergency care does not aid in providing dignity or comfort.

REFERENCES

Belcher AE: Mosby's Clinical Nursing Series: Cancer Nursing. St. Louis, MO: CV Mosby, 1992.

Bergstrom N, Bennett MA, Carlson CE, et al: Treatment of Pressure Ulcers, Clinical Practice Guideline. Rockville, MD: U.S. Department of Health and Human Services, Agency for Health Care Policy and Research, 1994.

Bildstein CY: Head and neck malignancies. In Groenwald SL, Frogge MH, Goodman M, Yarbro CH (eds): Cancer Nursing Principles and Practice, 3rd ed. Boston: Jones and Bartlett, 1993, pp. 1145–1146.

Burkey JL, Weinberg C, Brenden RA: Differential methodologies for the evaluation of skin and wound cleansers. Wounds 5(6):284–291, 1993.

Cutright LH: Head and neck cancers. In Clark JC, McGee RF (eds): Oncology Nursing Society Core Curriculum for Oncology Nursing, 2nd ed. Philadelphia: WB Saunders Co, 1992, pp. 514–516.

Foresman PA, Payne DS, Becker D, et al: A relative toxicity index for wound cleansers. Wounds 5(5):226–231, 1993.

Schwartz SS, Yuska CM: Common patient care issues following surgery for head and neck cancer. Semin Oncol Nurs 15(3):191–194, 1989.

CHAPTER 9

DIABETES INSIPIDUS

Susanne Vendlinski, BSN, MSN, RN, OCN

CHAPTER OBJECTIVES

At the completion of this chapter, the reader will be able to:

Define diabetes insipidus (DI).

Identify risk factors associated with DI occurrence in the client with cancer.

Describe the presenting signs and symptoms of DI.

Describe medical management of DI.

Describe nursing care of the oncology client with DI.

Anticipate and prepare the client with DI for future care needs.

OVERVIEW

ANTIDIURETIC hormone (ADH), a small tripeptide hormone produced in the supraoptic and paraventricular nuclei of the hypothalamus, is transmitted to and stored in the posterior lobe of the pituitary (neurohypophysis). ADH is stored in the axon terminals and is released into the perivascular space in response to subtle increases in plasma osmolality, hypotension, or reduced plasma volume. When released, ADH causes renal tubular cells to reabsorb water, thus preventing diuresis. ADH also causes vascular and gastrointestinal smooth muscle contraction and is sometimes referred to as arginine vasopressin (AVP). Central DI occurs when any part of the ADH regulatory pathway is disrupted (Chaudhuri, Twelves, Cox, and Bingham, 1992) (Fig. 9–1).

DESCRIPTION

DI is a syndrome of altered water balance in which ADH is deficient or there is renal resistance to its effects. It is characterized by polyuria (50 ml/kg body weight) leading to dehydration, in which urine specific gravity is usually 1.001 to 1.005 and the urine osmolality is less than 300 mOsm/kg of water. DI is caused primarily by inadequate secretion of

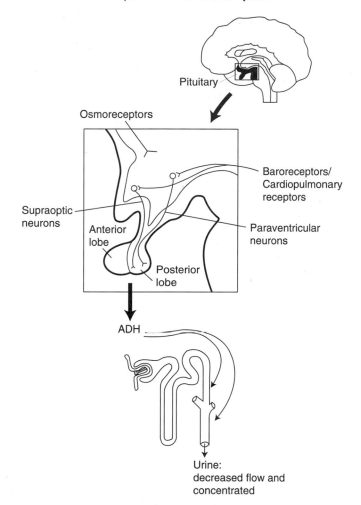

Figure 9–1 Neuroanatomy of the hypothalamus, where ADH is synthesized, and the posterior pituitary gland, where ADH is released. (From Guyton AC: Textbook of Medical Physiology. Philadelphia, WB Saunders, 1994, p. 360.)

ADH, often referred to as *neurogenic, cranial,* or *central DI,* or by renal collecting tubule resistance to the antidiuretic effect of AVP, referred to as *nephrogenic* or *renal DI.* DI also results from excessive water intake, generally referred to as primary polydipsia. This occurs secondary to physiologic changes in the thirst mechanism or psychogenic polydipsia. Gestational DI may result from the increase in metabolic clearance that normally occurs during pregnancy and generally resolves within 3 weeks postdelivery (Robertson, 1995). The reader is also referred to Chapter 21 on hypernatremia.

Neurohypophyseal or central DI

Central DI is caused by insufficient hypothalamo-neurohypophyseal axis release of ADH in response to appropriate osmotic stimuli. The decreased ADH production primarily results from destruction of the magnocellular neurons in the posterior pituitary (neurohypophysis) (Robertson, 1995), often from various primary or metastatic malignancies, surgery in the hypothalamic pituitary area, or trauma such as basilar skull fracture. The deficiency of ADH causes a failure of water reabsorption by the kidney distal tubules and collecting ducts, resulting in dilute urine and extracellular fluid (ECF) hyperosmolality. This ECF hyperosmolality does not trigger the usual response of increased ADH, due to the damaged area of production or release. However, it does stimulate the thirst mechanism, resulting in increased fluid intake, continuing the cycle of high urinary output and serum hyperosmolality (Lemone and Burke, 1996). Central DI is sometimes called vasopressin-sensitive DI because it responds well to vasopressin administration (Metheny, 1996).

Nephrogenic DI

Impairment of the renal antidiuretic response to ADH is secondary to kidney abnormalities in the collecting tubules or medulla, the structures most involved in urine concentration. Among the acquired forms of nephrogenic DI, lithium is the most frequent causative agent, but other drugs also contribute significantly, as well as electrolyte abnormalities (see Risk Profile). It appears that these agents interfere with postreceptor biochemical mechanisms that mediate ADH's effect on the hydro-osmotic permeability of collecting duct epithelium (Robertson, 1995).

Dipsogenic DI is sometimes caused by diseases, injuries, or drugs that affect multiple areas in the central nervous system (see Risk Profile below).

RISK PROFILE

Cancers: Leukemia (especially acute myelogenous), lymphoma, hypothalamic neoplasms, metastatic lesions to the hypothalamus, or posterior pituitary (lung [1 to 6%], breast [1 to 2%], leukemia, lymphoma, pancreas) (Chaudhuri, Twelves, Cox, and Bingham, 1992; Ko et al., 1994; Robertson, 1995).

Conditions

Central DI: Infections of the meninges or parenchyma; head injury, including clients having surgery in the pituitary-hypothalamic area (4 to 8% post craniotomy); amyloidosis; tuberculosis; neurosarcoid granuloma. Twenty-five to 50 percent of cases are idiopathic (Blumberg, Sklar, Wisoff, and David, 1994; Robertson, 1995; Metheny, 1996).

Nephrogenic DI: Sarcoma; electrolyte disturbances such as hypercalcemia, hypercalciuria, and hypokalemia. (The reader is referred to Chapters 18 and 19 for further information on the pathophysiology leading to the presence of hypercalcemia and hypokalemia in the oncology client.)

Dipsogenic DI: Head trauma, multiple sclerosis, tuberculosis meningitis.

Pediatrics: Suprasellar tumors, Langerhans histiocytosis, postcraniotomy for brain tumor (especially craniopharyngioma).

Environment: None.

Foods: None.

Drugs: Aminoglycosides, foscarnet, lithium, amphotericin B, cisplatin, demeclocycline, rifampin, methoxyflurane (Robertson, 1995; Metheny, 1996).

PROGNOSIS

Transient DI, of 12 to 36 hours duration following removal of pituitary adenomas (96% via the transsphenoidal route), occurs in up to one-third of clients and is managed with desmopressin. This complication is usually temporary because ADH can be secreted directly from the hypothalamus without pituitary storage (Donehower, 1993). If the client is capable of drinking, the hypernatremia can generally be corrected by increasing water intake. Chemotherapy and radiation therapy may be effective in resolving DI secondary to hypothalamic/pituitary area metastasis.

TREATMENT

Surgery: Craniotomy to resect primary tumors if feasible.

Chemotherapy: Agents appropriate to tumor type, if known to be responsive to chemotherapy, and when recurrence is likely. Decrease or discontinue amphotericin B, cisplatin.

Radiation: Use depends on radiosensitivity of tumor type.

Medications

In total ADH deficiency, replacement therapy with demopressin (intramuscularly [IM], nasally), lysopressin (nasally), or vasopressin (subcutaneously, IM). Desmopressin is the drug of choice due to its prolonged action, convenience of administration (intranasal), and minimal side effects (very little pressor activity). When rapid-acting, short-duration ADH replacement is needed, such as after cranial surgery, vasopressin is useful.

Chlorpropamide and carbamazepine may be used in clients with some capacity to secrete ADH, as both drugs increase its release or enhance its renal response, respectively.

Procedures

Stereotactic radiosurgery may be indicated for brain metastasis. Stereotactic biopsy followed by radiation may be indicated (Wegmann, 1993).

Other

Temporary osmotic disruption of the blood brain barrier concurrent with chemotherapy administration may be effective in primary central nervous system (CNS) lymphomas (Wegmann, 1993).

Correct underlying cause if possible.

Encourage fluid intake if feasible, or administer normal saline. Total body water (TBW) is approximately 60% of total body weight (50% in elderly). Calculate TBW deficit by the following formula:
- Step 1: Note mEq elevation of sodium.
- Step 2: What percentage (%) of elevation above 140 is this?
- Step 3: Percentage (%) of elevation × TBW = liters of body water needed.

Note: Correction of hypernatremia that is too rapid can result in cerebral edema, seizures, permanent neurologic damage, and death. Chronic (>2 days) hypernatremia should not be corrected faster than 0.7 mEq/L/hour or approximately 10% of the serum sodium concentration daily. Acute hypernatremia may be reduced by 6 to 8 mEq/L/hour the first 3 to 4 hours, but should not decline by more than 1 mEq/L/hour thereafter (Metheny, 1996).

ASSESSMENT CRITERIA: DIABETES INSIPIDUS

Vital signs	
Temperature	Elevated if dehydrated
Pulse	Possibly rapid, weak if dehydration severe
Respirations	Possibly increased
Blood pressure	Decreased if dehydrated
History	Thirst, mental confusion, polyuria.
	Removal of pituitary tumors (via transsphenoidal or cranial routes); primary tumors of lung, breast, pancreas, lymphoma, leukemia, with metastasis to hypothalamic-pituitary region.
Weight pattern	Decreased, correlated to amount of fluid loss.
Hallmark physical signs and symptoms	*Polyuria* (often >200 ml/hour); intense thirst in the alert client with resultant *polydipsia;* dry, sticky tongue and oral mucosa.
Additional physical signs and symptoms	Altered mental status, restlessness, and weakness in moderate hypernatremia; muscle irritability and convulsions in severe hypernatremia (high-pitched cry in infants); weight loss.

ASSESSMENT CRITERIA: DIABETES INSIPIDUS *(continued)*

Psychosocial signs	May become fatigued, depressed if polyuria/polydipsia interfere with other activities.
	Possible confusion, apprehension, disorientation related to hypernatremia.

Lab values	
Urine specific gravity	<1.005
Urine osmolality	<200 mOsm/L
Serum osmolality	>295 mOsm/kg
Serum sodium	Elevated (>145 mEq/L, >145 mmol/L SI Units)
Other	Hypokalemia may result in nephrogenic DI.

Diagnostic tests	MRI or CT scans of the brain

Other	Failure of fluid restriction to result in increased urine concentration.

NURSING DIAGNOSIS

Confusion, acute, related to hypernatremia.

Fatigue related to nocturia and polyuria.

Fluid volume deficit, risk for, related to polyuria from decreased production of, or renal response to, ADH.

Health maintenance, altered, risk for, related to insufficient knowledge of the disease process.

Injury, risk for, related to hypernatremia-related mental status changes.

Knowledge deficit related to diagnostic tests and drug therapy.

Sleep pattern disturbance related to nocturia.

NURSING INTERVENTIONS

Immediate nursing interventions

Assess vital signs and neurologic status q1h until sodium levels are within normal limits, then q 4 to 8 hours.

Establish patent IV access and obtain volumetric infusion pump.

Provide oral fluids to conscious, alert client or administer parenteral fluids to the confused or comatose client.

Maintain an accurate hourly intake and output (I and O). Insert indwelling urinary catheter, if needed.

Prepare for long-line catheter/access device placement for frequent blood sampling.

Anticipated physician orders and interventions

Spot urine electrolytes and osmolality.

Serum sodium levels q1–2h.

Water deficit is replaced over 48 hours. Normal saline is administered if client is hypotensive and hypernatremic until vascular volume is adequate; then free water is given. If hypernatremia is slight, 0.25% sodium chloride is used for fluid replacement (Blevins and Cassmeyer, 1995).

Ongoing nursing assessment, monitoring, and interventions

Assess:
- Level of consciousness q8h and PRN. Seizures may occur with serum sodium increase of 15 to 20 mEq/L in 24 hours or less, and usually occur at a level > 160 mEq/L (> 160 mmol/L SI Units).
- Mucous membranes q8h.

Measure:
- Blood pressure, pulse, temperature, and respirations q4h after acute hypernatremia is resolved.
- I and O q1h × 24h, then q8h.

Send:
- Serum sodium and potassium while acute hypernatremia being corrected q1h × 4, then q2h × 8, then q4h × 2. *If administering vasopressin replacement, be aware that rebound hyponatremia may occur.*
- Urine specific gravity qd.

Implement:
- Free water intake and/or IV fluid replacement as ordered.
- Reporting of urine volume greater than 200 ml in each of 2 consecutive hours or more than 500 ml in a 2-hour period (especially in the postoperative neurosurgical client) (Metheny, 1996).
- Seizure precautions until serum sodium is ≤160 mEq/L (≤160 mmol/L SI Units).

TEACHING/EDUCATION

Intranasal desmopressin: *Rationale:* Your body is not producing enough of a substance called antidiuretic hormone, which helps keep your body water in balance. Desmopressin is a form of this hormone that will replace the amount your body lacks. You should call your doctor if you develop drowsiness, listlessness, or headache while taking this medication. These are signs you may need a dosage adjustment. You also should reduce your water intake once you begin taking it, because your body's response will be to "hang on" to water now instead of losing it.

Decrease/discontinue chemotherapy or other medication: *Rationale:* Certain drugs can cause your body to get rid of too much water. Some of your drugs may be changed or alternated with other drugs.

IV blood samples and urine samples: *Rationale:* Several blood and urine samples will be taken over the next day. They are needed to track the amount of salt and water in your body.

IV line placement: *Rationale:* The IV line allows us to give you any necessary fluid treatments and to take blood samples easily, so you will not have to be "stuck" with needles repeatedly.

Indwelling urinary catheter placement: *Rationale:* Accurate urine measurement is very important for people with altered salt levels. The catheter prevents urine from spilling before it is measured and will also keep you from having to make numerous trips to the bathroom throughout the day and night until your condition is corrected.

IV fluid replacement or encouragement of oral fluid intake: *Rationale:* Encouraging you to drink if you can, or giving you IV fluids if you can't drink, keeps you from dehydrating while your body is unable to save water. This also helps to lower your body's salt level.

Signs and symptoms of hypernatremia (high salt) or hyponatremia (low salt): *Rationale:* You and your significant others need to watch for signs of low or high salt levels because early treatment and correction will help you feel better and live a higher quality of life. Signs include any of the following: fatigue, weakness, confusion, irritability, muscle cramps, muscle-twitching convulsions, nausea, vomiting, severe thirst, dry mouth, rapid heart beat, dizziness.

EVALUATION/DESIRED OUTCOMES

1. Serum sodium level decreases to 145 mEq/L (145 mmol/L SI Units) within 48 hours (for acute hypernatremia).
2. Serum sodium level decreases to normal values at a rate comparable to the time over which the hypernatremia developed.
3. Urine sodium level and urine osmolality return to normal within 72 hours.
4. Serum potassium level increases to normal values (3.5 to 5.0 mEq/L, 3.5 to 5.0 mmol/L SI Units) within 24 hours.
5. Systolic blood pressure returns to baseline within 72 hours.
6. Client is free of signs of water intoxication at 48 hours throughout fluid replacement.
7. The indwelling urinary catheter is discontinued within 72 hours.
8. Medication administration, fluid intake alterations, and reportable signs of altered salt levels are understood by client/caregiver prior to discharge.

DISCHARGE PLANNING

DI client may need:

Short-term IV fluids or long-term enteral nutrition if unable to take oral fluids to maintain fluid/electrolyte balance.

Intermediate care facility, daily home nursing visits, or family caregivers to manage the administration of intake.

Education of client and/or significant others in I and O measurement and documentation.

Education of client and/or significant others in signs of hypernatremia and dehydration that should be reported.

Consideration of palliative care or hospice if DI is caused by nontreatable brain metastasis of advanced disease.

FOLLOW-UP CARE

Anticipated care

Physician office visit within 1 week.

Outpatient lab testing for serum electrolytes within the next week.

Other blood work as appropriate.

Continuation of dietary/fluid restrictions or regimen.

Daily home nursing visit for clients discharged home with enteral or parenteral fluids.

Anticipated client/family questions and possible answers

Will this problem with high salt/low water in my blood happen again?

"It is possible this will happen again. It is important for you to take your medication as instructed. It is also important that you know the signs of diabetes insipidus, which are due to high body salt and low body water. If you start to put out a lot of urine again, your urine output greatly decreases, you become very tired, you have a fever, or your thinking becomes unclear, you or your caregiver needs to call your doctor right away. These could be signs of changes in your body's salt level. You should weigh yourself every day and measure the amount of fluids you drink and the amount of urine, vomit, or diarrhea your body puts out each day. Write these numbers down and call your doctor if you gain or lose more than a pound a day or if your body fluid output differs by more than 900 ml from your fluid intake by mouth each day. Be sure to keep your follow-up appointments with your doctor and follow his or her instructions."

CHAPTER SUMMARY

DI is a syndrome that occurs in some persons with primary or metastatic cancerous lesions of the hypothalamus/pituitary region or surgical trauma to this area (central DI), causing decreased ADH production. DI can also be caused by decreased renal response to ADH (nephrogenic DI), which can occur secondary to certain drugs or electrolyte imbalances. Whatever the cause, the result is increased urinary output and increased serum sodium if the person is unable to drink sufficient water to keep up with the fluid loss. Hypernatremia is considered mild at > 145 mEq/L (> 145 mmol/L SI Units) and severe at > 165 mEq/L (> 165 mmol/L SI Units). Treatment is aimed at eliminating the cause if possible, replacing fluids, and slowly replacing sodium if necessary. An understanding of water and sodium balance and the role of ADH in maintaining this homeostasis is essential to providing proper treatment and care.

TEST QUESTIONS

1. Diabetes insipidus (DI) is primarily caused by:
   A. Oversecretion of antidiuretic hormone (ADH)
   B. Oversecretion of insulin
   C. Undersecretion of ADH
   D. Increased renal sensitivity to ADH

1. Answer: C
Central DI, also known as hypophyseal DI, is the major type of DI, most often occurring secondary to brain trauma or tumors.

2. Inadequate antidiuretic hormone (ADH) secretion results in:
   A. Concentrated urine
   B. Dilute urine
   C. Decreased thirst
   D. Decreased serum osmolality

2. Answer: B
Lack of ADH results in lack of reabsorption of water by renal tubules, with subsequent diuresis.

3. Antidiuretic hormone (ADH) is produced in the:
   A. Anterior pituitary gland
   B. Renal collecting tubules
   C. Posterior pituitary gland
   D. Hypothalamus

3. Answer: D
ADH is primarily produced in the supraoptic nuclei of the hypothalamus and is transmitted to and stored in the posterior lobe of the pituitary.

4. Hallmark symptoms of DI are:
   A. Decreased thirst and oliguria
   B. Increased weight and skin turgor
   C. Nonpitting edema
   D. Polyuria and polydipsia

4. Answer: D
Increased diuresis leads to increased thirst, which is the body's normal mechanism for replacing water loss.

5. Nephrogenic DI can be caused by:
   A. Insufficient ADH
   B. Excess ADH
   C. Lithium and cisplatin
   D. Vasopressin

5. Answer: C
Lithium can decrease renal response to ADH (decreased urine-concentrating ability), resulting in a large output of dilute urine. Chronic cisplatin therapy can result in renal failure.

6. The drug of choice for central DI ADH replacement is:
   A. Chlorpropamide
   B. Carbamazepine
   C. Desmopressin
   D. Amphotericin

6. Answer: C
Desmopressin, a synthetic analog of natural human arginine vasopressin (AVP), has longer duration of action, lower incidence of allergic reactions, and no vasopressor action at therapeutic doses, and it is easy to administer (intranasally or IM).

7. Correction of hypernatremia in persons with DI should occur:
   A. Quickly, over 1 to 2 hours
   B. Slowly, decreasing no more than 1 mEq/L/hour
   C. At a rate of 2 mEq/L/hour
   D. Until serum sodium is decreased by 20%

7. Answer: B
Serum sodium levels should be corrected slowly to prevent cerebral edema or hemorrhage, which can result in death.

8. Assessment criteria for DI include:
   A. Elevated blood pressure and low respiratory rate
   B. Elevated temperature and pulse
   C. Increased weight and urine specific gravity
   D. Moist oral mucosa

8. Answer: B
Severe dehydration results in increased body temperature and symptoms of shock.

9. Primary nursing interventions for acute DI include:
   A. Provide oral fluids to the conscious alert client
   B. Restrict fluids to 1500 cc per day
   C. Assess vital signs q8h
   D. Assess neurologic status q8h

9. Answer: A
The conscious client should have plenty of fluids in easy reach. Oral intake that matches urine output will usually maintain the serum sodium within normal limits. Frequent vital-sign and neurologic checks can detect signs of dehydration and hypernatremia.

10. Side effects of vasopressin may include:
  A. Increased urinary output
  B. Decreased pulse rate
  C. Decreased blood pressure
  D. Decreased urinary output and headache

10. Answer: D
Decreased urinary output is the desired therapeutic response to ADH administration. Headache is a transient pressor side effect that may occur.

REFERENCES

Balmaceda CM, Fetell MR, Selman JE, Seplowitz AJ: Diabetes insipidus as first manifestation of primary central nervous system lymphoma. Neurology 44(2):358–359, 1994.

Bartuska DG, Kleinman DS, Kodroff KS, Piatok DJ: The sellar/parasellar endocrinopathies: A brief clinical overview. Semin Ultrasound CT MRI 14(3):178–181, 1993.

Bell TN: Diabetes insipidus. Crit Care Nurs Clin North Am 6(4):675–685, 1994.

Blevins, DR, Cassmeyer VL: Management of persons with problems of the pituitary, thyroid, parathyroid and adrenal glands, In Phipps WJ, Cassmeyer VL, Sands JK, Lehman MK (eds): Medical-Surgical Nursing: Concepts and Clinical Practice. St. Louis: Mosby Year Book, 1995.

Blumberg DL, Sklar CA, Wisoff J, David R: Abnormalities of water metabolism in children and adolescents following craniotomy for a brain tumor. Child's Nerv Syst 10:505–508, 1994.

Bryant WP, O'Naraugh AS, Lefger GA, Zimmerman D: Aqueous vasopressin during chemotherapy in patients with diabetes insipidus. Cancer 74(9):2589–2592, 1994.

Castagnola C, Morra E, Bernasconi P, Astori C, Santagostina A, Bernasconi C: Acute myeloid leukemia and diabetes insipidus: Results in 5 patients. Acta Hematol 93(1):1–4, 1995.

Chaudhuri R, Twelves S, Cox TCS, Bingham JB: MRI in diabetes insipidus due to metastatic breast carcinoma. Clin Radiol 46:184–188, 1992.

Donehower MG: Endocrine cancers. In Groenwald SL, Frogge MH, Goodman M, Yarbro CH (eds): Cancer Nursing Principles and Practice. Boston: Jones and Bartlett, pp. 984–1003, 1993.

Genka S, Sieda H, Takahashi M, Katikami H, Sanno N, Osamura Y, Fuchinoue T, Teramoto A: Acromegaly, diabetes insipidus, and visual loss caused by metastatic growth hormone-releasing hormone-producing malignant pancreatic endocrine tumor in the pituitary gland. J Neurosurg 83(10):719–723, 1995.

Gregoire JR: Adjustment of the osmostat in primary aldosteronism. Mayo Clin Proc 69(11):1108–1110, 1994.

Kanabar DJ, Betts DR, Gibbons B, Kingston JE, Eden OB: Monosomy 7, diabetes insipidus, and acute myelogenous leukemia in childhood. Pediatr Hematol Oncol 11(1):111–114, 1994.

Ko JC, Yang PC, Huang TS, Yeh KH, Kuo SH, Luh KI: Panhypopituitarism caused by solitary parasellar metastasis from lung cancer. Chest 105(3):951–953, 1994.

Lehne RA, Moore LA, Crosby L, Hamilton D: Pharmacology for Nursing Care, 2nd ed. Philadelphia: WB Saunders Co, 1994.

Lemone P, Burke KM: Medical Surgical Nursing: Critical Thinking in Client Care. Menlo Park, CA: Addison-Wesley, 1996.

Luk KH, Lam KSL, Kung AWC, Fung CF, Leung SY: Suprasellar ectopic pituitary adenoma presenting as cranial diabetes insipidus. Postgrad Med J 68:467–469, 1992.

Metheny NM: Fluid and Electrolyte Balance: Nursing Considerations. Philadelphia: JB Lippincott, 1996.

Ra'anani P, Shipberg O, Berezin M, Ben-Bassat I: Acute leukemia relapse presenting as central diabetes insipidus. Cancer 73(9):2312–2315, 1994.

Robertson GL: Diabetes insipidus. In Dluhy RG (ed): Endocrinology and Metabolism Clinics of North America: Clinical Disorders of Fluid and Electrolyte Metabolism. Philadelphia: WB Saunders Co, 1995, pp. 549–572.

Suganuma H, Yoshimi T, Kita T: Rare case with metastatic involvement of hypothalamo-pituitary and pineal body presenting as hypopituarism and diabetes insipidus. Intern Med 33(12):795–798, 1994.

Wang LC, Cohen ME, Duffner PK: Etiologies of central diabetes insipidus in children. Pediatr Neurol 11(4):273–277, 1994.

Wegmann JA: Central nervous system cancers. *In* Greenwald SL, Frogge MH, Goodman M, Yarbro CH (eds): Cancer Nursing Principles and Practice. Boston: Jones and Bartlett, pp. 959–983, 1993.

CHAPTER 10

DISSEMINATED INTRAVASCULAR COAGULATION

Kathleen Murphy-Ende, RN, PhD, FNP, OCN

CHAPTER OBJECTIVES

At the completion of this chapter, the reader will be able to:

Describe the pathophysiology of disseminated intravascular coagulation (DIC).

List the etiology, risk factors, and incidence of DIC.

Depict the treatment options available for DIC and their side effects.

Characterize the nursing assessment, diagnosis, and interventions involved in the care of clients with DIC.

Describe the evaluation criteria, discharge plans, and follow-up care to be provided to clients with DIC.

OVERVIEW

DISSEMINATED intravascular coagulation (DIC) is a hypercoagulable state in which inappropriate overstimulation of normal coagulation causes a simultaneous thrombosis and hemorrhage. There are two forms of DIC, acute and chronic, and although most cases of chronic DIC are caused by an underlying malignancy, this chapter will be limited to the discussion of acute DIC, which also occurs with malignancy but has a more favorable prognosis. The incidence of DIC in the oncology population is difficult to estimate and varies depending on the type of neoplasm, but is estimated to occur in 10% of all cancer patients (Chernecky and Ramsey, 1984); however, most of these cases usually go undetected. Abnormal blood coagulation studies have been reported in up to 92% of those with cancer, with the most commonly associated malignancies being acute promyelocytic

Table 10–1
Causes of DIC

Infections	Gram-negative sepsis (*Pseudomonas, Meningococcus, Enterobacteriaciae, Salmonella, Hemophilus*), gram-positive sepsis (*Pneumococcus, Staphylococcus*), viremias (cytomegalovirus, hepatitis, varicella, HIV), aspergillosis, postsplenectomy sepsis, purpura fulminans, Rocky Mountain spotted fever, malaria, and others
Obstetric complications	Abruptio placenta, amniotic fluid embolism, abortion, eclampsia, retained fetus
Neoplasms	Leukemias (acute promyelocytic, acute myelogenous, chronic myelogenous, acute lymphoblastic), pancreas, lung, prostate, gastric, acute leukemia, colon, unknown primary, ovary, gallbladder, breast (rarely melanoma, and lymphoma)
Vascular disorders	Malformations such as aortic aneurysm, and hemangiomas, vasculitis, grafts
Prosthetic devices	LaVeen shunts, aortic balloon assist device
Hepatic complications	Obstructive jaundice, fulminant hepatic failure
Massive tissue injury	Head trauma, burns, electric shock, and others
Transfusions	Multiple transfusions of whole blood, hemolytic transfusion reaction
Miscellaneous	Acute pancreatitis, snakebite, heat stroke, fat embolism, malignant hyperthermia, immune complexes, glomerulonephritis

leukemia (APL) and the adenocarcinomas (Rickles and Edwards, 1983). DIC is always secondary to a well-defined clinical entity, with infection being the most common cause, and disseminated malignancy being only one of many possible underlying conditions (see Table 10–1). A broad clinical spectrum of symptoms is seen in DIC, including multiple organ system dysfunction, which makes this disorder confusing and difficult to treat. The mortality rate from DIC ranges from 54 to 68% (Wintrobe, 1981). Death from DIC is generally caused by the inability to control the underlying cause of the DIC. Therefore, the initial and optimal treatment is directed toward treating the underlying condition.

DESCRIPTION

Physiology of coagulation

Under normal conditions, the body maintains a precisely balanced and steady state between clot formation (thrombosis) and clot dissolution (fibrinolysis). This balance is regulated by endogenous activators and inhibitors of coagulation. All human tissue has procoagulant factors, the most significant of which is tissue factor (TF), which is a cofactor to coagulation. When a vessel is severed or ruptured in an injury, the anticoagulant endothelial surface is disrupted, and the procoagulant subendothelium is exposed. The circulating platelets are activated by exposure to the subendothelial surface and adhere to this surface via a receptor for von Willebrand factor (glycoprotein Ib). This process represents the beginning of formation of a clot. Procoagulants are released from the damaged vascular wall, and the adhering platelets, which cause further platelet aggregation and activation of the clotting cascade, form a fibrin clot (Fig. 10–1).

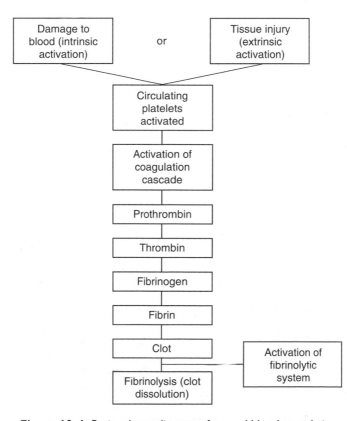

Figure 10–1 Basic schema diagram of normal blood coagulation.

There are numerous clotting factors necessary for normal clotting, which can be initiated by the intrinsic or extrinsic mechanism. The intrinsic mechanism is initiated when trauma or infection cause inflammatory proteins to be released, causing the activation of coagulation factor XII. The extrinsic mechanism is initiated when there is tissue injury and the release of factor VII. Once a clot has formed, in order to control the size of the clot and eventually reopen the healed vessel, the fibrinolytic system is activated; this process of fibrin clot dissolution is called fibrinolysis. During the fibrinolytic process, tissue plasminogen activator converts plasminogen to plasmin, and the release of plasmin causes enzymatic lysis of the fibrin clot. If fibrinolysis becomes uncontrolled, there is an accumulation of breakdown products

Table 10–2
Common Lab Findings in DIC Associated with Malignancy

Lab Test	Result	Cause of Abnormality
Platelets	Decreased < 100,000/mm³	Platelets are consumed.
Fibrinogen	Decreased < 150 mg/dl	Consumption and fibrinogenolysis
Prothrombin time (PT)	Prolonged > 12.5 seconds	Increase of fibrin split products Consumption of vitamin K-dependent factors
Thrombin time (TT)	Prolonged > 15 seconds	Heparin therapy and fibrin split products (hypofibrinogenemia)
Activated partial thromboplastin time (APTT)	Prolonged > 30 seconds	Consumption of clotting factors
Fibrin split products (FSPs)*	Positive	The breakdown of intravascular clots (fibrinolysis). (FSPs act as an anti-coagulant.)
Fibrin degradation products (FDPs)	Elevated > 40 µg/ml	Fibrinolysis
D-dimer assay*	Elevated > 500 µg/L	From the formation and breakdown of clots (antigen that forms when plasmin digests fibrin)
Antithrombin III assay	Decreased < 80%	Consumption of clotting factors
Peripheral smear (red blood cells)	Schistocytes	Intravascular clots shear the red blood cells (microangiopathic hemolytic anemia).
Hemoglobin	Decreased < 12 g/dl	Bleeding
Hematocrit	Decreased < 37%	Bleeding

*In chronic DIC associated with malignancy, the FSP and D-dimer tests are frequently elevated, with the rest of the lab results within normal limits.

called fibrinogen split, or degradation, products (FSPs or FDPs). FSPs have an anticoagulant activity and in elevated amounts can cause bleeding. Under normal conditions, there is a balance between blood coagulation and fibrinolysis (see Table 10–2).

There are systems to regulate the extent and location of coagulation. For example, the protein C, protein S system causes the inactivation of factors V and VIII when thrombin comes in contact with normal endothelium. Antithrombin III interacts with endogenous heparin or other similar substances to control coagulation by inactivation of thrombin.

Pathophysiology of DIC

DIC is a progressive and abnormal overstimulation of the coagulation process, manifested by rapid formation of fibrin thrombi, consumption of clotting factors, and activation of clot dissolution (fibrinolysis), resulting in varying degrees of diffuse microvascular obstruction and hemorrhage. The circulating, unopposed free thrombin causes platelet activation, fibrin clot formation, and factors V, VIII, and XIII to be activated, resulting in systemic thrombosis. The circulating, unopposed free plasmin causes lysis of fibrinogen and fibrin into high levels of serum fibrin and fibrinogen split products, resulting in hemorrhage. Therefore, these two main events result in concomitant systemic thombosis and hemorrhage.

The risk of bleeding rises when the prothrombin time (PT) rises 4 to 5 seconds above normal, the fibrinogen falls below 50 to 100 mg/dl, or the platelet count drops below 10,000 to 20,000/mm^3. Thrombotic complications may occur in small vessels, leading to microangiopathic hemolytic anemia and dysfunction of the liver, kidneys, or cerebral functions. Gastrointestinal bleeding may occur due to microthrombi causing mucosal damage in the stomach or duodenum.

DIC in the oncology population is essentially always related to either the malignancy or some other underlying entity such as infection. More than fifty underlying conditions have been identified as causing DIC, as seen in Table 10–1. APL is the malignancy most commonly associated with DIC, which occurs in 85% of those with this type of hematologic malignancy (Bick, 1988). Adenocarcinomas, such as those of the pancreas, lung, prostate, stomach, and breast, are the next most frequent causes of malignancy-related DIC, which is caused in this setting by an unidentified tumor procoagulant that directly stimulates the clotting cascade. It is important to realize that breast and prostate cancer are probably the most commonly seen DIC-associated malignancies in practice, because the incidence of these cancers is significantly higher than that of APL.

DIC often occurs in those with malignant conditions because tumor cells produce and release TF or other procoagulant substances that act directly on coagulation factors and plasminogen. These proteolytic enzymes produced by tumor cells act on the coagulation proteins or plasminogen, causing proenzyme activation. In APL, a procoagulant material is released either from granules of the promyelocyte, or during a large cell kill from chemotherapy. Necrotic promyelocytes release TF directly and/or release cytokines such as interleukin 1, which causes the endothelial cells to release TF (Kitchens, 1995). The promyelocytes also release a substance that directly activates plasminogen, yielding plasmin and thus resulting in uncontrolled fibrinolysis. Chemotherapeutic agents may induce DIC by damaging tumor and normal cells, or the endothelium, causing the release of procoagulants. Clients undergoing a chemotherapy regimen that causes a large cell kill are at risk for DIC because of the release of granule procoagulant from the dead cells into the systemic circulation (Bick, 1988).

Persons with cancer, leukemia, or those undergoing chemotherapy are at risk for infection and sepsis, which can lead to DIC. Sepsis, especially from gram-negative bacteria, is the most frequently recognized cause of DIC. A variety of infections may cause DIC, as seen in Table 10–1. The primary mediator in gram-negative sepsis is endotoxin (Lankiewicz and Bell, 1993), which is the procoagulant that activates factor XII and initiates a platelet release response. TF from endotoxin-damaged endothelium may also be a primary mediator in sepsis-associated DIC (Warr, Rao, and Rapaport, 1990). Certain peptidoglycans, which are primary structural components of bacterial cell walls, have been implicated to be important factors in determining the ability of specific organisms to produce DIC (Kessler, Nussbaum, and Tuazon, 1991). It is noteworthy that antibiotic therapy can alter coagulation by eliminating intestinal flora as a source of vitamin K, which is required for the coagulation process. Additionally, some antibiotics in the cephalosporin and penicillin families are antagonists of the vitamin K process (Lankiewicz and Bell, 1993).

Hepatic failure secondary to metastasis can increase the risk for developing DIC. The liver synthesizes most of the coagulation factors and inhibitors of coagulation. In addition, activated coagulation factors and fibrinolytic degradation products are cleared from the systemic circulation by the liver. The normal balance of coagulation can thereby be significantly disrupted in primary liver disease and liver metastasis, leading to DIC.

Peritoneovenous shunts are sometimes used to infuse ascitic fluid into the intravascular system in a variety of malignant conditions. Collagen and other procoagulants in the ascitic fluid, when shunted into the general circulation, can cause DIC (Lankiewicz and Bell, 1993). The client who has both a peritoneovenous shunt and hepatic disease may be even more prone to DIC, since normal liver function is imperative in fighting the challenge of the procoagulants.

Trousseau's syndrome is a syndrome of recurrent arterial or venous thrombosis that occurs in those with an underlying malignancy, particularly the mucin-producing adenocarcinomas such as those in the gastrointestinal tract or in hepatic and renal adenocarcinomas. Frequently, these clients will respond to heparin, but relapse when placed on therapeutic warfarin anticoagulation (Lankiewicz and Bell, 1993; Williams and Mosher, 1995).

Massive whole-blood transfusions or hemolytic transfusion reactions may result in DIC. The etiology of DIC after massive transfusions is unknown (Clavarella et al., 1987). Acute hemolytic reactions may be due to the generalized endothelial injury caused by activated complement, cytokines, and neutrophil products (Butler, Parker, and Pillai 1991). The ruptured red blood cells may produce platelet aggregation and the release of platelet factor 3, which causes coagulation to be activated. It is also thought that a protein may be released from the red blood cell membrane, which then initiates the clotting process (Wintrobe, 1981). This is more likely to occur in immune-mediated intravascular hemolysis.

RISK PROFILE

Cancer: APL; mucin-producing adenocarcinomas such as gastric, lung, pancreas, and prostate tumors (may be occult) and unknown primary, colon, ovary, gallbladder, and breast tumors, melanoma, and lymphomas. Any tissue injury directly from the tumor that causes procoagulant material to be released can initiate DIC. Certain solid tumors develop new vasculature with an abnormal endothelial lining that activates the procoagulant system, which may cause DIC.

Pediatrics: Children with infection, particularly meningococcemia, are at risk for developing purpura fulminans. Purpura fulminans is a cutaneous manifestation of DIC accompanied by skin lesions that are initially hemorrhagic, appearing as ecchymotic lesions, then progress to dermal necrosis. The pathologic process in this condition is a microvascular thrombosis (Lankiewicz and Bell, 1993).

Conditions: Infection and septicemia, toxic shock syndrome, obstetric complications, pancreatitis, aortic aneurysms, massive transfusions or transfusion reactions, hepatic failure, peritoneovenous shunts, collagen vascular diseases, snake or other animal bites, heat stroke, fat embolism, malignant hyperthermia, immune complexes, surgical procedures involving the liver or cardiopulmonary bypass, Kawasaki disease, amyloidosis, and pulmonary embolism (rare). See Table 10–1.

Environment: None.

Foods: Low vitamin K diet in a person with liver failure.

Drugs: Administration of hetastarch (Spearing, Hickton, Sizeland, Hannah, and Bailey, 1990), quinine (Chang, Gross, and Jang, 1990), and activated prothrombin complex preparations (Chistolini et al., 1990).

PROGNOSIS

The prognosis of DIC depends on the etiology and severity of the underlying condition. The mortality rate of DIC is approximately 54 to 68%, with an increase in mortality with age, number of clinical manifestations, and the severity of laboratory abnormalities (Wintrobe, 1981). DIC is considered a life-threatening condition because the hemorrhage and diffuse thrombosis, which are difficult to stop or reverse, can lead to irreversible end-organ damage and death. Providing effective therapy in a sequential and logical manner may help to control DIC and treating the underlying malignancy may result in complete cessation or significant improvement in DIC (Bick, 1992), prevent multiorgan failure, and improve survival (Kitchens, 1995). The mortality associated with DIC in those with acute promyelocytic leukemia has decreased significantly over the past 20 years (Kurtz, 1993) because of new antileukemia agents, combined therapy (heparin and antifibrinolytic therapy), and platelet transfusions (Lisiewicz, 1988).

TREATMENT

The treatment of DIC depends on the severity and etiology, but the treatment goal is to eliminate or ameliorate the underlying disorder. The actual treatment of DIC consists of coagulation factor replacement and drug therapy (see Table 10–3).

Surgery: Surgical resection of the tumor.

Chemotherapy: Any agent, combination chemotherapy, or hormonal treatment that is effective in treating the underlying malignancy.

Radiation: Radiation of the tumor site.

Medications

Any drug that treats the underlying disorder should be initiated to interrupt the pathologic production of the thrombin and plasmin. For example, aggressive antibiotic therapy for sepsis can be lifesaving. Heparin infusion is controversial, the benefit being that it enhances thrombin neutralization, the risk being that it may enhance bleeding. Heparin may be beneficial in DIC with APL; carcinoma, when thrombosis is present; and with chronic DIC (Trousseau's syndrome). It is unclear from the literature how useful heparin is in purpura fulminans. The recommended dose of heparin by most experts is 5 to 10 U per kilogram per hour by continuous IV infusion, a relatively low dose (Williams and Mosher, 1995).

Epsilon-amino-caproic acid (EACA), an antifibrinolytic therapy, may be given (combined with heparin) to inhibit the activity of circulating plasmin during uncontrolled life-threatening bleeding. Prior to giving EACA, heparin is administered to prevent uncontrolled life-threatening coagulation. After the heparin is given, EACA is infused as a loading dose of 4 g, followed by 1 g per hour (Kitchens, 1995). Another

Table 10–3
Treatment of DIC

BLOOD PRODUCT REPLACEMENT

Lab Test	Value	Deficient Factors	Replacement
Prothrombin time (PT)	> 16 seconds	II, V, VII, IX, X	Fresh frozen plasma: 2 units Vitamin K
Fibrinogen	< 100 mg/dl	Fibrinogen	Cryoprecipitate: 8–10 bags
Platelet count	< 20,000/mm³ or < 50,000/mm³ accompanied by significant bleeding	Platelets	Random donor platelets: 10 units Pheresed platelets: 1 unit

MEDICATIONS

Medication	Indication	Lab Test Follow-up
Heparin	Excessive coagulation	Antithrombin III (consumed in coagulation), activated partial thromboplastin time (APTT)
Amicar (aminocaproic acid) (to be given only with heparin in DIC)	Excessive fibrinolysis	Plasminogen, alpha-w plasmin inhibitor (both are consumed in fibrinolysis)

OTHER BLOOD COMPONENT THERAPY

Blood Component	Indication	Lab Test Follow-up
Packed red blood cells	Hemorrhage	Hematocrit and hemoglobin
Platelets	Platelet count < 20,000/mm³ or hemorrhage	Platelet count
Fresh frozen plasma	Hemorrhage, coagulation factor deficiency, volume expansion, and thrombotic thrombocytopenic purpura.	Coagulation factors
Cryoprecipitate	Hypofibrinogenemia, factor VIII deficiency	Fibrinogen and factor VIII
Antithrombin III	To neutralize thrombin, plasmin, and activated forms of factors VII, X, XI, and XII	Antithrombin III levels

antifibrinolytic agent used for the treatment of DIC caused by APL is tranexamic acid (Williams and Moser, 1995). Antithrombin III, which is a natural inhibitor for circulating thrombin, may be ordered to replenish exhausted supplies of antithrombin III (Kitchens, 1995).

Vitamin K and folate may be ordered, since clients with DIC are at risk of deficiency of these vitamins.

Experimental therapy consists of broad-spectrum protease inhibitors such as gabexate, nafamostat, trasylol, and alpha-1 antitrypsin; protein C concentrate, monoclonal antibody to bacterial endotoxin, and recombinant thrombomodulin.

Procedures

Assist in eradicating the source of infection, such as abscess drainage or removal of intravascular catheter.

Provide aggressive fluid administration to maintain blood pressure.

Other

Fresh frozen plasma and cryoprecipitate infusion to provide procoagulant materials to control hemostasis (Kitchens, 1995). The fresh frozen plasma and cryoprecipitate are usually given in a ratio of about 10 U of cryoprecipitate for every 2 or 3 U of plasma to achieve a PT within 2 to 3 seconds of the control value, and a fibrinogen level > 100 mg/dl.

Plasma factors and fibrinogen may be used in clients with liver disease, and platelet transfusions given for those with impaired platelet production, such as can be seen in leukemia.

Platelet transfusions are usually given at 1 to 3 U/10 kg/day if the platelet count is < 10,000–20,000/mm^3 or if bleeding is significant and the platelet count is < 50,000/mm^3 (Williams and Mosher, 1995).

Maintain blood pressure and blood volume to augment blood flow to the liver for clearance.

Correct acid-base balance, dysrhythmias, altered vascular resistance, decreased urine output, and electrolyte imbalances.

ASSESSMENT CRITERIA: DISSEMINATED INTRAVASCULAR COAGULATION

Vital signs

Temperature	Normal or abnormal secondary to underlying cause of DIC or intracranial bleeding.
Pulse	Increased secondary to compensatory response to bleeding and/or underlying cause of DIC.
Respirations	Increased secondary to compensatory response to bleeding.
Blood pressure	Decreased secondary to bleeding.
History	History of malignancy, hematologic disorder, recent chemo--therapy, transfusions, or drug treatment that interferes with coagulation; personal or family history of bleeding abnormalities; signs of bleeding tendency such as bruising, petechiae, nosebleeds, gingival bleeding, hematuria, or melena.
Hallmark physical signs and symptoms	*Early signs of bleeding*, such as anxiety, restlessness, confusion, petechiae, purpura, epistaxis, diffuse ecchymoses, hematomas,

ASSESSMENT CRITERIA: DISSEMINATED INTRAVASCULAR COAGULATION *(continued)*

	bleeding gums, conjunctival bleeding, joint pain, bleeding from wounds or previous injection sites, menstrual prolongation or heavy menses or spotting, hematuria. *Internal bleeding,* including intracranial (headache), pulmonary (hemoptysis, tachypnea, dyspnea, chest pain, tachycardia, and cough), gastrointestinal (melena, rectal bleeding, abdominal tenderness, and increase in abdominal girth).
Additional physical signs and symptoms	Assess for adrenal insufficiency in clients with sepsis and high-grade DIC (hemorrhagic necrosis of the adrenal glands).
Psychosocial signs	Anxiety, anger, and confusion.
Lab values	See Table 10–2. No single lab test is available to date that is absolutely diagnostic of DIC; however, several lab tests, along with certain clinical findings, support the diagnosis. It is important to recognize that due to the dynamic nature of DIC, lab results will change patterns and, therefore, can be very difficult to interpret. There are no data that provide a guideline for the diagnosis and prognosis of DIC. The following tests may help to establish the diagnosis and monitor the prognosis: Thrombin time (TT), prothrombin time (PT), fibrinogen level, partial thromboplastin time (PTT), platelet count, estimation of fibrin/fibrinogen split products (FSPs) or fibrin/fibrinogen degradation products (FDPs), D-dimer assay, and peripheral blood smear. Prolonged TT may indicate hypofibrinogenemia (in the absence of heparin), but is often normal in DIC. PT, which may be prolonged in acute DIC, provides a guide for plasma replacement. Fibrinogen and platelets may be decreased in acute severe DIC, but often, fibrinogen levels are normal. Platelet counts can become severely decreased in DIC associated with leukemia. Thrombocytopenia and a low fibrinogen level increase the risk of bleeding. Fibrinogen levels should be monitored every 12 hours because the level can be normal in DIC due to infection. A positive FSP and D-dimer assay (a specific type of fibrin split product) are often indicative of acute DIC; however, these assays can be too time consuming for routine use (Kitchens, 1995). A blood smear positive for schistocytes indicates microangiopathic hemolysis, seen in chronic DIC, but also seen in about 50% of those with acute DIC (Bick, 1988) (see Table 10–2).
Diagnostic tests Biopsy	A specimen showing microvascular deposition of fibrin clots is a strong indicator of DIC.
Other	Monitor oxygenation and hemodynamic parameters.

NURSING DIAGNOSIS

The nursing diagnoses will differ, depending on the cause, severity, and organ involvement related to the DIC. The following are examples of common diagnoses for the client with DIC.

Risk for trauma related to widespread thrombosis (purpura fulminans).

Altered tissue perfusion associated with organ hypoxia from hemorrhage and/or microthrombosis, anemia, or hypotension.

Risk for infection secondary to necrosis and tissue ischemia.

Risk for impaired skin integrity related to bed rest and impeded blood flow.

Risk for injury due to thrombocytopenia.

Impaired gas exchange secondary to respiratory distress (pulmonary microemboli, adult respiratory distress syndrome, or pulmonary embolism) and/or cardiac decompensation.

Risk for fluid volume deficit due to hemorrhage or massive fluid resuscitation.

Acute pain associated with thrombosis.

Knowledge deficit associated with diagnosis and treatment of DIC.

NURSING INTERVENTIONS

Immediate nursing interventions

Maintain circulation and oxygenation; assess tissue perfusion; monitor sites and amount of bleeding.

Initiate recommended treatment for the underlying malignancy.

Obtain and send blood cultures if infection is suspected.

Institute antibiotic and antipyretic (acetaminophen) therapy if the client is septic.

Monitor the client for bleeding and thrombosis. Institute bleeding precautions.

Provide educational and emotional support to the client and significant others.

Anticipated physician orders and interventions

Laboratory tests (see Table 10–2 and the Assessment Criteria section).

Initial treatment (see Table 10–3).

Maintain blood pressure by administering Ringer's lactate, normal saline, or albumin.

Oxygen at 2 L/minute.

Ongoing nursing assessment, monitoring, and interventions

The frequency of the following assessments will vary depending on the severity of the client's condition; therefore, the following recommendations should be used only as a general guideline. In conjunction with the physician, the nurse should establish specific observation parameters for signs, symptoms, and lab values for which the physician should be notified.

Assess:

- Neurologic status q4h—Perform neurologic checks; check level of consciousness; assess for seizure, strokelike symptoms such as blurred vision, tremors, disorientation, and headaches, which may indicate central nervous system (CNS) bleeding or clotting.
- Cardiovascular status q4h—Monitor for signs of decompensation such as increased heart rate, increased respirations, decreased blood pressure, and abnormal lung findings such as rales, rhonchi, and decreased breath sounds. Assess for neck vein distention, extra heart sounds, and murmurs.
- Respiratory status q4h—Assess for signs of respiratory distress such as chest pain, dyspnea, cyanosis, pupillary dilation, rapid irregular pulse, profuse perspiration, anxiety, and tachycardia.
- Peripheral vascular status q4h—Assess for acral cyanosis (gray purple mottling), decreased or absent pulse, cold extremity, unilateral swelling, or pain. Mark and measure any swollen extremity daily.
- For signs of bleeding q4h—Monitor for bleeding from the sclera; gums; old injection and IV sites; and nasal, oral, rectal, urethra, and vaginal orifices. Examine oral mucosa for ulceration and gingival bleeding. Assess the skin for petechiae, bruising, pallor, and ecchymosis. Assess for symptoms of dyspnea, dizziness, tachycardia, hypotension, lethargy, irritability, and fatigue. Test for occult blood in emesis, urine, and stool.
- Renal status q4h: intake and output (I and O), results of blood urea nitrogen (BUN) and creatinine tests.
- Gastrointestinal status–abdominal assessment.
- Monitor any sites of thrombosis for red indurated areas along vessels; muscle turgor, tenderness, and warmth over the thrombosis site; slight fever or chills; decreased pulses; and venous distention, which is increased with weight bearing.

Measure:

- Vital signs q2–4h. Monitor blood pressure, using an arterial line if present.
- I and O q8h (report urine output < 30 ml/hour).
- Weight qd.
- Abdominal girth q4h.
- Liver function tests, BUN, and serum creatinine qd.
- The time and amount of bleeding, weighing dressings, and estimating blood loss.
- Hematest urine, stools, and emesis.
- I and O q1h.

Send:

- Blood samples: Platelets, fibrinogen, TT, PT, PTT, FSPs, D-dimer assay, antithrombin III assay, peripheral smear, ABGs, culture, BUN, creatinine, liver functions, and electrolytes. Draw minimum volumes permitted to prevent iatrogenic anemia.
- Blood cultures for temperature $> 38°C$ ($> 100.4°F$).
- Urine for urinalysis, culture, and sensitivity.

Implement:

- *Measures to control bleeding:* Apply direct manual pressure to bleeding sites. Apply pressure dressings and/or sandbags to bleeding sites, and elevate bleeding extremities.
- *Bleeding precautions:* Pad side rails if raised; provide soft toothbrush; take oral instead of rectal temperature; no aspirin products; no razors; no enemas or suppositories; use oral stool softeners; avoid adhesive tape; have client wear shoes when out of bed. Avoid injections when possible, otherwise use the smallest-gauge needle and then apply direct pressure to injection site for several minutes. Topical thromboplastin may be required to stop bleeding from the injection site. Use the arterial line to monitor blood pressure and avoid excess use of the blood pressure cuff. Lubricate catheters and tubes to decrease friction on mucous membranes.
- *Administer blood and IV products* as prescribed.
- *Skin care:* Implement skin care protective measures such as gently turning the client every 2 hours, and avoid unnecessary pressure or friction on skin, padding side rails. Use mild, nondrying soap and keep the skin well lubricated with mild lotion. Remove any constrictive devices and clothing and apply elastic stockings as ordered.
- *Oral care:* Use soft toothbrush or toothette along with normal saline for oral care. Avoid using mouthwash, which has alcohol or irritants.
- *General comfort measures:* Offer pain medication and implement pain medication schedule as needed. Minimize requests for clients to move, and assist with activities of daily living. Offer frequent rest periods. Provide diversional activities. Supplemental oxygen as prescribed.
- *Prevent complications of bed rest:* Turn every 2 hours, perform gentle range of motion exercises twice a day, administer oral stool softeners and laxatives as needed, instruct client to perform deep-breathing exercises every 2 hours while awake, use incentive spirometer if needed.
- *Relaxation techniques:* Provide information, emotional support, and reassurance to decrease fear and anxiety. Offer relaxation techniques such as soft music, meditation, biofeedback, gentle massage, or other methods that the client has found helpful in the past.

TEACHING/EDUCATION

Define DIC: *Rationale:* DIC is a serious complication of cancer in which the body's ability to maintain the normal balance between clotting and bleeding is temporarily altered. In this condition, the body may form clots in some areas or may bleed in other areas, or may clot and bleed at the same time.

Signs and symptoms of DIC: *Rationale:* The symptoms, which are due to either clotting or bleeding, include: change in the color of the skin; swelling of arms, legs, abdomen, or neck; fatigue; confusion; irritability; anxiety; headaches; change in vision; chest pain; difficulty breathing; swollen joints; blood in the urine, from the nose, mouth, vagina, or rectum.

Purpose of lab tests: *Rationale:* Many types of blood tests are needed to diagnose DIC and help guide the health care team to the best treatment program. Once treatment is started, some of these tests are repeated periodically to evaluate how well the treatment is working.

Goal of nursing care: *Rationale:* The nurses will frequently assess for signs and symptoms of bleeding and clotting in order to evaluate your condition and response to treatment. These assessments may involve asking you a lot of questions, as well as physical examination.

Treatment program (medications, blood products): *Rationale:* Heparin is a drug given to prevent blood clots from forming and to prevent the extension of existing clots. It will not dissolve clots. The major adverse reaction is bleeding. The side effects of heparin to report are bleeding of the gums, under the skin, or in the urine or stool, and back pain. Aminocaproic acid (Amicar) is a drug that hastens clot formation to reduce bleeding. The major adverse reaction is blood clot formation. The side effects of aminocaproic acid to report are sudden headache, chest or leg pain, shortness of breath, visual changes, extremity weakness or swelling, or decrease in urinary output. The blood products are given by transfusion to replace the blood cells or factors that have been destroyed or depleted from the DIC.

Prevention of thrombus: *Rationale:* In order to prevent a clot from forming in the arms or legs, it is helpful to avoid constrictive clothing or devices, keep the legs elevated and straight, and move toes, feet, and legs frequently to help the blood flow back to the heart.

Prevention of bleeding: *Rationale:* It is important to take precautions against accidental bleeding. Minor bumps or scrapes could result in bleeding, so it is important to have assistance as needed to prevent falls or injury.

Reporting symptoms of bleeding: *Rationale:* It is important to notify your health care provider immediately if you have any of the following: bruising, red rash, headache, black stools, blood in the urine or stools, and bleeding from the gums, nose, eyes, vagina, or rectum.

EVALUATION/DESIRED OUTCOMES

1. The client or significant others will describe DIC, the symptoms, prognosis, and follow-up treatment plan prior to discharge.
2. No signs of hemorrhage will occur. Clotting studies are maintained within therapeutic range.
3. Extension of the thrombus or embolization of thrombi does not occur.
4. Tissue perfusion is maintained, as evidenced by alert and oriented state; pink, warm skin; palpable peripheral pulses; urine output > 30 ml/hour; and stable vital signs.
5. Infection will be prevented or controlled with the absence of fever and normal white blood cell count.
6. Skin integrity is maintained, as evidenced by intact skin free of open lesions.
7. The client will state that he or she is comfortable and pain free.
8. The client will be free of injury.
9. Fluid volume will be maintained or restored to normal, as manifested by normal vital signs, specific gravity, and clear lung sounds.

DISCHARGE PLANNING

Most of the health care needs of the client with acute DIC will be taken care of during the period of hospitalization. Depending on the individual's condition and home situation, the following items should be addressed:

Assess the client's functional status to determine if he or she is able to return home and live independently.

Evaluate the client's home situation in terms of the physical environment and availability of support people to assist as needed.

Arrange for a home care nurse to provide nursing care and to assess the client's status.

Review medications that the client will be taking at home with the client and significant others.

Review the early signs and symptoms of DIC, and the importance of seeking immediate medical care if these should occur. Include information on signs and symptoms related to excessive bleeding or clotting.

If the client is going home with a deep vein thrombosis, teach him or her about the use of antiembolic stockings, appropriate positioning and activity level, anticoagulant therapy, and the signs and symptoms to report to the health care provider.

Arrange for consultation with clergy and social services.

FOLLOW-UP CARE

Anticipated care

Outpatient office or clinic visit in 1 week.

Outpatient lab testing of complete blood count, platelets, chemistry, and coagulation studies.

Explain and offer a list of support groups for people with cancer.

Severe complications of DIC may result in organ dysfunction and activity limitations, causing lifestyle changes that may require additional resources such as home equipment or assistance.

Anticipated client/family questions and possible answers

Will the DIC occur again?

"Since the underlying malignancy or infection has been successfully treated, and the clotting and bleeding problem controlled, the DIC has been resolved. It is possible that in the future another problem with DIC could occur if the cancer relapses, or if you developed an infection in the blood."

How will I know if I am developing DIC again, and what can I do to prevent this from happening?

"The signs and symptoms of DIC that should be reported and that indicate bleeding or clotting are as follows. The signs of bleeding are bruising, red rash, headache, black stools, blood in the urine or stools, and bleeding from the gums, nose, eyes, vagina, or rectum. The signs of clotting are shortness of breath, dizziness, rapid pulse, low blood pressure, lethargy, irritability, and fatigue. The symptoms of a clot in an arm or leg include a red raised area along vessels, tenderness and warmth over a red or swollen area, and slight fever or chills. Stroke-like symptoms to be reported are blurred vision, tremors, disorientation, and headaches. There is no guaranteed method of preventing DIC; however, it is helpful to keep the cancer under control with the prescribed treatment and it is helpful to avoid a serious infection. Early detection and treatment of DIC allows for a more effective treatment, better prognosis, and fewer complications."

Is DIC a hereditary condition?

"People who have certain hereditary blood disorders may be more prone to developing DIC; however, DIC in and of itself is always due to some underlying problem and is not a hereditary condition."

Is DIC a fatal disease?

"DIC is a very serious, life-threatening condition that can cause death. The earlier it is diagnosed and treated, the better the chance of total recovery."

Are there any long-term effects from DIC?

"Depending on the extent and severity of the DIC, there may or may not be any long-term effects. For example, if there has been permanent damage to the kidneys, dialysis might be necessary. If there is reversible damage to an organ or tissue, then the body will heal with time."

CHAPTER SUMMARY

DIC is a life-threatening condition that demands complex and intensive nursing care. A thorough understanding of the pathophysiology and clinical manifestations is critical for effective nursing care. Nurses are in a prime position to detect the early signs and symptoms of DIC, allowing for prompt diagnosis and treatment, which will help to improve the client's chances of survival. The client with suspected or actual DIC requires accurate and thorough assessment and monitoring. Since there is no single definitive diagnostic test for DIC, the nursing assessment, along with the abnormal coagulation studies, is important in making an accurate diagnosis.

The initial treatment of DIC is directed at treating the underlying malignancy or infection. Medications as well as blood component therapy are given to control the bleeding and thrombotic complications of DIC. The primary care nurse is responsible for identifying signs of improvement or deterioration through continual assessment and evaluation. Health information and emotional supportive care is provided to the client and family to decrease anxiety and assist in coping. Oncology nurses should be familiar with the disease process and the numerous treatment options available in order to provide the emergency care required to save the life of those who suffer this disastrous complication.

TEST QUESTIONS

1. DIC is primarily a disorder of:
   A. The autoimmune system
   B. The cardiovascular system
   C. The bone marrow
   D. Overstimulation of the coagulation process

1. Answer: D
DIC is a progressive and abnormal overstimulation of the coagulation process, manifested by rapid formation of fibrin thrombi, consumption of clotting factors, and activation of clot dissolution, resulting in simultaneous clotting and hemorrhaging.

2. DIC in the client with cancer may be caused by:
   A. A mental health psychosis
   B. Massive blood transfusions or transfusion reaction
   C. Cardiac failure
   D. Polycythemia vera

2. Answer: B
DIC can be caused by an underlying disease process such as malignancy as well as by massive blood transfusions or a transfusion reaction.

3. The most common cause of DIC is:
   A. Solid tumor malignancy
   B. Hepatic failure
   C. Infection
   D. Complication of anticoagulant therapy

3. Answer: C
Infection is the most common cause of DIC, and disseminated malignancy is only one of many possible underlying conditions causing DIC.

4. A basic pathophysiologic process in DIC is:
   A. Rapid formation of microemboli, causing vascular system reconstruction
   B. Activation of clot dissolution, resulting in hemorrhage
   C. Endotoxin (in infection), which activates factor XII and initiates leukocytosis
   D. A decrease in fibrinolysis

4. Answer: B
DIC consists of formation of microemboli, causing microvascular obstruction; activation of clot dissolution, causing hemorrhage; activation of factor XII, which initiates a platelet release response; and an increase in clot dissolution (fibrinolysis).

5. The nursing diagnosis of highest priority for a client with DIC is:
   A. Altered tissue perfusion
   B. Acute pain
   C. Knowledge deficit
   D. Impaired skin integrity

5. Answer: A
Although all of the nursing diagnoses listed are important, preventing organ hypoxia is the most urgent, and should be given priority.

6. Bleeding precautions for a client with DIC include all of the following *except:*
   A. Use a soft toothbrush
   B. Avoid use of razor
   C. Pad side rails
   D. Avoid products with acetaminophen

6. Answer: D
Aspirin products should be avoided. Acetaminophen is not contraindicated in persons with bleeding disorders.

7. The malignancies most commonly associated with DIC include all *except:*
   A. Acute promyelocytic leukemia
   B. Gastric adenocarcinoma
   C. Breast cancer
   D. Glioblastomas

7. Answer: D
Acute promyelocytic leukemia is the malignancy most commonly associated with DIC, although the incidence of leukemia is lower than other malignancies. DIC is also seen in breast, pancreas, gastric, prostate, and colon cancer. Glioblastoma is not associated with DIC.

8. When assessing for CNS bleeding or clotting, an important sign to report is:
   A. Disorientation
   B. Fatigue
   C. Chest pain
   D. Acral cyanosis

8. Answer: A
Although all of the signs and symptoms should be reported, disorientation is a possible indication of CNS involvement.

9. The blood test least useful in the diagnosis of DIC is:
   A. Alkaline phosphatase
   B. Liver function tests
   C. Platelet count
   D. Prothrombin time

9. Answer: A
Alkaline phosphatase is of no clinical value in the diagnosis of DIC.

10. The primary treatment of DIC is directed toward:
   A. Restoring the platelet count to normal levels
   B. Treating the underlying malignancy
   C. Controlling the acute pain
   D. Anticoagulation

10. Answer: B
Treating the underlying malignancy is the most effective means of correcting the coagulation abnormality associated with DIC.

REFERENCES

Bick RL: Disseminated intravascular coagulation and related syndromes: A clinical review. Semin Thromb Hemost 14(4):299, 1988.

Bick RL: Disorders of Thrombosis and Hemostasis: Clinical and Laboratory Practice. Chicago: American Society of Clinical Pathologists Press, 1992, pp. 137–173.

Butler J, Parker D, Pillai R: Systemic release of neutrophil elastase and tumor necrosis factor alpha following ABO incompatible blood transfusion. Br J Hematol 78:525, 1991.

Chang JC, Gross HM, Jang NS: Disseminated intravascular coagulation due to intravenous administration of hetastarch. Am J Med Sci 300:301, 1990.

Chernecky C, Berger B: Laboratory Tests and Diagnostic Procedures. Philadelphia: WB Saunders Co, 1997.

Chernecky C, Ramsey P: Critical Nursing Care of the Client with Cancer. Norwalk, CT: Appleton-Century-Crofts, 1984.

Chistolini A, Mazzucconi MG, Tirindelli MC, LaVerde G, Ferrarri A, Mandelli F: Disseminated intravascular coagulation and myocardial infarction in a haemophilia B patient during therapy with prothrombin complex concentrates. Acta Haematol (Basel) 83(3):163–165, 1990.

Clavarella D, Reed R, Counts R, Baron L, Pavlin E, Heimbach DM, Carrico CJ: Clotting factor levels and the risk of diffuse microvascular bleeding in the massively transfused patient. Br J Haematol 67(3):365–368, 1987.

Kessler CM, Nussbaum ES, Tuazon CU: Disseminated intravascular coagulation associated with Staphylococcus aureus septicemia is mediated by peptidoglycan-induced platelet aggregation. J Infect Dis 164:101, 1991.

Kitchens CS: Disseminated intravascular coagulation. *In* Brain MC, Carbone PP, Kelton JG, Schiller JH (eds): Current Therapy in Hematology–Oncology. St. Louis, MO: Mosby, 1995, pp. 182–187.

Kurtz A: Disseminated intravascular coagulation with leukemia patients. Cancer Nurs 16(6):456–463, 1993.

Lankiewicz MW, Bell WB: Disseminated intravascular coagulation. *In* Bell WR (ed): Hematologic and Oncologic Emergencies. New York: Churchill Livingstone, 1993, p. 110.

Lisiewicz J: Disseminated intravascular coagulation in acute leukemia. Semin Thromb Hemost 14:339–347, 1988.

Rickles FR, Edwards RL: Activation of blood coagulation in cancer: Trousseau's syndrome revisited. Blood 63:14–31, 1983.

Spearing RL, Hickton DM, Sizeland P, Hannah A, Bailey RR: Quinine-induced disseminated intravascular coagulation. Lancet 336:1535–1537, 1990.

Warr TA, Rao VM, Rapaport SI: Disseminated intravascular coagulation in rabbits induced by administration of endotoxin or tissue factor: Effect of anti-tissue factor antibodies and measurement of plasma extrinsic pathway inhibitor activity. Blood 75:1481, 1990.

Williams EC, Mosher DF: Disseminated intravascular coagulation. *In* Hoffman R, Benz DJ, Shattil SJ, Furie B, Cohen HJ, Silberstein LE (eds): Hematology: Basic Principles and Practice. New York: Churchill Livingstone, 1995, pp. 1758–1769.

Wintrobe M: Clinical Hematology. Philadelphia: Lea and Febiger, 1981.

Chapter 11

ESOPHAGEAL VARICES

Melissa Manojlovich, MS, RN, CCRN

CHAPTER OBJECTIVES

At the completion of this chapter, the reader will be able to:

Define esophageal varices.

State risk factors associated with esophageal varices in the oncology client.

Differentiate between various treatment options available to clients with esophageal varices.

Describe nursing care as it relates to oncology clients with esophageal varices.

Prepare the client with esophageal varices for future care needs.

OVERVIEW

ESOPHAGEAL varices have been defined as "a complex of longitudinal, tortuous veins at the lower end of the esophagus, enlarged and swollen as the result of portal hypertension. These vessels are especially susceptible to hemorrhage" (Anderson, Anderson, and Glanze, 1994, p. 575). They develop in a majority of clients with cirrhosis of the liver, which is responsible for the development of portal hypertension. Cirrhosis arises from a variety of causes, primary liver cancer being among them. Varices can rupture suddenly or gradually leak, but in either case bleeding varices are life-threatening. They require immediate intensive care intervention and monitoring. Clients can be overwhelmed by the amount and duration of bleeding. Therefore, expert nursing care is needed to provide emotional support while attending to highly technical interventions. A newer treatment option that simplifies management has emerged, but in many institutions bleeding esophageal varices are still treated with mechanical tamponade and vasopressin infusions. These treatments have many complications associated with them, which are compounded by the fact that there is a high mortality rate, 25% in the first 48 hours and 50% within 6 weeks, associated with bleeding varices. Even after the acute episode of hemorrhage has been successfully stopped, there is a high risk of rebleeding unless measures are taken to permanently lower portal pressure. In clients whose liver disease is a result of cancer, options may be limited. However, all clients need to be taught the signs and symptoms of recurrent bleeding, as well as behaviors to avoid increasing intra-abdominal pressure.

DESCRIPTION

The sudden, painless hemorrhage of esophageal varices is a medical emergency. Two main theories have been proposed to explain what leads to the bleeding of esophageal varices—the erosive and the eruptive theories. According to the erosive theory, damage to the overlying mucosa causes bleeding. The eruptive theory claims that pressure within the varices is the critical variable, and when it reaches a certain point, the variceal wall ruptures with a resulting hemorrhage. The erosive theory has fallen out of favor because it has now been well documented that esophageal varices will not bleed if the pressure within the varices is reduced below 12 mmHg (Mackay and Henderson, 1992).

Although varices may arise from a variety of causes, in the United States most result from alcohol-induced cirrhosis. Cirrhosis refers to fibrous tissue changes in the liver brought on by chronic injury. The term is not specific to any one liver disease but, rather, describes the pathologic tissue changes associated with many liver diseases in the final stages, including cancer. Most of the signs and symptoms of cirrhosis are similar, regardless of the cause. Although the liver is unique in its ability to regenerate after an acute injury, chronic injury causes regenerating nodules to form. These nodules, the chief characteristic of cirrhosis, alter liver structure and cause irreparable functional damage (Butler, 1994). A process of hepatic injury develops, with subsequent scarring, which increases post sinusoidal resistance. These changes inhibit portal venous outflow and raise portal pressure. As outflow resistance and portal hypertension rise, collateral pathways emerge to redirect portal flow to the lower-pressure systemic venous circulation. Eventually, however, pressure rises in the collateral vessels too so that gastric and esophageal varices develop. Varices are irregularly shaped and thin-walled. Spontaneous hemorrhage occurs when venous inflow and portal outflow resistance combine to generate pressures that exceed the bursting level of a varix (White, Milazzo, and Comerota, 1985).

The care of a client with ruptured esophageal varices can be divided into three phases. Priorities in the emergent phase are to correct hypovolemia, achieve hemostasis at the bleeding site, and prevent pulmonary aspiration (Kerber, 1993). These interventions are carried out in an intensive care environment. During the second phase, which is completed by discharge, the goals are to prevent recurrent hemorrhage and build the client's knowledge base about the disease process and long-term care. Treatment then continues in the community, where the client is followed on an outpatient basis. This third phase involves annual endoscopies, vigilant monitoring for signs or symptoms of rebleeding, and reinforcement of behaviors that decrease the probability of bleeding.

Emergency endoscopy should be performed as soon as possible to confirm the diagnosis of bleeding varices and isolate the source of bleeding. The first line of treatment is sclerotherapy. It can be performed emergently at the time of the first endoscopy or delayed until after variceal bleeding has been controlled by pharmacologic agents or balloon tamponade. Sclerotherapy controls acute variceal bleeding in 90 to 95% of clients and is considered more effective than balloon tube tamponade or treatment with vasopressin. Sclerosant solution is injected directly into the lumen of the varix or into the submucosa around it and causes contraction of the varix and, usually, cessation of bleeding. An inflammatory reaction produced by the sclerosant solution causes a venous thrombus to form, which is eventually converted to a fibrous band. Repeated sclerotherapy results in the development of supportive scar tissue around the vessel. This treatment is believed to help lower the risk of recurrent hemorrhage by strengthening the wall and decreasing tension on the vessel (Kerber, 1993).

Vasopressin, given systemically, is an effective pharmacologic agent used to lower portal pressure and thus control variceal bleeding. It works by constricting vessels in the splanchic bed, thereby reducing blood flow and decreasing or stopping variceal bleeding. Unfortunately, it also constricts coronary arteries, causing reduced coronary blood flow and increased blood pressure. This creates an imbalance between myocardial oxygen supply and demand (Burns and Martin, 1990). Therefore, vasopressin must be given cautiously to clients with a history of cardiac disease. Other adverse effects include decreased heart rate, cool/pulseless extremities, and skin color changes or mottling (Burns, Martin, Merrill, Luer, and Stone, 1993). These deleterious effects can be lessened by using simultaneous IV nitroglycerin with vasopressin infusions (Burns et al., 1993). Mechanical tamponade is often necessary if the client cannot be stabilized by either of the two methods described above. This is accomplished by the insertion of a Sengstaken-Blakemore tube, which will temporarily control bleeding in over 90% of clients. However, it too can be a dangerous treatment option. See Table 11–1 for complications associated with the use of this device.

Since the early 1990s, at least in major medical centers, a new procedure has emerged that relieves pressure on esophageal varices. Known as TIPS (transjugular intrahepatic portosystemic shunt), this procedure involves placement of a stent between the portal and hepatic veins. Performed by a radiologist in the x-ray department, it replaces the surgical creation of a portosystemic shunt and reduces postoperative recovery time from 10 to 14 days to 2 to days (Doherty and Carver, 1993). Briefly, a catheter is guided through the jugular vein into the liver parenchyma, where a new pathway for blood is created. A stent is deployed after radiographic confirmation of proper placement is made. General anesthesia is not used, and although clients are

Table 11–1
Complications of the Sengstaken-Blakemore Tube

Complication	Potential Causes	Prevention
Esophageal rupture	Inflation of gastric balloon within the esophagus balloon	Obtain chest x-ray to document proper position of the balloon below the gastroesophageal junction prior to inflation.
	Overinflation of esophageal balloon	Inflate esophageal balloon to the lowest pressure that will prevent bleeding (25–40 mmHg). Monitor pressure in esophageal balloon q2h. Deflate esophageal balloon for 20 minutes q12h.
Aspiration pneumonia	Aspiration of oropharyngeal secretions	Evacuate secretions with an NG tube above the esophageal balloon. Keep oral airway and suction apparatus set up at the bedside. Maintain HOB elevation of 30–45 degrees. Consider oral intubation and mechanical ventilation for airway protection if mental status deteriorates.
Airway obstruction	Upward migration of esophageal balloon with occlusion of the epiglottis	Securely anchor the tube and avoid deflation of the gastric balloon while the esophageal balloon is inflated. Keep scissors taped to the head of the bed. Mark insertion point of the tube with tape at the nostril or lip.
Esophageal erosion	Prolonged or excessive pressure on the esophageal mucosa	Maintain esophageal balloon pressure between 25 and 40 mmHg. Deflate and remove the esophageal balloon as soon as possible (preferably within 24–48 hours).

given analgesics and sedatives, they require continuous reassurance and support from an attentive nurse. The TIPS procedure is superseding the use of a Sengstaken-Blakemore tube in major centers across the United States.

Special care is required to keep the client from aspirating blood clots, which may occur from large-volume hematemesis. A safe airway can usually be maintained by placing the client in a left lateral decubitus position during lavage and keeping a suction apparatus ready near the client's mouth. At times, though, endotracheal intubation is necessary, such as when the client has copious bleeding, acute respiratory distress, or obtundation. Clients with active hemorrhage will require supportive care for shock as well as careful monitoring of the extent of hemorrhage. A Foley catheter will be placed to assess urinary output. A central line may be necessary, with eventual placement of a pulmonary artery catheter, to monitor cardiac hemodynamics and to provide information about circulatory volume (Gervin, Gostout, and Zinner, 1991). Fluid resuscitation is achieved with isotonic IV fluids and blood products. Ringer's lactate solution is not recommended for fluid resuscitation in clients with liver dysfunction because they may be unable to convert lactate to bicarbonate, leading to an accumulation of lactate in the serum (Kerber, 1993). Clients may refuse blood products for religious or cultural reasons. In such instances, dextran and hetastarch (Hespan, Volex) may be used to expand plasma volume in conjunction with crystalloid solutions. Packed red blood cells (RBCs) are administered to keep the hematocrit at approximately 30%. Although this may seem low, overtransfusion can contribute to portal hypertension and potentiate variceal rupture (Kerber, 1993). Hemoglobin and hematocrit (H and H) determinations should be regularly obtained, but remember that these levels may not be accurate until complete volume restoration and equilibration occur over several hours. Checking for coagulation defects and correcting clotting abnormalities will also be necessary, particularly if the client has received 4 to 6 units of blood (Gervin et al., 1991).

RISK PROFILE

Identification by screening endoscopy of clients at high risk for bleeding is justified, according to one source. Clients with cirrhosis should undergo endoscopic examination on a yearly basis. High-risk clients should be considered for prophylactic management (Mackay and Henderson, 1992).

Cancers: Primary and metastatic liver cancer.

Conditions: Cirrhosis (develops in about 60% of clients). In one study, clients with cirrhosis who did not have varices were followed for 2 years. At the end of that time, more than half had developed the abnormality. Approximately 30% of clients with varices experience gastrointestinal (GI) hemorrhage, usually within 2 years of their diagnosis. Thrombocytopenia, which accompanies treatment for many cancers, also places the client at increased risk for esophageal bleeding. When variceal rupture occurs, about one-third of clients die within 6 weeks (most of them within 48 hours), and another third die by the end of 1 year (Resnick, 1993). High-risk varices are predominantly determined by their size and the presence of visible signs. At the time of endoscopy, varices that are noticeably widened (> 5 mm) with red markings (the so-called red color sign) or that are thin and blue are considered to be at high risk for bleeding. Other risk factors include multiple, large, dilated varices and coexisting gastric varices. Alcoholism and poor liver function independently raise the likelihood of bleeding by two to three times (Resnick, 1993).

Environment: None.

Foods: None.

Drugs: See discussion of alcoholism under "Conditions" in this section.

PROGNOSIS

The mortality rate for cirrhotic clients within 6 weeks of the first episode of variceal hemorrhage is about 50% (Kerber, 1993). Without intervention, 70% of survivors rehemorrhage within 1 year of the initial episode. When sclerotherapy is used, rebleeding rates fall to 48 to 58% (Resnick, 1993). Only 25% survive 2 years (Pierce, Wilkerson, and Griffiths, 1990). The Child-Pugh classification system is widely used to predict long-term survival (Table 11–2).

TREATMENT

Surgery: A portosystemic decompressive procedure, such as a portacaval or mesocaval shunt.

Chemotherapy: Not indicated.

Radiation: Not indicated.

Medications

Vasoconstrictors such as vasopressin (Pitressin) and octreotide (Sandostatin) to temporarily lower the portal flow and allow the client to stabilize while the team determines the best permanent option.
IV nitroglycerin.
Aquamephyton given intramuscularly.
Beta-blocker therapy with propranolol.

Procedures

Endoscopic variceal sclerotherapy.
TIPS.
Sengstaken-Blakemore tube.

Table 11-2
Modified Child-Pugh Classification System

Class	Serum Albumin	Serum Bilirubin	Prothrombin time (secs)	Ascites	Encephalopathy	3-Year Survival (%)	5-Year Survival (%)
A	>3.5	<2.0	1–3	None	Absent	62	47
B	3.0–3.5	2.0–3.0	4–6	Slight	Minimal	20	11
C	<3.0	>3.0	>6	Moderate	Advanced	8	8

Other

Replace clotting factors.

Replace blood to keep hematocrit at about 30% to avoid overtransfusion, which can contribute to portal hypertension and potentiate variceal rupture (Kerber, 1993).

Fluid resuscitation with isotonic fluids. *Note:* Ringer's lactate solution is not recommended for fluid resuscitation in clients with liver dysfunction, because they may be unable to convert lactate to bicarbonate, leading to an accumulation of lactate in the serum and subsequent lactic acidosis (Kerber, 1993).

Substitute dextran and hetastarch (Hespan, Volex) for plasma volume expansion in place of blood products for clients who refuse for religious or cultural reasons.

Supportive care for shock and careful monitoring of the extent of the hemorrhage.

ASSESSMENT CRITERIA: ESOPHAGEAL VARICES

Vital signs	
Pulse	Rapid, thready
Blood pressure	Initially high, secondary to vasoconstrictive compensatory response, then drops quickly to hypotensive level.
Respiratory rate	Rapid, gasping
Temperature	Normal to low
Central venous pressure (CVP)	Low
Pulmonary artery pressure (PAP)	Low
History	Cirrhosis, liver cancer, or thrombocytopenia. Often sudden onset of vomiting bright red blood, or recent black and tarry bowel movements. Recent weakness, dizziness, abdominal cramping, and nausea.
Hallmark physical signs and symptoms	Coughing and choking if blood is entering the airway faster than the client can clear it, cool clammy skin, dusky color.
Additional physical signs and symptoms	If prior cirrhosis, client will have distended abdomen; jaundiced skin and sclera; peripheral edema; and thin, friable skin scattered with petechiae and ecchymoses.
Mentation	Varies from alertness to obtundation.
Urine output	Decreased
Psychosocial signs	Fright

ASSESSMENT CRITERIA: ESOPHAGEAL VARICES (continued)

Lab values

Alanine aminotransferase (ALT)	High
Aspartate aminotransferase (AST)	High
Hemoglobin and hematocrit	Low
Occult blood, stool	Positive
PT/PTT	Prolonged

Red blood cell indices

Mean corpuscular hemoglobin (MCH)	Normal
Mean corpuscular hemoglobin concentration (MCHC)	Normal
Mean corpuscular volume (MCV)	Normal
Urine specific gravity	High

Diagnostic tests

Upper GI endoscopy	Eroded or ruptured varix (varices) with active bleeding.

Other	None

NURSING DIAGNOSIS

Fluid volume deficit related to massive hemorrhage, resulting from rupture of esophageal varices.

Decreased cardiac output related to hemorrhage, resulting from rupture of esophageal varices.

Tissue perfusion, altered, related to decreased circulating blood volume, resulting from hemorrhage.

(Potential for) ineffective airway clearance related to unprotected airway, resulting from obtundation.

Anxiety related to observation of bright red blood, resulting from rupture of esophageal varices.

NURSING INTERVENTIONS

Immediate nursing interventions

Place suction equipment and oral airway at bedside.

Assess pulse, respirations, and blood pressure q1h until bleeding is stopped, then q2h × 24 hours.

Monitor respiratory status q2h, including assessment of cough and gag reflexes. Prepare for intubation if depressed.

Assess temperature q2h × 24 hours, then q4h × 48 hours.

Establish two peripheral IVs of 18 gauge or larger. If not possible, prepare for physician to insert central line.

Obtain volumetric infusion pumps and isotonic crystalloids such as 0.9% saline.

Send blood sample for STAT H and H and type and crossmatch or screen.

Obtain blood warmer, if more than 2 units of blood are anticipated for transfusion.

Prepare for arterial line insertion for frequent blood sampling and continuous arterial pressure monitoring.

Insert nasogastric (NG) tube and attach to low intermittent suction.

Insert indwelling urinary catheter.

Measure hourly intake and output (I and O).

Anticipated physician orders and interventions

STAT H and H.

Arterial line insertion.

Indwelling urinary catheter.

Upper GI endoscopy with sclerotherapy.

0.9% NaCl IV infusion at 150 ml/hour.

0.9% NaCl lavage until clear.

Transfuse packed RBCs to maintain hematocrit at about 30%.

Transfuse platelets to maintain platelet count above 20,000. After every 6 units of RBCs, transfuse 2 units of fresh frozen plasma and 6 units of platelets.

Begin vasopressin infusion: Loading dose is 15 units of vasopressin in 50 ml D5W over 15 minutes. Then infuse 250 units of vasopressin in 250 ml D5W at 0.4 to 0.6 U/minute.

Intubation for the client with copious bleeding, acute respiratory distress, or obtundation.

Central line for large-volume infusions.

Pulmonary artery catheter to monitor hemodynamics and obtain information about circulatory volume (Gervin et al., 1991).

Gastroesophageal endoscopy and possible sclerotherapy.

Prepare for Sengstaken-Blakemore tube insertion if bleeding is not controlled.

Ongoing nursing assessment, monitoring, and interventions

Assess:
- Level of consciousness q2h and PRN.
- Cough and gag reflexes q2h and PRN.
- Color and amount of drainage from NG tube q8h and PRN.
- For signs of bleeding from sites other than esophagus q8h.

- For edema and skin turgor q4h.
- For fluid volume overload q4h (rales, tachycardia, tachypnea, S_3.
- IV sites for redness, edema, bleeding, and pain q4h and PRN. Increase observations to q1h for vasopressin infusion.

Measure:

- Blood pressure, pulse, and respirations q1h × 24 hours, then q2h × 24 hours.
- Temperature q2h until bleeding stopped, then q4h.
- I and O q1h × 24 hours, then q4h and PRN
- Weight qd.

Send:

- H and H q4h until bleeding stops, then q6h × 24 hours. *Note:* Levels will not be accurate until complete volume restoration and equilibration occur over several hours, particularly if the client has received more than 3 units of blood (Gervin et al., 1991).
- Complete blood count (CBC), including platelet count, q24h.
- Clotting factors q12h × 24 hours.

Implement:

- Measures to protect the airway: oral airway and suction apparatus at bedside, head of bed elevated to 30 degrees.
- During gastric lavage, protect client from aspiration of clots by positioning in left lateral decubitus position and keeping a suction cannula close to the mouth.

TEACHING/EDUCATION

Select items, based on client's pathophysiology:

Intravenous blood samples: *Rationale:* Several blood samples will be taken every day. They are needed to track the amount of bleeding and your body's response to transfusions and treatment.

IV line placement: *Rationale:* The IV line allows us to easily take blood samples and to give you necessary treatments with fluids and medications.

Indwelling urinary catheter placement: *Rationale:* Accurate urine measurement is very important for people who are bleeding. The catheter prevents any urine from spilling before it is measured. We may also give you medicine that will cause your kidneys to make more urine, so the catheter keeps you from having to get up frequently to go to the bathroom.

IV site symptoms: *Rationale:* We are giving you a medicine through your veins to stop the bleeding. This IV may hurt you if it starts to leak out into the tissues of your (hand, arm, etc.). Your nurse will be checking how well this IV is working every hour, but if it starts hurting you or swells at any time, call your nurse right away.

Blood transfusions: *Rationale:* You have lost so much blood that it is necessary to replace some by transfusion. The blood is tested for HIV and hepatitis, so the risk of these diseases being transmitted to you is very small. You will only receive enough blood to prevent you from having major symptoms of anemia. Your body will continue to manufacture its own blood, though, so that in the next few weeks the anemia should resolve.

Mechanical ventilation: *Rationale:* You cannot talk right now because a breathing tube passes through your vocal cords. It is attached to a ventilator and is helping you to breathe. The nurse-call button is right here, so you can get help when you need it. Also, we can communicate for now with a pad and pen, or flashcards if you prefer. As you become more awake, you will no longer need the ventilator, and it will be removed. Then you will be able to talk again.

Signs and symptoms of rebleeding: *Rationale:* You and significant others need to watch for signs or symptoms of rebleeding because early treatment may preclude the need for blood transfusions and may prevent serious complications. Signs and symptoms include any of the following: weakness, dizziness, "coffee ground" vomit, black tarry stools, maroon or frankly bloody stools, abdominal cramping, "black and blue" marks easily obtained, a low platelet count.

Identification of behaviors that increase the chance of bleeding: *Rationale:* You will need to avoid alcohol, medication containing aspirin (salicylates), and other medications that irritate gastric and esophageal mucosa. You must also avoid activities that increase intra-abdominal pressure, such as heavy lifting, straining to stool, vomiting, and the ingestion of a large meal.

Safety considerations: *Rationale:* While you are in the hospital, we will be taking precautions to ensure your safety. The amount of blood you have lost will make you weak, and you may not be able to think very clearly, so you are prone to injury. The safety measures include checking on you closely and frequently, putting the call light within easy reach, instructions not to get out of bed without someone to help you, and perhaps applying soft wrist restraints while the breathing tube is in place. When you are ready to be discharged, your nurse will discuss safety measures you can use at home to prevent falls or injury.

EVALUATION/DESIRED OUTCOMES

1. Cessation of bleeding immediately after sclerotherapy.
2. No recurrence of bleeding during hospital stay.
3. Hematocrit of ≥30% within 24 hours.
4. Platelet count > 20,000 within 24 hours.
5. Clotting factors return to normal values within 24 hours.
6. Systolic blood pressure returns to baseline within 24 hours.
7. Adequate urine output of about 0.5 to 1 ml/kg/hour within 24 hours.
8. Lungs are clear to auscultation within 48 hours.

9. Ventilatory support is discontinued within 48 hours.
10. Mentation returns to baseline within 48 hours.
11. Vasopressin infusion is discontinued within 48 hours.
12. Client does not experience complications from TIPS procedure.
13. Follow-up care and discharge teaching are understood by the client and/or caregiver prior to discharge.

DISCHARGE PLANNING

Client with esophageal varices may need:

Repeated sclerotherapy.
Beta-blocker therapy.
Preparation for TIPS procedure, if indicated.
Portosystemic shunting, if TIPS is not feasible.
Training of the client and significant others in the signs and symptoms of repeat bleeding.

FOLLOW-UP CARE

Anticipated care

Home health nursing visits.
Physician office visit within 1 week.
Outpatient lab testing for hemoglobin, hematocrit, and platelet count within the next week.
Other blood work as appropriate (liver enzymes, ammonia, serum bilirubin, etc.).
Continuation of dietary regimen of avoiding aspirin, alcohol, and large meals.
Continued monitoring for signs of rebleeding.
Repeat sclerotherapy within 1 year.

Anticipated client/family questions and possible answers

Will I start throwing up blood again?
"Probably. That is why it is so important for you to have repeat sclerotherapy injections. They can prevent bleeding from recurring."
"Yes, it is highly likely that you will bleed again, which is why your doctor has recommended the TIPS procedure. This procedure will permanently lower the pressure in your veins so that the risk of rebleeding is very small."
"It is very possible that you will experience another bleeding episode. Let's talk about ways to prevent it from happening until you have the TIPS procedure."

Is there any way I can tell if I'm bleeding before it gets too bad?
"That is a good question. It is very important for you to detect bleeding early

so that you get prompt medical attention. Yes, there are ways to tell. Inspect every bowel movement for color. Black, tarry-looking stools should be reported to your doctor. Any bowel movement that is maroon or frankly red needs immediate medical attention. Sometimes when you begin to throw up, the emesis has a 'coffee ground' appearance. This indicates bleeding, as does bright red blood. If this happens, you should either notify your doctor at once or go directly to a hospital emergency department. Feeling weak or dizzy can sometimes mean that you have begun to bleed again, even when there are no overt signs of it. If this happens, lie down until the feeling passes, then get up slowly and call your doctor. If the feeling persists, you should seek immediate medical attention."

Is there any way to prevent the bleeding from happening again?

"The only way to permanently stop the bleeding is to have the TIPS procedure or surgery. Until then, though, there are things you can do to lower the chances of bleeding again. You should not take medicine like aspirin or drinks like alcohol because they irritate your esophagus and stomach lining. You should also avoid activities that raise the pressure inside your abdomen. These activities include heavy lifting, straining to have a bowel movement, or vomiting. Having a large meal also increases the pressure in the abdomen, so rather than eating three large meals a day, you may find it more comfortable to eat five or six smaller meals."

CHAPTER SUMMARY

Bleeding esophageal varices are a catastrophic, life-threatening event, associated with a 50% mortality rate within 6 weeks of the initial bleed. Treatment can be divided into three phases, the first of which requires intensive care monitoring. Highly technical equipment and new procedures represent some of the efforts directed toward stopping the bleeding. It is a truly skilled nurse who can blend technical proficiency with the empathy necessary to meet the needs of a frightened client. Once bleeding has stopped, the prevention of further bleeding episodes becomes the focus of therapy. The importance of follow-up visits and client education is imperative to maintaining a significant quality of life.

TEST QUESTIONS

1. The term "cirrhosis" refers to:
   A. Alcoholic liver disease
   B. Fibrous tissue changes in the liver
   C. Carcinoma of the liver
   D. Acute inflammatory changes in the liver

1. Answer: B
Although the liver has the ability to regenerate after an acute insult, chronic injury causes scarring, which increases resistance to portal blood flow.

2. Esophageal varices occur when:
   A. Blood in the cardiac system is shunted away from a cirrhotic liver.
   B. Blood in the gastric system is shunted away from a cirrhotic liver.
   C. Blood in the portal system is shunted away from a cirrhotic liver.
   D. Blood in the esophagus is shunted away from a cirrhotic liver.

2. Answer: D
Scarring of a cirrhotic liver inhibits portal venous outflow and raises portal pressure. Collateral vessels in the esophagus and stomach develop in an attempt to reroute the flow of blood. As pressures continue to rise, however, these vessels too become distended and engorged.

3. The first line of treatment for bleeding esophageal varices is:
   A. Sclerotherapy
   B. Vasopressin
   C. Sengstaken-Blakemore tube
   D. Blood transfusions

3. Answer: A.
Sclerotherapy is the quickest way to achieve hemostasis at the bleeding site, which is the primary objective of treatment.

4. Vasopressin should be used with caution in clients with:
   A. Liver disease
   B. Metastatic cancer
   C. Carotid artery disease
   D. Coronary artery disease

4. Answer: D.
Vasopressin causes an imbalance between myocardial oxygen supply and demand that can be harmful to clients with pre-existing coronary artery disease.

5. The TIPS is a nonsurgical procedure that lowers portal pressure by creating a path between:
   A. Splenic and portal veins
   B. Portal and hepatic veins
   C. Gastric and portal veins
   D. Renal and hepatic veins

5. Answer: B
An artificially created shunt between the portal and hepatic veins lowers resistance to blood flow through the liver, with a net result of lowering pressure in the portal venous system, including veins in the esophagus.

6. A priority nursing assessment during the emergent phase of bleeding esophageal varices is for:
   A. Heart sounds
   B. Adequate urine output
   C. A patent airway
   D. Breath sounds

6. Answer: C
Remembering the "ABCs" of basic resuscitation and of treatment for copious bleeding, acute respiratory distress, or obtundation may include using oral intubation to maintain an adequate airway. Respiratory distress or obtundation may call for using oral intubation to maintain an adequate airway.

7. The primary nursing diagnosis of clients with bleeding esophageal varices is:
   A. Fluid volume deficit
   B. Anxiety
   C. Body temperature, altered
   D. Breathing pattern, ineffective

7. Answer: A
Massive hemorrhage causes a blood volume deficit inadequate enough to meet needs or sustain life. Because of the lab time between the start of the bleeding and initiation of fluids, there is at first inadequate fluid resuscitation as well.

8. Once the client with bleeding esophageal varices has stabilized and is out of danger, teaching is directed to the identification of:
   A. Safety considerations
   B. Maintenance of adequate nutrition
   C. Appropriate coping mechanisms
   D. Signs and symptoms of rebleeding

8. Answer: D
By recognizing when bleeding resumes, the client can seek early treatment, which may preclude the need for blood transfusions and may prevent serious complications.

9. The client with a history of esophageal varices must also be taught to avoid activities that will increase intra-abdominal pressure. These include:
   A. Stair climbing, bending, deep breathing
   B. Heavy lifting, straining to pass a stool, eating large meals
   C. Running, dancing, brisk walking
   D. Coughing, kneeling, streching

9. Answer: B
Increasing intra-abdominal pressure may precipitate the rupture of esophageal varices.

10. An important intervention in the outpatient phase that should be stressed for the client with esophageal varices to seek is:
    A. Annual endoscopy
    B. Monthly endoscopy
    C. Biannual endoscopy
    D. No further endoscopy is needed

10. Answer: A
The physician is able to monitor the progress of the varices with an annual endoscopy and treat them with sclerotherapy if necessary. An annual schedule represents both the safest and most cost-effective option.

REFERENCES

Anderson K, Anderson L, Glanze W (eds): Mosby's Medical, Nursing, and Allied Health Dictionary, 4th ed. St. Louis, MO: Mosby Year Book, 1994.

Burns S, Martin M: VP/NTG therapy in the patient with variceal bleeding. Crit Care Nurs 10(9):42–49, 1990.

Burns S, Martin M, Merrill P, Luer J, Stone D: Evaluation and revision of vasopressin/nitroglycerin protocol for use in variceal bleeding. Am J Crit Care 2(3):202–207, 1993.

Butler R: Managing the complications of cirrhosis. Am J Nurs 9:46–49, 1994.

Conn H: Transjugular intrahepatic portal-systemic shunts: The state of the art. Hepatology 17(1):148–158, 1993.

Doherty M, Carver D: New relief for esophageal varices. Am J Nurs 8:58–63, 1993.

Edling JE, Bacon BR: Pleuropulmonary complications of endoscopic variceal sclerotherapy. Chest 99(5):1252–1257, 1991.

Ellis P, Cunningham D: Management of carcinomas of the upper gastrointestinal tract. Br Med J 308:834–838, 1994.

Gervin A, Gostout C, Zinner M: Upper GI bleeding: Treatment options. Patient Care 25(2):59–77, 1991.

Gruber M: Endoscopic injection sclerotherapy: Nursing responsibilities. Crit Care Q 7(4):73–80, 1985.

Jacoby AG, Weigman MV: Cardiovascular complications of intravenous vasopressin therapy. Focus Crit Care 17(1):63–66, 1990.

Kerber K: The adult with bleeding esophageal varices. Crit Care Nurs Clin North Am 5(1):153–162, 1993.

Mackay GJ, Henderson JM: Update on the management of variceal bleeding. J Am Acad Physician Assist 5(3):165–175, 1992.

Nurses' Drug Alert. Beta-blocker prophylaxis in patients with cirrhosis. Nurses' Drug Alert 15(7):55, 1991.

Pierce JD, Wilkerson E, Griffiths S: Acute esophageal bleeding and endoscopic injection sclerotherapy. Crit Care Nurse 10(9):67–72, 1990.

Resnick RH: Management of varices in cirrhosis. Hosp Pract (November 15):123–129, 1993.

White JV, Milazzo JV, Comerota AJ: Management of massive hemorrhage from esophageal varices. Crit Care Q 8(2):69–79, 1985.

CHAPTER 12

FEVER

Roger Carpenter, RN, MSN

CHAPTER OBJECTIVES

At the completion of this chapter, the reader will be able to:

Describe the pathophysiologic processes of fever.

Identify risk factors that predispose a client to fever.

List assessment data vital in diagnosing fever.

Select appropriate nursing diagnoses and care for the client experiencing fever.

Give examples of education relevant to the client at risk for or experiencing fever.

Anticipate home-going needs for the client at risk for developing fever.

OVERVIEW

FEVER is one of the oldest known medical ailments, and antipyresis is one of the oldest, most common, and most automatic interventions (Henker and Shaver, 1994). Fever is recognized as the most common manifestation of disease. Although considered a disease, fever is actually a sign or indicator of disease activity. It accompanies many illnesses and serves as an indicator or response to disease activity. It is often debated whether clinicians should focus on treating the fever itself, rather than focusing on what is the actual pathophysiologic process that is causing the fever.

Also referred to as "hyperpyrexia," fever is a product of thermoregulation. It is a state in which the body temperature is elevated above normal but regulated by the usual body temperature control mechanism—the thermoregulatory ability remains intact (Henker and Shaver, 1994; Holtzclaw, 1992). This differs from hyperthermia, in which the body temperature is elevated and there is dysfunction of the thermoregulatory ability, characterized by failure of the compensatory cooling mechanisms (Holtzclaw, 1992).

For the cancer client, fever is the most frequently occurring complication experienced, either as a result of disease process and/or the treatment of cancer.

DESCRIPTION

Maintenance of body temperature

A constant body temperature is needed to provide the optimal environment for physiologic and metabolic processes in the body. Although no single body temperature can be considered normal due to variations in body temperature in healthy persons, the normal *range* of temperature (orally) is 36.7 to 37.0° C (98.0 to 98.6° F) and approximately 0.6° C (1.0° F) higher when measured rectally (Guyton, 1991) and 0.6° C (1.0° F) lower when measured tympanically.

The prevailing explanation for the cause of fever (in spite of competing explanations, conflicting data, and proposed models of fever) involves the effects of endogenous pyrogens on the hypothalamic thermosensitivity affecting the set point range. Endogenous pyrogens such as interleukin 1, interleukin 6, tumor necrosis factor (TNF), and interferon are produced by host cells such as macrophages and monocytes (Henker and Shaver, 1994; Bruce and Grove, 1992). Mediators of endogenous pyrogens can include noninfectious agents such as toxic drugs, chemical compounds, blood products, neoplastic cells, and foreign bodies, or infectious agents such as bacteria, viruses, and fungi.

The set point is the preferred body temperature level around which temperature is regulated. It is the optimum temperature for the individual's cellular metabolism and neurotransmission (Holtzclaw, 1992). Body temperature is regulated by the hypothalamus. When body temperature rises above or falls below the set point, the hypothalamus institutes compensatory warming or cooling measures to restore the set point temperature (Henker and Shaver, 1994; Holtzclaw, 1992; Guyton, 1991; Styrt and Sugarman 1990).

In fever, endogenous pyrogens displace the body's hypothalamic set point and cause it to reset at a higher than normal level. When the set point is shifted upward to a warmer level, heat-conserving mechanisms are brought into place to elevate body temperature to the new set point range. Heat-conserving mechanisms of the body include shivering (the friction of muscle spindle fibers generates heat), vasoconstriction (conserves heat by diminishing blood supply to the surface of the body), increased metabolic rate, and heat-seeking behaviors such as putting on extra blankets or drinking hot liquids (Holtzclaw, 1992; Styrt and Sugarman, 1990).

Conversely, when the hypothalamic set point is shifted downward, as occurs with antipyretic therapy, compensatory cooling mechanisms are brought into place. Cooling mechanisms include vasodilation (brings blood closer to the skin surface, thus heat is lost through conduction, convection, and radiation), sweating (when water evaporates, it takes heat with it), and heat-reducing behaviors such as shedding layers of clothes or moving to a cooler environment (Holtzclaw, 1992).

Causes of fever in oncology clients

Oncology clients present with fever that is usually a result of one of the following five causes: infection, tumor-associated fever, drug side effects, allergic reaction to a drug or to blood products, or treatment with a biologic response modifier. Infectious, inflammatory, and immunologic processes are the most frequently cited causes of fever (Bruce and Grove, 1992).

Infection

Infection should always be the first suspected cause of fever in an oncology client because immunosuppression and neutropenia place such clients at high risk for this complication. Fever has special significance in oncology because 55 to 75% of fevers in cancer clients are caused by infection (Pizzo, 1989). Infection is significant because it is the major cause of mortality in the cancer client, especially when immunocompromised (Burke, Wilkes, Berg, Bean, and Ingwersen, 1991).

Tumor-Associated Fever

For clients with hematologic malignancy, fever is a common manifestation at the time of diagnosis. Other cancers that commonly present with fever are included below, in the Risk Profile. The onset and degree of the febrile response may correlate with tumor activity (Gucalp, 1991). Theories of the cause of tumor-associated fever include an allergic response to the presence

---

Table 12–1
Drugs That Can Cause a Febrile Response

Acyclovir	Ganciclovir
Allopurinol	Immunoglobulins
Amphotericin B	Interferons
Bacillus Calmette Guerin (BCG) vaccine	Interleukin 2
Bleomycin	Interleukin 3
Busulfan	Interleukin 4
Cladribine	Methotrexate
Dacarbazine	Molgramostim
Dactinomycin	Pamidronate
Daunorubicin	Phenytoin
Femcitabine	Procarbazine
Filgramostim	Sargramostim
Fluconazole	Varicella vaccine
5-Flucytosine	Venorelbine
Fludarabine	Vindesine
Gallium nitrate	

---

of the tumor, direct release of toxins by the tumor itself, and blockage of drainage routes from secretory tumors (Young, 1988).

Drug Side Effects

Many drugs, acting as noninfectious agents, can be recognized by the body as foreign and thus can elicit an immune response and trigger a febrile response. Some of the more common drugs that elicit the febrile response are listed in Table 12–1.

Allergic Reaction to Drug or Blood Products

White blood cells (WBCs) pose the highest risk for allergic reaction in oncology clients receiving blood products. Measures to reduce this risk include removing WBCs from administered blood, administering only irradiated blood products, and premedicating with antipyretics, hydrocortisone, and/or an antihistamine prior to transfusion.

Treatment with Biologic Response Modifiers

Biologic response modifers create a flulike syndrome that is thought to be caused by the actions of cytokines on the hypothalamic temperature center. This action includes the release of prostaglandins and histamine, which increase the body temperature, causing fever.

Phases of the febrile response

The febrile response can be described in three phases: the chill phase, the plateau or hot phase, and the defervescence phase (Holtzclaw, 1992; Bruce and Grove, 1992). In the chill phase, there is a sensed discrepancy between the existing body temperature and the new set point. Shivering and vasoconstriction and a hypermetabolic state begin. In the plateau or hot phase, normal thermoregulation is maintained, but at the new set point level. In the defervescence phase, heat loss mechanisms are initiated and a significant cooling response occurs as endogenous pyrogen levels fall (Holtzclaw, 1992).

The (oral) temperature range of fever is between 38.0 and 41.0° C (100.4 and 105.8° F). True fevers rarely exceed 41.0° C (104.8° F) due to feedback mechanisms and their action on the hypothalamus, and fevers greater than 41.0° C (104.9° F) are usually caused by additional activities (such as seizure activity), whereby additional heat is generated through muscle activity (Bruce and Grove, 1992).

RISK PROFILE

All risk factors are greater when occurring in an immunocompromised client.

Cancers

Underlying malignancies: tumors that infarct and become necrotic, secondary infections in a necrotic tumor; Hodgkin's disease, acute leukemias, lymphomas, hypernephromas (renal cell carcinoma), bone sarcoma, atrial myxoma, and adrenal carcinoma/pheochromocytoma.

Malignancies that involve abnormalities in humoral immunity, cellular immunity (Hodgkin's and non-Hodgkin's lymphoma).

Malignant tumors that produce antigens that elicit immune responses (renal cell carcinoma).

Primary or metastatic tumors of the thermoregulatory areas of the brain.

Hepatic metastases from primary sites of the colon, lung, or breast.

Obstructive solid tumors of the gastrointestinal, genitourinary, or respiratory systems.

Conditions: Infection (bacterial, viral, fungal):

Neutropenia (< 50,000 polymorphonuclear neutrophils or band forms/mm³).

Immunosuppression (impairment of cellular and humoral immune systems).

Alterations in physical defense barriers such as mucositis, perirectal excoriation (clients at highest risk have a history of hemorrhoids combined with neutropenia), indwelling lines, and catheters.

Impaired phagocyte function.

Bone marrow transplant and peripheral stem cell transplant treatment that result in profound neutropenia or graft vs. host disease (GVHD).

Surgery.

Splenic dysfunction.

Frequent receipt of blood products.

Radiation therapy, which impairs T-lymphocyte and mononuclear phagocyte function.

Dehydration. (The thermostatic control in the hypothalamus is sensitive to dehydration from sodium excess or dessication from water loss.)

Head injury (thrombocytopenia-induced).

Environment: As it affects the immunocomprised or potentially immunocompromised client:

Within health care environments, microbial flora that colonize in the nasopharynx, small and large bowel, and the skin of the client.

Recent travel outside of the country to Third World countries, parts of North, Central, and South America, and to tropics and subtropics.

Presence of household members at high risk for tuberculosis, varicella virus, cytomegalovirus, or influenza in the home or work environment.

Exposure to microorganisms from farm or other animals.

Allergic response to environmental allergens or iatrogenically introduced allergens, such as blood products.

(R. E. White's Manual of Oncologic Therapeutics, 1991/1992)

Foods: As it affects the immunocompromised or potentially immunocompromised client: The ingestion of fresh vegetables, fresh fruits, or plant products such as spices and tobacco is prohibited.

Drugs: See Table 12–1.

Other: None.

PROGNOSIS

The prognosis for a febrile client depends on the cause of the fever and the client's response to treatment for both the fever and the underlying cause of the febrile response. It has been debated extensively whether fever is beneficial or harmful. Benefits from fever include an enhanced immune response of the host, ranging from activation of T-lymphocytes to secretion of antibacterial chemicals. A harmful effect of fever is increased metabolic expenditure. It has been estimated that fever can raise the metabolic rate approximately 13% for each degree Celsius of body temperature elevation (Holtzclaw, 1992).

Infection is the major cause of death in the cancer client. Fevers left untreated can result in death within 48 hours in up to 50 to 70% of neutropenic clients with fever, because of rapidly developing sepsis (Burke et al., 1991; Pizzo, 1989). The reader is referred to Chapter 38 for further information on this complication.

TREATMENT

Two major categories of therapy exist in clinical practice for the management of fever: pharmacologic agents and the use of physical modalities to reduce fever.

Surgery: Not indicated.

Chemotherapy: Indicated for treatment of the cause of tumor-associated fever.

Radiation: Indicated as appropriate for cancer type to treat the cause of tumor-associated fever.

Medications

Antibiotic therapy for the immunosuppressed client: empirical broad-spectrum antibiotic therapy that provides coverage for gram-negative bacteria such as *Escherichia coli, Klebsiella pneumonias,* or *Pseudomonas aeruginosa,* and gram-positive bacteria such as *Staphylococcus aureus* and streptococcal species. Empirical antifungal therapy may be added for fungal infections such as *candida* and *aspergillus* if the febrile state continues while the client continues on broad-spectrum antibiotics (Pizzo, 1993).

Antibiotic therapy for the nonimmunosuppressed client may be used, based on the client's risk for infection, risk for immunosuppression, or past history of infections.

Antibiotic therapy may also be provided when an infectious process and the organism have been identified.

Antipyretic therapy: Antipyretic drugs, primarily acetaminophen, are given primarily for comfort or to reduce potentially damaging temperature. Nonsteroidal antipyretic drugs, such as aspirin and acetaminophen, reduce fever by affecting the hypothalamic response to pyrogens (Holtzclaw, 1992). However, aspirin is usually contraindicated in persons with cancer due to its potential side effect of bleeding. In immunosuppressed clients, fever is often the only reliable sign of infection or of response to antimicrobial treatment. Antipyretic drugs are used only if the client is extremely uncomfortable or cannot tolerate the hypermetabolic state accompanying fever (Holtzclaw, 1992).

Procedures

Fluid replacement: Fluid imbalances such as dehydration are known to cause changes in body temperature. Fluid replacement that improves hydration and imbalance directly affects hypothalamic sensitivity (Holtzclaw, 1992).

Application of cooling blankets and ice packs should be used only when the core temperature is rising uncontrollably to potentially damaging levels. However, there is no empirical research to define that these interventions are effective.

Other

Increased oral fluid intake.

Minimal use of clothing and blankets.

Possible use of ice packs or a cooling blanket to induce hypothermia (Styrt and Sugarman, 1990). Not well supported in the literature, this treatment is reserved for conditions in which temperatures are at risk for rising uncontrollably to potentially dangerous levels.

Increase in caloric intake to supply increased metabolic demand.

Provision for adequate rest.

ASSESSMENT CRITERIA: FEVER

	Chill Phase	Hot/Plateau Phase	Defervescence Phase
Vital signs*			
Temperature**	>38.0° C (>100.4° F)	>38.0° C (>100.4° F)	<38.0° C (<100.4° F)
Pulse	Increased	Increased	Normalizing
Respiration	Increased	Increased	Normalizing
Blood pressure	Increased	Increased	Normalizing

*Fever causes increased basal metabolic rate and increased oxygen consumption by tissues. This results in increased cardiac output and workload. The body compensates by increasing the heart rate and respiratory rate (Bruce and Grove, 1992).

**Temperature changes can occur rapidly in response to endogenous pyrogens. Also, clients may vary in their ability to sense and express temperature changes (Holtzclaw, 1992).

ASSESSMENT CRITERIA: FEVER *(continued)*

History	Past medical illness or recent surgery, recent ingestion of medications, exposure to infectious or chemical agents, allergies, presence of indwelling lines or catheters.		

Hallmark physical signs and symptoms

Subjective feeling	Feels cold.	Feels hot, loss of appetite, myalgia, restlessness, headache, weakness, drowsiness, photophobia (Bruce and Grove, 1992).	Feels warm or hot.
Shivering***	Present	Absent	Absent
Skin	Cool, pale, and dry	Warm, flushed; diaphoretic	Warm, flushed; diaphoretic
Nail beds	Cyanotic (due to vasoconstriction) (Bruce and Grove, 1992)	Normal	Normal

Additional physical signs and symptoms	Assess carefully for breaks in skin integrity at sites of infection, including line sites, all body orifices, skin folds, and perirectal area. Tender abdomen may indicate internal abscess or peritonitis.

Psychosocial signs and symptoms	Heat-seeking behaviors such as using extra blankets or wraps, and changes in body posture that decrease the amount of body surface area through which heat is lost (Henker and Shaver, 1994)	Behaviors that cool the body, such as removing wraps, fanning, and changes in posture that increase surface area (i.e., stretching) (Henker and Shaver, 1994).	Same as hot/ plateau phase.

Lab values

Sodium, serum	High, secondary to dehydration
Hematocrit	High, secondary to dehydration
Osmolality, serum	High
Osmolality, urine	Low
Culture, wound, blood, urine and line tips/ports	Positive results for infectious causes of fever.

Diagnostic tests

Chest x-ray	May be normal or show evidence of underlying disease process or show evidence of pulmonary embolus as cause of fever.

***Shivering occurs when environmental temperatures are sensed as being too cool. A compensatory warming mechanism of the body, it is stressful and increases energy expenditure at a time when metabolic rate is already high (Holtzclaw, 1992).

NURSING DIAGNOSIS

The nursing diagnoses will vary, depending on the cause(s) of fever. Some of the common diagnoses and etiologies are as follows:

Risk for altered body temperature related to:
- Brain tumor, hypothalamic tumor, underlying malignancy.
- Infection.
- Myelosuppression (anemia, neutropenia).
- Medications.
- Blood product administration.
- Surgery.
- Dehydration.

Fluid volume deficit (potential for) related to:
- Anorexia that may accompany fever, or as a side effect of treatment.
- Diaphoresis during the febrile response.

Knowledge deficit related to:
- Signs and symptoms of fever and infection.
- Technique for assessing body temperature.
- Management of the febrile response.

NURSING INTERVENTIONS

Observation and client monitoring are often the most appropriate nursing interventions. In the noncritical client, many authorities believe fever has immunomodulatory benefits. For the critically ill and the immunosuppressed client, fever is an emergency. The client, who may not be able to tolerate the increased basal metabolic rate, may be at risk for cardiopulmonary instability and hypoxia.

Immediate nursing interventions

Assess temperature in critically ill clients and in clients at risk for fever.
Assess pulse, blood pressure, and respiratory rate.
Prevent shivering by avoiding drastic changes in skin-to-core temperatures.

Anticipated physician orders and interventions

Medical treatment of fever depends on the cause or suspected cause. Various health care practitioners may vary in their diagnostic workup and treatment of fever, based on the perceived risks and benefits of both the fever itself and the available treatments. Interventions to determine cause and treatment can include:

Cultures of blood, sputum, urine, stool, and any discharge or drainage noted.
Cultures of any invasive line and/or catheter.

Complete blood count (CBC) with differential.

Chemistry panel.

Radiographic or ultrasonic scanning of common sites of infection, which include but are not limited to the peritoneum, pharynx, lower esophagus, lung, perineum, anus, nail beds, and any skin lesions.

IV hydration with isotonic crystalloids (0.9% saline), which may be preceded by hypotonic crystalloids, depending on the degree of dehydration accompanying the fever.

Antipyretic therapy (refer to "Medications" in Treatment section).

Organism-specific antimicrobial therapy if the source of infection is known.

Additional Interventions for the Immunosuppressed Client

STAT blood cultures from two peripheral sites, or a peripheral site and a central venous access site (*always* culture an invasive line in the febrile immunosuppressed client).

Chest x-ray—posteroanterior and lateral.

Urine culture and sensitivity.

Serologies and cultures for viral diseases.

Begin empiric antibiotics STAT after culturing (see Treatment section). Antipyretics, however, can be given before blood cultures are drawn.

Repeat fever evaluations q24h if fever is unresolved, or whenever oral temperature ≥39.5° C (103.1° F) or if the client develops rigors unrelated to medications or blood product administration.

Ongoing nursing assessment, monitoring, and interventions

Assess:

- Head-to-toe physical assessment qd. Thorough inspection of skin, mucous membranes, skin folds, and body orifices for breaks in integrity and signs of infection.
- For signs of dehydration: poor skin turgor, dry mucous membranes, weight loss, lethargy, increased serum osmolality (norm is 280 to 300 mOsm/L). Severe signs of dehydration include electrolyte imbalance and confusion progressing to seizures as brain cells become dehydrated.
- CBC results qd for evidence of neutrophil recovery.

Measure:

- Vital signs, including temperature q4h while the client is febrile or is at risk for fever. Avoid rectal temperatures.
- Intake and output q8h.

Send:

- CBC with differential qd.
- Electrolyte panel qd.

- Serum osmolality qd, or it may be calculated by the following formula:

  For client with a normal glucose value:

  (serum sodium) × 2 = serum osmolality

  For a client with hyperglycemia:

  (serum sodium × 2) – (glucose/18) + (BUN/2.4) = osmolality

Implement:

- Measures to reduce febrile reaction:

  Administer antipyretic as prescribed.

  Administer antihistamine or hydrocortisone premedication as prescribed before blood infusions or infusions of drugs expected to cause febrile response.

  Reduce ambient room temperature.

  Remove clothing and reduce number of blankets covering the client.

  (*Note:* Sponge baths and cooling with electric fans should be avoided. Alcohol baths should never be used to treat fever because of the health risk posed by the fumes [Holtzclaw, 1992]).

- Measures to prevent shivering:

  Add clothing or blankets.

  Keep a supply of dry blankets to replace those moistened by diaphoresis.

  Increase ambient room temperature and minimize drafts.

TEACHING/EDUCATION

Description of febrile response: *Rationale:* A fever is a body temperature taken by mouth that is higher than normal (greater than 99.5° F or 37.5° C). Many things can cause a fever, such as medicine, dehydration, and being sick, but the most common cause of a fever is infection by bacteria and viruses. A fever isn't always harmful. It is one way of helping your body fight off infection. However, if your blood counts are low, a fever is usually the most reliable sign of an infection.

Avoidance of infection: *Rationale:* An infection, if not treated quickly, can be life-threatening if your blood counts are low. When you go home, you should take it easy, not overexert yourself, and avoid large crowds and people you know who may be sick with a cold, flu, or some other infection like chicken pox or measles, or infants and adults who have been recently vaccinated with a live vaccine. You will have to take your temperature at home to watch for another fever. Your doctor will tell you what temperature you should call him or her about right away.

Change in use of chemotherapy: *Rationale:* Chemotherapy drugs can cause your blood counts to fall too low, putting you at greater risk for infection and anemia. Your chemotherapy may be decreased in dose, held until further notice, or discontinued based on your blood counts. If you have a fever, your chemotherapy may be decreased, held, or stopped until the cause of the fever is determined and/or treated.

Blood work: *Rationale:* Your blood counts will be checked often while your counts are low. Blood may also be drawn if you have a fever to help find out the cause of the fever. Also, if you have a central venous catheter, blood will also be drawn from it to test for infection.

Fluids: *Rationale:* If you have a fever while in the hospital, you may be placed on IV fluids to give you extra body water. If you have a fever or are at risk for one while you are at home, drinking a glass of water every hour may help to reduce or prevent a fever.

IV site symptoms: *Rationale:* IV sites and IV catheters, such as a central venous catheter, are at risk for becoming infected and causing a fever. If you have a fever, watch these areas closely for pain, redness, swelling, warmth, or drainage. Call your doctor or nurse right away if you notice these changes.

Medications: *Rationale:* Your doctor may prescribe medication, such as acetaminophen, for your fever. Take this medicine only as directed.

EVALUATION/DESIRED OUTCOMES

1. The fever will resolve within 24 hours after institution of pharmacologic and physical interventions.
2. The client will be free of signs and symptoms of fever within 24 hours after initiation of interventions.

DISCHARGE PLANNING

The client at risk for recurrent fever will need:

Oral temperature taken at home every 4 hours while at risk for recurrence.
Instruction related to proper technique for taking an oral temperature and caution against taking a rectal temperature.
Instructions to immediately report recurrence of fever to a nurse or physician.

FOLLOW-UP CARE

Anticipated care

If the client is not neutropenic and the cause of the fever is known or suspected:
• Physician visit within 1 week.

- Fever workup for each new fever.

If the client is neutropenic or potentially neutropenic:

- Same-day home visit by a nurse.
- Outpatient or home visits several times per week for blood testing or IV antibiotics.

Anticipated client/family questions and possible answers

Does having a fever mean I have an infection?

"Many things cause a fever; however, infection is one of the most common and most serious causes of a fever. Your fever will need to be evaluated to determine its cause so that you will receive the right treatment."

How serious is a fever, anyway?

"It can be very serious. Depending on what is causing your fever, the results can be fatal, if it is left untreated. Fevers are treated very safely and effectively if caught early."

Should I take acetaminophen to keep from having a fever?

"Take any medicine only as your doctor tells you to take it. Fever does serve as a signal that something is wrong. If you have a fever, your nurse and doctor want to know about it. You may be told to take medicine, such as acetaminophen, only after the cause of your fever has been found. Do not try to hide a fever or prevent your body from having one, and attempt such prevention only if your nurse or doctor tells you to take the acetaminophen."

Will a fever prevent me from receiving more chemotherapy?

"Your chemotherapy may be placed on hold until the cause of your fever is found. Once the cause is known and treated, your treatment schedule will most likely resume where you left off."

CHAPTER SUMMARY

Fever is one of the most common symptoms experienced by clients with cancer and by the client receiving treatment for cancer. Although fever can have many causes, it has special significance in the oncology client because 55 to 75% of fevers in this population are caused by infections, the sequelae of which may result in death. Whatever the cause, fever does serve as a valuable, and sometimes the only, signal that something is wrong or that an infection may be present. Suppression of fever without a proper diagnostic workup may prevent the clinician from identifying the cause of the fever, which can significantly alter favorable outcomes for the client.

TEST QUESTIONS

1. Which of the following is an endogenous pyrogen?
   A. Monocyte
   B. Interferon
   C. Neoplastic cells
   D. Bacteria

1. Answer: B
As an endogenous pyrogen, interferon is produced by host cells such as macrophages and monocytes. Monocytes, neoplastic cells, and bacteria are mediators of endogenous pyrogens.

2. During which phase or stage of fever do compensatory warming measures take place?
   A. Chill
   B. Plateau/Hot
   C. Defervescence
   D. Vasodilatation

2. Answer: A
During the chill phase, the set point temperature is shifted upward. A discrepancy is sensed between the new higher set point and the existing body temperature. The existing body temperature is sensed as cold, thus compensatory warming measures begin.

3. Which of the follow statements is *not* true of the pathophysiologic processes of fever?
   A. Fever is a product of thermoregulation.
   B. Fever is characterized by failure of compensatory cooling mechanisms.
   C. The body's thermoregulatory ability remains intact during the febrile response.
   D. Fever is a response to disease activity.

3. Answer: B
Failure of compensatory cooling mechanisms during a state of elevated body temperature is a characteristic of hyperthermia. In fever, also known as hyperpyrexia, thermoregulatory ability remains intact.

4. Nonsteroidal, antipyretic drugs reduce fever by:
   A. Affecting hypothalamic response to pyrogens
   B. Decreasing metabolic rate
   C. A vasodilation effect
   D. Secondary antimicrobial effects

4. Answer: A
Nonsteroidal antipyretic drugs, such as aspirin and acetaminophen, reduce fever by affecting hypothalamic response to pyrogens.

5. Clinical presentation of fever may include:
   A. Tachycardia, apnea
   B. Bradycardia, tachypnea
   C. Tachycardia, tachypnea
   D. Tachycardia, bradypnea

5. Answer: C
Fever causes increased basal metabolic rate and increased oxygen consumption by tissues. This results in increased cardiac output and workload. The body compensates by increasing the heart rate and increasing the respiratory rate.

6. Nursing interventions for the client with fever include all of the following *EXCEPT:*
   A. Hypothermia blankets
   B. Antipyretic drug therapy
   C. Alcohol baths
   D. Antimicrobial therapy

6. Answer: C
Alcohol baths should never be used because of the harmful effects of fumes.

7. Client teaching for the person at risk for developing fever at home may include:
   A. Oral temperature monitoring every 4 hours at home while the client is at risk.
   B. Instructions to notify a doctor or nurse within 72 hours if a fever is detected while at home.
   C. The warning that a fever with associated bradycardia could be the only reliable sign of an infection the client may have or be developing.
   D. Adding a humidifier to liquify air in order to decrease tachypnea and ultimately to decrease the basal metabolic rate.

7. Answer: A
For the client who is at risk for developing fever while at home, an oral temperature q4h is appropriate for detecting the early sign of fever, which should be reported immediately to the physician or nurse.

8. A fever may be the only reliable sign of _____ in the immunocompromised client.
   A. Immune status
   B. Allergic response
   C. Potential infection
   D. Drug reaction

8. Answer: A
In immunosuppressed clients, fever is often the only reliable sign of actual infection or sign of response to antimicrobial treatment. For this reason, antipyretic drugs are used only if the client is extremely uncomfortable or cannot tolerate the hypermetabolic state accompanying fever (Holtzclaw, 1992).

9. Although fever has many causes, it has special significance in
oncology because _____
of fevers in the cancer client are
caused by infections.
A. 10 to 20%
B. 25 to 45%
C. 30 to 50%
D. 55 to 75%

9. Answer: D
Infection is the cause of the majority of fevers in cancer clients. The
incidence of this complication is
reported as 55 to 75%.

10. Fever should be treated immediately in every client with
antipyretics and
antibiotics/antifungals because
the effects of untreated fever
are harmful.
A. True
B. False

10. Answer: B
It has been debated extensively
whether fever is beneficial or harmful. The benefits from fever include
an enhanced immune response of
the host, ranging from the activation of T-lymphocytes to the secretion of antibacterial chemicals. The
harmful effects of fever include
increased metabolic expenditure.

REFERENCES

Bruce JL, Grove SK: Fever: Pathology and treatment. Crit Care Nurse 12(1):40–49, 1992.

Burke MB, Wilkes GM, Berg DB, Bean CK, Ingwersen K: Cancer Chemotherapy: A Nursing Process Approach. Boston: Jones and Bartlett, 1991.

Gucalp R: Management of the febrile neutropenic patient with cancer. Oncology 5(7):137–144, 1991.

Guyton AC: Body temperature, temperature regulation, and fever. In Textbook of Medical Physiology, 8th ed. Philadelphia: WB Saunders Co, 1991, pp. 797–808 (Chap 73).

Henker R, Shaver J: Understanding the febrile state according to an individual adaptation framework. AACN Clin Iss in Crit Care 5(2):186–193, 1994.

Holtzclaw BJ: The febrile response in critical care: State of the science. Heart Lung 21(5):482–501, 1992.

Pizzo PA: Evaluation of fever in the patient with cancer. Eur J Cancer Clin Oncol 25(Suppl 2):s9–s16, 1989.

Pizzo PA: Management of fever in patients with cancer and treatment-induced neutropenia. New Engl J Med 328(18):1323–1330, 1993.

Pizzo PA, Meyers J: Infections in the cancer patient. In DeVita VT, Hellman S, Rosenberg SA (eds): Cancer Principles and Practice of Oncology, 3rd ed. Philadelphia: JB Lippincott, 1989, pp. 2088–2133.

Styrt B, Sugarman B: Antipyresis and fever. Arch Intern Med 150(8):1589–1597, 1990.

Wittes RE (ed): Manual of Oncologic Therapeutics, 2nd ed. Philadelphia: JB Lippincott, 1991–1992

Young LS: Fever and septicemia. In Rubin RH, Young LS (eds): Clinical Approach to Infection in the Compromised Host, 2nd ed. New York: Plenum Medical Book Company, 1988, pp. 75–114.

Chapter 13

GRAFT VS. HOST DISEASE

Margaret Quinn Rosenzweig, CRNP-C, MSN, AOCN

CHAPTER OBJECTIVES

At the completion of this chapter, the reader will be able to:

Define graft vs. host disease (GVHD).

Differentiate acute graft vs. host disease from chronic graft vs. host disease.

State identified risk factors associated with GVHD acute and chronic; morbidity; and mortality.

Describe nursing assessment and interventions for GVHD.

Anticipate present and future care needs in the client with acute and chronic GVHD.

OVERVIEW

GVHD is an immunologic reaction manifested in allogeneic bone marrow transplant (BMT) clients in response to their transplanted marrow. GVHD is manifested in two time frames in the post-transplant population: acute GVHD, seen in the first 100 days following transplantation, and chronic GVHD seen in the post-100-day time period. Of all allogeneic BMT clients up to 80% will manifest some form of acute graft vs. host disease and approximately 25% will succumb to this complication of transplantation (Vogelsanng, 1993).

Acute GVHD is a complication of marrow transplantation. The donor's lymphocytes recognize the client as "foreign" and attack the client. This is manifested in skin rash or in liver and gastrointestinal (GI) involvement (Shulman, 1993). Chronic graft vs. host disease, resembling a collagen vascular disorder, occurs in up to 50% of marrow transplants in which the human leukocyte antigens (HLAs) are identical (Atkinson, 1995). This usually occurs within 100 to 400 days following marrow transplantation. The overall incidence of GVHD increases with mismatched transplantation.

This chapter will discuss the risks, assessment, treatment, and prognosis along with specific nursing interventions for both chronic and acute graft vs. host disease.

DESCRIPTION

Indications for transplantation

Bone marrow transplantation is a revolutionary field within oncology care, used for a wide variety of hematologic and nonhematologic malignancies, including metabolic and immunologic causes. The underlying principle of marrow transplantation is very straightforward. Chemotherapy and radiation therapy utilized singly or in combination to ablate malignancies are administered in high doses. Without a regenerative source, bone marrow would be unable to rejuvenate, and the client would succumb to the complications of pancytopenia. Infusion of a marrow source serves as the precursor to marrow regeneration, serving essentially as "marrow rescue." In nonhematologic malignancies autologous marrow, or stem cells obtained from peripheral blood of the client prior to ablative therapy, can serve as the marrow source. In hematologic malignancies, concern regarding disease relapse triggers the search for alternative sources of marrow stem cells. Approximately one-quarter of the general population has an HLA-matched sibling donor, which allows allogeneic or "donor" transplantation (Rowe and Segel, 1993).

For the three-quarters of the population without a matched donor, other options exist. More hazardous treatment options include the use of mismatched siblings with "purged" marrow, or matched but unrelated donors (obtained through a national registry). Overall, GVHD increases with the degree of incompatibility. Interestingly, allogeneic transplantation, while offering fewer relapses, has the same 50% long-term survival rate as autologous marrow transplantation. Despite less disease relapse due to the complications of GVHD, the immunosuppression and infection seen in allogeneic transplant clients create significant morbidity and mortality.

Acute GVHD

GVHD is manifested in two forms: acute and chronic. While similar in risk potential, the entities are separate in pathogenesis and timing of occurrence. Acute GVHD is seen in identically and nonidentically HLA-matched allogeneic transplants. The knowledge regarding the pathophysiology is still evolving. Conventional thinking has been that GVHD is caused by donor immune cells reacting against antigens of the immunodepleted recipient. The pathophysiologic process is essentially the opposite of the solid organ "rejection" seen in traditional organ transplants. Conventional wisdom has held the mediator of this pathophysiologic process to be T-cells. Current research still implicates T-cells but also points to a "cytokine storm" secreted by T-cells. These cytokines mediate an inflammatory process and ultimately tissue damage that result in the clinical manifestations of GVHD (Theobald, 1995). A new understanding of the pathophysiologic role of cytokines in GVHD may lead to improved predictive indices and treatment (Ochs et al., 1994).

Graft vs. leukemia

Acute GVHD is not without perceived benefit. Relapse rates in leukemics are significantly higher in the autologous transplant group. In the allogeneic populations, relapse has occurred in 75% of leukemics with no GVHD and in 39% of those who developed GVHD, supporting a "graft vs. leukemia" (GVL) effect.

Clinical Manifestations

Typically, acute GVHD occurs, at its earliest, within 2 to 5 weeks following allogeneic transplantation. Acute GVHD is manifested clinically by skin rash, elevation in liver enzymes, and GI involvement, primarily manifested as diarrhea. Although not classic target organs, the mucous membranes, lungs, and bone marrow may be involved. Accurate assessment and grading are essential. Symptoms may present singularly or in constellation.

1. *Skin:* Macular rash appears anywhere on the skin surface, primarily the face, abdomen, and extremities. The skin initially appears as if it has been "sunburned," and the patient may complain of pruritus. Following the initial manifestations and depending on severity, the skin may form bullae and ultimately desquamate. Depending on the severity of the skin presentation, the desquamation and loss of skin integrity may present serious management issues for heat and fluid conservation and increase infection risks (see Table 13–1).

Table 13–1
Acute GVHD: Staging

Organ	Parameters	Stage
Skin	Rash	
	<25% BSA	I
	25–50% BSA	II
	Erythroderma	III
	Bullae/desquamation	IV
Liver	Total bilirubin (mg/dl)	
	2.0–3.5	I
	3.5–8.0	II
	8.0–15.0	III
	>15.0	IV
Gut	Diarrhea (volume)	
	500–1000 ml	I
	1000–1500 ml	II
	1500–2000 ml	III
	>2500 ml	IV

Source: Reprinted with permission, from Vogelsanng G: Acute graft vs. host disease following marrow transplantation. Marrow Transplant Rev 2(4):49–55, 1992/1993.

Table 13–2
Acute GVHD: Overall Clinical Stage

Stage	Description
0	Stage I clinical skin GVHD with grade II histology
I	Stage II clinical skin GVHD with grade > II histology
II	Stage II–III clinical stage GVHD with grade II histology and stage I clinical gut *and/or* liver
III	Stage II–IV clinical skin GVHD with grade II or greater histology and grade II–IV clinical liver and/or gut GVHD. Only one system stage III or greater.
IV	Stage III–IV clinical skin GVHD with grade II or greater histology and stage II–IV clinical liver and/or gut GVHD. Two or more systems stage III or greater.

Source: Reprinted with permission, from Vogelsanng G: Acute graft vs. host disease following marrow transplantation. Marrow Transplant Rev 2(4):49–55, 1992/1993.

2. *Liver:* The patient with acute GVHD presents classically with an elevated alkaline phosphatase and elevated bilirubin. In fractionation of the bilirubin, there is usually a pattern of indirect elevation, indicating increased liver metabolism (see Table 13-1). In more severe forms, liver involvement may lead to coagulopathies, hepatic failure, or metabolic encephalopathy. Early after transplantation the symptoms of veno-occlusive disease and hepatic GVHD may be difficult to delineate. Hepatic GVHD does not usually lead to the more systemic ascites or weight gain as in the clinical scenario of veno-occlusive disease (Vogelsanng, 1993).

3. *GI Tract:* Acute GVHD is manifested by acute, watery, explosive diarrhea. Quantity of output indicates severity. A recent consensus conference regarding the grading of GVHD recommended scoring persistent nausea without diarrhea as grade I GVHD if there is histologic confirmation (Przepiorka et al., 1995) (see Table 13-1).

Clients may develop one or all of the symptoms with varying levels of severity. The combined scores of skin, liver, and gut are then tabulated to give the overall grade, indicating the severity of the acute GVHD. It is imperative for the sake of data collection regarding incidence and treatment that accurate grading be completed (see Table 13-2).

Chronic GVHD

Chronic GVHD, while similar to acute GVHD in pathogenesis and treatment, is very dissimilar in timing after transplantation and clinical manifestations. Chronic GVHD develops within 3 to 24 months following allogeneic marrow transplantation in up to 50% of long-term survivors of allogeneic transplantation (Ochs et al., 1994).

Clinical manifestations are similar to autoimmune diseases, such as scleroderma, Sjögren's syndrome, and rheumatoid arthritis. They are present in the skin, oral mucosa, and liver as in acute GVHD but differ distinctly in manifestations involving the eye, oral mucosa, joints, and lungs. The classification of chronic GVHD is based on the client's previous experience with acute GVHD and extent of involvement. "De-Nova" characterizes clients with no documented acute GVHD, "quiescent" those with previous acute GVHD with complete resolution and then development of chronic GVHD, and "progressive" those with a history of acute GVHD who have progressed into chronic manifestations without complete resolution of the acute form. This last group represents by far the most common manifestation of chronic GVHD (Atkinson, 1995).

Staging is based on *limited* or *extensive* organ involvement (see Table 13–3). Chronic GVHD most commonly involves the skin (73%), oral mucosa (48%), liver (40%), GI tract (26%), eye (18%), lung (15%), and joints (12%) (Atkinson, 1995).

Immunosuppression resulting from chronic GVHD as well as the required immunosuppressive therapy, is significant. The most common bacterial infections are encapsulated gram-positive organisms. Viral varicella infections occur in up to 80% of clients with chronic GVHD. Late interstitial pneumonia can also be seen. While chronic GVHD may be less acutely life-threatening than acute GVHD, the quality-of-life issues involved with the symptom profile and the side effects of long-term treatment are significant.

Table 13–3
Criteria for the Diagnosis of Graft vs. Host Disease

Limited

Either or both:
1. Localized skin involvement.
2. Hepatic dysfunction due to chronic GVHD.

Extensive

1. Generalized skin involvement.
2. Localized skin involvement and/or hepatic dysfunction due to chronic GVHD, plus:
   a. Liver histology showing chronic aggressive hepatitis, bridging necrosis or cirrhosis, *or*
   b. Involvement of the eye: Schirmer's test with less than 5 mm wetting, *or*
   c. Involvement of the minor salivary glands or oral mucosa demonstrated by labial biopsy specimen, *or*
   d. Involvement of any other target organ.

Source: Used with permission, from Sullivan K: Acute and chronic graft vs. host disease in man. Int J Cell Cloning 4:42–93(Suppl 1), 1986.

RISK PROFILE

Not all allogeneic transplant clients develop GVHD. Allogeneic clients without some degree of immunosuppression will develop acute GVHD. The necessary commitment of all allogeneic clients to immunosuppression and its potential risks makes the "risk profile" of such clients increasingly important in marrow transplantation research. The potential to limit immunosuppression in clients with less GVHD risk is promising. The most critical risk factors for acute GVHD include:

1. Histoincompatability.
2. Allosensitization of both donor and recipient.
3. Age of both donor and client.
4. Sex mismatch of donor and recipient.
5. Omission of GVHD prophylaxis.
6. Infusion of viable donor leukocytes.
7. Intensity of the conditioning regimen.

As the understanding of the molecular basis of the pathophysiology of GVHD grows, the measurement of GVHD-mediating or GVHD-suppressing T-cells through cytokine assay analysis becomes increasingly important. The current direction of research is to preserve or increase GVL-mediating T-cells, while suppressing or ablating GVHD-mediating cells (Theobald, 1995).

The risk factors for chronic GVHD include all of the preceding risks, combined with the presence of acute GVHD. Seventy percent of clients with advanced acute GVHD develop chronic GVHD. Male recipients with female donors over the age of 18 years are also at high risk for chronic GVHD. Alloimmunization of the donor through pregnancy or transfusion is also a predominant risk factor. T-cell depletion has proved to be implicated more often than GVHD prophylaxis *in vivo* with standard immunosuppressive regimens. The presence of cytomegalovirus (CMV) or herpes seropositivity is implicated but not distinctly proven (Atkinson, 1995).

PROGNOSIS

The prognosis is variable for both acute and chronic GVHD and depends on grading and severity. Complete responses to treatment with high-dose corticosteroid as the cornerstone of therapy is 25%, with partial responses in 40% to 50% of clients treated with acute GVHD of stage II to IV severity (Deeg and Huss, 1994). Survival is poor for clients unresponsive to initial therapy. Infection is overwhelmingly the cause of death (Aschan, 1994).

The prognosis for clients with chronic GVHD, who have received an adequate course of immunosuppressive therapy is much better. Up to 90% of clients treated have reportedly been disease-free. Adequacy of the treatment is key. Thirty-five percent of clients treated adequately became disease-free with no long-term sequelae (Atkinson, 1995).

TREATMENT

The most optimal, indeed the imperative, treatment for GVHD is prophylaxis. All clients with HLA-matched transplants would develop GVHD without some post-transplant prophylaxis. Immunosuppression is the gold standard for prophylaxis utilizing methotrexate, cyclosporine, corticosteroids, antithymocyte globulin (ATG), and Fk-506 as single agents or in a multidrug regimen (Aschan, 1994). While multidrug regimens result in an overall decreased incidence of acute GVHD, the combination of drugs results in a higher toxicity profile (Deeg and Huss, 1994).

T-cell depletion, through *in vitro* removal of GVHD-mediating T-cells by means of mechanical or antibody processes, is the most effective method of GVHD prophylaxis. T-cell depletion, however, results in a higher incidence of graft failure and in increased incidence of disease relapse, particularly chronic myelogenous leukemia. This phenomenon again supports the necessary component of the GVHD mediators for engraftment and prevention of disease recurrence (Deeg and Huss, 1994).

Surgery: Not indicated.

Chemotherapy: Not indicated, unless used as an immunosuppressive.

Radiation: Not indicated.

Medications

Prophylaxis is the goal: Long-term cyclosporine therapy should be initiated following allogeneic transplantation with a slow taper. This dosing regimen is less likely to cause chronic GVHD (Atkinson, 1995). The treatment for established chronic GVHD is first a full dose of cyclosporine, then a high dose of prednisolone, tapered to a medium dose for 9 months. Thalidomide has shown great promise in early clinical studies.

Immunosuppressive agents: Once acute GVHD has been identified, aggressive immunosuppressive therapy needs to be initiated, based on the grading and severity of acute or chronic GVHD. Immunosuppressive medications utilized chronically as prophylaxis are usually intensified, depending on the severity of the GVHD. Performance status, immune status, and concurrent or potential infection are critical indications for re-admission of an outpatient.

Antibiotics: Infection prophylaxis is an important ingredient in the prevention and treatment of GVHD. Because of the combination of immunosuppression mediated from the chronic GVHD and the immunosuppressive drug therapy, infection prophylaxis against encapsulated gram-positive organisms, pneumocystis carinii pneumonia (PCP), and fungus is essential (Atkinson, 1995). As immunosuppression increases, so does infection risk. Viral and fungal organisms are of particular concern, and appropriate prophylactic antibiotics are often initiated with the onset of GVHD therapy.

IV immunoglobulin: Classically utilized in the BMT populations for infection prophylaxis, IV immunoglobulin may serve as GVHD prophylaxis, perhaps through interference with the recognition of antibodies to cellular antigens (Deeg and Huss, 1994).

Procedures: Other agents that have been utilized have been Psolorens and high-intensity ultraviolet A (PUVA) phototherapy for resistant chronic GVHD of the mouth and skin.

ASSESSMENT CRITERIA: GRAFT VS. HOST DISEASE

Assessment for GVHD, both acute and chronic, needs to be consistent and systematic. A complete review of systems for both the inpatient and outpatient will point to symptoms that may indicate GVHD. For acute GVHD the assessment should be focused on the target organs involved. Questions dealing with skin changes, changes in stool (color or consistency), or abdominal pain can denote beginning symptomatology. The classic seven questions pertaining to any symptom (timing, alleviating or exacerbating factors, setting, location, quality, quantity, and associated manifestations) will help to clarify the symptom and indicate severity (Bates, 1995).

Physical assessment for acute GVHD should be focused on the target organs. All BMT clients need to have thorough head-to-toe physical assessments. For skin assessment, acute GVHD initially has the appearance of sunburn progressing to desquamation. The extent of disease is determined by applying the "Rule of 9s," which is used primarily to determine the extent of burned body surface.

Assessment for hepatic GVHD involvement is based on liver function test analysis. The physical exam is essentially noncontributory. Liver tenderness or enlargement is not a common physical finding in acute GVHD.

Gut GVHD is graded according to the severity of diarrhea. Upper GI involvement may be manifested by persistent nausea. If GI symptoms are present in an allogeneic transplant client, the use of endoscopy to confirm GVHD is warranted.

Chronic GVHD presents in a similar fashion to a collagen-vascular disorder. The disease can involve any body system, manifesting itself in complaints of "dryness" of the mucous membranes to grittiness of the eyes. Physical exam findings are characteristic of the organs involved. Skin involvement may reveal pigmentary changes or patchy erythema with eventual thickening of the skin, which results in joint deformities. Involvement of the oral mucosa produces, in the earliest manifestations of GVHD, stria resembling lichen planus. If salivary glands are destroyed, dysphagia may be present, with resultant weight loss and decline in performance status. Liver involvement is manifested in an obstructive jaundice pattern. The sinuses, esophagus, intestines, lungs, and virtually all the organ systems can exhibit manifestations of chronic GVHD (Atkinson, 1995). (See the following table for a summary of assessment criteria for GVHD.)

Assessment Criteria: Graft vs. Host Disease

	Acute GVHD	Chronic GVHD
History	Usually skin rash followed by . diarrhea Feelings of malaise.	Quiescent or progressive acute GVHD.
Vital signs	Low-grade temp, hypovolemia with fluid depletion.	No significant changes.
Hallmark physical signs and symptoms		
Skin	Sunburnlike rash, progressive to blistering and desquamation.	Leathery, "scleroderma"-like skin. May be limited or extensive.
Liver	Elevation in bilirubin.	
Gut	Liquid diarrhea, measured in liters.	Constipation or diarrhea.
Other	Crampy abdominal pain, persistent nausea.	
Lab values		
Blood counts	Not usually affected.	
Chemistries	Elevated LFT. Albumin, electrolytes, magnesium may be low.	Abnormal LFT.
Diagnostic tests		
Endoscopy	Also sigmoidoscopy, colonoscopy for histologic confirmation of GVHD.	If dysphagia present.
Biopsy	Liver—if abnormal bilirubins, unclear etiology.	Liver—if abnormal LFT; lacrimal gland if indicated.
Pulmonary function tests		D_{CO}—diminished with obstructive pattern if pulmonary manifestations.

NURSING DIAGNOSIS

Because acute and chronic GVHD are manifested in a variety of symptoms, the nursing diagnosis will need to be tailored to each client. The most likely clinical scenarios are described in the following diagnoses.

Fatigue related to clinical manifestations of GVHD, both acute and chronic.

Fluid volume deficit related to diarrhea or loss of skin integrity with severe acute GVHD manifested in the skin and GI tract.

Diarrhea related to lower GI tract involvement of acute GVHD or GI manifestations of chronic GVHD.

Altered protection related to:

- Immunosuppression secondary to both acute and chronic GVHD.
- Loss of skin integrity.
- Gut involvement of GVHD, allowing alteration in GI mucosa.

Body image disturbance related to clinical manifestations of both acute and chronic GVHD and long-term steroid side effects.

Infection related to immunosuppression intrinsic to the pathology of GVHD.

Impaired physical mobility related to:

- Steroid effects.
- Possible contracture from chronic GVHD skin manifestations.
- Demands of treatment or illness, or both.

Knowledge deficit related to:

- Demands of the illness.
- Lack of knowledge base regarding pathophysiology and treatment.

NURSING INTERVENTIONS

Immediate nursing interventions

Vital signs, q2–4h immediately and then q6h.

Prepare client for biopsy procedure (endoscopy, skin).

NPO if necessary.

STAT chemistry panel.

Establish patent IV access.

Maintain strict intake and output (I and O); measure stool output.

Send stool for *Clostridium difficile.*

Anticipated physician orders and interventions

IV fluids, aggressively if dehydrated, then at 100 ml/hour.

Stool culture and sensitivity.

Strict I and O maintained; quantify stool.

Chemistry, complete blood count (CBC), with differential (DIFF), immunoglobulin levels.

Prophylactic amphotericin to be considered with confirmed GVHD of the gut.

Antidiarrheal and/or antiemetic medications.

Increase in immunosuppressive agents or change to continuous infusion rather than oral or intermittent dosage.

Medication regimens will vary but will generally include, initially, high-dose steroids.

Ongoing nursing assessment, monitoring, and interventions

Assess:
- Skin closely for progression of skin involvement.
- Skin for evidence of desquamation, breakdown.
- For nausea, diarrhea, GI dysfunction.
- Vital signs for evidence of dehydration.
- Temperature, vital signs, and other evidence of infection.

Measure:
- Vital signs q2h and PRN.
- Urine output.
- Stool output and associated symptoms.
- All fluid intake.
- Calorie count.

Send:
- Repeat liver function tests (LFTs) qd until trend is established.
- Daily electrolytes until stable.
- Stool cultures.
- Blood cultures if indicated.
- Appropriate pathology if biopsies obtained at bedside.

Implement:
- IV fluid replacement as prescribed.
- Antidiarrheal medications.
- Antibiotics as prescribed.
- Skin care: Do appropriate cleansing, lubrication, allowing debridement of loosened skin, then apply hydrogel dressings and secure with gauze (Ezzone and Camp-Sorrell, 1994).

TEACHING/EDUCATION

Increased immunosuppression: *Rationale:* When GVHD occurs T-lymphocytes may need to be suppressed in order to stop the inflammation reaction. Your drug treatment may need to be changed by using different drugs or by using the same drugs in larger doses or by giving them through a vein.

Accurate I and O: *Rationale:* When GVHD occurs you are at risk for dehydration. It is very important to carefully measure all your urine and stool output. Careful measurement helps us know how severe your GVHD is, if you are getting enough fluids, and how well the treatment is working.

Skin assessment: *Rationale:* Constant assessment of the skin is necessary in order to judge if the treatment is working. It is also important to quickly find and treat skin breakdown.

IV medications and fluids: *Rationale:* At first the treatment for GVHD has to be aggressive in order to get the process reversed. This initial treatment may require IV fluids and/or medicines.

Neutropenic precautions (if necessary): *Rationale:* GVHD can reduce your body's ability to fight infection. If your white count drops, neutropenic precautions may need to be instituted. These precautions generally include limitation of fresh fruits and vegetables, strict hand washing, and perhaps your visitors wearing masks.

Preparation for diagnostic procedures/biopsies: *Rationale:* It is very important to have tissue confirmation of the diagnosis of GVHD because the pathologist is able to determine its severity based on tissue analysis. The treatment of GVHD includes medicines with side effects. We do not want to commit a client to a treatment with potential side effects without tissue confirmation.

Preparation for long-term treatment with slow taper of immunosuppression: *Rationale:* The treatment of GVHD often involves a long-term commitment to steroids. This may require many months of steroids, with a slow taper in order to avoid recurrence.

EVALUATION/DESIRED OUTCOMES

1. The client will be in a neutral fluid balance within the first 24 hours.
2. The client will have documentation of involved sites and extent of involvement.
3. Increased immunosuppression will not result in iatrogenic infection.
4. The client and significant others will have an increased understanding of potential immunosuppression.

DISCHARGE PLANNING

The client with GVHD may need:

Teaching, upon discharge, about prophylaxis for recurrent GVHD.
Teaching regarding:
   • Signs and symptoms of GVHD, both acute and chronic.
   • Potential treatment of GVHD if GVHD develops.
Follow-up office, laboratory/diagnostic testing, and clinic appointments.

FOLLOW-UP CARE

Anticipated care

For early identification of GVHD:
   • Immediately following discharge from the BMT unit, most allo-

geneic clients are followed twice weekly, or more often in the BMT clinic. The outpatient clinic personnel need to be very familiar with the signs and symptoms of GVHD, both acute and chronic, in order to adequately triage clients in the clinic or by telephone.

- Most allogeneic clients are followed one to two times weekly in the first 100 days following transplantation, this period being considered the most critical for the development of graft rejection, acute GVHD, or infection.

After GVHD has occurred:

- If the client has been treated for acute or chronic GVHD and is in follow-up, he or she will need to be followed at least one or two times weekly during the steroid taper.
- If the client has a history of acute GVHD, he or she will need to be followed at least weekly after day 100 through the first year for chronic GVHD.

Anticipated client/family questions and possible answers

What is GVHD?

"GVHD is a process specific to clients with poor immune systems. It is caused by parts of your donor's immune system rejecting detected components of your immune system. Because your donor's immune system is "stronger," a reaction occurs. We are not sure why GVHD comes out in the skin, GI tract, or liver, but in the first 100 days after transplant, this development is likely to be seen. There is also a form of GVHD that is seen after 100 days, called chronic GVHD. This can develop almost anywhere, and the symptoms are related to the body part involved."

What can I do to avoid GVHD?

"The most important thing is to follow your medication and blood work schedule as you have been taught. Although we can predict somewhat who is more likely to get GVHD, any allogeneic transplant client may develop some form of it."

If I develop GVHD, is it reversible?

"Yes! It is very important to report any symptom immediately, particularly a skin rash or diarrhea. Depending on the severity of the GVHD, you may be admitted to the hospital or followed as an outpatient. Most likely your immunosuppressive medications will be increased and you will be watched closely."

CHAPTER SUMMARY

GVHD is a fascinating phenomenon that manifests primarily in the allogeneic BMT population. It has two forms, acute and chronic. Risk factors include age, degree of HLA mismatch, sex mismatch, and degree of alloimmunization. The best treatment for GVHD is prevention through immunosuppression. Intrinsic risks are present in immunosuppression. Through a better understanding of risk factors, a subset of allogeneic clients may have their immunosuppressive regimens safely reduced.

Assessment for GVHD or of documented GVHD must be systematic and thorough in order to gauge treatment effectiveness. Every assessment should include thorough skin assessment, quantification of stool output, and evaluation of liver enzymes. Treatment is directed toward aggressive immunosuppression. The prognosis is completely dependent on the stage of GVHD at presentation. Nursing focus, including client and family education, should be centered on fluid and electrolyte status, infection prophylaxis, long-term steroid effects, and psychosocial factors related to the chronicity of the disease.

TEST QUESTIONS

1. GVHD is a pathophysiologic reaction of graft and host tissue mediated by:
   A. T-cells only
   B. T-cells and cytokines
   C. Viruses
   D. Immunosuppressive agents

1. Answer: B
Until recently, conventional wisdom held that only T-cells mediated GVHD, but it is now known that many cytokines are released as part of the immunologic/inflammatory reaction that occurs.

2. The most commonly utilized immediate treatment option for clients with progressive acute or chronic GVHD is:
   A. Watchful waiting
   B. Increase in immunosuppressive therapy
   C. Decrease in infection prophylaxis
   D. Decrease in immunosuppressive therapy

2. Answer: B
If the GVHD increases in clinical significance, an immediate attempt to boost immunosuppression is almost always made. Infection prophylaxis may be augmented as well.

3. The most significant risk factor for GVHD is:
   A. Degree of histoincompatibility
   B. Sex mismatch
   C. Age
   D. ABO red cell typing

3. Answer: A
Histocompatibility is by far the most important risk factor. The degree of GVHD can be predicted based on histocompatibility. Although the other options are considered, they are not as singularly predictive.

4. Understanding the risk factors for GVHD has implications for:
   A. Increase in infection prophylaxis for all clients
   B. Potential decrease in immunosuppressive therapy for all clients
   C. Potential decrease in immunosuppressive therapy for some clients
   D. Potential elimination of immunosuppressive therapy in some clients

4. Answer: C
Understanding the risk factors will never eliminate the need for immunosuppression. The goal is a decrease in immunosuppression in appropriately chosen populations.

5. A common nursing diagnosis formed for all clients with GVHD is:
   A. Inability to meet fluid volume needs
   B. Hypokalemia
   C. Hypernatremia
   D. Inability to maintain coping mechanisms

5. Answer: A
Dehydration resulting from inability to maintain fluid intake is common in acute and chronic GVHD. It is a common nursing and medical concern.

6. A client requests information regarding the best way to avoid GVHD. Your best response would be:
   A. There is nothing you can do. It is really fate.
   B. Following a neutropenic diet and strict hand washing may assist you.
   C. Avoiding all contact with family and friends is an important step.
   D. Following your treatment regimen is the best preventative step.

6. Answer: D
Compliance with, in particular, immunosuppressive medications is the most important intervention in the prevention of GVHD. The other options are not true or are not particularly relevant to the prevention of GVHD.

7. The relationship between GVHD and possible prevention of leukemic reccurrence is best described as follows:
   A. The occurrence of GVHD is related totally to the patient's risk of disease relapse.
   B. The graft vs. leukemia (GVL) effect that may be present from GVHD is only present in autologous transplant recipients.
   C. There may be a protective or GVL effect in the cytokines that cause GVHD that assists with engraftment.
   D. GVHD treatment prevents recurrence of leukemia.

7. Answer: C
Because relapse rates among allogeneic transplant populations of leukemics who developed GVHD are significantly lower than among those with no GVHD, a GVL effect has been postulated, though it has yet to be fully explained.

8. How is the extent of involvement of skin GVHD measured?
   A. Any rash is described.
   B. Body surface area with any desquamation is evaluated.
   C. Histological analysis alone is used.
   D. The "Rule of 9" is applied to the body surface area for all involved skin.

8. Answer: D
The "Rule of 9" is applied to quantify the degree of skin involvement.

9. How is *chronic* GVHD quantified?
   A. By the degree of gut, liver, and skin involvement
   B. By the measurement that determines whether it is "limited" or "extensive"
   C. By grading the degree of skin rash
   D. By the degree of stool output

9. Answer: B
Quantification can only be completed through measurement determining "limited " or "extensive" involvement. Choices A, C, and D are appropriate for *acute* GVHD.

10. A determination of *acute* GVHD is based on what parameter(s)?
    A. Grading of skin, liver, and gut involvement
    B. Total amount of stool output
    C. Pathology results of skin biopsy
    D. Grading of BUN/creatinine toxicity

10. Answer: A
All three parameters must be considered in the assessment for acute GVHD.

REFERENCES

Aschan J: Treatment of moderate to severe acute graft vs. host disease: A retrospective analysis. Bone Marrow Transplant 14:601–607, 1994.

Atkinson K: Chronic Graft vs. Host Disease. *In* Atkinson K. (ed): Clinical Bone Marrow Transplantation. Cambridge: University Press, 1995, pp. 312–322.

Bates B: An Approach to Symptoms: A Guide to History Taking and Physical Examination. Philadelphia: JB Lippincott, 1995, pp. 31–61.

Bearman S: Bone marrow tranplantation. *In* Wood M, Bunn P (eds): Hematology/Oncology Secrets. Philadelphia: Hunley and Belfus, 1994, pp. 213–217.

Deeg HJ, Huss R: Acute graft vs host disease. Marrow Transplant 14(Suppl 4):297–309, 1994.

Ezzone S, Camp-Sorrell D (eds): Manual for Bone Marrow Transplant Nursing: Recommendations for Practice and Education. Pittsburgh: Oncology Nursing Society, 1994, p. 13.

Mangan K, Klump T, Rosenfeld CS, Shadduck R: Bone marrow transplantation. *In* Makowka L (ed): The Handbook of Transplantation Management. Austin, Tx: RG Landes,1991, pp. 322–400.

Ochs LA, Miller WJ, Fillipovich RJ, et al.: Predictive factors for chronic graft vs. host disease after histocompatible sibling donor marrow transplantation. Bone Marrow Transplant 13:455–460, 1994.

Przepiorka D, Weisdorf D, Martin P, Klingemann HG, Beatty P, Hows J, Thomas ED: Meeting Report. Consensus Conference on acute care grading. Bone Marrow Transplant 15:825–828, 1995.

Rowe JM, Segel GB: The leukemias. *In* Rubin P (ed): Multidisciplinary Approach for Physicians and Students. Clinical Oncology. Philadelphia: WB Saunders, 1993, pp. 455–486.

Shulman L: The normocytic anemias. *In* Robinson S, Reich P (eds): Hematology, Pathophysiologic Basis for Clinical Practice. Boston: Little, Brown, 1993, pp. 109–126.

Theobald M: Allorecognition and graft vs. host disease. Bone Marrow Transplant 15:489–498, 1995.

Vogelsanng G: Acute graft vs. host disease following marrow transplantation. Marrow Transplant Rev 2:(4):49–55, 1993.

CHAPTER 14

HEMORRHAGE SECONDARY TO CERVICAL CANCER

Patricia Novak-Smith, MS, RN, OCN

CHAPTER OBJECTIVES

At the completion of this chapter, the reader will be able to:

Identify risk factors for the development of hemorrhage in the presence of cervical cancer.

Identify the initial interventions to control bleeding in hemorrhage from cervical cancer.

Describe the nursing interventions appropriate to the care of the client with hemorrhage secondary to cervical cancer.

Anticipate the supportive and learning needs of the client newly diagnosed with cervical cancer.

OVERVIEW

HEMORRHAGE secondary to cervical cancer is a rare condition. It is usually associated with the presence of bulky necrotic tumor, which is characteristic of advanced stages of disease. Surface erosion of the cervix, which results secondary to the growth of cancer cells, exposes underlying capillary networks (Hatch, 1994). The surface of the tumor becomes irregular, friable, and prone to bleeding with contact. Spontaneous bleeding is more likely to occur with increasing tumor size and the associated process of neovascularization required to support growth. The risk of hemorrhage is greater in individuals who have not had routine gynecologic care on a regular basis because cervical cancer is more likely to reach an advanced stage without detection in this population.

DESCRIPTION

Risk for hemorrhage in cervical cancer may be anticipated from the knowledge of preinvasive and early invasive disease. Invasive cervical cancer is preceded by a lengthy period of cellular abnormality. Although the cellular appearance resembles malignancy, the abnormality is limited to the surface layers and does not penetrate the basement membrane. These preinvasive conditions, referred to as either cervical intraepithelial neoplasia (CIN) or squamous intraepithelial lesions (SILs) of low or high grade, are amenable to detection with routine exfoliative sampling by Papanicolaou (PAP) smear (Yoder and Rubin, 1992). Magnification of the cervix during colposcopic examination for preinvasive disease commonly reveals increased vascularity of the cervical microcirculation (Wiggins, Granai, Steinhoff, and Calabresi, 1995). As the cancer invades the cervical tissue, abnormal branching vessels, which arise in the cervical stroma, are pushed to the surface. The contour of the cervix becomes irregular and friable secondary to the loss of surface epithelium. Ulceration occurs as intercellular cohesiveness is lost (Hatch, 1994). Continued tumor growth results in a more expansive erosive surface. The tumor, which is now clearly visible, is classified as either (a) an ulcerative lesion, which creates a defect in the cervix or upper vagina; (b) an exophytic lesion, which protrudes from the cervix and may appear to replace it; or (c) an endophytic lesion, which distends the endocervix (Hoskins, Perez, and Young, 1993).

Sustained tumor growth is dependent on the development of new blood vessels. Angiogenesis is the process whereby blood vessels in the surrounding normal tissues are stimulated to increase in number. Subsequent infiltration of the expanding tumor mass by newly formed blood vessels supplies oxygen and nutrients necessary to sustain growth. Release of polypeptide angiogenic growth factor by tumor cells is thought to be the initiating mechanism for neovascularization (Liotta and Stetler-Stevenson, 1993; Templeton and Weinberg, 1995). The newly vascularized tumor is now capable of more rapid growth through local expansion and metastasis. Increased vascular supply, combined with a highly erosive cervical surface, contribute to the potential of hemorrhagic events.

Abnormal vaginal bleeding is frequently the initial symptom of cervical cancer that prompts the client to seek medical attention. Vaginal bleeding associated with earlier stages of disease is painless and intermittent, with postcoital spotting being the most frequently reported symptom (Hatch, 1994; Hoskins et al., 1993). Bleeding becomes more significant if tumor growth continues unabated and erosion into collateral branches of the extensive arterial network or the newly formed blood vessels occurs. Profuse spontaneous bleeding, or hemorrhage, may occur when an untreated and, in most cases, previously undiagnosed cervical cancer is present. On rare occasions, bleeding may be substantial, requiring the employment of resuscitative measures (Harwood-Nuss, Benrubi, and Nuss, 1987).

RISK PROFILE

Cancers: Cervical cancer (squamous cell histology most common, followed by adenocarcinoma and adenosquamous carcinoma).

Conditions: Lack of routine gynecologic exam with PAP smear; previous untreated or undertreated abnormal PAP smear.

Environment: Decreased access to health care; lower socioeconomic class.

Foods: None.

Drugs: Anticoagulants (heparin, warfarin, ticlopidine); aspirin, ibuprofen, and other nonsteroidal anti-inflammatory drugs (NSAIDs), which cause inhibition of platelet aggregation and prolonged bleeding time.

PROGNOSIS

Control of hemorrhage secondary to cervical cancer through the use of firm vaginal packing and the initiation of external radiation are successful in almost 95% of cases. Four to 5% of clients may experience recurrence of bleeding when vaginal packing is removed, thus necessitating repacking with continuation of radiation until higher cumulative dosing has been achieved. Less than 1% of clients may have uncontrolled bleeding.

TREATMENT

Surgery: Not indicated.

Chemotherapy: Radiation sensitization with 5-fluorouracil, cisplatin, or hydroxyurea may be initiated.

Radiation: External beam radiation to pelvis in daily fractions of 300 to 400 cGy for 3 to 4 days followed by decreased daily fractions of 180 to 200 cGy to maximum dosage to promote tumor shrinkage and damage to hemorrhagic surface blood vessels. Treatment is administered over 5 to 6 weeks and is followed by intracavitary radiation (brachytherapy). Radiation therapy produces cell death directly through damage to deoxyribonucleic acid (DNA) and ribonucleic acid (RNA) and indirectly through the production of cell-toxic free radicals (Hilderley, 1992).

Medications

IV isotonic, crystalloid, and colloid solutions for hypovolemia.
IV pressors for hypotension.
Supplemental oxygen for hypoxemia secondary to blood loss.
Transfusion with packed red blood cells (RBCs) to maintain hematocrit above 30% to maximize tissue oxygenation during radiation therapy.
Fresh frozen plasma and/or vitamin K intramuscularly or intravenously for correction of coagulopathy.
IV broad-spectrum antibiotic coverage for prevention of sepsis/toxic shock syndrome (TSS).

Procedures

Insertion of vaginal gauze packing to promote hemostasis. Ferric subsulfate solution may be applied to proximal end of gauze packing for chemical cautery effect.

Insertion of indwelling urinary catheter to monitor urine output and alleviate pressure on bladder secondary to vaginal pack.

Placement of triple lumen IV catheter to monitor central venous pressure (CVP) and to facilitate administration of blood products, IV fluids, and antibiotics.

Placement of Swan-Ganz catheter to monitor cardiovascular status in the case of hypovolemic or septic shock.

Arteriogram with potential arterial embolization in the event of massive, uncontrolled bleeding.

Other: Use of medical antishock trousers (MAST) to improve cardiac blood supply.

The majority of clients with hemorrhage from cervical cancer experience initial control of bleeding with the insertion of vaginal packing and the immediate initiation of external beam radiation therapy. In very rare instances, hemorrhage may continue unabated despite these measures. The use of arterial embolization for the successful control of pelvic hemorrhage has been suggested (Yamashita et al., 1994). Despite the reported efficacy of this procedure, it is not widely used. The resulting reduction in vascularization of the primary tumor can decrease the efficacy of subsequent radiation therapy treatments. Radiation therapy produces greater cell-kill when the tumor is more vascular and well oxygenated (Shingleton and Orr, 1995). Since embolization produces the opposite effect, attempts to control bleeding with pressure and radiation therapy are preferred whenever possible.

ASSESSMENT CRITERIA: HEMORRHAGE SECONDARY TO CERVICAL CANCER

Vital signs

Temperature	Subnormal or normal
Pulse	Tachycardia (>100 per minute); weak and/or thready
Respirations	Shortness of breath, tachypnea
Blood pressure	Decreased (systolic BP <90 mm Hg)
CVP	Decreased (<8 mm Hg)

History

Symptoms, conditions	Lack of routine gynecologic care for ≥5 years
	Previous untreated abnormal PAP smear
	Irregular, intermenstrual, postcoital bleeding
	Heavier menses
	Underlying coagulopathy
	Increased use of aspirin, ibuprofen products

Hallmark physical signs and symptoms	Agitation; cold, clammy skin; confusion; diaphoresis; disorientation; pallor; profuse vaginal bleeding.

ASSESSMENT CRITERIA: HEMORRHAGE
SECONDARY TO CERVICAL CANCER (continued)

Additional physical signs and symptoms	Fatigue

Psychosocial signs	Anxiety, confusion, disorientation, fear

Lab values

Hemoglobin and hematocrit	Decreased
Potassium	Decreased
PT, PTT	Normal or increased

Diagnostic tests

Cervical biopsy	Confirm diagnosis of cervical cancer; confirm histology (squamous cell, adenocarcinoma, adenosquamous).
Pelvic exam	Determine degree of tumor extension (stage). May be performed under anesthesia.
Cystoscopy and/or proctoscopy	Evaluate for bladder or bowel invasion if suspected. May be performed at time of exam under anesthesia.
Chest x-ray	Evaluate for lung metastasis.
Abdominal/pelvic CAT scan	Evaluate for ureteral obstruction, lymphadenopathy, and distant metastasis. Also used for radiation planning.

NURSING DIAGNOSIS

Risk for fluid volume deficit secondary to blood loss, which may be of a chronic and irregular nature over a period of months or an acute process with sudden, profuse bleeding.

Risk for infection secondary to necrotic tumor mass in which vaginal colonization with bacteria has access to systemic circulation.

Decreased cardiac output related to acute blood loss and fluid volume depletion.

Fatigue associated with acute or chronic blood loss and subsequent bone marrow toxic radiation treatment.

Fear related to:
- News of cancer diagnosis.
- Administration of radiation therapy.
- Recurrence of bleeding.

(Potential for) acute confusion secondary to hypoxemia associated with hypovolemia and possible sepsis.

NURSING INTERVENTIONS

Immediate nursing interventions

Assess temperature, pulse, respirations, and blood pressure q15min × 2 hours, then q1h × 8 hours.

Establish peripheral IV access with large-bore catheter.

Send STAT complete blood count (CBC), electrolytes, prothrombin time (PT), partial thromboplastin time (PTT).

Draw blood sample for type and crossmatch in anticipation of blood transfusion.

Insert indwelling urinary catheter.

Initiate hourly intake and output (I and O).

Anticipated physician orders and interventions

STAT CBC, chemistry panel, PT, PTT.

Serial hemoglobin and hematocrit q6h.

Typing and crossmatching for 2 units packed RBCs; keep 2 units ahead at all times.

Transfusion of 2 units packed RBCs if hematocrit < 30% or uncontrolled and profuse bleeding is present.

Cervical biopsy followed by insertion of vaginal packing with rolled gauze.

Central venous catheter placement to monitor fluid status and to administer blood, IV fluids, and antibiotics.

CVP q4h. Notify physician if < 8 cm H_2O or > 15 cm H_2O.

I and O measurement. Notify physician if urinary output < 30 ml/hour.

Indwelling urinary catheter to gravity drainage.

IV fluids (D5 0.9% NaCl or D5 0.45% NaCl) at 100 to 200 ml/hour until CVP indicates adequate intravascular volume, then change to 10 ml/hour to keep vein open or saline lock IV access.

Oxygen per nasal cannula—titrate to maintain 0_2 saturation > 90%.

Triple antibiotic coverage for prevention of sepsis/TSS.

Vaginal packing in place—notify physician for breakthrough bleeding.

STAT radiation therapy consult.

Ongoing nursing assessment, monitoring, and interventions

Assess:
- For breakthrough vaginal bleeding q1h × 24 hours.
- For signs of hypovolemia (CVP < 8, tachycardia, decreased blood pressure [BP], decreased urine output < 30 ml/hour, hematocrit < 30%).
- For fluid overload (CVP > 15 cm H_2O, increased BP, jugular vein distention [JVD], peripheral edema, dyspnea, tachypnea, rales).
- For signs of sepsis or TSS (CVP < 8 cm H_2O, tachycardia, decreased BP, subnormal or elevated temperature, O_2 desaturation, confusion, agitation).

Measure:
- Temperature, pulse, respirations, blood pressure q4h.
- CVP q4h.

- I and O q1h × 8 hours, then q8h.
- Arterial blood gas (ABG) q8h until hematocrit > 30, then pulse oximetry q8h.
- Weight qd.

Send:
- CBC q6h × 4 hours.
- Repeat serum electrolytes qd.
- Blood cultures, urine culture if temperature ≥38° C or ≥100.4° F.

Implement: bedrest.

TEACHING/EDUCATION

Cervical cancer: *Rationale:* You have a tumor on the cervix, which is the opening to the uterus. Your doctor thinks this is probably a cancer. We will know for sure when the biopsy report comes back. The tumor is large, and it is bleeding because the tissue around it is damaged.

Vaginal packing: *Rationale:* The gauze has been inserted in the vagina to put pressure on the cervix to stop the bleeding, just as you would hold pressure on a cut you could see. The gauze will need to stay in place for a few days to make sure the bleeding has stopped.

Indwelling urinary catheter: *Rationale:* The gauze in the vagina puts pressure on the bladder and will make you feel as though you have to urinate all the time. The tube will drain the urine from the bladder so you won't be so uncomfortable. It also helps us measure how much urine your kidneys are making so we can make sure you are getting the right amount of fluid back into your body through your IV catheter.

IV central catheter: *Rationale:* This is a special catheter that can measure the fluid pressure in your heart so the doctors know whether you need more or less fluid. You have been losing large amounts of blood, and we will need to replace it along with some IV fluid. We can also give you other medications and draw blood samples from it.

Blood transfusion: *Rationale:* You have lost a large amount of blood over a short period of time. Your body will not be able to replace it as rapidly as you have lost it. The blood transfusions help to replace this lost volume, bring your pulse and blood pressure back to normal, and replace the red blood cells that carry oxygen in the body.

Radiation therapy: *Rationale:* X-ray therapy will be used to shrink the tumor. The radiation damages the tumor cells, causing them to die. Once this happens, the tumor will start to get smaller. This will also help to stop and control the bleeding. External radiation is given 5 days a week for about 5 to 6 weeks. This is followed by internal radiation treatments in which the radioactive source is inserted into the vagina and placed next to the cervix. You will be re-admitted to the hospital for a few days for this treatment.

Oxygen: *Rationale:* Since you have lost a lot of blood, there are fewer red blood cells to carry oxygen in your body. This may be why you feel tired. You probably won't need this for more than a few days—just until the bleeding stops and your blood level is stable.

EVALUATION/DESIRED OUTCOMES

1. The client has no breakthrough vaginal bleeding for 72 hours with packing in place.
2. Blood pressure, pulse, respirations, and CVP are within normal limits for client within 24 hours.
3. Hematocrit stable at ≥30% within 48 hours.
4. Radiation therapy initiated within 24 hours of client admission.
5. The client has no evidence of sepsis or TSS for duration of vaginal packing.
6. The client has no recurrence of vaginal bleeding for 24 hours after the packing has been removed.

DISCHARGE PLANNING

The client with hemorrhage secondary to cervical cancer may need:

Social service consultation for assessment of financial status for continued treatment.
Arrangement of transportation for daily outpatient radiation therapy.

FOLLOW-UP CARE

Anticipated care

Daily radiation therapy for 5 to 6 weeks followed by intracavitary radiation.
Possible outpatient chemotherapy.
Weekly outpatient CBC.
Weekly office visit and pelvic exam with radiation oncologist.
Office visit with gynecologic oncologist in 3 to 4 weeks.
Support group referral.

Anticipated client/family questions and possible answers

Will there be any more bleeding?
"Although the acute bleeding will be under control before you leave the hos-

pital, you could possibly have more episodes of hemorrhage within the next week or two. This will be less of a threat as you continue the radiation therapy treatments and the tumor shrinks."

"You may continue to have some light vaginal bleeding or spotting throughout the time you receive the radiation treatments. This happens as the tumor cells die and are shed from the body."

Will I need to receive more blood transfusions?

"You may require additional blood transfusions if the vaginal bleeding continues during the radiation treatments."

"Radiation treatments to the pelvis can interfere with the ability of the bone marrow in the pelvis to produce red blood cells. You may need a blood transfusion if the bone marrow can't keep up with the normal process of replacement of red blood cells even if the bleeding has stopped."

Why does the radiation take so long?

"Only a small portion of the total amount of radiation needed to kill the cancer can be given daily. Larger doses of radiation will cause more damage to the healthy tissue of the pelvis. Smaller daily doses of radiation given over several weeks will still kill the cancer cells, but the damage to noncancerous tissue is less."

Will I be radioactive?

"Receiving external radiation treatments does not make your body radioactive. The radioactivity comes from the machine that delivers the treatment."

"When you are hospitalized for the internal radiation treatments, a radioactive source is placed next to the cervix. The radioactivity comes from this source. Once it is removed, there is no possibility that your body can give off radiation."

Why can't the cancer be removed surgically?

"The cancer is too large to remove with surgery. Since it has probably been there for a long time, it has had a chance to spread to the tissue around the cervix. This reduces the possibility that the whole tumor could be removed without leaving cancer cells at the edge that was cut."

"The cancer is large and has spread all the way to the pelvic bone. It is not possible to surgically remove all the involved tissue or bone."

"The cancer has spread to lymph nodes outside the pelvis. They cannot all be removed with surgery."

CHAPTER SUMMARY

Hemorrhage in cervical cancer is the result of unabated tumor growth with the commensurate development of supporting vascularization. It may be the mechanism by which the client becomes aware of the presence of an advanced malignancy. Treatment modalities and nursing interventions are aimed at

achieving hemostasis, replacing lost fluid volume, and preventing septic complications. Radiation therapy is initiated urgently for long-term stasis through the
reduction in tumor bulk and damage to hemorrhagic surface blood vessels.

TEST QUESTIONS

1. Hemorrhage in cervical cancer is:
   A. Common with preinvasive dis-
      ease
   B. Associated with advanced stages
      of disease
   C. Precipitated by PAP smear sam-
      pling
   D. Related to normal menstruation

1. Answer: B
Spontaneous, profuse bleeding is
associated with large, bulky tumor
that has spread to surrounding tissues and that stimulates the growth
of new and extensive blood vessels.

2. Abnormal vaginal bleeding is
   most commonly reported by the
   client with cervical cancer:
   A. Following intercourse
   B. As soon as it occurs
   C. As intermittent and painful
   D. As a variance of menstrual
      bleeding

2. Answer: A
Postcoital bleeding is the most common pattern of abnormal bleeding
that prompts women to seek medical care.

3. Tumor angiogenesis contributes to
   the potential for hemorrhage in
   cervical cancer by:
   A. Releasing polypeptide angio-
      genic growth factor
   B. Increasing ulceration of the
      surface of the cervix
   C. Decreasing the vascular supply
      to the cervix
   D. Increasing the vascular supply
      to the cervix

3. Answer: D
Angiogenesis is the process whereby blood venules and capillaries in
surrounding normal tissue are stimulated to grow and form new vessels. Increased blood vessel growth
results in a vascular tumor surface
prone to spontaneous bleeding and
hemorrhage.

4. The main factor that contributes
   to the development of advanced
   cervical cancer is:
   A. Treatment for a previous
      abnormal PAP smear
   B. Family history of cervical cancer
   C. Absence of routine gynecologic
      exam including PAP smear for
      ≥5 years
   D. Dysmenorrhea

4. Answer: C
Cervical cancer is preceded by a
lengthy preinvasive state that is
amenable to detection with routine
PAP smear screening. Advanced disease is more common in clients
who have not had routine gynecologic care.

5. Treatment of hemorrhage in cervical cancer is directed at:
   A. Immediate control of the bleeding and initiation of external beam radiation therapy
   B. Identification of the bleeding vessel(s) through arteriography
   C. Arterial embolization of the pelvic vasculature
   D. Maintaining nutrition to the tumor

5. Answer: A
The insertion of vaginal packing promotes hemostasis of the bleeding tumor mass. Initiation of radiation therapy promotes tumor shrinkage and subsequent occlusion of hemorrhagic surface blood vessels.

6. IV antibiotics are administered for the duration of the vaginal packing because:
   A. Gauze packing is no longer sterile once it is placed in the vagina
   B. Septic shock may develop secondary to colonization of the vagina with bacteria
   C. Antibiotics act as radiation sensitizers
   D. Indwelling urinary catheter placement may introduce bacteria to the urinary tract

6. Answer: B
In the presence of superabsorbent packing, bacteria that colonize the vagina proliferate. Access to the systemic circulation through an erosive cervical surface and the process of tumor angiogenesis may lead to the development of sepsis or toxic shock syndrome.

7. Radiation therapy causes cell death through:
   A. Reduction in the delivery of cell nutrients
   B. Increased oxygenation of intracellular medium
   C. Damage to DNA and RNA
   D. Interference with the production of free radicals

7. Answer: C
Radiation therapy directly causes cell death through damage to DNA and RNA, thus preventing cell replication.

8. *Initial* nursing interventions for clients with hemorrhage in cervical cancer are directed at:
   A. Preventing septic shock
   B. Assessment of psychosocial support
   C. Preparing the patient for cervical biopsy
   D. Preventing hypovolemic shock

8. Answer: D
Initial nursing interventions in hemorrhage secondary to cervical cancer are concerned with correction of sudden volume depletion.

9. Follow-up care for the client with hemorrhage secondary to cervical cancer is most significant for:
   A. Adherence to the radiation treatment plan
   B. Initiation of chemotherapy
   C. Continuation of oral antibiotics
   D. Completion of diagnostic procedures to determine the extent of disease

9. Answer: A
The control of bleeding in cervical cancer is contingent on reduction of tumor bulk through the continuation of daily radiation therapy.

10. The desired outcome for a hospitalized client with hemorrhage secondary to cervical cancer is:
   A. Prevention of thrombotic events
   B. Absence of bleeding for 24 hours after vaginal packing has been removed
   C. Initiation of radiation therapy within 72 hours of admission
   D. Utilization of arterial embolization to control bleeding

10. Answer: B
Spontaneous, profuse bleeding is associated with large, bulky tumor that has spread to surrounding tissues and that stimulates the growth of new and extensive blood vessels. To stop this bleeding, vaginal packing is inserted, then removed when bleeding has stopped; a waiting period of 24 hours ensues for assessment of further bleeding. The goal is absence of bleeding 24 hours after the vaginal packing has been removed, at which time the client is discharged.

REFERENCES

Harwood-Nuss AL, Benrubi GI, Nuss RC: Management of gynecologic emergencies. Emerg Med Clin North Am 5(3):577–599, 1987.

Hatch KD: Cervical cancer. In Berek JS, Hacker NF (eds): Practical Gynecologic Oncology, 2nd ed. Baltimore: Williams and Wilkins, 1994, pp. 243–283.

Hilderley LJ: Radiation oncology: Historical background and principles of teletherapy. In Dow KH, Hilderley LJ (eds): Nursing Care in Radiation Oncology. Philadelphia: WB Saunders Co, 1992, pp. 3–15.

Hoskins WJ, Perez CA, Young RC: Gynecologic tumors. In DeVita VT, Hellman S, Rosenberg SA (eds): Cancer Principles and Practice of Oncology, 4th ed. Philadelphia: JB Lippincott, 1993, pp. 1152–1225.

Liotta LA, Stetler-Stevenson WG: Principles of molecular cell biology of cancer: Cancer metastasis. In DeVita VT, Hellman S, Rosenberg SA (eds): Cancer Principles and Practice of Oncology, 4th ed. Philadelphia: JB Lippincott, 1993, pp. 134–149.

Shingleton HM, Orr JW: Cancer of the Cervix. Philadelphia: JB Lippincott, 1995.

Templeton, DJ, Weinberg RA: Principles of cancer biology. In Murphy GP, Lawrence W, Lenhard RE (eds): American Cancer Society Textbook of Clinical Oncology, 2nd ed. Atlanta: American Cancer Society, 1995, pp. 164–177.

Wiggins DL, Granai CO, Steinhoff MM, Calabresi P: Tumor angiogenesis as a prognostic factor in cervical carcinoma. Gynecol Oncol 56(3):353–356, 1995.

Yamashita Y, Harada M, Yamamoto H, Miyazaki T, Takahashi M, Miyazaki K, Okamura H: Transcatheter arterial embolization of obstetric and gynaecological bleeding: Efficacy and clinical outcome. Br J Radiol 67(798):530–534, 1994.

Yoder L, Rubin M: The epidemiology of cervical cancer and its precursors. Oncol Nurs Forum 19(3):485–493, 1992.

CHAPTER 15

HEMORRHAGIC CYSTITIS

Jane Stearns, RN, MSN

CHAPTER OBJECTIVES

At the completion of this chapter, the reader will be able to:

Explain hemorrhagic cystitis and its significance for oncology clients.

State the risk factors associated with hemorrhagic cystitis in the oncology client.

Discuss treatment options for hemorrhagic cystitis.

Describe nursing care as it relates to oncology clients with hemorrhagic cystitis.

Anticipate and prepare the client with hemorrhagic cystitis for future care needs.

OVERVIEW

HEMORRHAGIC cystitis is an irritation of the bladder that ranges from microscopic hematuria to acute exsanguinating hematuria. When discussing hemorrhagic cystitis in the oncology client, it is important to know that it is a condition primarily induced by oxazaphosphorine alkylating chemotherapeutic drugs such as cyclophosphamide (Cytoxan), ifosfamide (Ifex), and radiation. It can also be caused by other chemicals, such as dyes, insecticides, and recreational drugs. Antibiotics, viruses, thrombocytopenia, and idiopathic etiologies such as rheumatoid arthritis have also been known to cause hemorrhagic cystitis (DeVries and Freha, 1990). The onset of hemorrhagic cystitis is variable. It can occur immediately after the first dose of chemotherapy or be delayed for several months or even years after treatment has been discontinued. Long-term treatment with Cytoxan or ifosfamide can lead to chronic fibrosis or hemorrhage. It has been reported that the incidence of hemorrhagic cystitis ranges from 4% to approximately 24% of those treated with the chemotherapeutic compounds mentioned earlier (Stillwell, Benson, and Burgert, 1988). Additionally, bone marrow transplant (BMT) clients treated with high doses of Cytoxan are at increased risk for developing hemorrhagic cystitis with an incidence of approximately 13 to 56% (Thomas, Patterson, Prentice, et al.,

1987). The occurrence of hemorrhagic cystitis has been associated with increased length of hospitalization, mortality, and morbidity.

DESCRIPTION

Chemically induced hemorrhagic cystitis is caused by the metabolites of cyclophosphamide (Cytoxan) and its structural analogue ifosfamide (Ifex). Cytoxan is broken down or metabolized by hepatic microsomal enzymes to the compound phosphoamide mustard, an active antineoplastic metabolite and acrolein, an inactive urinary metabolite (Schoenike and Dana, 1990) (see Table 15-1). Ifosfamide is metabolized to ifosfamide mustard and acrolein.

The alkylating agents do not have specific action on the bladder, but their metabolites do affect it. The entire urothelium can be affected by these metabolites, but the bladder is the most frequently involved organ. The major source of urothelial toxicity is urinary excretion of the acrolein (Cox, 1979). The binding of the acrolein to the bladder mucosa can result in inflammation, erythema, partial or complete ulceration, necrosis, hemorrhage, and reduced bladder capacity (Stillwell and Benson, 1988).

Glutathione, a naturally occurring thiol, protects cells by allowing the cells to break down chemotherapeutic metabolites and diminish the toxic effects. In urine, however, glutathione is present in very low levels (Cox, 1979; Shaw and Graham, 1987). Mesna, a thiol compound and a uroprotectant, was developed to bind with toxic metabolites and form nontoxic compounds in the urine. Urinary cytology studies commonly indicate that clients who develop Cytoxan-induced hemorrhagic cystitis display abnormal, atypical epithelial cells, characterized by increased nuclear size and strangely shaped cytoplasm.

Cystitis normally improves within several days after discontinuation of the toxic chemotherapeutic drug, but occasionally it can persist for months to years. When therapy is not stopped, according to Shepherd and colleagues (1991), up to 55% of clients can have persistent symptoms. Clients with

---

Table 15–1
Cyclophosphamide Metabolic Breakdown

Cytoxan
↓
Hydroxycyclophosphamide
↓
Aldophosphamide
↓
Phosphoamide mustard and acrolein
(active antineoplastic metabolite)   (inactive urinary metabolite)

Table 15-2
Grades of Hematuria

0 = None
1 = Micro only
2 = Gross, no clots
3 = Gross, with clots
4 = Gross, exsanguinating

hemorrhagic cystitis can present with any one or a combination of the following symptoms: dysuria, frequency, urgency, suprapubic discomfort, blood clots, and microscopic-to-gross exsanguinating hematuria. Hematuria is graded on a scale of 0 to 4 (see Table 15–2). Shepherd et al. (1991) also report that extensive chronic bleeding can lead to long-term cystitis, bladder fibrosis, bladder contraction, and an increased risk for bladder cancer.

RISK PROFILE

Cancers: Clients undergoing radiation for cervical, uterine, bladder, prostate, or rectal cancer can suffer direct or indirect damage to the bladder that could result in hemorrhagic cystitis. The risk is increased if a client has had multiple radiation treatments or high-dose radiation, previous surgery, persistent urinary tract infections, or intravenous Cytoxan in combination with radiation (Jayalakshamamma and Pinkel, 1976; DeVries and Freha 1990). According to Levenback, Eifel, Burke, Morris, and Gershenson (1994), the median time from the beginning of radiation treatments to the onset of hemorrhagic cystitis was approximately 35 months.

Conditions

Intravesical phototherapy: Treatment for superficial bladder tumors often involves the administration of an IV photosensitizer, which can lead to irritation, suprapubic discomfort, urgency, urge incontinence, acute and chronic inflammation, and hemorrhage (Prout et al., 1987).

Conditioning regimens for BMT: Regimens with high doses of Cytoxan increase the risk of hemorrhagic cystitis 13 to 56%. Prior treatment with busulfan also increases the risk compared to clients on the same regimen without prior exposure to busulfan (Thomas et al., 1987). Other contributing factors that may lead to hemorrhagic cystitis during a BMT are prior radiation treatments, bladder catheterization, infections, medications, or thrombocytopenia.

Viruses: Viruses have been associated with hemorrhagic cystitis in BMT clients, either as new infections, viral reactivations, or latent forms of the virus (Ambinder et al., 1986). Clients who have had viruses can develop hematuria approximately 55 days after transplantation, compared to 27 to 29 days for those with idiopathic hemorrhagic cystitis. The viral type of cystitis has a longer duration than idiopathic cystitis (Arthur, Shak, Baust, Santos, and Saral, 1986). Hemorrhagic cystitis has also been associated with the excretion of the BK type of polyomavirus in clients following a BMT (Bedi et al., 1995) (see Table 15–3).

Pediatrics: Sterile urine, accompanied by irritative voiding symptoms and hematuria could be caused by viral cystitis (Devries and Frehas 1990).

Environment: Insecticides and dyes have been known to cause hemorrhagic cystitis.

Foods: None.

Drugs

Cyclophosphamide (Cytoxan) and ifosfamide (Ifex) are the two major chemicals responsible for hemorrhagic cystitis in oncology clients. Damage to the bladder can be cumulative but dose-limiting. Cystitis occurs frequently and early after IV chemotherapy treatments, especially in high-dose regimens. Oral Cytoxan can cause hemorrhagic cystitis to develop weeks after treatment, but it has also been observed after just one or two doses. Long-term therapy often produces both acute hemorrhagic cystitis and chronic bladder fibrosis.

DeVries and Freha (1990) report that other chemotherapeutic agents can cause hemorrhagic cystitis even though they are not normally associated with bladder toxicity. Busulfan and bleomycin are two of these agents. The researchers also report that cisplatin, VM-26, and vincristine can have a synergistic effect and result in similar bladder toxicities.

Intravesical treatment for superficial bladder cancer with chemotherapy or biologic modifiers such as thiotepa, doxorubicin, mitomycin C, and bacillus Calmette-Guérin can also cause cystitis with or without hematuria (DeVries and Freha 1990; Lamm, Stogdill, Stogdill, and Crispen, 1986).

Pediatrics: Bladder fibrosis, severe hematuria, and telangiectasis are more common in pediatric clients receiving cyclophosphamide (Stillwell, Benson, and Burgert, 1988). Children undergoing chemotherapy with Cytoxan develop hemorrhagic cystitis with lower doses and shorter durations of treatment (Stillwell et al., 1988).

Antibiotics: Another source of hemorrhagic cystitis can be antibiotics used to treat chemotherapeutic-related infections. The incidence of antibiotic related hemorrhagic cystitis is 4% for oncology clients (DeVries and Freha, 1990).

PROGNOSIS

Although there are many factors that contribute to hemorrhagic cystitis (see Table 15–3), the majority of clients can be treated successfully. In particular, prevention of hemorrhagic cystitis occurs through the use of uroprotectors, hyperhydration, and diuresis. Stillwell and Benson (1988) studied 100 clients with hemorrhagic cystitis and noted that 32 died from their disease, 10 clients from exsanguinating hemorrhage, and 1 from a postoperative cystectomy.

TREATMENT

No established protocol or set method of treatment for hemorrhagic cystitis is available. When hemorrhagic cystitis develops, the chemotherapeutic drug

---

Table 15-3
Factors Contributing to Hemorrhagic Cystitis

Antineoplastics

Cyclophosphamide (Cytoxan)
Ifosfamide (Ifex)
Busulfan
Bleomycin
Thiotepa
Epodyl
Doxorubicin
Mitomycin C
Bacillus Calmette-Guérin

Viruses

Adenovirus
Cytomegalovirus
Polyomavirus BK
Papovarius
Influenza A

Antibiotics

Methicillin
Nafcillin
Ticarcillin
Carbenicillin
Penicillin G
Piperacillin

---

or antibiotic is normally discontinued (Shepherd et al., 1991). Stopping or reducing the amount of the drugs the client is receiving can help manage hemorrhagic cystitis.

Surgery: *Suprapubic cystotomy:* Surgical treatment for severe hemorrhagic cystitis increases mortality rates for those who require surgery, but not those who respond to medical treatment alone. Those who need surgery also have greater transfusion requirements than those who respond to medical treatment. Surgery should only be used after failure of medical treatment has been established (Baronciani et al., 1995).

Chemotherapy: Not indicated.

Radiation: Not indicated.

Medications

Hydration and diuresis: Diuretics and hydration are routinely used to prevent or reduce effects of chemotherapeutic-induced hemorrhagic cystitis by diluting the metabolites in the urine, which minimizes toxicity. Furosemide may also be given for clients with urine output of less than 100 ml every 2 hours to prevent the possible complications (hyponatremia, seizures, death) of the oxazaphosphorine side effect of free water accumulation.

Investigational regimens: In an attempt to prevent or reduce antineoplastic-induced hemorrhagic cystitis, the following drugs have been investigated to decrease the toxicity by inactivating acrolein in the bladder:

• *Mesna:* Chemoprotective agents such as 2-mercaptoethane sulfonate sodium (mesna) have been developed to provide site-specific protection against antineoplastic-related tissue toxicity, without compromising antitumor activity and has been used to protect the bladder against hemorrhagic cystitis and other detrimental effects of chemotherapy (Lewis, 1994). Chemotherapy with an oxazaphosphorine, such as ifosfamide and Cytoxan, is often limited by unacceptable urotoxicity. Without uroprotection, hemorrhagic cystitis becomes dose-limiting. Dose-limiting toxicity is principally caused by the inability of the antineoplastic drugs to differentiate between normal and malignant cells. The consequences include serious adverse effects and the inability to deliver adequate dose-intensive therapy against the cancer. Mesna is a drug that is able to bind to the toxic metabolites forming nontoxic compounds in the urine. Mesna is normally given at the same total dose as the Cytoxan or ifosfamide. Studies cite several standard protocols for administering mesna (see Nursing Interventions section), and all the methods have the same efficiency. Timing of the dosages of mesna is important, because its half-life is 35 minutes (Katz et al., 1995; Schoenike and Dana, 1990). It is not clear if the addition of mesna therapy versus bladder irrigation with IV hydration and diuresis alone provides greater protection against antineoplastic-induced hemorrhagic cystitis. In BMT clients, studies show that mesna has no adverse effects on engraftment, since it is hydrophilic and activates only in the kidneys. Because it is inactive in the bloodstream and unable to penetrate cell membranes, it does not interfere with the action of chemotherapy (Haselberger and Schwinghammer, 1995).

- *Prostaglandin E2 (PGE2):* Intravesical instillation of PGE2 directly into the bladder by irrigation has been shown to inactivate the acrolein, which results in a complete resolution of hematuria within 4 to 5 days. In some clients, urine has cleared within 24 hours after initial treatment. PGE2 caused no systemic circulatory or respiratory problems. Bladder spasms are a side effect of PGE2 in most clients and can be treated with sedative drugs and morphine (Lazio et al., 1995).

- *Other:* Solutions such as saline, potassium aluminum sulfate, silver nitrate, and formalin cause a protein precipitate to form over bleeding surfaces. Aminocaproic acid, a vasopressin that can be administered intravenously or orally, may decrease clotting.

Procedures

Bladder irrigation: If cystitis occurs, bladder irrigation through a three-way indwelling urinary catheter is performed at a rate of 1 liter per hour during treatment with high-dose Cytoxan (5626 mg/m^2 over 3 days) and for 24 hours after the treatment. Continuous irrigation clears clots from the bladder. Studies by Meisenberg et al. (1994) indicate that hyperhydration and continuous bladder irrigation result in a low incidence of microscopic hematuria, and no reported cases of visible hematuria were noted when IV fluids were administered at 200 ml/m^2/hour during chemotherapy infusions. Additional fluid boluses were given if urine output fell below 200 ml/hour.

Prophylactic continuous bladder irrigation for clients receiving Cytoxan and/or busulfan in preparation for BMT significantly decreased the frequency of hemorrhagic cystitis. Turkeri et al. (1995) reported that 23% of those receiving continuous bladder irrigation experienced hemorrhagic cystitis, as opposed to 53% of those who do not receive continuous bladder irrigation prophylactically. The researchers also stated that there was no difference in the frequency of hemorrhagic cystitis when clients underwent continuous irrigation, even if they received different preparative regimens for their BMT.

Hyperbaric oxygen therapy (HBO): HBO has been used since 1985 to treat radiation-induced hemorrhagic cystitis. Results show that macroscopic hematuria diminished in the majority of clients treated with HBO. Cystoscopic findings before and after HBO showed significant decreases in hemorrhagic sites and telangiectasis of the bladder mucosa. Studies (Lee, Liu, Chiao, and Lin, 1994) indicate that HBO can be an effective and safe form of treatment for radiation-induced hemorrhagic cystitis.

Other

If oral cyclophosphamide is prescribed, it must be taken early in the morning and followed by a 2 to 3 L/day of oral fluid intake, if not medically contraindicated. The bladder must be emptied every 2 to 3 hours so that the cyclophosphamide urinary metabolites are not in constant contact with the bladder mucosa.

Cystoscopy may be necessary to cauterize bleeding vessels if continuous bladder irrigation proves to be ineffective in evacuating clots within 24 hours.

Pediatrics: Intravesical administration of 1% alum irrigation and aluminum-containing antacids can cause mental status changes in an immunosupressed child. Even mildly elevated aluminum levels of 14 to 22 (norm = 0 to 6) can lead to mental status changes. Resolution of levels occurs within a 9-week course of IV deferoxamine (Kanwar, Jenkins, Mandrell, and Furman, 1996).

For refractory hemorrhagic cystitis: Carboprost at 1 mg/dl every 6 hours for a maximum of 7 days is a possible treatment for refractory hemorrhagic cystitis. Evacuation of clots prior to the administration of Carboprost may be required to achieve full benefit of the treatment (Ippoliti et al., 1995).

For life-threatening hemorrhagic cystitis: Formalin instillation of 1 to 4% is standard therapy for life-threatening cystitis that is refractory to conservative treatments. Intravesical treatment with formalin is painful and requires general or regional anesthesia. All blood clots must be evacuated prior to formalin treatment in order to prevent ureteral reflux, which can cause injury to the kidney or ureters. The client should be placed in reverse Trendelenburg position to prevent ureteral reflux. Usually 1% formalin is used via bladder irrigation for approximately 20 minutes through a urethral catheter. If bleeding is not controlled with 1% formalin, higher concentrations up to 4% can be used. Results with formalin are usually immediate, but owing to the side effects of severe bladder fibrosis and contraction, it is used only when other treatments have failed (Donahue and Frank, 1989).

ASSESSMENT CRITERIA:
HEMORRHAGIC CYSTITIS

Vital signs	
Temperature	Elevated secondary to infection and/or inflammation.
Pulse	Increased secondary to compensatory response to bleeding and/or temperature elevation.
Respirations	May be increased secondary to compensatory response to bleeding.
Blood pressure	May be increased secondary to the body's compensatory response to hypovolemia from bleeding or later decreased as the capacity of the compensatory response is exceeded.
History	Leukemia.
	Genitourinary, gastrointestinal, or gynecologic cancer.
	Radiation to the pelvic area.
	History of viral infection, thrombocytopenia, or rheumatoid arthritis.
	Oxazaphosphorine alkylating chemotherapy (cyclophosphamide, ifosfamide).
	Use of bacillus Calmette-Guérin, chemotherapy.
	Use of busulfan, bleomycin, cisplatin, doxorubicin, epodyl, mitomycin-C, thiotepa, VM-26 and/or vincristine.
	Use of antibiotics, dyes, insecticides and/or recreational drugs.
Hallmark physical signs and symptoms	Hematuria: red blood cells in urine, pink-tinged urine, sediment, blood clots. Assess grade of hematuria (see Table 15–2).
Additional physical signs and symptoms	Dysuria, burning, frequency, urgency, hematuria, incontinence, nocturia, suprapubic discomfort/pain. Complications: urosepsis, obstructive uropathy.
Psychosocial signs	Anxiety.
Lab values	
Urinalysis	See Table 15–2 for grading of hematuria.
BUN and creatinine	Increased with obstructive uropathy present.
Serum potassium	May be low secondary to furosemide side-effect.
Hemoglobin and hematocrit	Low secondary to bleeding.
	Low secondary to hemodilution from reduced urine output.
Electrolytes	May be abnormal secondary to furosemide side effect.
Urine for cytology	Red blood cells count > 3.
	May show tumor cells if bladder cancer is present.
	High numbers of normal cells may be present owing to tissue sloughing.

ASSESSMENT CRITERIA: HEMORRHAGIC CYSTITIS *(continued)*

Diagnostic tests

Cystoscopy	Shows bleeding capillaries, diffuse mucosal ulceration, hemorrhage, and necrosis.
Excretory urography	Bladder may appear normal or abnormally small. May show urinary tract outflow obstruction or nodular filling defects.

Other	Onset can be months or years after chemotherapy treatment is discontinued.
Urinary I and O	Less than 100 ml/hour.
Weight (twice a day)	Increased.

NURSING DIAGNOSIS

Some of the common diagnoses for hemorrhagic cystitis are as follows:

Altered urinary elimination related to:
- Hyperhydration.
- Bladder catheterization.
- Diuretic therapy.
- Hemorrhagic cystitis complicated by obstructive uropathy.

Impaired physical mobility related to three-way indwelling urinary catheter.

Knowledge deficit related to:
- Side effects of chemotherapy and/or radiation.
- Prevention of hemorrhagic cystitis.
- Signs and symptoms of hemorrhagic cystitis.
- Unfamiliarity with complications and treatment of hemorrhagic cystitis.

Anxiety related to:
- Sight of blood and/or clots in urine.
- Fear of blood transfusions.
- Placement of three-way indwelling urinary catheter.

NURSING INTERVENTIONS

Immediate nursing interventions

Preventive measures during administration of chemotherapy:

Administer uroprotectant prior to chemotherapy as prescribed. Several standard protocols for administering mesna exist:

1. Loading dose of mesna IV approximately 20% (wt/wt) of ifosfamide, or 60 to 120% of Cytoxan, followed by two similar doses in 4 and 8 hours.
2. IV mesna in three equal doses 15 minutes before and 4 hours and 8 hours following the chemotherapy.

3. Mesna IV in two equal doses 15 minutes before and 4 hours following. Some studies have indicted that mesna can be given by continuous infusion, beginning 24 hours before and finishing 24 hours after the administration of chemotherapy.

Administer chemotherapy early in the day.

Monitor urine for blood by observation and dipstick.

Measure hourly intake and output (I and O).

Insert three-way indwelling urinary catheter, if necessary.

Irrigate urinary catheter, if necessary.

Increase rate of hydration or bolus fluids.

Insert three-way indwelling urinary catheter for continuous irrigation to ensure that the chemotherapeutic agents are continuously being cleared from the bladder.

Administer furosemide if urine output is less than 100 ml/hour.

Monitor for mesna toxicity (diarrhea, headache, limb pain).

Anticipated physician orders and interventions

Insertion of three-way catheter with continuous bladder irrigation.

Urine cytology to determine degree of cystitis.

Urinalysis to determine hematuria.

Cystoscopy—shows bleeding capillaries, diffuse mucosal ulceration, hemorrhage, and necrosis that allows for cauterization of bleeding.

Blood sampling for measurement of hematocrit, hemoglobin, blood urea nitrogen (BUN), and electrolytes.

Type and screen for potential blood transfusion(s).

Ongoing nursing assessment, monitoring, and interventions

Assess:
- Urine for blood qd.
- For signs and symptoms of transfusion reaction if blood replacement products are given.
- For signs of hypovolemia secondary to bleeding q4h.
- For pain and suprapubic discomfort, as well as pain relief received from interventions q4–8h.

Measure:
- I and O. Measure urine output q1h, and add diuretics as needed.
- Vital signs q4h.

Send:
- Blood samples for hemoglobin and hematocrit q6h.
- Blood samples for BUN and creatinine qd. Add electrolytes or potassium if the client is receiving furosemide.
- Urine for urinalysis q 2 days until there is no longer evidence of microscopic hematuria.

Implement:
- Pain management for suprapubic discomfort. (Refer to Chapter 33.)
- Fluid administration (by mouth, IV) of 2 to 3 L/day (when not contraindicated).
- Teaching regarding the potential for reoccurrence of hemorrhagic cystitis in the future.
- Teaching related to home urine dipstick testing for hematuria.

TEACHING/EDUCATION

Hemorrhagic cystitis: *Rationale:* Hemorrhagic cystitis is an inflammation of your bladder that can be caused by chemotherapeutic agents such as Cytoxan or ifosfamide. It can also be caused by radiation treatments. Sometimes the inflammation can lead to bleeding.

Decreased/discontinued chemotherapy: *Rationale:* The chemotherapy drugs you are taking have byproducts that can damage the lining of your bladder and cause serious bleeding—a condition known as hemorrhagic cystitis. Stopping the drugs can prevent or reverse the damage that might have been caused by them.

Medication timing: *Rationale:* Your doctor has prescribed oral Cytoxan to treat your cancer. It is important to take the medication early in the day to prevent the accumulation of the drug in your bladder. Taking the medication early allows you to drink and urinate frequently during the day without keeping you up at night.

Increase dietary fluids/diuresis: *Rationale:* It is important to make sure that you empty your bladder on a regular basis and urinate adequate amounts so that the byproducts of the chemotherapy don't remain in your bladder. It is important that you drink at least 2 to 3 liters of fluid a day while you are taking your chemotherapy so that you will urinate often. Your doctor will also prescribe drugs, such as Lasix, that will help you urinate and wash the chemotherapy byproducts out of your bladder.

Indwelling three-way urinary catheter placement: *Rationale:* While you are in the hospital receiving chemotherapy it may be necessary to insert a catheter into your bladder. This catheter will have fluids flowing through it so the chemotherapy will be flushed out of your bladder, and this will decrease your risk of hemorrhagic cystitis. The placement of the catheter will allow us to accurately measure your urine output. In case you develop hemorrhagic cystitis that results in blood clots, the catheter will allow us to irrigate (flush) the catheter so that we can remove the clots.

I and O: *Rationale:* While you are in the hospital, we will be measuring your urine output every hour to make sure that you are flushing the chemotherapy out of your bladder. It will be important for you to save all your urine so that we can measure it.

Signs and symptoms of hemorrhagic cystitis: Rationale: If you develop hemorrhagic cystitis you may notice some symptoms. You may see pink-tinged urine, or you may see actual blood or clots. You may also have the need to urinate more frequently, especially at night, and you may experience some burning and pain in your lower abdomen right above your bladder

Treatment regimens for hemorrhagic cystitis: Rationale: You will receive an IV medication right before you get your chemotherapy. This medication is called mesna. It will help protect your bladder and reduce the side effects of chemotherapy. You will also get this medication 4 and 8 hours after the chemotherapy. You may experience some nausea, vomiting, and/or diarrhea. Your doctor will prescribe medicine to prevent or reduce these side effects.

Follow-up care: Rationale: Hemorrhagic cystitis can recur. It can also be a delayed complication of chemotherapy or radiation treatments. It will be important for you to notify your physician immediately if you see any blood in your urine, or if you notice any other signs and symptoms such as a change in voiding patterns or pain. It will also be necessary to have annual checkups by your physician.

EVALUATION/DESIRED OUTCOMES

1. The indwelling urinary catheter is discontinued within 24 to 48 hours after chemotherapy treatment.
2. Urine will be clear and free of red blood cells.
3. Urine output will be within normal limits.
4. Side effects from mesna therapy will be minimized through use of medication.
5. The client will be free of symptoms of hemorrhagic cystitis.
6. The client will follow up consistently with physician appointments.
7. The client will notify physician immediately if delayed symptoms of hemorrhagic cystitis are noted.

DISCHARGE PLANNING

The client with hemorrhagic cystitis may need:

Education about keeping oral liquid intake at 2 to 3 liters a day for at least 48 hours after completion of chemotherapy.

Education about recognition of signs and symptoms of hemorrhagic cystitis, about which the client must immediately notify his or her physician.

Encouragement to have routine annual physical checkups because hemorrhagic cystitis can occur again, even after many years.

FOLLOW-UP CARE

Anticipated care

Routine physician visits, with frequency determined by type of oncologic problem.

Continuation of increased fluids if oral chemotherapy treatment continues.

Routine urine dipsticking during continued treatment.

Annual urinalysis, urine cytology, and cystoscopy.

Periodic excretory urography.

Anticipated client/family questions and possible answers

What do I have to do to reduce my chances of getting hemorrhagic cystitis?

"If you are talking oral chemotherapy, it is important that you take the chemotherapy early in the day and drink at least 2 to 3 liters of fluid a day."

"While on chemotherapy make sure you empty your bladder at least every 2 to 3 hours and before bedtime."

"If you are not urinating on a regular basis or you notice signs and symptoms of hemorrhagic cystitis such as pain by your bladder, burning, urgency, frequency, or blood in your urine, notify your physician immediately."

What will reduce my chances of getting hemorrhagic cystitis during my bone marrow transplant?

"When you are in the hospital preparing for your BMT, you will have an IV that will provide fluids through your veins. You may also receive a diuretic. The fluids and diuretic will ensure that you urinate and prevent urine from remaining in your bladder. You may also have a three-way urinary catheter. This catheter will allow fluids to flow through your bladder and flush out the chemotherapy drugs. It will also allow the nurses to measure your urine to make sure that your fluid intake and output is adequate. You will also get a medication called mesna. This medication will protect your bladder from the negative effects of the chemotherapy."

Can I get hemorrhagic cystitis again?

"Hemorrhagic cystitis can recur, even after many years have passed. It can also be a delayed complication of chemotherapy or radiation. It will be important for you to have routine physical examinations and notify your physician if you notice any signs and symptoms indicating recurrence."

CHAPTER SUMMARY

Hemorrhagic cystitis is primarily found in clients treated with oxazaphosphorine alkylating agents, particularly cyclophosphamide and ifosfamide. It is also caused by radiation treatment. Clients undergoing high-dose chemotherapy regimens in preparation for a BMT are at a greater risk for hemorrhagic cystitis. Radiation effects can appear for the first time 15 to 20 years after the first radiation treatment. Iatrogenic causes can be related to viruses, antibiotics, recreational drug use, or conditions such as rheumatoid arthritis. Although there is no standard treatment, hemorrhagic cystitis has been prevented by hyperhydration, diuresis, and the prophylactic use of uroprotectors such as mesna. The use of three-way urinary catheters may also reduce or prevent hemorrhagic cystitis. Nursing assessment and client education is very important to help the client deal with the acute and chronic symptoms of hemorrhagic cystitis.

TEST QUESTIONS

1. Hemorrhagic cystitis is a condition that affects the:
   A. Prostate gland
   B. Urethra
   C. Bladder
   D. Bone marrow

1. Answer: C.
Hemorrhagic cystitis can occur when metabolites of certain chemotherapeutic agents accumulate in the bladder and bind to the mucosal lining.

2. The primary nursing diagnosis of clients with hemorrhagic cystitis is:
   A. Impaired physical mobility
   B. Altered urinary elimination
   C. Alteration in tissue perfusion
   D. Fluid volume deficit

2. Answer: B.
Altered urinary elimination can occur as a result of treatment modalities used for the client's primary disease as a result of the interventions used to prevent complications from the treatments, and/or as a result of complications from the treatments.

3. Which chemotherapeutic drugs induce hemorrhagic cystitis?
   A. Carmustine and idarubicin
   B. Cisplatin and ifosfamide
   C. Cytoxan and idarubicin
   D. Cyclophosphamide and ifosfamide

3. Answer: D.
The metabolites from cyclophosphamide (Cytoxan) and ifosfamide are toxic to the epithelium of the bladder and cause irritation of the bladder that ranges from microscopic hematuria to frank bleeding.

4. A client receiving cyclophosphamide would most likely be taught about:
   A. Restriction of water intake
   B. Alopecia
   C. Hyperhydration and diuresis
   D. Self-administration of antiemetics

4. Answer: C.
To prevent or reduce the effects of hemorrhagic cystitis, it is important to teach the client to drink at least 2 to 3 liters of fluid per day and to empty the bladder every 2 to 3 hours and especially at bedtime in order to prevent the urine that contains the cyclophosphamide metabolites from remaining in contact with the lining of the bladder.

5. The uroprotector mesna protects the bladder by:
   A. Transforming endocrine cells in the bladder by diminishing myelotoxicity
   B. Interfering with synthesis of DNA, thus inhibiting DNA repair
   C. Activating microsomes in the bladder
   D. Binding with the chemotherapeutic metabolites, resulting in their detoxification

5. Answer: D.
Mesna binds with acrolein, the toxic metabolite of Cytoxan and ifosfamide, and provides site-specific protection against tissue toxicity without compromising the antitumor activity of the chemotherapy.

6. The major signs and symptoms of hemorrhagic cystitis are:
   A. Dysuria, urgency, hematuria, suprapubic pain
   B. Hematuria, nausea, vomiting, diarrhea
   C. Thrombocytopenia, neutropenia, hematuria
   D. Ascites, upper quadrant pain, urticaria

6. Answer: A.
Hemorrhagic cystitis is an irritation of the bladder and can present with symptoms such as suprapubic discomfort, urgency, frequency, dysuria, and incontinence. Symptoms can range from microscopic hematuria to frank bleeding.

7. Clients taking oral cyclophosphamide are taught to:
   A. Take the medication on an empty stomach
   B. Restrict their oral intake
   C. Take the drug early in the day
   D. Report signs of dyspnea, stomatitis, and myelotoxicity

7. Answer: C.
Clients are instructed to take oral cyclophosphamide early in the day so that the large amounts of fluid intake required to cause frequent urination can be taken before bedtime.

8. The monitoring of which laboratory value will best indicate a change in the amount of bleeding from hemorrhagic cystitis?
   A. Serum creatinine
   B. Hematocrit
   C. Bilirubin
   D. Factor VIII

8. Answer: B.
The hematocrit is the percentage of red blood cells in a volume of whole blood, which is a good indicator of the amount of bleeding.

9. Intake and output should be measured in the client with hemorrhagic cystitis:
   A. Every 12 hours
   B. Every 8 hours
   C. Every hour
   D. Every 5 minutes for 1 hour

9. Answer: C.
Hourly measurements of intake and output are the best indicators regarding hydration and elimination status.

10. Bladder irrigation, one of the treatments used for hemorrhagic cystitis, is best accomplished through a:
    A. Rectal tube
    B. Single-lumen urinary (Foley) catheter
    C. Three-way urinary (Foley) catheter
    D. Laparotomy-placed nephrostomy tube

10. Answer: C.
Use of a multilumen urinary catheter allows for instillation of solution, irrigation, and output.

REFERENCES

Ambinder RF, Burnes W, Forman M, Charache P, Arthur R, Beschorner W, Santos G, Saral R: Hemorrhagic cystitis associated with adenovirus infection in bone marrow transplantation. Arch Intern Med 146:1400, 1986.

Arthur RR, Shak KV, Baust SJ, Santos GW, Saral R: Association of BK virus with hemorrhagic cystitis in recipients of bone marrow transplants. New Engl J Med 315:230-234, 1986.

Baronciani D, Angelucci E, Erer B, Fabrizi G, Galimberti M, Gardini C, Milella D, Montesi M, Polchi P, Severini A, et al.: Suprapubic cystotomy as treatment for severe hemorrhagic cystitis after BMT. Bone Marrow Transplant 16:267–270, 1995.

Bedi A, Miller CB, Hanson JL, Goodman S, Ambinder RF, Charache P, Auther RR, Jones RJ: Association of BK virus with failure of prophylaxis against hemorrhagic cystitis following bone barrow transplantation. J. Clin Oncol 13:1103–1109, 1995.

Cox PJ: Cyclophosphamide cystitis: Identification of acrolein as the causative agent. Biochem Pharmacol 28:2045–2049, 1979.

DeVries CR, Freha FA: Hemorrhagic cystitis: A review. J Urol 143:1–9, 1990.

Donahue LA, Frank IN: Intravesical formalin for hemorrhagic cystitis: Analysis of therapy. J Urol 141:809–812, 1989.

Haselberger MB, Schwinghammer TL: Efficacy of mesna for prevention of hemorrhagic cystitis after high-dose cyclophosphamide therapy. Ann Pharmacother 29:918-921, 1995.

Ippoliti C, Prezepiorka D, Mehra R, Neumann J, Wood J, Claxton D, Gajewski J, Khouri I, Van Besien K, Anderson B, et al.: Intravesicular carboprost for the treatment of hemorrhagic cystitis after marrow transplantation. Urology 46(6):811–815, 1995.

Jayalakshamamma B, Pinkel D: Urinary-bladder toxicity following pelvic irradiation and simultaneous cyclophosphamide therapy. Cancer 38:701–707, 1976.

Kanwar VS, Jenkins JJ, Mandrell BN, Furman WL: Med Pediatr Oncol 27:64-67, 1996.

Katz A, Epelman S, Anelli A, Gorender EF, Cruz SM, Oliverira RM, Marques LA: J Cancer Res Clin Oncol 121(2):128–131, 1995.

Lamm DL, Stogdill VD, Stogdill BJ, Crispen RG: Complications of bacillus Calmette-Guérin immunotherapy in 1,278 patients with bladder cancer. J Urol 35:272-274, 1986.

Lazio D, Bopsi A, Guidi S, Saccardi R, Vannucchi AM, Lombardini L, Longo G, Fanci R, Azzi A, De Santis R. et al.: Prostaglandin E2 bladder instillation for the treatment of hemorrhagic cystitis after allogeneic bone marrow transplantation. Haematologica 80:421–425, 1995.

Lee HC, Liu CS, Chiao C, Lin S: Hyperbaric oxygen therapy in hemorrhagic radiation cystitis: A report of 20 cases. Undersea Hyperb Med 21:321–327, 1994.

Levenback D, Eifel PJ, Burke TW, Morris M, Gershenson DM: Hemorrhagic cystitis following radiotherapy for stage Ib cancer of the cervix. Gynecol Oncol 55:206–210, 1994.

Lewis C: A review of the use of chemoprotectants in cancer chemotherapy. Drug Saf 11:153–162, 1994.

Meisenberg B, Lassiter M, Hussein A, Ross M, Vredenburgh JJ, Peters WP: Prevention of hemorrhagic cystitis after high-dose alkylating agent chemotherapy and autologous bone marrow support. Bone Marrow Transplant 14(2):287–291, 1994.

Prout GR Jr, Lin GW, Benson R Jr, Nseyo UO, Daly JJ, Griffin PP, Kinsey J, Tian ME, Lao YH, Mian YZ, et al.: Photodynamic therapy with hematoporophrin derivative in the treatment of superficial transitional cell carcinoma of the bladder. New Engl J Med 317:1251–1255, 1987.

Schoenike SE, Dana WJ: Ifosfamide and mesna. Clin Pharm 9:179–191, 1990.

Shaw JC, Graham MI: Mesna: A short review. Cancer Treat Rev 14:67–86, 1987.

Shepherd JD, Pringle LE, Barnett M, Klingemann HG, Reece DE, Phillips GL: Mesna versus hyperhydration for the prevention of cyclophosphamide-induced hemorrhagic cystitis in bone marrow transplantation. J Clin Oncol 9(11):2026–2020, 1991.

Shoenike SE, Dana WJ: Infosfamide and mesna. Clin Pharm 9:179–191, 1990.

Stillwell TJ, Benson RC: Cyclophosphamide-induced hemorrhagic cystitis: A review of 100 patients. Cancer 61:451–457, 1988.

Stillwell TJ, Benson RC Jr, Burgert EO Jr: Cyclophosphamide-induced hemorrhagic cystitis in Ewing's sarcoma. J. Clin Oncol 6:76–82, 1988.

Thomas AE, Patterson J, Prentice HG, Brenner MK, Ganczakowski M, Hancock JF, Pattinson JK, Blacklock HA, Hopewell JP: Haemorrhagic cystitis in bone marrow transplantation patients: Possible increased risk associated with prior busulfan therapy. Bone Marrow Transplant 1: 347–355, 1987.

Turkeri LN, Lum LG, Uberti JP, Abella E, Momin F, Karanes C, Sensenbrenner LL, Haas GP: Prevention of hemorrhagic cystitis following allogeneic bone marrow transplant preparative regiments with cyclophosphamide and busulfan role of continuous bladder irrigation. J Urol 153(3):637–640, 1995.

CHAPTER 16

HEPATIC ENCEPHALOPATHY

Barbara J. Berger, MSN, RN, CCRN
Michael Wrigley, RN, MA
AND
J. Christopher Ladaika, BSN, RN, CCRN

CHAPTER OBJECTIVES

At the completion of this chapter, the reader will be able to:

Define hepatic encephalopathy.

State the risk factors for hepatic encephalopathy in an oncology client.

Describe nursing care as it relates to oncology clients with potentially reversible hepatic encephalopathy.

Anticipate and prepare the client with reversible hepatic encephalopathy for future care needs and follow-up.

Anticipate and prepare the client with irreversible hepatic encephalopathy and his or her family for hospice care.

OVERVIEW

HEPATIC ENCEPHALOPATHY is a term used to describe a syndrome that includes symptoms of personality and behavior changes, altered neuromuscular coordination and control, and progressively diminishing level of consciousness (LOC). Clients with cancer are at higher risk (than the general population) for hepatic encephalopathy due to the possibility of primary or metastatic liver cancer and due to the presence of oncologic complications that can precipitate encephalopathy symptoms in a person with pre-existing cirrhosis. In the oncology client, the appearance of hepatic encephalopathy symptoms can signal either an acute oncologic emergency or further deterioration in an irreversible disease process. The type and intensity of intervention will depend on the client's history, the causative factors of the disease(s), and the client's treatment preferences.

DESCRIPTION

Causes

Hepatic encephalopathy in a client with cancer can be caused by malignant primary tumors of the liver, by fulminant hepatic failure secondary to massive malignant infiltration of the liver (Bernau, Rueff, and Benhamou, 1986), or by the superimposition of oncologic complications such as graft vs. host disease (GVHD) (see Chapter 13), sepsis, alkalosis, veno-occlusive disease (see Chapter 17), or hypovolemia in a client who has pre-existing cirrhosis. In addition, acute hepatic failure can occur with failing liver transplant primary grafts (Bernau et al., 1986) accompanied by the presence of encephalopathy. Hepatotoxic chemotherapeutic drugs and benzodiazepines are other potential causes of hepatic encephalopathy in oncology clients.

In an oncology client without pre-existing liver disease, the onset of hepatic encephalopathy may occur within the first 8 weeks after liver dysfunction symptoms appear (Bonnice, 1985). In a client with pre-existing cirrhosis, encephalopathy symptoms may develop quickly after the onset of any of the oncologic complications listed above.

Pathophysiology

The physical presence of liver tumor or metastatic cancer to the liver blocks the normal hepatic blood flow, leading to the development of alternate (collateral) circulation pathways where venous blood bypasses portal circulation. These alternate circulation pathways allow substances, usually metabolized hepatically, to bypass the liver and accumulate in the blood and cross the blood-brain barrier, where they become toxic to brain cells. Clients with pre-existing liver damage from cirrhosis have gradually developed such alternate circulation pathways, but may not have reached the point of encephalopathy. Because these pathways are already present, increased ammonia production common in many oncologic complications can rapidly precipitate hepatic encephalopathy in the oncology client with a history of cirrhosis (Table 16–1).

The exact mechanisms leading to the symptoms of hepatic encephalopathy are not completely understood. The literature proposes a multifactorial pathogenesis for this condition that includes the formation of "false neurotransmitters," impaired deamination leading to abnormal amino acid and neurotransmitter balance, an altered Krebs cycle, and possibly a deficiency of some type of protective substance that has not yet been identified. A major toxin thought to influence the degree of hepatic encephalopathy symptoms is ammonia, which is thought to alter the normal hydroxylation of precursor amino acids, producing "false neurotransmitters" that occupy norepinephrine receptors at synaptic junctions, preventing normal neurotransmission and leading to sedation. Reduced deamination of aromatic amino acids by

Table 16-1
Common Causes of Increased Ammonia Levels in Oncologic Complications

Complication	Mechanism
Graft vs. host disease	Research points to a "cytokine storm" by T-cells, which results in an inflammatory process and hepatic and other tissue damage after bone marrow transplant (Theobald, 1995).
Sepsis	Hypermetabolic state increases deamination of amino acids and their ammonia metabolite accumulates in the blood at an increased rate.
Alkalosis secondary to hypoxia	Alkalosis promotes the growth of intestinal bacteria that produce ammonia.
Veno-occlusive disease	Tumor necrosis factor-alpha release triggers coagulation and consequent obstruction of the hepatic sinusoids and venules. Sinusoids are engorged with hepatocytes and red blood cells, which impairs the hepatic microcirculation, leading to hepatic cellular toxicity (Shulman and Hinterberger, 1992).
Hypovolemia	Reduced renal perfusion leads to retention of nitrogenous waste that should normally be excreted in the urine (uremia).

the liver leads to higher than normal levels of aromatic amino acids and lower than normal levels of excitatory neurotransmitters in the bloodstream. As these neurotransmitters become imbalanced, neurotransmission is reduced, and sedation develops. The combination of these two problems may explain the pathogenesis of hepatic coma (Mosseau and Butterworth, 1994). Injection of high doses of ammonium acetate into animal brains has been shown to interfere with the Krebs cycle, leading to reduced levels of adenosine triphosphate (ATP) required for energy. This effect may play a role in cerebral damage and produce a negative neurologic outcome in clients who reach the stage of hepatic coma (Felipo et al., 1994).

Symptoms

The symptoms of hepatic encephalopathy include changes in behavior, personality, and neuromuscular abilities. Hallmark symptoms include reduced LOC; asterixis, or flapping tremor of the hands when outstretched; and fetor hepaticus, which is a musty breath odor caused by respiratory excretion of mercaptans left in the bloodstream after bypassing the liver, which normally performs mercaptan removal (Smith, 1993 p. 995). See Table 16-2 for a detailed list of symptoms. The severity of encephalopathy in clients with cirrhosis is categorized by four commonly referenced stages, or grades, in the literature. No separate categorization of symptoms was found for non-cirrhotic encephalopathy, and thus Table 16-3 is included as a general reference for evaluating the degree of deterioration in any client.

Table 16-2
Symptoms of Hepatic Encephalopathy

Changes in Behavior and Neurologic Status	Changes in Personality
Decreased self-care ability	Forgetfulness
Agitation	Disorientation
Decreased alertness and responsiveness	Confusion
Daytime sleepiness	Delirium
Progressive stupor	Dementia
Seizures (rare)	Mood changes
Coma	
Positive Babinski reflex	
Decerebrate posturing	

Changes in Movement and Neuromuscular Coordination	Physical Changes
Ataxia	Jaundice
Apraxia	Ascites
Abnormal deep tendon reflexes	Fetor hepaticus
Reduced fine motor coordination	Musty odor from urine
Asterixis during purposeful movement	Gynecomastia
Muscle stiffness or rigidity	Malnourished state
Speech impairment—slurring, sluggishness	

Diagnosis

Four major factors should be present for diagnosis:

1. Acute or chronic hepatocellular disease and/or extensive portal-systemic collateral shunts.
2. Disturbances of awareness and orientation, which may progress from forgetfulness to stupor and, finally, to coma.
3. Shifting combinations of neurologic signs, including asterixis; rigidity; hyperreflexia; extensor plantar signs; and, rarely, seizures.
4. A characteristic, nonspecific, high-voltage, slow-wave (2- to 5-second) pattern on the electroencephalogram.

(See Podolsy and Isselbacher, 1991, p. 1349.)

Hepatic encephalopathy is diagnosed after other causes of newly developed neuropsychiatric symptoms have been ruled out. Other causes may include intracranial bleeding or tumor, drug-induced personality changes, metabolic encephalopathy, and psychiatric abnormalities. Electroencephalography (EEG) is used to identify characteristic changes of hepatic encephalopathy and also to rule out encephalopathy as a cause of the neuropsychiatric changes.

Table 16-3
Clinical Assessment of Hepatic Encephalopathy

Stage	LOC and Orientation	Intellectual Functioning	Behavior	Mood	Neuromuscular Signs	EEG
I (Prodrome)	Awake; total orientation, with progression to confusion, followed by loss of orientation to time and place.	Mental clouding; lack of attention to detail; slowing in response to questions; impaired handwriting; constructional apraxia.	Personality changes; forgetfulness and restlessness; irritability; untidiness; apathy; disobedience; sleep inversion (night into day).	Euphoria; depression; crying.	Muscular incoordination; tremors; yawning; insomnia; presence or absence of asterixis	Mild-to-moderate abnormalities.
II (Impending coma)	Lethargic; opens eyes spontaneously; experiences disorientation to time and place; severely confused.	Further intellectual and personality deterioration; amnesia of past events; poor psychosomatic test scores.	Inappropriate behavior; lessened inhibitions; lethargy.	Apathy to paranoia.	Asterixis; hyporeactive reflexes; ataxia; slurred speech.	Moderate-to-severe abnormalities.

Stage	LOC and Orientation	Intellectual Functioning	Behavior	Mood	Neuromuscular Signs	EEG
III (Stupor)	Asleep; no spontaneous eye-opening; rouses to verbal stimuli; experiences complete disorientation when roused.	Confused; unable to make computations.	Bizarreness; rage; possible combativeness.	Increased apathy.	Asterixis; inability to cooperate with instructions; incoherent speech; nystagmus; positive Babinski response; clonus; decorticate and decerebrate posturing.	Severe abnormalities.
IV (Coma)	Comatose; initial response to painful stimuli, then no response to painful stimuli.	Comatose.	Asleep; comatose.	Comatose.	Seizures; absence of asterixis; dilated pupils; rigidity progressing to flaccidity.	Severe abnormalities.

Source: Modified from Davidson CS: Hepatic coma. *In* Backus HL (ed): Gastroenterology, vol 2, 3rd ed. Philadelphia: WB Saunders Co, 1976, and from Smith SL: Patients with liver dysfunction. *In* Clochesy JM, Breu C, Cardin S, Rudy EB, Whitaker AA (eds): Critical Care Nursing. Philadelphia: WB Saunders Co, 1993.

RISK PROFILE

Cancers

Primary malignant liver tumors include hepatocellular carcinoma and cholangiocarcinomas (bile duct cancer). Clients with a history of cirrhosis, hepatitis B infection, or hepatitis C infection are at highest risk for development of hepatocellular carcinoma (NCI, 1996; Tsukuma et al., 1993).

Metastatic cancers: gastric, colorectal, breast, lung, lymphoma, pancreatic, biliary tree and small intestine, and testicular.

Pediatrics: *Hepatoblastoma* (usually occurs before age 3).
Hepatocellular carcinoma (incidence peaks at ages 0 to 4 years and ages 12 to 15 years (NCI, 1996). Children who have had hepatitis B or C infections have an increased incidence of developing hepatocellular carcinoma, a primary malignant liver tumor. The incidence is highest in children with perinatally acquired virus (Tsukuma et al., 1993).

Conditions: The following conditions precipitate the symptoms of hepatic encephalopathy more quickly in the oncology client with pre-existing cirrhosis: Constipation, electrolyte loss, gastrointestinal (GI) bleeding, GVHD, hepatitis B carrier, hypokalemia, hypoxia, infection, metabolic alkalosis, primary graft nonfunction after liver transplantation, renal failure, sepsis, venoocclusive disease, vomiting.

Environment: Exposure to the dust of vinyl chloride has been associated with increased risk of subsequent hepatic sarcoma (NCI, 1996).

Foods: A high-protein diet in the oncology client with pre-existing cirrhosis; ingestion of food containing aflatoxin (a mycotoxin) is associated with the incidence of primary liver cancer (Alpert, Hutt, and Wogan, 1971).

Drugs: Alcohol, analgesics, anesthetics, barbiturates, benzodiazepines, carboplatin, diuretics (causing hypovolemia), FIFO regimen (fluorouracil/folinic acid/ifosfamide), floxuridine, sedative-hypnotics (Kattan, Culine, Theodore, and Droz, 1995; Ettinger, Krailor, Gaynon, and Hammond, 1993).

PROGNOSIS

Mortality statistics for the condition of hepatic encephalopathy are not directly available. The condition carries a mortality rate of approximately 80% if symptoms become so severe that coma develops. The presence of hepatic dysfunction and encephalopathy places the client at increased risk of developing cerebral edema with transtentorial herniation; permanent neurologic damage; sepsis; and respiratory, cardiovascular, and renal failure.

Prognosis when symptoms are associated with hepatocellular carcinoma

In the small number of clients who have a localized resectable form of hepatocellular carcinoma, the 5-year survival rate ranges from 10 to 30%. Cure rates are highest in the fibrolamellar variant (Lack, Neave, and Vawter, 1983). Clients may be considered for liver transplantation if hepatocellular carcinoma is localized but considered unresectable. Transplantation carries a chance for reversal of hepatic encephalopathy symptoms if transplant occurs before coma develops. In advanced (inoperable) hepatocellular carcinoma, the median length of survival after diagnosis is 2 to 4 months.

Prognosis when symptoms are associated with hepatic metastases

Eras and Sherlock (1971) reported that 21 of 427 (7.2% of autopsied) clients with hepatic metastases died in hepatic coma.

> **Pediatrics:** Children and adolescents with hepatoblastoma have a better chance of survival than those with adult-type hepatocellular carcinoma, which has a cure rate of only 25%. Hepatoblastoma is associated with a 70% survival rate (Ortega et al., 1994) unless it is the small-cell histologic variant, for which treatment is relatively unsuccessful. Like adults, those children with the fibrolamellar form of hepatocellular carcinoma have the best prognosis (Lack, Neave, and Vawter, 1983).

Potential liver transplant candidates

In clients otherwise eligible for liver transplantation (described above), uncorrectable low cerebral perfusion pressure (CPP) (< 40 mmHg) is associated with a poor chance of reversal of neurologic changes and may serve as a contraindication to liver transplantation. In addition, clients who reach stage IV hepatic coma are not likely to survive the surgery required for transplant (Smith, 1993, p. 982).

TREATMENT

The development of symptoms of hepatic encephalopathy in an oncology client signals an acute condition requiring hospitalization, unless the client has chosen hospice care. The goals of immediate treatment for the symptoms are to (1) attain positive nitrogen balance; (2) prevent development or worsening of increased intracranial pressure (ICP); (3) decrease circulating ammonia and other toxins; (4) protect the airway; and (5) prevent or control bleeding.

Surgery

Liver transplant for localized hepatocellular carcinoma (a small portion of clients) (Di Bisceglie, Rustgi, Hoofnagle, Dusheiko, and Lotze, 1988). Hepatic resection for resectable colorectal hepatic metastases.

Pediatrics: Stage I   Initial treatment for stage I childhood liver
cancer is complete removal of tumor by
wedge resection, lobectomy, or extended
lobectomy.

Stage II   Treatment for stage II childhood liver cancer
is gross resection of tumor with microscopic
residual disease (i.e., positive margins).

Stage III   In stage III childhood liver cancer, the disease
is initially considered unresectable or is
resectable with gross residual tumor, positive
lymph nodes, or spilled tumor.

Stage IV   In stage IV childhood liver cancer, there are
distant metastases regardless of the extent of
liver involvement.
(Douglass et al., 1994).

Chemotherapy: Chemotherapy such as floxuridine (FUDR) alone or in combination with other drugs has been used systemically and through portal vein or regional arterial infusion to treat primary and metastatic liver cancer responsible for the symptoms of hepatic encephalopathy. Systemic fluorouracil has also been used. No clear improvement in survival has been demonstrated in repeated trials of either method (Chang et al., 1987; Kemeny et al., 1987; Patt, 1991). It is important to note that regional arterial infusion is contraindicated in clients with portal hypertension or jaundice.

Pediatrics: *Stage I and stage II hepatoblastoma:* After complete surgical excision, combination cisplatin-based chemotherapy (cisplatin/doxorubicin, cisplatin/vincristine/fluorouracil) has shown > 90% survival (Ortega et al., 1994; Douglass et al., 1993)

Radiation: Radiation has been used alone and in combination with chemotherapy to palliatively treat the cancer causing the symptoms. External beam radiotherapy and chemotherapy in combination with subsequent polyclonal antiferrin antibody has produced improvement in symptoms in up to half of the subjects with advanced hepatic metastases (Order et al., 1985).

Medications

Lactulose to prevent intestinal ammonia absorption and increase peristalsis.
Neomycin to reduce the quantity of intestinal bacteria, which produces ammonia.
Discontinuation of drugs that require a functioning liver for metabolism and that contain ammonium, such as antacids.

Mannitol to provide an osmotic diuresis if the client (with adequate renal function) develops cerebral edema.

Procedures: Hepatic artery ligation and hepatic artery embolization have been shown to stimulate a short-term necrotic process and size reduction in hepatic tumors. Exchange transfusions intended to reduce blood ammonia levels have been shown to be ineffective. A current experimental procedure involves injection of alcohol directly into the hepatic tumor (Ensminger, 1990). Other experimental procedures for metastatic liver cancer include tumor vaccine (Hoover, 1991), biologic response modifiers, and cryotherapy (Ravikumar, Steele, Kane, and King, 1991).

Other

Reduce protein diet or branched-chain amino acid enteral or parenteral nutrition.

Head-of-bed (HOB) elevation and hyperventilation for cerebral edema.

The progression of symptoms to hepatic coma in a client considered a liver transplant candidate or a client without liver cancer but experiencing an oncologic complication is a medical emergency, requiring mechanical ventilation and intensive care. The development of hepatic coma in a client with inoperable liver cancer is an expected sequella of the disease process, and resuscitation provides no hope for reversal of neurologic changes.

ASSESSMENT CRITERIA: HEPATIC ENCEPHALOPATHY

Vital signs

Pulse	Usually increased and unrelated to fever. May be decreased with increased ICP.
Blood pressure	Hypotension common secondary to:
	1. Hypovolemia caused by third-spacing (due to hypoalbuminemia), sepsis, hemorrhage, pre-renal state.
	2. Cerebral edema.
Respirations	Increased due to hyperemia, pulmonary edema, aspiration, atelectasis, metabolic acidosis (<10%) or metabolic alkalosis.
	Decreased due to increased ICP, worsening hepatic encephalopathy, deepening level of coma.
Temperature	Not affected by hepatic encephalopathy.
ECG pattern	May see heart block or PVCs with electrolyte disturbances. Nonspecific S-T segment and T wave changes with acidemia. Sinus tachycardia secondary to decreased fluid volume and hypotension.

(continued)

ASSESSMENT CRITERIA: HEPATIC ENCEPHALOPATHY *(continued)*

History	
Symptoms, conditions	Common precipitants to hepatic encephalopathy:
	1. Increased nitrogen load due to GI bleeding, excess dietary protein, azotemia, or constipation.
	2. Electrolyte imbalance (hypokalemia, alkalosis, hypoxia, hypovolemia).
	3. Drugs (narcotics, benzodiazepines, sedatives; diuretics that cause alkalosis).
	4. Infection.
Other history	Cirrhosis, hepatitis, cancer, alcohol intake, weight loss or gain, inappropriate behavior, lethargy, forgetfulness, jaundice, bruising, difficulty in stopping bleeding, difficulty in breathing.

Hallmark physical signs and symptoms	Coagulopathy, jaundice, hypoglycemia, metabolic acidosis, asterixis (stage-dependent II and III).

Additional physical signs and symptoms	See Tables 16–2 and 16–3.

Psychosocial signs	See Tables 16–2 and 16–3.

Lab values	
Albumin, serum; and total protein, serum	Low secondary to loss to the interstitium through increased capillary permeability.
Bilirubin (direct and indirect), serum	High secondary to reduced hepatic conjugation of bilirubin and glucuronic acid.
Ammonia, serum	High secondary to reduced ability of liver to convert ammonia to urea for renal excretion. Increased levels reflect disruption of the pathways of urea synthesis. A marked increase usually reflects severe hepatocellular necrosis.
Alanine aminotransferase (ALT), serum	High. May rise prior to jaundice. Reflects acute hepatocellular damage.
Alkaline phosphatase, serum	High. Primary indicator of space-occupying hepatic lesions, but is not diagnostic without concurrent levels of other liver enzymes.
Gamma glutamyl transferase (GGT), serum	High. Rises in acute hepatic disease. Sharpest increase occurs with hepatic metastatic infiltrations and obstructive jaundice.
Aspartate aminotransferase (AST), serum	High secondary to hepatic cellular damage, but is nonspecific for liver damage as it can also indicate cardiac, kidney, or skeletal muscle damage.
Lactate dehydrogenase isoenzymes (LD_4, LD_5), serum	High secondary to hepatic cellular damage.
Cholesterol, serum	Low due to impaired hepatic synthesis.
Glucose, blood	Low.
Arterial blood gas (ABG)	Metabolic acidosis (carries higher mortality rate) (may be compensated by the respiratory buffer system). Metabolic alkalosis.

ASSESSMENT CRITERIA: HEPATIC ENCEPHALOPATHY *(continued)*

Prothrombin time (PT), blood	High secondary to inability of liver to synthesize clotting factors. Will not correct with aquamephyton.
Partial thromboplastin time (PTT), blood	High. Will not correct with fresh frozen plasma.
Isocitrate dehydrogenase (ICD), serum	High. Rises in acute hepatic cell damage. May help distinguish between cardiac and hepatic damage when AST is elevated, but essentially offers no advantage over ALT and is rarely used.
Leucine aminopeptidase (LAP), serum	High. May be helpful in distinguishing between skeletal and hepatic disease, but is rarely used.
5′ Nucleotidase (5'NT), serum	High in hepatic metastases, hepatic carcinoma, biliary tract obstruction.
	Normal in skeletal damage.
	More specific for hepatic dysfunction than alkaline phosphatase or LAP. Most often used to differentiate the cause of elevated alkaline phosphatase.
Ornithine carbamoyl transferase (OCT), serum	High.
	Found almost exclusively in the liver. OCT levels are one of the most sensitive indicators of acute hepatocellular dysfunction.
Platelets, blood	Possibly low due to chemotherapy side effects.
White blood cells (WBC), blood	Low.

Diagnostic tests

Computed tomography (CT) Scan	CT evidence of cerebral edema correlates with intracranial hypertension in 60–75% of cases.
	May detect cerebral atrophy.
	CT with arterial portography (Karl, Morse, and Halpert, 1993) or dynamic CT and MRI to help determine surgical resectability of hepatocellular carcinoma.
	Cystic lesions are readily identified, and abscesses can be distinguished from tumors.
EEG	Shows characteristic abnormalities, which include symmetric, high-voltage, slow-wave (2–5 per second) pattern.
Lumbar puncture	Cerebrospinal fluid (CSF) analysis to identify WBC elevations (indicating infection) or red blood cell (RBC) elevations (indicating intracranial bleeding).
Angiography	For distinguishing certain vascular lesions of the liver, i.e., hemangiomas, adenomas, focal nodular hyperplasia, hemangioendotheliomas, and hepatocellular carcinomas.
	Valuable in assessing surgical resectability of isolated lesions.
	For placement of transjugular intrahepatic portosystemic shunt (TIPS).
Percutaneous needle biopsy of the liver	Useful in diagnosing cirrhosis, hepatitis, drug reactions, granulomas, and tumor infiltrates.

(continued)

ASSESSMENT CRITERIA: HEPATIC ENCEPHALOPATHY *(continued)*

Other

Pulmonary artery catheter readings *(Note: insertion of a pulmonary artery catheter is likely to be contraindicated in clients with hepatic encephalopathy due to, or accompanied by, impaired coagulation.)*

Pulmonary artery pressure (PAP), pulmonary vascular resistance (PVR), and systemic vascular resistance (SVR)	Low, secondary to poor vasomotor tone from hypoalbuminemia.
Pulmonary capillary wedge pressure (PCWP) and central venous pressure (CVP)	Low, secondary to low circulating volume.
Cardiac output (CO)	High, secondary to compensation for low SVR.
Intracranial pressure (ICP) monitoring	ICP monitoring can more accurately detect and monitor cerebral edema than can CT. ICP > 15 mmHg and CPP < 50 mmHg indicates cerebral edema. 75 to 80% of clients with encephalopathy demonstrate increased ICP.

NURSING DIAGNOSIS

The most common diagnoses for the client with hepatic encephalopathy are listed here. Typically, all of theses diagnoses apply concurrently.

Ineffective airway clearance related to diminishing LOC.
Ineffective breathing pattern related to ICP.
Altered tissue perfusion, cerebral, related to compensatory cerebral vasodilation in response to hypotension and hypercarbia.
(Potential for) fluid volume deficit related to side effects of osmotic diuresis used to reduce ICP.
Altered nutrition, less than body requirements, related to impaired hepatic metabolism.
Altered bowel elimination, diarrhea, secondary to lactulose administration
(Potential for) impaired skin integrity related to immobility secondary to obtundation.
Impaired verbal communication related to cerebral clouding.
Self-care deficit, all activities of daily living (ADL) related to obtundation.
Potential for injury related to confusion and agitation.

NURSING INTERVENTIONS

Immediate nursing interventions

Assess vital signs and oxygen saturation.
Ensure a patent airway for the client who is obtunded, and administer oxygen as needed to keep oxygen saturation > 90%.

Assess neurologic status (LOC, pupils, ability to follow commands).
Implement aspiration precautions. Elevate HOB 10 to 30 degrees.
Implement seizure precautions. Place oral airway at bedside.
Reduce stimulation present in client's surrounding environment.
Provide frequent observation to ensure client safety.

Anticipated physician orders and interventions

Intubation to protect airway and prevent aspiration.
Complete blood count (CBC), PT/PTT, serum iron, ammonia, and ALT
  levels, urine and serum osmolality.
Nasogastric lavage to rule out GI bleeding.
Discontinuation of benzodiazepines and chemotherapy drugs that can
  potentiate hepatotoxicity.
ICP monitoring (bolt, ventriculostomy) for direct ICP measurement.
For high ICP (normal < 15 mmHg) or low CPP (< 50 mmHg):
- Mannitol 20% 0.5 to 1.0g IV bolus. May repeat hourly to maintain
  a high serum osmolality 310 to 320 mOsm/L.
- Hyperventilate to keep $PaCO_2$ 30 to 32 mmHg (if ventilated and
  client demonstrates an acute change in mental status).
- Keep HOB elevated 10 to 30 degrees.
- Ultrafiltration via dialysis/continuous arteriovenous hemofiltration
  (CAVH) if diuresis with mannitol is unsuccessful.
Intake and output (I and O) q1h.
Discontinuation of drugs that are hepatically metabolized.
For elevated serum ammonia:
- Lactulose 10 to 30 ml q6–8h to produce three to four stools per day.
- 20% lactulose enema if deep coma is present.
- Neomycin 4 to 6g orally qd in divided doses (used short-term only
  due to risk for nephrotoxicity and ototoxicity).
- Diet: *For all clients:* 10% dextrose in water (D10W) by IV.
    For awake client: 0.6–1.0 g/kg/day protein and 35 to 40
      kCal/kg/day.
    For client in light coma with functioning gut: tube feeding
      with standard amino acid levels or a branched-chain
      enriched amino acid formula and 35 to 40 kCal/kg/day.
    For client in deep coma or with ileus: total parenteral nutri-
      tion with standard levels of amino acids or a branched-
      chain enriched amino acid formula and 35 to 40
      kCal/kg/day.
    (Terran, McCullough, and Mullen, 1995.)
Blood transfusion to keep hemoglobin > 10 g/dl to maximize oxygen-
  carrying capacity.
Consultation with liver transplant team about criteria for clients who
  potentially require transplant.

Ongoing nursing assessment, monitoring, and interventions

Assess:
- For increased urine output after mannitol diuresis.
- For desired frequency of stooling q4–6h.
- Skin for breakdown after each bowel movement.
- Neurologic status q1h.
- For dangerous trends downward in CPP:
  < 60 mmHg = pathologic.
  < 50 mmHg = ischemia and production of anoxic byproducts.
  < 40 mmHg = cerebral blood flow reduced by 25%.
  < 30 mmHg = brain death.
- For signs of progressive increase in ICP and risk for brain stem herniation:
  Deteriorating level of consciousness.
  Ipsilateral pupil with motor changes on the opposite side.
  Signs of bleeding: (petechiae, hemoccult + stool, delayed clotting).

Measure:
- ICP q1h.
- MAP q1h.
- CPP q1h (CPP = MAP – ICP).
- I and O q1h.

Send:
- Blood cultures drawn from two sites for temperature > 38.5° C (> 101.3° F) each 24-hour period.
- Blood sample for levels: serum ammonia, CBC, electrolytes, osmolality, ALT, glucose, PT/PTT qd.
- Blood sample for ABG q4h and PRN to assess CO_2 level.

Implement:
- Measures to reduce the chance of increasing ICP:
  Tape endotracheal tube to the peri-oral area instead of using circumferential ties.
  Keep head of bed elevated 10 to 30 degrees.
  Reduce environmental stimulation from lights, noise, and activity.
  Space interventions to leave the client undisturbed for blocks of time.
  Provide family teaching about minimizing stimulation.
- Skin care protocol to prevent skin breakdown consequential to diarrhea.
- Oral care: HCO_3/H_2O mouth rinse PRN.
- Passive range-of-motion exercises q4–5h in comatose clients.
- Hospice, home care, or social work consultation to plan discharge for clients who respond to treatment.
- Physical therapy evaluation and instruction related to mobility and safety.
- Pastoral care consultation for client's family/significant others.

TEACHING/EDUCATION

For the oncology client experiencing hepatic encephalopathy, incidental explanations and reassurances related to procedures and care are appropriate. More detailed explanations (below) should be given to the client's family or significant others, and to any client experiencing a reversal of symptoms.

Changing LOC: *Rationale:* The liver normally keeps ammonia and other toxins from traveling through the blood to the brain. When the liver is not working as well as it normally should, these substances reach the brain and cause your family member to become confused and drowsy and to possibly go into a coma. We can try to slow down the process with medicine, and it might help him or her to wake up temporarily for a period of time. However, this is not usually a reversible symptom.

ICP monitoring: *Rationale:* The liver cannot make enough protein, which acts like a magnet to hold body water in the arteries and veins. When there are not enough proteins in the blood, the body water soaks out of the arteries and veins and into the body cells, including the brain cells. This increases the pressure in the brain, which is very dangerous and can cause death. The ICP monitor lets us monitor the brain pressure so that we can detect rising pressure and give medicine to try to prevent damage.

Mechanical ventilation: *Rationale:* We know that hepatic encephalopathy will cause your family to become so drowsy and confused that he (or she) will not be able to keep an open path for the air to reach the lungs, and he (or she) is at risk for having stomach fluids go into the lungs. Because we can predict that this will happen, we prevent the damage it could cause by putting in a breathing tube before it happens.

Lactulose administration: *Rationale:* The lactulose will help pull the ammonia from the bloodstream into the gut and allow it to leave the body in the bowel movement. This helps prevent the ammonia from traveling to the brain and making the symptoms of confusion and drowsiness worse.

Noise reduction: *Rationale:* Loud noises, bright lights, and activity can each increase the pressure in the brain. We keep the room quiet and dark because it helps keep your family member's brain pressure as low as possible. It is important to talk in calm, quiet tones and about topics that won't excite or upset your family member.

EVALUATION/DESIRED OUTCOMES

1. Improved hepatic function: return to baseline cognitive level.
2. The client demonstrates no further deterioration of hepatic function.
3. The client tolerates increased dietary protein, while maintaining a positive nitrogen balance.

4. Resolution of azotemia.
5. Potassium level increases to >3.5 mEq/L (>3.5 mmol/L SI Units)
6. Glucose level stabilizes within normal range.
7. The client is free of GI bleeding and coagulopathy.
8. The client is free of infection.
9. Families of clients with a poor prognosis (e.g., grade IV hepatic coma) understand the likelihood that the client will die, and support mechanisms for them are in place throughout the dying process.
10. Clients who survive, and their families, can describe the early signs of encephalopathy to watch for at home.
    (See Scharschmidt, 1992.)

DISCHARGE PLANNING

The client who is not a candidate for liver transplant may need:

Hospice referral.
Social work referral to volunteer services that provide in-home caregiver relief.
Home health aid around-the-clock for assistance with ADLs.
Equipment ordered: hospital bed, wheelchair, walker, bedside commode.
Family/significant other teaching related to skin or wound care, suctioning, dressing changes, oral care, medication administration, urinary catheter care, bowel care, and pain management.

The client who is a candidate for liver transplant may need:

2 to 4 weeks in the hospital after the transplant.
Teaching related to symptoms of infection and transplant rejection.
Home care referral for daily weight and vital sign monitoring.
Capillary glucose monitoring.
Teaching related to homegoing medication information and regimen.
Teaching about avoidance of the use of ethanol, which can prevent adequate evaluation of the success of the liver transplant.
Referral for mental health, reproductive, dependency counseling. The client should avoid pregnancy for at least 1 year after transplant.
Nutrition/dietician consultation.
Avoidance of travel to high-risk areas, due to immunosuppression.
Ability to keep follow-up appointments.
(See Zetterman, 1994.)

FOLLOW-UP CARE

Anticipated care (for clients discharged to hospice care)

Communication to hospice nurse of in-hospital plan of care for the client and family.

Communication to hospice nurse about ethical issues and resolution during hospital stay.

Social work referral for evaluation of client's home situation.

Pastoral care referral.

Assistive equipment such as a hospital bed, a wheelchair, a walker, and a bedside commode.

Anticipated client/family questions and possible answers

Will the confusion get worse?

"The confusion is likely to worsen. Because there is no way to get the liver to start working again, the symptoms will eventually progress to coma, and normally death will follow."

Will I have pain because of the liver damage?

No. Liver damage does not cause pain. Any pain you might have would be caused by other reasons, such as tissue damage from the cancer. The hospice nurse and your doctor will work out a plan with medicine to stop your pain.

Anticipated care
(for clients discharged after liver transplant)

Chemotherapy (adriamycin) is given prior to and after transplant.

Acyclovir prophylaxis for cytomegalovirus infection × 3 months.

Trimethoprim-sulfamethoxazole prophylaxis for pneumocystis infection × 1 year.

Rigorous lab testing. A typical schedule includes blood chemistries (Chem 23), CBC, and cyclosporin levels:

- q week × 2 weeks coordinated by the surgeon, then
- q week × 4 weeks coordinated by the hepatologist, then
- q month × 6 months coordinated by the hepatologist, then
- Staggered visits and measurements coordinated by the hepatologist, based on the client's progress, then
- Annual physicals, eye examination, and evaluation by the hepatologist for the remainder of the client's life.

Ultrasound may be needed if biliary obstruction is suspected.

Endoscopic retrograde cholangiopancreatography (ERCP) to relieve obstruction.

Liver biopsy if the client is unresponsive to antirejection treatment.

Long-term preventive health measures, including immunizations, screening for malignancy, screening for cardiac risk factors (i.e., hypertension, hypercholesterolemia, obesity, diabetes mellitus), and nutritional management (i.e., low-sodium diet for hypertension, American Diabetes Association [ADA] diet for pre- or post-transplant diabetes mellitus).

Management of the many metabolic side effects and treatment of the many complications (listed in Table 16-4) that may arise.

(See Sherman et al., 1995; Zetterman, 1994.)

Anticipated client/family questions and possible answers

Could I have hepatic encephalopathy again?

"Yes. This could happen again if your body rejects the transplanted liver."

How can I avoid getting an infection?

"By keeping yourself as healthy as possible, and by avoiding other people who are sick. This means you must get plenty of rest, eat a balanced diet, and keep as active as your doctor advises. If your family members have a cold, virus, or other problem that might be contagious, avoid touching or kissing them until they are better. Wash your hands frequently and always before touching your nose, mouth, or eyes. Your family members should always wash their hands well with soap after coughing or blowing their noses."

Table 16-4
Potential Metabolic Side Effects and Complications after Liver Transplant

Metabolic Side Effects	Complications
Diabetes (occurs in as high as 13% of clients . secondary to high-dose steroids)	Opportunistic infection
	Drug interaction
Hypertension (occurs in as high as 60% of clients).	Acute allograft rejection
Hypercholesterolemia	Chronic allograft rejection
Renal dysfunction	Biliary obstruction, stricture, or leakage
Immunosuppression	Intraabdominal abscess
Fever	Hepatitis
Headache	Depression

Source: Data from Munoz SJ: Long-term management of the liver transplant recipient. Med Clin North Am 80:1103–1116, 1996 and Stegall MD, Everson G, Schroeter G, Bilir B, Karrer F, Kam I: Metabolic complications after liver transplantation. Diabetes, hypercholesterolemia, hypertension, and obesity. Transplantation 60(9), 1057–1060, 1995.

CHAPTER SUMMARY

Although hepatic encephalopathy may be precipitated by many factors, the goals for the treatment of symptoms are the same: protecting the airway, controlling bleeding, decreasing the levels of circulating ammonia and other toxins, preventing and reducing increased intracranial pressure, and maintaining a positive nitrogen balance. Recognizing the signs and symptoms of hepatic encephalopathy can help the nurse anticipate and implement both immediate and long-term care needs, whatever the future might hold: comfort care during the dying process, reversal of the cause through liver transplantation, or discharge to hospice care.

TEST QUESTIONS

1. Hallmark symptoms of hepatic encephalopathy include all *except:*
   A. Decreased level of consciousness (LOC)
   B. Asterixis
   C. Pain
   D. Fetor hepaticus

1. Answer: C
Hallmark symptoms include reduced LOC; asterixis, or flapping tremor of the hands when outstretched; and fetor hepaticus, which is a musty breath odor caused by respiratory excretion of mercaptans left in the bloodstream after bypassing the liver, which normally performs mercaptan removal.

2. Conditions that may precipitate the symptoms of hepatic encephalopathy in the oncology client with pre-existing cirrhosis include all of the following *except:*
   A. GI bleeding
   B. Hypokalemia
   C. High-protein diet
   D. Low-protein diet

2. Answer: D
Oncology clients with pre-existing liver damage from cirrhosis have gradually developed alternate circulation pathways that allow ammonia, produced commonly in many oncologic complications, to bypass the liver, accumulate in the blood and cross the blood-brain barrier, and rapidly precipitate hepatic encephalopathy.

3. The goal(s) of immediate treatment for the symptoms of hepatic encephalopathy is/are to:
   A. Protect the airway
   B. Decrease circulating ammonia levels
   C. Decrease intracranial pressure (ICP)
   D. All of the above

3. Answer: D
Because the symptoms of hepatic encephalopathy may progress to obtundation, coma, and increased ICP, airway protection, and prevention of progression are the highest priorities.

4. What is the medication used to prevent intestinal ammonia absorption in clients with hepatic encephalopathy.
   A. Lactulose
   B. Vancomycin
   C. Metronidazole
   D. Nystatin

4. Answer: A
Lactulose given through a nasogastric tube prevents intestinal ammonia absorption and increases peristalsis, which moves the ammonia out of the body.

5 Anticipated interventions for increased ICP in the client with hepatic encephalopathy include all of the following *except:*
   A. Mannitol 20% 0.5 to 1.0 g IV
   B. Hypoventilation
   C. Maintain head-of-bed elevation of 10 to 30 degrees
   D. Decrease environmental stimuli

5. Answer: B
Hyperventilation is used to keep the client's $PaCO_2$ 30 to 32 mmHg and cause vasoconstriction, which reduces intracranial blood flow, thus preventing further increase in ICP.

6. Causes of hypovolemia in the oncology client with hepatic encephalopathy are *least likely* to include:
   A. Cardiogenic shock
   B. Hemorrhage
   C. Fluid shift to the interstitium secondary to hypoalbuminemia
   D. Fluid shift to the interstitium secondary to sepsis

6. Answer: A
Oncology clients with hepatic encephalopathy are at risk for hemorrhage due to impaired production of clotting factors. They are at risk for interstitial shifts of fluid due to impaired albumin production leading to decreased colloid osmotic pressure. They are also at risk for sepsis due to immunosuppression.

7. Hallmark *physical* signs of hepatic encephalopathy include:
   A. Hypertension, hemorrhage, hyperammonemia, and decreased urine output
   B. Jaundice, renal failure, neutropenia, and third-degree heart block
   C. Coagulopathy, jaundice, hypoglycemia and metabolic acidosis
   D. Hyperglycemia, metabolic alkalosis, thrombocytopenia, and hyperalbuminemia

7. Answer: C
See Assessment Criteria table.

8. The mortality rate in clients with hepatic encephalopathy who reach coma has been reported to be:
   A. 30%
   B. 45%
   C 65%
   D. 80%

8. Answer: D
Although mortality statistics for oncology clients with hepatic encephalopathy are not available, the condition in all clients carries a mortality rate of approximately 80% if symptoms become so severe that coma develops. The presence of hepatic dysfunction and encephalopathy places the client at increased risk of developing cerebral edema with transtentorial herniation, permanent neurologic damage, sepsis, respiratory, cardiovascular and renal failure.

9. Decorticate posturing appears in which stage of hepatic encephalopathy?
   A   Stage I (prodrome)
   B. Stage II (impending coma)
   C. Stage III (stupor)
   D. Stage IV (coma)

9. Answer: C
Neuromuscular signs that may appear in stage III of hepatic encephalopathy include asterixis, inability to cooperate with instructions, incoherent speech, nystagmus, positive Babinski response, clonus, decorticate and decerebrate posturing, rigidity and seizures.

10. All of the following serum lab values are usually *elevated* in the oncology client when hepatic encephalopathy is present, *except:*
    A. Alkaline phosphatase, GGT, ALT
    B. Direct bilirubin, indirect bilirubin, and total bilirubin
    C. Ammonia, PT, and PTT
    D. Glucose, cholesterol, and albumin

10. Answer: D
Glucose, cholesterol, and albumin are usually decreased in clients with hepatic encephalopathy secondary to impaired hepatic function.

REFERENCES

Alpert ME, Hutt MS, Wogan GN: Association between aflatoxin content of food and hepatoma frequency in Uganda. Cancer 28(1):253–260, 1971.

Bernuau J, Rueff B, Benhamou JP: Fulminant and subfulminant liver failure: Definitions and causes. Semin Liver Dis 6(97), 97–106, 1986.

Bonnice CA: Fulminant hepatic failure. *In* Rippe JM, Irwin RS, Alpert JS et al. (eds): Intensive Care Medicine. Boston: Little, Brown, 1985, pp. 747–754.

Chang AE, Schneider PD, Sugarbaker PH, Simpson C, Culnane M, Steinberg SM: A prospective randomized trial of regional versus systemic continuous 5-fluorodeoxyuridine chemotherapy in the treatment of colorectal liver metastases. Ann Surg 206(6):685–693, 1987.

Davidson CS: Hepatic coma. In Bockus HL (ed): Gastroenterology, vol 2, 3rd ed. Philadelphia: WB Saunders and Co, 1976.

Di Bisceglie AM, Rustgi VK, Hoofnagle JH, Dusheiko GM, Lotze MT: NIH Conference: Hepatocellular carcinoma. Ann Intern Med 108(3):390–401, 1988.

Douglass EC, Reynolds M, Finegold M, Cantor AB, Glicksman A: Cisplatin, vincristine, and fluorouracil therapy for hepatoblastoma: A Pediatric Oncology Group study. J Clin Onc 11(1): 96–99, 1993.

Douglass E, Ortega J, Feusner J, Reynolds M, King D, Finegold M, Haas J, Krailo M: Hepatocellular carcinoma (HCA) in children and adolescents: Results from the Pediatric Intergroup Hepatoma Study (CCG 8881/POG 8945). Proc Am Soc Clin Onc 13:A-1439, 420, 1994.

Ensminger WD: Phase I Study of Hepatic Arterial Yttrium-90 Glass Microsphere Therapy in Patients with Primary and Metastatic Liver Cancer (Summary last modified October 1988). University of Michigan Comprehensive Cancer Center, Ann Arbor: MICH-0785, clinical trial, closed, September 1, 1990.

Eras P, Sherlock P: Hepatic coma secondary to metastatic disease. Ann Intern Med, 74:591, 1971.

Ettinger LJ, Krailo MD, Gaynon PS, Hammond GD: A phase I study of carboplatin in children with acute leukemia in bone marrow relapse: A report from the children's cancer group. Cancer 3(72): 917–922, 1993.

Felipo V, Kosenko E, Minana MD, Marcaida G, Grisolia S: Toxicity and its prevention by L-carnitine. In Felipo V, Grisolia S (eds): Hepatic Encephalopathy, Hyperammonemia, and Ammonia Toxicity. New York: Plenum Press, 1994.

Hoover HC,: Phase II/III Randomized Study of Surgery Followed by No Further Treatment vs BCG-Tumor Vaccine with vs without Cyclophosphamide in Patients with Totally Resectable Liver Metastases from Colorectal Carcinoma (Summary last modified September 1988). Massachusetts General Hospital Cancer Center, Boston: MGH-CR1, clinical trial, closed, February 1, 1991.

Karl RC, Morse SS, Halpert RD, Clark RA: Preoperative evaluation of patients for liver resection: Appropriate CT imaging. Ann Surg 217(3):226–232, 1993.

Kattan J, Culine S, Theodore C, Droz JP: Phase II trial of ifosfamide, fluorouracil, and folinic acid (FIFO regimen) in relapsed and refractory urothelial cancer. Cancer Invest 3(13):276–279, 1995.

Kemeny N, Daly J, Reichman B, Geller N, Botet J, Oderman P: Intrahepatic or systemic infusion of fluorodeoxyuridine in patients with liver metastases from colorectal carcinoma. Ann Intern Med 107(4):459–465, 1987.

Lack EE, Neave C, Vawter GF: Hepatocellular carcinoma: Review of 32 cases in childhood and adolescence. Cancer 52(8):1510–1515, 1983.

Mousseau DD, Butterworth RF: Current theories on the pathogenesis of hepatic encephalopathy. Proc Soc Exp Biol Med 206(4):329–344, 1994.

Munoz S J: Long-term management of the liver transplant recipient. Med Clin North Am 80:1103–1116, 1996.

Ni YH, Chang MH, Hsu HY, Hsu HC, Chen CC, Chen WJ, Lee CY: Hepatocellular carcinoma in childhood: Clinical manifestations and prognosis. Cancer 68(8):1737–1741, 1991.

Order SE, Stillwagon GB, Klein JL, Leichner PK, Siegelman SS, Fishman EK, Ettinger DS, Haulk T, Kopher K, Finney K: Iodine 131 antiferritin, a new treatment modality in hepatoma: A Radiation Therapy Oncology Group study. J Clin Onc 3(12):1573–1582, 1985.

Ortega JA, Douglass E, Feusner J, Reynolds M, King D, Quinn J, Finegold M, Haas J, Krailo M: A randomized trial of cisplatin (DDP)/vincristine (VCR) 5-fluorouracil (5FU) vs. DDP/doxorubicin (DOX) i.v. continuous infusion (CI) for the treatment of hepatoblastoma (HB): Results from the Pediatric Intergroup Hepatoma Study (CCG-8881/POG-8945). Proc Am Soc Clin Onc 13:A-1421, 416, 1994.

Patt YZ: Phase I/II Trial of Pulse Hepatic Arterial FUDR Infusion Using the Medtronic Syn-chroMed Pump for Colorectal Cancer Metastatic to the Liver (Summary last modified January 1989). University of Texas—M.D. Anderson Cancer Center: MDA-ID-88006, clinical trial, closed, September 1, 1991.

Podolsy D, Isselbacher K: Cirrhosis of the liver. *In* Wilson JD, Harrison TR (eds): Principles of Internal Medicine, 12th ed. New York: McGraw-Hill, 1991.

Ravikumar TS, Steele G, Kane R, King V: Experimental and clinical observations on hepatic cryosurgery for colorectal metastases. Cancer Res 51(23, Part 1):6323–6327, 1991.

Scharschmidt B F: Acute and chronic hepatic failure. *In* Wyngaarden JB, Smith LH, Bennett JC, (eds): Cecil Textbook of Medicine, 19th ed. Philadelphia: W B Saunders Co. 1992.

Sherman S, Jamidar P, Shaked A, Kendall BJ, Goldstein LI, Busuttil RW: Biliary tract complications after orthotopic liver transplantation. Transplantation 60(5), 467–470, 1995.

Shulman H, Hinterberger W: Hepatic veno-occlusive disease—Liver toxicity syndrome after bone marrow transplantation. Bone Marrow Transplant 10(3): 197–214, 1992.

Smith SL: Patients with liver dysfunction. *In* Clochesy JM, Breu C, Cardin S, Rudy EB, Whittaker AA (eds): Critical Care Nursing. Philadelphia: WB Saunders Co, 1993, pp 970–1008.

Stegall MD, Everson G, Schroter G, Bilir B, Karrer F, Kam I: Metabolic complications after liver transplantation: Diabetes, hypercholesterolemia, hypertension, and obesity. Transplantation 60(9), 1057–1060, 1995.

Terran JC, McCullough AJ, Mullen KD: A three-step nutritional approach to patients with hepatic encephalopathy: How to correct malnutrition without worsening mental status changes. J Crit Illness 10(5):309–315, 1995.

Theobald M: Allorecognition and graft vs. host disease. Bone Marrow Transplant 15:489–498, 1995.

Tsukuma H, Hiyama T, Tanaks S, Nakao M, Yabuuchi T, Kitamura T, Nakanishi K, Fujimoto I, Inoue A, Yamakazi H: Risk factors for hepatocellular carcinoma among patients with chronic liver disease. New Engl J Med 328(25):1797–1801, 1993.

Zetterman RK: Primary care management of the liver transplant patient. Am J Med 96 (Suppl 1A): 1A-10S–1A-17S, 1994.

CHAPTER 17

HEPATIC VENO-OCCLUSIVE DISEASE

Helen Foley, MSN, RN

AND

Wendy Rowehl Miano, MSN, RN, AOCN

CHAPTER OBJECTIVES

At the completion of this chapter, the reader will be able to:

Differentiate risks associated with hepatic veno-occlusive disease (VOD).

Describe pathophysiology of hepatic VOD.

Discuss medical management specific to prevention of hepatic VOD and supportive therapies as a result of hepatic VOD.

Discuss nursing assessment and supportive therapies employed in treating hepatic VOD.

Provide teaching interventions for the client with hepatic VOD.

OVERVIEW

HEPATIC VOD is a major threat to the long-term survival of bone marrow transplant (BMT) recipients. It is a common and serious complication due to the preparative chemotherapy regimens used in BMT. This syndrome results in hepatomegaly, jaundice, fluid retention, and abdominal pain. VOD can progress to failure of major organ systems, specifically, renal and pulmonary systems. Severe VOD is frequently fatal. This chapter discusses the pathophysiology, risk factors, etiology, and the medical prevention and management of the disease. Important aspects of nursing assessment, treatment, support, and education of the client with VOD will be discussed.

DESCRIPTION

Pathophysiology

VOD is a syndrome of liver damage characterized by injury to hepatocytes and endothelium in zone 3 of the liver acinus. The exact sequence of molecular events leading to VOD is not known. However, it is thought by most experts that this cellular toxicity is associated with tumor necrosis factor-alpha release, which in turn triggers coagulation and consequent obstruction of the hepatic sinusoids and venules. Sinusoids are engorged with hepatocytes and red blood cells. This impairment in the hepatic microcirculation results in water retention, weight gain, elevation of serum bilirubin, and painful hepatomegaly. McDonald et al. (1993) reported initial symptoms of weight gain and hepatomegaly on the day of transplant in many clients, and subsequent hyperbilirubinemia between days T + 2 (Transplant plus 2 days) and T + 9 post-transplant. That symptoms appear so soon after transplant in hepatic VOD distinguishes this syndrome from other hepatic complications associated with BMT, such as graft vs. host disease, which initially appears after engraftment.

Diagnosis

The diagnosis of hepatic VOD is often difficult to determine, given the myriad of complications that may cause similar symptoms. These BMT complications often appear concomitantly. An individual undergoing BMT is not a good candidate for invasive diagnostic procedures, such as liver biopsy due to myelosuppression (specifically, thrombocytopenia). Most transplant physicians make the diagnosis of VOD based on the presence of two or more symptoms appearing within the first 20 days post-transplant (McDonald et al., 1993). An individual diagnosed with VOD can be classified retrospectively as having mild, moderate, or severe VOD. The classification is based on the extent of symptoms, which include hepatomegaly, sudden weight gain of more than 2% body weight, and hyperbilirubinemia greater than 2 mg/dL that is not attributable to other causes.

Individuals with severe VOD are much more likely to die than those with mild symptomatology. More than 50% of clients with severe VOD develop multiorgan failure, most commonly renal failure, pleural effusions, and pulmonary failure (McDonald et al., 1993).

RISK PROFILE

Etiology: The precise etiology of VOD remains obscure. Research over the past 5 years has been directed at determining predisposing factors. Because VOD occurs when chemotherapy is given as conditioning, it is suspected that it is related to the hepatic toxicities of specific preparative regimens. This view is supported by the evidence that hepatic VOD occurs just as frequently in clients receiving their own bone marrow as it does in those given well-matched donor marrow. Also, symptoms may appear before the marrow is administered.

Conditions: Many factors are thought to increase the risk of developing hepatic VOD. Clients with a history of and/or active hepatitis C infection

(Frickhofen et al., 1994) and those individuals receiving mismatched or matched unrelated allogeneic transplant grafts seem more likely to develop VOD. Elevated serum transaminase at the time of transplant correlates to an increased risk for developing the disease. The higher the serum transaminase, the higher the risk of hepatic VOD (McDonald et al., 1993).

Environment: None.

Foods: None.

Drugs: While conditioning with busulfan appears most clearly correlated with hepatic VOD (Essell et al., 1992), Meresse et al. (1992) and Shulman and Hinterberger (1992) observed that the syndrome may be seen in clients receiving a wide variety of preparative regimens, including those with total body irradiation. Clients being treated with antifungal agents, such as amphotericin, and antibiotic therapy, such as vancomycin, at the time of transplant have an increased risk of developing hepatic VOD. Individuals with fever at the time they receive the conditioning chemotherapy exhibit the same increased risk. It has not been established whether this predisposition is due to the toxicity of the concomitant drug therapy or results from the presumed underlying infection.

PROGNOSIS

In a comprehensive study of 355 subjects in a large transplant center, 190, or 54%, developed hepatic VOD. Forty-four of the clients were classified as having mild hepatic VOD, which did not require analgesics for painful hepatomegaly or diuresis. Ninety-two clients had moderate disease requiring sodium restrictions, diuresis, and analgesics, but it was eventually reversible. Fifty-four individuals had severe disease, or disease in which laboratory values and symptoms did not resolve before day 100 post-transplant. Seventy-nine of the 190 clients with hepatic VOD died before day 100 post-transplant. Of those, 54 deaths appeared to be directly related to liver complications. Mortality progressively increased according to the severity of hepatic VOD: 9%, 23%, and 98% of those with mild, moderate, and severe disease, respectively, did not survive past day 100 post-transplant. Thus, it was concluded that the more severe the disease, the more likely it was that the client would not survive the post-transplant period.

TREATMENT

Surgery: Not indicated.

Chemotherapy: Individual adjustment of busulfan doses based on pharmacokinetics is now available for clients who present with elevated serum transaminase levels. This strategy is currently under investigation and may prevent some of the liver injury that clients currently experience.

Radiation: Not indicated.

Medications: Heparin, which interferes with the initiation of the clotting cascade, has been investigated as a preventive strategy (Attal et al., 1992; Cahn et al., 1992). In a randomized trial of 161 clients, half of whom received 100 U/kg/day of heparin from the first day of conditioning through day T + 30 or discharge from laminar flow, this drug therapy appeared helpful in preventing hepatic VOD (Attal et al., 1992). In this preventive trial, of the 81 clients receiving heparin therapy, 2 clients developed hepatic VOD in this first month, as compared with 18 clients in the control group. Additional studies are under way to measure the safe and effective use of heparin as a preventive drug therapy. While treatment with recombinant tissue plasminogen activator (tPA) shows promise, more investigation is warranted. Another drug, ursodeoxycholic acid (ursodiol), whose mechanism of action includes protecting hepatocytes from cholestatic injury, is well tolerated and is currently under investigation as a protective agent (Berman, 1995).

Other medications are used whose goals are palliation and treatment of hepatic VOD. Diuretics may diminish ascites. Spironolactone (Aldactone) is the diuretic of choice, as it is relatively free of side effects. By inhibiting aldosterone, sodium and water excretion occur, whereas potassium is spared. Short-acting narcotics (morphine and hydromorphone) may be employed as analgesics. Meperidine is contraindicated because normeperidine, the metabolite of meperidine, may accumulate and cause central nervous system irritability. Lactulose may be used to reduce serum ammonia (thereby decreasing blood urea nitrogen) and the production of ammonia in the intestinal tract.

Procedures: Paracentesis may be performed to relieve ascites. Some individuals require hemodialysis and mechanical ventilation. Clients who do require hemodialysis and/or mechanical ventilation do not have a good prognosis.

Other: Prevention of hepatic VOD is especially important as conditioning chemotherapy regimens become increasingly more aggressive and potentially more toxic. Minimizing risk factors and careful selection of transplant candidates is an additional goal. Whenever possible, BMT in individuals with fever and/or those being treated with systemic antifungals and antibiotics should be delayed.

ASSESSMENT CRITERIA:
HEPATIC VENO-OCCLUSIVE DISEASE

Vital signs

Temperature	May be elevated.
Pulse	May be tachycardic.
Respirations	Tachypneic with pleural effusions.
Blood pressure	Systolic blood pressure may be elevated (secondary to portal hypertension).

(continued)

ASSESSMENT CRITERIA: HEPATIC VENO-OCCLUSIVE DISEASE *(continued)*

History	Due to the many associated risks for this condition, and unknown specific etiology, please refer to the Description and Risks Profile sections of this chapter.
Hallmark physical signs and symptoms	RUQ pain, ascites, hepatomegaly. Sudden weight gain. Nausea and vomiting with decreased appetite.
Additional physical signs and symptoms.	Pleural effusions.
Psychosocial signs	Lethargy; hepatic encephalopathy, which can result in traumatic mental status changes.
Lab values	Bilirubin (elevated). Serum sodium (elevated).
Diagnostic tests	None.
Other	Jaundice.

NURSING DIAGNOSIS

The nursing diagnoses specific to hepatic VOD and contributing factors are as follows.

Fluid volume, excess, related to abdominal ascites.

(Potential for) pain related to right upper quadrant (RUQ) tenderness, ascites.

(Potential for) altered nutrition: less than body requirements related to nausea and vomiting, and anorexia.

(Potential for) ineffective airway clearance related to pleural effusions.

(Potential for) knowledge deficit related to BMT complications/subsequent treatments and supportive therapy required to manage complications.

NURSING INTERVENTIONS

Immediate nursing interventions

Measure weight.
Take strict intake and output (I and O) measurement.
Monitor serum electrolytes, liver function enzymes, and bilirubin.
Measure abdominal girth.

Anticipated physician orders and interventions

Anticoagulant therapy may be initiated.
Implement diuretic therapy.

Implement sodium restriction (500 mg oral intake/day) to reduce fluid
   excess. Eliminate sodium from parenteral nutrition and IV additives.
Plasma expanders may be ordered to maintain adequate intravascular
   volume and renal perfusion.
Assess serum electrolytes.

Ongoing nursing assessment, monitoring, and interventions

Assess:
  • Level of consciousness, energy, strength.
  • Pain.
  • Nutrition status: nausea/vomiting, anorexia.
  • For respiratory compromise (shortness of breath, tachypnea due to
    effusions, diminished breath sounds, and/or crackles).

Measure:
  • Weight twice a day.
  • I and O (4-hour increments; 24-hour totals).
  • Abdominal girth qd.

Send: Serum electrolytes.

Implement: 2 g sodium restriction.

TEACHING/EDUCATION

Prevention of hepatic VOD: *Rationale:* Given pre-disposing conditions, you
may be at an increased risk for developing liver toxicity.

Management of ascites: *Rationale:* Limiting salt and salty foods helps to
reduce fluid overload. Checking your weight twice daily and carefully measuring your intake and output helps the health care team to accurately assess
and manage your fluid status.

Nutritional support: *Rationale:* IV nutrition may be needed to better control
your fluid balance and provide the nutrients your body needs.

Comfort: *Rationale:* Careful body positioning will be offered to improve comfort. Careful use of pain medications to relieve pain will be offered. An important goal with pain medication is to prevent further damage to the liver.

Coping: *Rationale:* It is very important that you and your family or significant other understand about the supportive care you will need because of
hepatic VOD. Understanding the reasons for each part of your care will help
you to cope better during this time.

EVALUATION/DESIRED OUTCOMES

1. Fluid volume returns to client's baseline. Weight returns to baseline.
2. Nausea, vomiting, and anorexia diminish with appropriate nutritional
   support.

3. Pain is diminished with appropriate intervention and analgesics.
4. The lungs remain clear to auscultation.
5. The client states understanding of supportive therapies: salt restriction, diuretics (as needed), anticoagulant therapy (as selected to decrease the severity of the syndrome), and nutritional support.

DISCHARGE PLANNING

The client experiencing VOD may need:

Ongoing assessment of liver function, post-BMT.
Short-term nutritional support to normalize fluid and electrolytes.
Family and significant others will require emotional support throughout the course of the syndrome, especially if the hepatic VOD progresses to a severe or potentially fatal state.

FOLLOW-UP CARE

Anticipated care

Liver toxicity may take weeks or months to completely resolve. Liver function tests and weight may be elevated, and abdominal swelling and liver enlargement may still be present for several months.
Nutrition and electrolyte supplementation should be ongoing until symptoms resolve and electrolytes are normal.
Follow-up transplant care will include weekly (or more frequent) visits through the first 3-month period.
Weekly lab work (to include liver function, electrolytes, blood counts).

Anticipated client/family questions and possible answers

What are my chances of survival with this condition?
"This is an important question to ask your physician. The condition may be mild to severe. Watching your symptoms and giving you adequate support throughout this condition are important treatment measures. Managing your liver symptoms through nutrition support, relief of swelling, pain management, and fluid/salt restrictions are the treatments your doctor uses to support you through this condition."

When might this condition happen and how long will it be present?
"This liver syndrome happens within the first few weeks (sometimes days) of transplant. The signs are quick: weight gain; changes in your labs; swelling in your right abdomen (liver) and possible pain; and nausea/vomiting, with loss of appetite. The syndrome, with supportive care, has to run its course. That may take an additional 1 to 2 weeks. Symptoms could be pres-

ent for several months, and we will continue to monitor them and treat you as long as they exist. You will likely return home before recovery from hepatic VOD is complete.

When I recover from VOD, can it recur?

"Generally VOD occurs in the first several weeks after transplant. Once the liver has recovered the syndrome does not recur."

"VOD is a specific liver problem after transplant. Once it has run its course, it is not likely to return. There are other liver problems that we carefully watch for, and treat, depending on what the underlying cause is."

CHAPTER SUMMARY

Hepatic VOD is a potentially fatal liver disorder specific to BMT recipients. Current research is aimed at preventative measures. Understanding of predisposing factors and proper medical management and nursing assessment are critically important in distinguishing VOD from other liver toxicities. Vigilant assessment and supportive therapies are imperative to ensure a favorable outcome for this complication.

TEST QUESTIONS

1. Hepatic VOD is a complication associated with bone marrow transplantation. This syndrome is best described as:
   A. An engraftment rejection
   B. An autoimmune dysfunction of the liver, as a result of the preparative regimen
   C. Liver damage characterized by injury to the hepatocytes
   D. An irreversible destruction of the liver endothelium

2. A risk factor associated with the development of hepatic VOD includes:
   A. History of hepatitis C
   B. Hematologic malignancy, such as acute or chronic leukemia
   C. Age
   D. Preparative regimen that includes alkylating chemotherapeutic agents

1. Answer: C
Injury occurs to both the hepatocytes and endothelium in zone 3 of liver acinus. The exact sequence of this syndrome is unclear. Hepatic VOD appears to result because of release of tumor necrosis factor-alpha, which in turn, triggers coagulation and consequent obstruction of hepatic sinusoids and venules.

2. Answer: A
A history of hepatitis C (current or previous exposure) has been implicated in the development of hepatic VOD.

3. A primary nursing diagnosis associated with the care of a client with hepatic VOD is:
   A. Fluid deficit related to hypovolemia
   B. Ineffective airway clearance related to pleural effusions
   C. Skin integrity, risk of impairment, related to capillary leak syndrome
   D. Infection, risk for development, due to neutropenia

3. Answer: B
Ineffective airway clearance related to pleural effusions can occur as a result of portal hypertension, ascites, and fluid overload.

4. A preventative drug used in BMT clients to decrease likelihood of developing VOD is:
   A. Aspirin
   B. Bumex
   C. Heparin
   D. Amphotericin B

4. Answer: C
Heparin, which interferes with the clotting cascade, has been investigated as a preventive strategy.

5. Signs and symptoms associated with hepatic VOD include:
   A. Anxiety, irritability, weight loss
   B. Lethargy, sudden weight gain, tachypnea
   C. Increased appetite, hypertension, decreased level of consciousness
   D. Nausea and vomiting, weight loss, hypokalemia

5. Answer: B
Lethargy (as a result of elevated liver enzymes and hepatic encephalopathy in severe cases); sudden weight gain (secondary to portal hypertension, ascites, obstruction of liver sinusoids and venules); and tachypnea (in response to pleural effusions) are hallmark signs of hepatic VOD.

REFERENCES

Attal M, Huguet F, Rubie H, Huynh A, Charlet J, Payen J, Voigt J, Brousset P, Selves J, Muller C, Pris J, Laurent G: Prevention of hepatic veno-occlusive disease after bone marrow transplantation by continuous infusion of low dose heparin: A prospective, randomized trial. Blood 79(11):2834–2840, 1992.

Berman S: The syndrome of hepatic veno-occlusive disease after marrow transplantation. Blood 85(11):3005–3020, 1995.

Berman S, Shuhart M, Hinds M, McDonald G: Recombinant human tissue plasminogen activator for the treatment of established severe veno-occlusive disease of the liver after bone marrow transplantation. Blood 80(10):2458–2462, 1995.

Cahn J, Flesch M, Brion A, Deconinck E, Leconte Des Floris M, Vuillat L, Plouvier E, Amsallem D, Tiberghien P, Fest T, Angonin R, Carbillet J, Herve P: Prevention of veno-occlusive disease of the liver after bone marrow transplantation: Heparin or no heparin? Blood 80(8):2149–2150, 1992.

Essel J, Thompson J, Harman G, Halvorson R, Snyder M, Johnson R, Rubinsak J: Marked increase in veno-occlusive disease of the liver associated with methotrexate use for graft-versus-host-disease prophylaxis in patients receiving busulfan/cyclophosphamide. Blood 79(10):2784–2788, 1992.

Frickhofen N, Wiesneth M, Jainta C, Hertenstein B, Heymer B, Bianchi L, Dienes H, Koerner K, Arnold R: Hepatitis C virus infection is a risk factor for liver failure from veno-occlusive disease after bone marrow transplantation. Blood 83(7):1998–2004, 1994.

Grandt N: Hepatic veno-occlusive disease following bone marrow transplantation. Oncol Nurs Forum 16(6):813–817, 1989.

McDonald G, Hinds M, Fisher L, Schoch H, Wolford J, Banaji M, Brugieres L, Lemerle J: Veno-occlusive disease of the liver and multiorgan failure after bone marrow transplantation: A cohort study of 355 patients. Ann Intern Med 118(4):255–267, 1993.

Meresse V, Hartmann O, Vassal G, Benhamou E, Valteau-Counanet D, Brugueres L, Lemerle J: Risk factors for hepatic veno-occlusive disease after high-dose busulfan-containing regimins followed by autologous bone marrow transplantation: A study of 136 children. Bone Marrow Transplant 10(3):197–214, 1992.

Shaffer S, Wilson J: Bone marrow transplantation: Critical care implications. Crit Care Nurs Clin North Am 5(3):531–541, 1993.

Shulman H, Fisher L, Schoch H, Henne K, McDonald G: Veno-occlusive disease of the liver after marrow transplantation: Histological correlates of clinical signs and symptoms. Hepatology 19(5):1171–1181, 1994.

Shulman H, Hinterberger W: Hepatic veno-occlusive disease—Liver toxicity syndrome after bone marrow transplantation. Bone Marrow Transplant 10(3):197–214, 1992.

Wujcik D, Ballard B, Camp-Sorrell D: Selected complications of allogeneic bone marrow transplantation. Semin Oncol Nurs 10(1):28–41, 1994.

CHAPTER 18

HYPERCALCEMIA

Deborah Kryspin Meriney, RN, MN, OCN

AND

Sara J. Reeder, PhD, RN

CHAPTER OBJECTIVES

At the completion of this chapter, the reader will be able to:

Define normal calcium homeostasis.

Identify the pathophysiologic mechanisms associated with malignant hypercalcemia.

Discuss the signs and symptoms of hypercalcemia.

Describe nursing management for the client with hypercalcemia.

Discuss the teaching/learning needs of clients with hypercalcemia.

OVERVIEW

HYPERCALCEMIA occurs in approximately 0.5% of all hospitalized clients (Nussbaum, 1993). However, hypercalcemia is one of the most life-threatening disorders associated with cancer, occurring in an estimated 10 to 20% of clients (Kaplan, 1994). Malignant hypercalcemia is usually progressive and causes the client's condition to deteriorate rapidly (Lang-Kummer, 1993). Prompt identification and treatment of this complication by the nurse, physician, and client are imperative to allay symptoms and prevent death.

DESCRIPTION

Normal calcium homeostasis

Calcium concentration in the body is maintained within a range of 9 to 11 mg/dl under normal conditions (Moore, 1994; Huether, 1994). A delicate balance among three forms of body calcium—stored (bone), ionized, and albumin bound (in serum)—helps to maintain serum calcium within the narrow range of 9 to 11 mg/dl (Kaplan, 1994). Most calcium (99%) is located in bone, where it combines with phosphate (forming an organic compound that contributes to bone rigidity), and the remainder is in the plasma and body cells. The total fraction of calcium circulating in the blood is small. Of the calcium in plasma, 50% is bound to plasma proteins and about 40% is in the free or ionized form. The protein-bound form of serum calcium is not biologically active and has no clinical significance (Huether, 1994). However, ionized calcium has important physiologic functions, such as maintaining neuromuscular function.

Serum calcium is often reported and measured as total serum calcium. Currently, there are newer, more precise instruments that can calculate ionized calcium, which normally ranges from 1.16 to 1.32 mmol/L (Nussbaum, 1993; Edelson and Kleerekoper, 1995). It is important to interpret calcium in relation to serum proteins, specifically, albumin. If the serum albumin is reduced, which is likely to occur in cancer clients because of anorexia and catabolic wasting, less calcium is protein bound (Kaplan, 1994; Moore, 1993; Nussbaum, 1993). Hypercalcemia should be suspected when a normal calcium level is associated with a significant reduction in serum albumin, since this may result in an elevation of ionized calcium. It is therefore important to measure either serum ionized calcium or, if ionized calcium is not available, to correct the serum calcium for the serum albumin concentration. If the client has hypoalbuminemia (below 4.0 g/dl), a convenient formula to increase the serum calcium is by 0.8 mg/dL for every 1 g/dL of albumin below normal (see Table 18–1).

Calcium is a necessary ion for many metabolic processes. In addition to its role in maintaining bones and teeth, calcium also influences enzymatic cofactors for blood clotting, nerve impulse transmission, hormone secretion, muscle contraction, and cellular permeability (Heuther, 1994). The ionized portion must be maintained within narrow limits to ensure neuromuscular activity and hormone secretion.

Table 18–1
Correction of Serum Calcium Levels

Step 1	Step 2	Step 3	Step 4
Sample lab reports: Ca^{++} = 10.0 mg/dL Albumin = 1.6 g/dL Increase calcium by 0.8 mg/dL for each 1.0 g/dL of albumin below normal: $$\frac{0.8}{1.0} = \frac{X}{\text{Corrected albumin}}$$	Correct albumin: Subtract low normal serum albumin level from report level: Normal 4.0 g/dL minus reported − 1.6 g/dL 2.4 g/dL	To correct under-reported Ca^{++}: $$\frac{Ca}{\text{Albumin}} = \frac{X}{\text{Corrected albumin}}$$ $$\frac{0.8}{1.0} = \frac{X}{2.4}$$ $X = 1.92$ mg/dL	Corrected Ca^{++} = Reported Ca^{++} + correction factor: 10.0 mg/dL + 1.92 mg/dL 11.92 mg/dL

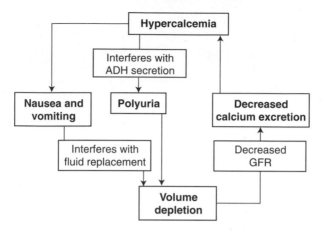

Figure 18–1 Negative feedback mechanism of hypercalcemia. Hypercalcemia interferes with antidiuretic hormone (ADH) secretion, causing a nephrogenic diabetes-insipidus-like syndrome that gives rise to polyuria. Despite the resulting extreme thirst, nausea and vomiting may interfere with fluid replacement, which leads to dehydration. Fluid volume depletion decreases the glomerular filtration rate (GFR), causing vasoconstriction of renal blood flow and further augmentation in calcium resorption.

In normal calcium homeostasis, the rate of bone formation is approximately equal to the rate of bone resorption, and calcium reabsorption from the gut is equal to the urinary excretion of calcium (Kaplan, 1994). Normal calcium is regulated by a negative feedback loop controlled by the concentration of three hormones: parathyroid hormone (PTH), vitamin D, and calcitonin (Kaplan, 1994; Heuther, 1994; Moore, 1993) (see Fig. 18–1).

PTH prevents serum calcium concentration from falling below a normal level by stimulating bone resorption (Lang-Kummer, 1994). PTH stimulates the activity of osteoclasts, which are multinucleated bone cells that break down bone tissue (Kaplan, 1994). Osteoclastic activity results in the release of calcium from storage in bone into the serum. The effect of PTH on the kidney is to regulate and fine-tune calcium balance. A fall in plasma calcium concentration stimulates the release of PTH and increases renal absorption of calcium (Lang-Kummer, 1993). PTH also stimulates the kidneys to convert vitamin D to an active form of 1,23-dihydroxy-vitamin D, which enhances the absorption of ingested calcium from the gastrointestinal (GI) tract (Huether, 1994). In addition, PTH regulates phosphorous levels in inverse proportion to calcium. Thus, if the concentration of one ion increases, that of the other decreases (Huether, 1994; Nussbaum, 1993). In the GI tract, 1,23-dihydroxyvitamin D stimulates the absorption of dietary calcium in response to low circulating levels of calcium, producing a net absorption of calcium from the gut equal to renal calcium excretion. Calcitonin inhibits bone resorption and thus acts as a counter-regulator to PTH.

Pathophysiology

In the past, cancer-related hypercalcemia was thought to be a consequence of bone metastasis. It is now known that the propensity of a tumor to develop hypercalcemia does not depend solely on the extent of skeletal involvement (Edelson and Kleerekoper, 1995). The reason for this is multifaceted and relates to factors that affect calcium transport at sites distant from metastases (Adami and Rossini, 1992). A host of etiologic factors have been described that have distant effects on calcium transport. Current evidence has shown that hypercalcemia is a complex metabolic complication in which the primary defect is an increase in bone resorption that exceeds both bone formation and the kidney's ability to excrete extracellular calcium. Three theories regarding malignant hypercalcemia will be presented below.

First, malignant hypercalcemia is thought to be caused by tumors that produce parathyroid-hormone-related protein (PTH-rP). PTH-rP is thought to reduce renal tubular reabsorption of phosphate, increase osteoclastic bone resorption, increase tubular reabsorption of calcium, and cause phosphate wasting (Lang-Kummer, 1993; Adami and Rossini, 1992). Hypercalcemia interferes with the action of antidiuretic hormone (ADH) on the kidney's collecting tubules, causing an inability to concentrate urine and polyuria (a syndrome similar to nephrogenic diabetes insipidus) (Lang-Kummer, 1993). PTH-rP appears to be the most common mediator of cancer-related hypercalcemia (Warrell, 1993). The discovery of this peptide in 1987 led to an understanding of the pseudo-hyperparathyroid features of a number of clients with malignant hypercalcemia.

Second, malignant hypercalcemia is thought to be caused by osteolytic prostaglandins of the E series. Research has shown that tumors grown in culture produce a bone-resorbing substance identified as prostaglandin E_2. Accelerated bone resorption results in increased serum calcium. The source of prostaglandin remains unclear; it may arise from the tumor, bone, or the renal medulla and remains an area of intensive investigation (Moore, 1994).

The third mechanism of hypercalcemia in malignancy is associated with the existence of osteoclast-activating factors. This activity is now understood to be associated with a variety of cytokines, including interleukin 1, lymphotoxin, and tumor necrosis factor (Warrell, 1993; Moore, 1994). Stimulation of osteoclasts, with resulting bone demineralization, increases serum calcium (Moore, 1994; Nussbaum, 1993). A critical factor in the immune response, interleukin 1 has been shown to stimulate bone resorption *in vitro* and hypercalcemia *in vivo* (Kaplan, 1994; Nussbaum, 1993). Lymphotoxin is a lymphocytic product with cytostatic effects on cancer cells. It has been shown to stimulate osteoclastic activity and induce hypercalcemia *in vivo*. Myeloma cells, which produce lymphotoxin, have been shown to be mediators of increased osteoclastic bone resorption and hypercalcemia. Tumor necrosis factor is a cytokine activated by the macrophages. It has been associated with malignant cachexia and chronic infections. Research indicates that tumor necrosis factor binds with lymphotoxin and is a powerful stimulator of bone resorption (Kinirons, 1993).

Clients with hypercalcemia can present with a wide variety of symptoms affecting multiple body systems. The clinical presentation of hypercalcemia is variable and does not correlate with serum calcium levels (see the Assessment Criteria section for summary of symptoms). However, there is some evidence to suggest that the rapidity of the development of hypercalcemia influences the degree and severity of symptoms.

RISK PROFILE

All of the following factors present greater risks when occurring in an elderly client.

Cancers: Breast, lung (commonly squamous cell carcinomas), multiple myeloma, renal cell, squamous cell carcinoma of the head and neck, adult T-cell leukemia/lymphoma, bladder, ovary, colon, prostate, seminomas, Ewing's sarcoma, thyroid.

Conditions: Hyperparathyroidism, milk-alkali syndrome, sarcoidosis, immobility, dehydration, renal dysfunction, skeletal fractures, acute osteoporosis, vitamin D intoxication, hyperthyroidism, Paget's disease, pheochromocytoma, tuberculosis, coccidioidomycosis, human immunodeficiency virus (HIV) infection, adrenal insufficiency.

Pediatrics: Infantile hyperphosphatasia.

Environment: None.

Foods: Excessive calcium, vitamin D intake. Foods containing calcium and vitamin D, which include almonds, broccoli, collards, dairy products, fortified orange juice, leafy green vegetables, milk, salmon, sardines, shrimp, soy beans, tofu.

Drugs: All-trans-retinoic acid, estrogens and antiestrogens, antacids containing calcium, calcium supplements, lithium, thiazide diuretics.

Pediatrics: 13-cis-retinoic acid.

PROGNOSIS

Without treatment, hypercalcemia is associated with a 50% mortality rate. The onset of hypercalcemia usually occurs late in the malignancy, when life expectancy is usually 1 to 6 months (Ralston, Gallagher, Patel, Campbell, and Boyle, 1990). The prognosis, then, is similar to the prognosis for that particular cancer. With malignancy, increased serum levels of PTH-rP indicate a decreased hypocalcemic response to bisphosphonates and an advanced tumor state and are thus associated with an extremely poor prognosis (Pecherstorfer et al., 1994). Despite a poor prognosis, the treatment of hypercalcemia may enhance the quality of life.

TREATMENT

Emergency measures to correct or decrease severe or life-threatening hypercalcemia must be instituted. The severity of the hypercalcemia depends on the underlying cause. Calcium levels are generally highest when related to malignancy or acute hyperparathyroidism. Treating the underlying cause is the most effective therapy for hypercalcemia. However, in cases of limited life span, where the malignancy is refractory and bone pain is intractable, the most compassionate course may be no treatment.

Surgery: For acute hyperparathyroidism and as indicated by the malignancy.

Chemotherapy: As indicated by the malignancy.

Radiation: As indicated by the malignancy.

Medications

   Avoid the use of drugs that may cause hypercalcemia, as indicated above.

   Give oral fluids 3 to 4 liters daily for clients with mild or asymptomatic hypercalcemia.

   Administer IV normal saline 5 to 8 L per day for moderate to severe hypercalcemia to replenish intravascular volume and restore the glomerular filtration rate, followed by 3 L daily to maintain hydration, unless such aggressive hydration is otherwise contraindicated.

   Administer IV loop diuretic therapy *after rehydration is complete* to enhance calcium excretion. Administration of diuretics prematurely will result in more profound dehydration and exacerbate the hypercalcemia.

   Administer drugs that inhibit bone resorption or increase bone formation (see Table 18–2).

   Provide analgesics for bone pain.

   Administer antiemetics and corticosteroids as indicated for chemotherapy and radiation therapy.

Procedures

   Hemodialysis for clients who develop renal failure.
   Placement of IV access for hydration and medication administration.
   Blood sampling to monitor lab values.

Table 18–2
Hypocalcemic Agents

Drug	Action	Comments
Calcitonin	Inhibits bone resorption.	Nontoxic; rapid onset and short duration of action. Tachyphylaxis quickly develops. Useful in decreasing calcium initially while more potent, longer-acting agents are taking effect.
Plicamycin (mithramycin)	Inhibits bone resorption.	One of the first recognized hypocalcemia agents. May cause nephrotoxicity, hepatotoxicity, and platelet defects. Potent tissue irritant; avoid extravasation.
Gallium nitrate	Increases bone formation.	Potent; hypocalcemic effect is sustained; causes dose-related nephrotoxicity.
Bisphosphonates First generation: Etidronate Second generation: Pamidronate Clodronate Third generation: Alendronate YM175 BM 21.0955	Inhibit bone resorption.	Lower serum calcium gradually over several days. Do not affect the renal component of hypercalcemia and therefore have limited efficacy in clients with elevated serum PTH-rP levels. *First generation:* Etidronate has little advantages over other therapies. *Second generation:* Presently pamidronate is the most effective therapy; clodronate may be an effective adjuvant therapy in breast cancer clients. *Third generation:* Presently these agents are under investigation.
Phosphate	Inhibits bone resorption.	May cause skeletal and potentially fatal soft tissue precipitation and are therefore not recommended.

Source: Adapted from Adami and Rossini, 1992; Fukumoto et al., 1994; Gulcalp et al., 1994; Kinirons, 1993; Nussbaum, 1993; Paterson et al., 1993; Wuster et al., 1993; Zysset et al., 1992.

Other

Increase mobility; if bedrest is necessary, perform active range-of-motion exercises.

During episodes of hypercalcemia, except for some lymphoma clients, calcium absorption from the gut is decreased; therefore, it is not necessary to restrict calcium in the diet of a client who may already have nutritional deficiencies.

ASSESSMENT CRITERIA: HYPERCALCEMIA

Vital signs

Temperature	Elevated
Pulse	Rapid and weak
Respirations	Tachypneic or normal
Blood pressure	Systolic blood pressure <90 mmHg or 20 mmHg below baseline

History

Symptoms	Decreased oral intake (nausea, vomiting, confusion, anorexia, stupor). Volume and electrolyte loss from GI tract (nausea, vomiting) and renal system (urine).
Conditions	Malignancy, hyperparathyroidism, milk-alkali syndrome, sarcoidosis, immobility, dehydration, renal dysfunction, skeletal fractures, acute osteoporosis, vitamin D intoxication, hyperthyroidism, Paget's disease, pheochromocytoma, tuberculosis, coccidiomycosis, HIV infection, adrenal insufficiency; clients receiving thiazide diuretics, lithium, estrogen, and antiestrogen therapy.
Weight pattern	Decrease of 1–2 kg/day.

Hallmark physical signs and symptoms

Anorexia, confusion, polydipsia, polyuria, weakness.

Additional physical signs and symptoms

Blurred vision, *bone pain,* cardiac arrest, coma, constipation, crystals on cornea, fatigue, hyporeflexia, hypotonia, ileus, increased digitalis sensitivity, muscle fatigue, *nausea and vomiting,* renal calculi, renal failure, seizures, stupor.

Psychosocial signs

Apathy, *disorientation,* lethargy, *personality changes.*

Lab values	**Adult Reference Range**	**Pediatric Reference Range**	**Result**
Calcium, serum	9–11 mg/dL	8.5–10.5 mg/dL	High
Calcium, urine	≤300 mg/day	≤300 mg/day	Low
Sodium, serum	135–147 mEq/L	136–146 mEq/L	Low
Potassium, serum	3.5–5.0 mEq/L	3.5–5.0 mEq/L	Low
Phosphorus, serum	2.5–5.0 mg/dl	2.5–4.5 mg/dl	Low
Creatinine, serum	0.6–1.2 mg/dl	0.5–1.4 mg/dl	High
BUN, serum	8–18 mg/dl	5–20 mg/dl	High

Diagnostic tests

Deep tendon reflexes	Diminished.
Electrocardiogram	Dysrhythmias, sinus bradycardia, short QT interval, wide PR interval.

Other

Consider serum calcium in relation to the albumin level and correct if the albumin is low: 0.8 mg% of calcium for every 1.0 g% of albumin (see Table 18–1).

NURSING DIAGNOSIS

The nursing diagnoses will vary, depending on the cause(s) of hypercalcemia. Some of the common diagnoses and etiologies are as follows.

Potential for injury related to:

- Seizure activity secondary to neurologic irritability.
- Confusion and mental status changes.
- Muscle fatigue.
- Pathologic fractures secondary to decreased bone density.
- Dysrhythmias secondary to hypercalcemia and hypokalemia.
- Blurred vision secondary to calcium crystals on the cornea.

Fluid volume deficit related to:

- Dehydration secondary to polyuria, nausea, and vomiting.
- Nausea and vomiting secondary to chemotherapy.

(Potential for) pain related to bone pain and pathologic fractures, secondary to decreased bone density.

Altered urinary elimination related to:

- Polyuria secondary to impaired ADH action on the kidneys.
- Renal failure secondary to decreased glomerular filtration rate.

Constipation related to dehydration.

(Potential for) ineffective individual and family coping related to:

- Unfamiliarity with sequelae and treatment for hypercalcemia.
- The onset of hypercalcemia signaling the recurrence of the cancer.

NURSING INTERVENTIONS

Immediate nursing interventions

Assess pulse, blood pressure, respirations, mental status, and neurologic status.

Initiate seizure precautions. Place suction equipment and oral airway at bedside.

Send STAT serum calcium, electrolytes, albumin, total protein, phosphate, blood urea nitrogen (BUN), and creatinine panel; urine calcium.

Obtain STAT electrocardiogram.

Establish patent IV access and obtain volumetric infusion pump.

Measure hourly intake and output (I and O). Insert indwelling urinary catheter, if necessary.

Institute safety precautions, including call bell within reach, side rails up and restraints, if necessary.

Anticipated physician orders and interventions

Decrease/discontinue medications that may cause hypercalcemia.
Reduce doses of digoxin.

Initiate chemotherapy or other treatments for the underlying malignancy or cause of the hypercalcemia.

Administer analgesics for bone pain.

Administer antiemetics as indicated for GI upset, chemotherapy premedication.

Administer laxatives and stool softeners as indicated for constipation.

Administer IV potassium chloride to correct hypokalemia.

Initiate dietary calcium restriction (lymphoma clients only).

Increase/encourage activity as tolerated qd, physical therapy PRN.

Asymptomatic/mild hypercalcemia: Encourage oral fluid intake 3 to 4 L daily.

Moderate to severe hypercalcemia:

- IV hydration with 5 to 8 L normal saline daily to promote sodium and calcium diuresis; 3 L daily to maintain hydration.
- Administer loop diuretic (usually furosemide) after rehydration is complete to promote calcium excretion.
- Initiate IV administration of hypocalcemia agents (see Table 18–2).
- Prepare for hemodialysis, as indicated.

Ongoing nursing assessment, monitoring, and interventions

Assess:

- Neurologic status q4h and PRN.
- For arrhythmias, bradycardia, tachycardia, cardiac arrest q4h and PRN.
- For nausea and vomiting and medicate with antiemetics as ordered PRN.
- For bone pain and medicate with analgesics as ordered PRN.
- For signs and symptoms of pathologic fractures.
- Urine for calcium crystals q4h and PRN.
- IV site for redness, edema, pain q4h and PRN, and throughout plicamycin infusion for signs and symptoms of extravasation.
- For signs and symptoms of fluid overload (due to treatment) q4h.
- For signs and symptoms of hypocalcemia (due to treatment) q4h.

Measure:

- Blood pressure, pulse, and respirations q4h.
- I and O q2h × 24 hours, then q4–8h thereafter.
- Weight qd.

Send:

- Serum calcium, albumin, phosphate, BUN, creatinine, and electrolyte panel in 24 hours and PRN.
- Repeat urine calcium in 24 hours and PRN.

Implement:

- Seizure precautions until serum calcium level is < 12 mg/dL.
- Dietary calcium intake restriction PRN (lymphoma clients only) as ordered.

- Safety precautions, including restraint devices—vest and wrist—as ordered PRN.
- Activity schedule—out of bed/ambulate at least three times a day, or active range-of-motion exercises if on bedrest.
- Treat plicamycin extravasation with cold compresses q2–4h and PRN.

TEACHING/EDUCATION

Maintain adequate hydration: *Rationale:* You can become dehydrated from frequent urination, vomiting, and loss of appetite. Report any changes, such as dry mouth, too little or too much urine, changes in bowel habits, or changes in your weight.

Mobilize when possible: *Rationale:* Moving around independently as much as possible is important to keep calcium in your bones. Report any pain over bony areas. Fractures can occur because calcium is leaving your bones.

Report changes in sensory status: *Rationale:* Report any changes in your ability to think clearly, drowsiness, or personality changes. Too much calcium can cause these types of changes.

Report changes in heart rate: *Rationale:* Calcium affects your heart muscle. Report any changes in your heart rate—if you feel it is beating too fast or too slowly.

Continue your usual diet: *Rationale:* A high blood calcium is usually caused by calcium leaving your bones, not by what you eat. Therefore, it is not necessary to avoid eating foods that contain calcium (except in the case of lymphoma clients).

EVALUATION/DESIRED OUTCOMES

1. Serum Ca^{++} decreases 2–3 mg/dl within the first 24 to 48 hours.
2. Serum Ca^{++} returns to normal range within 5 to 7 days.
3. Serum electrolytes return to and are maintained within the normal range.
4. The client is free from injury.
5. The client is free from the signs and symptoms of hypercalcemia or hypocalcemia.
6. The client is free from the signs and symptoms of dehydration or fluid overload.
7. The indwelling urinary catheter is discontinued within 72 hours.
8. Chemotherapy or other antineoplastic treatment is commenced within 72 hours.
9. The client's activity and mobilization are maximized, as his or her condition allows.

10. Constipation resolves within 5 days.
11. The signs and symptoms of hypercalcemia and preventative measures are understood by client and/or caregiver prior to discharge.

DISCHARGE PLANNING

The hypercalcemic client may need:

Intervention for volume deficit when having vomiting, polyuria, and decreased oral intake.

Home care nursing visits to assist with pain management and mobility from muscular weakness.

Training of the client and/or significant others regarding the signs and symptoms of hypercalcemia.

FOLLOW-UP CARE

Anticipated care

Physician office visit within 1 week.

Outpatient testing for serum electrolytes within the week.

Urine analysis within 1 week.

Continuation of dietary regimen.

Home health nursing visits on weekly basis for client to assist with pain management and mobility.

Anticipated client/family questions and possible answers

Will this problem with hypercalcemia happen again?

"It is likely that this problem will happen again. Knowing the signs and symptoms of hypercalcemia can help you determine when to call your doctor or nurse."

"Whenever you experience vomiting, frequent urination, constipation, or any change in personality, call your doctor. These may be early warning signs of hypercalcemia."

"Treatment of your cancer may prevent hypercalcemia from happening again, although you should still watch for signs of hypercalcemia."

Should I try to move even if I have pain?

"Yes, you should try to stay as active as possible. Moving around is good because it helps keep calcium in your bones."

"Yes, using pain medication before you get up may help."

"Yes, but be sure to have someone help you, since you may be weak and are at risk for falling."

"Yes, but if your pain continues even after taking medication, or if it gets worse, be sure to tell your doctor or nurse."

Should I change my diet?

"You should continue your regular diet. The source of calcium is from your bones, not what you eat. Drink plenty of fluids so that you won't become dehydrated."

"Drinking lots of fluid helps you get rid of excess calcium."

(For lymphoma clients:) "Yes, you should avoid foods high in calcium and vitamin D. The calcium you eat is one reason your blood calcium is high."

Should I avoid certain medications?

"Avoid taking antacids containing calcium and calcium pills. Remind your doctor that you have hypercalcemia. Some prescription drugs may also cause hypercalcemia."

CHAPTER SUMMARY

Hypercalcemia is one of the more common oncologic emergencies, occurring in about 10 to 20% of cancer clients. It causes rapid deterioration. Three mechanisms—tumors that produce PTH-rP, osteolytic prostaglandins, and osteoclast activating factors—are thought to be the cause of malignant hypercalcemia. Hypercalcemia affects all the body systems. The symptoms generally appear when the serum calcium exceeds 12 mg/dl and may be confused with the cancer or its treatment. The management of hypercalcemia focuses on attenuating acute symptoms and treating the underlying cause. An understanding of calcium and its role in the body are essential for effective treatment, care, and teaching.

TEST QUESTIONS

1. Hypercalcemia is most commonly associated with which type of cancer?
   A. Cervical
   B. Breast
   C. Melanoma
   D. Liver

1. Answer: B
Hypercalcemia is most common in persons who have breast cancer.

2. The signs of hypercalcemia include:
   A. Polyuria and polyphagia
   B. Increased urine calcium and weight loss
   C. Anorexia and hyperkalemia
   D. Confusion and dehydration

2. Answer: D
Confusion is due to the effect of calcium and electrolyte abnormalities on the central nervous system. Dehydration results from nausea, vomiting, and polyuria.

3. Which IV treatment is appropriate for a prolonged (over several days) hypocalcemic effect?
   A. Pamidronate
   B. Normal saline 5 to 8 L per day
   C. Calcitonin
   D. Phosphate

3. Answer: A
Pamidronate, a bisphosphonate, lowers serum calcium gradually over several days.

4. A client with multiple myeloma asks the nurse how hypercalcemia can be prevented. The best response is:
   A. "The plicamycin you are receiving will permanently prevent hypercalcemia."
   B. "Omit all dairy products from your diet when you go home."
   C. "Decrease your activity level to decrease the stress on your bones."
   D. "The chemotherapy to treat your cancer can help to prevent hypercalcemia."

4. Answer: D
Treating the underlying cancer is the only definitive means of preventing hypercalcemia.

5. In a client with cancer and bone metastases, which symptom should alert a nurse to the early presence of hypercalcemia?
   A. Muscle cramps
   B. Edema
   C. Dyspnea
   D. Polyuria

5. Answer: D
Polyuria is one of the presenting, early signs of hypercalcemia.

6. A client's serum calcium is 10.2 mg/dl (normal = 9 to 11 mg/dl), and the serum albumin is 2.0 g/dl (normal = 4.0 to 6.0 g/dl). The nurse correctly concludes that this client is:
   A. Normocalcemic
   B. Hypercalcemic
   C. Hypocalcemic
   D. Hyperalbuminemic

6. Answer: B
The corrected serum calcium indicates hypercalcemia. Result is 10.2 + 0.8 + 0.8 = 11.8 mg/dl.

7. Which of the following factors is not a mechanism of malignant hypercalcemia?
   A. Calcitonin
   B. Osteoclast activating factor
   C. Parathyroid-related protein
   D. Cytokines

7. Answer: A
Calcitonin inhibits bone resorption.

8. The pathophysiology of hypercalcemia includes:
   A. Fluid overload
   B. Anuria
   C. Sodium retention
   D. Hyperphosphatemia

8. Answer: C
Sodium and calcium are resorbed by the renal tubules during hypercalcemia.

9. Serum calcium must be considered in conjunction with:
   A. Serum potassium
   B. Serum albumin
   C. Serum phosphate
   D. Urine calcium

9. Answer: B
Serum calcium must be considered with serum albumin because calcium is 50% protein bound.

10. Nursing management for the client with hypercalcemia includes:
    A. Instituting seizure precautions
    B. Maintaining a 1000 ml fluid restriction
    C. Maintaining bedrest
    D. Administering thiazide diuretics

10. Answer: A
Instituting seizure precautions is an appropriate nursing intervention for the client with hypercalcemia.

REFERENCES

Adami S, Rossini M: Hypercalcemia of malignancy: Pathophysiology and treatment. Bone 13:S51–S55, 1992.

Edelson M, Kleerekoper M: Hypercalcemic crisis. Med Clin North Am 79:79–92, 1995.

Fukumoto S, Matsumoto T, Takebe TO, Onaya T, Eto S, Nawata H, Ogata E: Treatment of malignancy-associated hypercalcemia with YM175, a new bisphosphonate: Elevated threshold for parathyroid hormone secretion in hypercalcemic patients. J Clin Endocrinol Metab 79(1):165–170, 1994.

Gulcalp R, Theriault R, Gill I, Madajewicz S, Chapman R, Navari R, Ahmann K, Zelenakas K, Heffernan M, Knight RD: Treatment of cancer-associated hypercalcemia: Double-blind comparison of rapid and slow intravenous infusion regimens of pamidronate disodium and saline alone. Arch Intern Med 154:1935–1944, 1994.

Huether S: The cellular environment: Fluids and electrolytes, acids, and bases. In McCance K, Huether S (eds): Pathophysiology: The Biologic Basis for Disease in Adults and Children, 2nd ed. St. Louis, MO: Mosby, 1994, pp. 107–113.

Kaplan M: Hypercalcemia of malignancy: A review of advances in pathophysiology. Oncol Nurs Forum 21(6):1039–1047, 1994.

Kinirons MT: Newer agents for the treatment of malignant hypercalcemia. Am J Med Sci 305(6):403–406, 1993.

Lang-Kummer J: Hypercalcemia. In Goenwald S, Frogge M, Goodman M, Yarbro C (eds): Cancer Nursing: Principles and Practice. Boston: Jones and Bartlett, 1993, pp. 644–660.

Moore J: Metabolic emergencies. In Gross J, Johnson B (eds): Handbook of Oncology Nursing, 2nd ed. Boston: Jones and Bartlett, 1994, pp. 675–691.

Nussbaum SR: Pathophysiology and management of severe hypercalcemia. Endocrinol Metab Clin 22(2):343–362, 1993.

Paterson AHG, Powles TJ, Kanis JA, McCloskey E, Hanson J, Ashley S: Double-blind controlled trial of oral clodronate in patients with bone metastases from breast cancer. J Clin Oncol 11(1):59–65, 1993.

Pecherstorfer M, Schilling T, Blind E, Zimmer-Roth I, Baumgartner G, Ziegler R, Raue F: Parathyroid hormone-related protein and life expectancy in hypercalcemia cancer patients. J Clin Endocrinol Metab 78(5):1268–1270, 1994.

Ralston SH, Gallagher SJ, Patel U, Campbell J, Boyle IT: Cancer associated hypercalcemia: Morbidity and mortality. Ann Intern Med 112:499–504, 1990.

Warrell RP: Metabolic emergencies: Hypercalcemia. In DeVita VT, Hellman S, Rosenberg S (eds): Cancer: Principles and Practice of Oncology, 4th ed. Philadelphia: JB Lippincott, 1993, pp. 2128–2134.

Wuster C, Schoter KH, Thiebaud D, Manegole C, Krahl D, Clemens MR, Ghielmini M, Jaeger P, Scharla SH: Methylpentylaminopropylidenebisphosponate (BM 21.0955): A new potent and safe bisphosphonate for the treatment of cancer-associated hypercalcemia. Bone Miner 22(2):77–85, 1993.

Zysset E, Ammann P, Jenzer A, Gertz BJ, Portmann L, Rizzoli R, Jaquet-Muller F, Pryor-Tillotson S, Bonjour JP, Burckhardt P: Comparison of a rapid (2-h) versus a slow (24-h) infusion of alendronate in the treatment of hypercalcemia of malignancy. Bone Miner 17(3):237–249, 1992.

CHAPTER 19

HYPERKALEMIA

Wendy Cooper, RN, BSN, OCN

AND

Cynthia C. Chernecky, PhD, RN, CNS, AOCN

CHAPTER OBJECTIVES

At the completion of this chapter, the reader will be able to:

Define hyperkalemia.

Differentiate the three principle causes of hyperkalemia.

Define pseudohyperkalemia.

State the risk factors associated with hyperkalemia in the oncology client.

Describe nursing care as it relates to oncology clients with acute hyperkalemia.

Anticipate and prepare the client with hyperkalemia for future care needs.

OVERVIEW

HYPERKALEMIA is a condition that occurs when the serum potassium (K^+) concentration is 5 mEq/L (5 mmol/L SI Units) or greater (Chernecky and Berger, 1997). The normal serum concentration levels fall between the range of 3.5 to 5.0 mEq/L (3.5 to 5.0 mmol/L SI Units). This condition can induce catastrophic symptoms leading to death. The client with cancer has a greater risk for increased levels than the general hospital population in part because of the massive amounts of K^+ released from destroyed malignant cells during the course of cancer-related treatments (Shelton, Baker, and Skecher, 1996). The elderly cancer client has an additional risk for hyperkalemia due to the decrease in renal function associated with the general aging process (O'Donnell, 1995). The renal risk factor is also increased by the use of multiple medications, which place an additional burden on the kidneys.

DESCRIPTION

Potassium is sometimes referred to as the chief intracellular electrolyte. It serves several body functions, including controlling the vital transmission of electrical impulses, and is involved in the homeostatic mechanisms of acid-base balance (De Fronzo and Smith, 1994). It is essential in maintaining electrical conduction within the cardiac and skeletal muscles. Lethal cardiac dysrhythmias (ventricular tachycardia, ventricular fibrillation) are the most serious consequences of hyperkalemia. To complicate matters, in many clinical situations, initial K^+ deficit can slowly or abruptly shift into excess, and excess can shift back into deficit. The speed of development of this complication can be accelerated in the seriously ill client, whose homeostasis is already compromised. In some instances, cardiac arrest is the first sign of hyperkalemia.

Several bodily regulatory mechanisms maintain a K^+ balance: aldosterone production, dietary intake, gastrointestinal (GI) tract excretion, and renal elimination or retention. Three categories of causes of hyperkalemia exist: (1) factitious (pseudo-) hyperkalemia, (2) redistribution of K^+ from the intracellular to the extracellular compartment, and (3) decreased renal excretion of K^+.

Pseudohyperkalemia

Pseudohyperkalemia is a condition in which laboratory results show an elevated K^+ level without the systemic condition of hyperkalemia (see Table 19–1). This is the first cause of hyperkalemia that should be ruled out with ·every high K^+ level. A key element to differentiate between true hyperkalemia and pseudohyperkalemia is an elevated serum K^+ level without the expected electrocardiogram (ECG, EKG) changes. The major contributing cause of this problem is hemolysis of the blood sample due to use of a small-gauge needle, turbulence during collection, or rough handling of the specimen. Red blood cell trauma due to tight tourniquet placement or pumping of the hand can cause a 20% increase in serum K^+ level. Laboratory reports typically note whether specimen hemolysis was evident. In such instances, a repeat sample must be drawn before any treatment for potassium elevation is undertaken. False elevations may also be reported in clients with thrombocytosis or leukocytosis, if the blood sample coagulates and large amounts of K^+ are released from platelets or white blood cells.

Redistribution of K^+ from the intracellular to the extracellular compartment

Ninety-eight percent of K^+ is normally contained within the intracellular compartment. The extracellular fluid contains the other 2% of total body K^+.

Table 19–1
Causes of Pseudohyperkalemia

Hemolysis *in vitro*
Marked leukocytosis
Marked thrombocytosis
Traumatic phlebotomy
Rare familial conditions

Redistribution of K^+ is influenced by serum aldosterone, sodium, pH, and glucose sodium levels (Perez, 1995).

Influence of Aldosterone and Sodium

Aldosterone regulates the K^+ levels by influencing cellular uptake and renal excretion of this electrolyte. In normal persons, aldosterone promotes reabsorption of sodium and water by the kidneys in response to low intravascular volume. As sodium (a positive ion) is reabsorbed, potassium (another positive ion) is excreted in the urine to maintain ionic balance. An aldosterone deficiency promotes intracellular conservation of sodium and water and a shift of K^+ into the bloodstream from the intracellular space to maintain ionic balance as sodium is lost in the urine. Because a reciprocal relationship appears to exist between K^+ and sodium, a concurrent electrolyte abnormality may be serum sodium deficit (hyponatremia). The reader is referred to Chapter 25 for further information on this topic.

Influence of Acidic Blood pH (acidemia)

Respiratory and metabolic acidosis are the most common conditions causing a compensatory exchange of intracellular K^+ for extracellular hydrogen and are a significant cause of hyperkalemia in the oncology client. High levels of lactic acid can occur in the client with certain malignant cells when the condition of tumor lysis syndrome occurs. Toxic cell lysis releases massive amounts of K^+ and other substances from the destroyed malignant cells during treatment. (The reader is referred to Chapter 43 for further information on this condition.) Lactic acidosis can also result in the client with liver metastasis, because lactic acid cannot be sufficiently metabolized through the impaired hepatic system. Because hyperkalemia is potentially one of the most devastating consequences of rapid tumor lysis, K^+ is not normally administered to clients undergoing high-dose chemotherapy. (The reader is referred to Chapter 27 for further information.)

Influence of Glucose Level

Elevations of serum glucose in conditions such as diabetic ketoacidosis cause concomitant loss of serum K^+ through extracellular shifting of K^+ and osmotic diuresis.

Decreased renal excretion of K+

Daily dietary K^+ intake is usually about 40 to 100 mEq (40 to 100 mmol SI Units), equaling 1500 to 4000 mg. Almost all of dietary K^+ is excreted by the kidneys with a small percentage lost through the GI tract. The ability to retain or excrete K^+ in states of deficit or excess is influenced by the state of functioning of the distal convoluted tubules of the nephrons in the kidneys.

Sustained hyperkalemia can be prevented in clients with normal renal function because the excess K^+ is excreted at these tubules through diuresis. In acute or chronic renal impairment, however, potassium that is normally excreted is not able to be filtered out of the bloodstream into the urine. The possibility of renal impairment is increased in oncology clients receiving multiple drugs, which place an additional burden on the kidneys.

RISK PROFILE

Cancers: Burkitt's lymphoma, Hodgkin's disease, acute lymphoblastic leukemia, lymphosarcoma, oat cell lung carcinoma, adrenal metastasis.

Pediatrics: Burkitt's lymphoma, T-cell lymphoma, acute leukemia, severe dehydration.

Conditions: Acidosis, Addison's disease, adrenal hypofunction, acute renal failure, acute tubular necrosis, acute post–streptococcal glomerulonephritis, excessive IV infusion of K^+ (rare), severe tissue trauma, tumor lysis syndrome.

Environment: None.

Foods: Low-sodium diet, excessive intake of dietary potassium (rare). High levels of K^+ are contained in apricots, prunes, bananas, potatoes, dates, tomatoes, cantaloupe, peaches, scallops, veal, beans, mushrooms, squash, figs, orange juice, tomato juice, and prune juice.

Drugs: See Table 19–2.

Table 19–2
Common Drugs That Can Contribute to Elevated K^+ Levels

Drug	Mechanism
Amphotericin B	Renal tubular damage resulting in impaired K^+ excretion.
Cyclophosphamide	Unknown.
Diuretics, potassium-sparing: acetazolamide, amiloride, spironolactone, triamterene, and thiazides (chlorothiazide, hydrochlorothiazide, metolazone).	Hemoconcentration.
Diuretics, osmotic: Mannitol	Hemoconcentration.
Glucose	Osmotic diuresis and hemoconcentration.
Methicillin	Renal damage resulting in impaired K^+ excretion.
Nonsterile anti-inflammatory drugs (NSAIDs) (ibuprofen, naprosyn sodium)	Renal damage resulting in impaired K^+ excretion.
Penicillin G potassium	Contains potassium.
Potassium chloride	Direct serum infusion of K^+.

PROGNOSIS

Less severe symptoms may be present in the client who develops hyper-kalemia over a longer period of time, such as in chronic renal failure (Kelly, 1996), than in the client whose condition develops rapidly. The type and severity of symptoms also depend on how high the serum K^+ becomes. Serum K^+ levels of 6.6 to 8.0 mEq/L (6.6 to 8.0 mmol/L SI Units) are most likely to cause cardiac dysrhythmias, and levels >8 mEq/L (8 mmol/L SI Units) most often cause acute symptoms, which may include cardiac arrest. Such clients require immediate intensive medical and nursing interventions.

TREATMENT

Surgery: None.

Chemotherapy: Discontinue or decrease doses of chemotherapy.

Radiation: None.

Medications

Discontinue IV solutions containing K^+.
Administer IV 0.45% saline or 5% dextrose for dehydration.
Administer IV, K^+-wasting, diuretic therapy.
Initiate prescribed treatment of medications (see Table 19–3).

Procedures: Hemodialysis is the preferred method for quick reduction of potentially lethal K^+ levels.

Other: Dietary restriction of K^+-containing foods.

Table 19–3
Medications Used to Treat Hyperkalemia

Medication	Dose and Route	Action
Calcium gluconate	10–20 ml of 10% solution IV.	Stabilizes cardiac membranes; positive inotropic effect counteracts K^+'s effect on the cardiac muscle contractility.
Insulin with glucose	10 units regular insulin preceded by 1 ampule of 50% dextrose IV.	Shifts K^+ intracellularly.
Beta-adrenergic agonist	20 mg albuterol in 4 ml normal saline via nebulizer.	Shifts K^+ intracellularly.
Sodium bicarbonate	One 50 mEq ampule IV.	Shifts K^+ intracellularly.
Cation exchange resin	30 g by mouth *or* 50 g per rectum of sodium polystyrene sulfonate (Kayexalate).	Causes exchange of sodium for K^+ in the gut. K^+ leaves the body through the GI tract.

ASSESSMENT CRITERIA: HYPERKALEMIA

	Hyperkalemia	Pseudohyperkalemia
Vital signs		
Temperature	Normal	Normal
Pulse	Rapid, irregular	Normal
Respirations	Tachypneic	Normal
Blood pressure	Decreased	Normal
History	Excessive K+ intake	Leukocytosis, thrombocytosis
Hallmark physical signs and symptoms	Muscle weakness, nausea, diarrhea, heaviness of limbs, muscle irritability progressing to flaccid paralysis, oliguria, slowing of pulse (see ECG changes described below).	No changes
Additional physical signs and symptoms	Colicky pain, difficulty speaking, malaise, oliguria.	No changes
Psychosocial signs	Apprehension, disorientation, nervousness.	None
Lab values		
K^+, serum	High	High
K^+, urine	Low	Normal
Sodium, serum	Low	Normal
Sodium, urine	Low	Normal
WBC count, total, and/or platelet count, total	Normal or low	May be high
Arterial blood gas	May show acidemia if a contributing cause of hyperkalemia.	No change
Diagnostic tests		
ECG changes:		
K^+ = 5.5–7.8 mEq/L	Tall, narrow, symmetrically peaked T waves and short Q-T interval.	No changes
K^+> 7.8 mEq/L	Shortened P-R interval, disappearing P wave, and widened QRS complex with continued rise in serum K^+ levels. Bradycardia, ventricular tachycardia/fibrillation, or cardiac standstill may occur.	No changes
Other	None	None

NURSING DIAGNOSIS

Altered tissue perfusion, cardiopulmonary, related to possible lethal cardiac dysrhythmias resulting from cardiac muscle weakness.

Decreased cardiac output related to bradycardia.

Knowledge deficit related to the unknown occurrence and treatment for hyperkalemia.

Potential for injury related to muscle weakness and paresthesia.

(Potential for) altered urinary elimination, decreased, related to impaired renal function resulting in fluid retention.

NURSING INTERVENTIONS

Immediate nursing interventions

Send serum sample to laboratory for analysis STAT. Collect sample without hemolysis and leave tourniquet in place less than 1 minute.

Assess history for drugs that can raise serum K^+ level (see Table 19-2).

Initiate continuous cardiac monitoring, and monitor for bradycardia and ectopy.

Compare ECG T-wave height and morphology to baseline ECG, if available.

Establish patent IV access.

Implement bedrest to avoid falls, and prepare for possible cardiac arrest.

Anticipated physician orders and interventions

Decrease and discontinue chemotherapy that may cause hyperkalemia.

STAT serum K^+ and sodium.

Administer:
- Calcium gluconate 10 to 20 ml of 10% solution IV over 5 minutes.
- Regular insulin either IV push or IV over 4 hours.
- 1 ampule 50% dextrose IV prior to insulin.
- 50 mEq ampule of sodium bicarbonate IV.
- Kayexalate by enema or via nasogastric tube.
- K^+-wasting (loop) diuretics IV.
- Antiemetics, antidiarrheal medications.

Prepare client for hemodialysis.

Transfer client to critical care unit.

Ongoing nursing assessment, monitoring, and interventions

Assess:
- Diet for K^+-containing foods.
- For signs of nausea.
- ECG for peaked T-wave and/or ventricular fibrillation/tachycardia.

- For increased platelets and/or white blood cells (WBCs) for possible pseudohyperkalemia.
- For muscle weakness q4h × 24 hours.
- For colicky pain or abdominal cramps q4h × 24 hours.
- Serum venous samples for hemolysis.
- Deep tendon reflexes (DTRs) q8h until K$^+$ level normalizes.
- Skin temperature, color, moisture, and turgor q8h.
- Level of consciousness (LOC) q8h.
- For dependent edema q8h.

Measure:
- Blood pressure, pulse, respirations q4h.
- Intake and output (I and O) q1h × 24 hours.
- Weight qd.
- Peripheral pulses q8h.

Send: Repeat serum K$^+$ and sodium.

Implement:
- Low-K$^+$ diet, primarily for clients with renal impairment.
- Fall and/or safety precautions.
- Bedrest until K$^+$ level normalizes and signs of muscle weakness are gone.
- Adequate oral hydration.

TEACHING/EDUCATION

Decreased/discontinued chemotherapy: *Rationale:* Certain chemotherapy drugs can make your potassium so high in your body that you can have severe side effects. Therefore, your treatment may be stopped, changed, or delayed.

Dietary changes: *Rationale:* Since you have too much potassium in your body, you need to decrease eating foods that contain large amounts. These include prunes, bananas, potatoes, peaches, cantaloupe, apricots, dates, tomatoes, scallops, veal, dried beans, raw mushrooms, squash, dried figs, prune juice, orange juice, and tomato juice.

IV blood samples: *Rationale:* Several blood samples will be taken over the next several days. They are needed to track the amount of potassium in your body.

ECG diagnostic test: *Rationale:* The large amount of potassium in your body may cause changes in how your heart beats. Your heart will be checked with a machine that measures your heartbeat.

IV line placement: *Rationale:* The IV line allows us to easily give you medicines and fluids that you will need.

Signs and symptoms of hyperkalemia: *Rationale:* You (significant others) need to watch for signs of high potassium levels because early treatment helps you feel better and gives you a high quality of life. The signs include any of the following: muscle weakness, nausea, difficulty speaking, tiredness, abdominal cramps, diarrhea, heart fluttering, and decrease in frequency of normal urination.

EVALUATION/DESIRED OUTCOMES

1. Serum K^+ decreases to normal values (3.5 to 5.0 mEq/L, 3.5 to 5.0 mmol/L) within 2 hours for acute levels, greater than or equal to 7 mEq/L.
2. Serum K^+ level is maintained within normal range for extended period of time.
3. ECG normalizes.
4. The client verbalizes the importance of minimizing foods high in K^+.
5. Nausea and/or diarrhea subside within 24 hours.
6. Chemotherapy regimen will continue as prescribed.

DISCHARGE PLANNING

Hyperkalemic client may need:

Short-term IV fluids if oral intake inadequate.
Training of client on I and O measurement.
Reinforcement of dietary instructions.

FOLLOW-UP CARE

Anticipated care

Physician office visit within 1 week.
Outpatient lab testing for serum K^+ and sodium within 1 week.
Outpatient ECG within 1 week.
Continuation of dietary regimen.
Home health nurse for possible IV fluids and continuing evaluation.

Anticipated client/family questions and possible answers

Will this problem with high potassium in my blood happen again?
"It is possible for this problem to happen again. It is very important to know the signs of hyperkalemia, to stay on your special dietary regime, and to keep your follow-up appointments."

When can I continue my chemotherapy?
"When the potassium in your body returns to normal, your doctor will discuss with you options for continuing or changing your chemotherapy."

Will I have any heart problems because of this high potassium?

"High potassium causes heart problems that can usually be corrected. There are usually no lasting effects. However, it is advisable to maintain regular visits to your physician to have your blood and heart checked."

CHAPTER SUMMARY

Hyperkalemia is a metabolic complication with serious consequences that constitutes an acute oncologic emergency. Symptoms generally appear when K$^+$ levels rise above 5 mEq/L. Clients with impaired renal function are at increased risk for hyperkalemia due to impaired K$^+$ excretion, and clients with tumor lysis syndrome are at increased risk due to the release of large amounts of K$^+$ into the body. For the oncology client, ongoing nursing assessment must be maintained for detection and treatment of this potentially rapidly-developing complication, in order to prevent cardiac arrest and death. After ruling out pseudohypokalemia, the treatment and interventions selected for elevated levels are related to the cause(s) of hyperkalemia.

TEST QUESTIONS

1. The primary nursing diagnosis for clients with hyperkalemia is:
   A. Potential for infection
   B. Alteration in tissue perfusion, cardiopulmonary
   C. Fluid volume deficit
   D. Alteration in respiratory perfusion

1. Answer: B
Hyperkalemia can develop rapidly, with cardiac arrest sometimes being the first sign.

2. Pseudohyperkalemia is defined as:
   A. An increased serum K$^+$ without systemic hyperkalemia
   B. A false diagnosis due to hypernatremia
   C. A systemic infection of unknown etiology
   D. A decreased urine K$^+$ as a result of increased K$^+$ ingestion

2. Answer: A
Laboratory results show an elevated serum K$^+$ level due to hemolysis of the blood sample, when there is actually no systemic hyperkalemia.

3. What clinical clue might be used to differentiate true hyperkalemia from pseudohyperkalemia?
   A. Thrombocytosis
   B. Acidosis
   C. Elevated blood urea nitrogen (BUN)
   D. No electrocardiogram (ECG/EKG) changes

3. Answer: D
Both pseudohyperkalemia and true hyperkalemia would show an increase in serum K$^+$ levels. However, there would not be ECG changes in the client with pseudohyperkalemia.

4. Signs of hyperkalemia include:
   A. Increased serum sodium and decreased blood pressure
   B. Decreased serum K$^+$ and changes in the ECG
   C. Increased serum K$^+$ and hyperactive deep tendon reflexes
   D. Increased creatinine clearance and increased lymphocytes

4. Answer: C
Serum K$^+$ is greater than 5 mEq/L. Deep tendon reflexes are increased due to intracellular shift of K$^+$ to the extracellular compartment.

5. Teaching about the need to decrease the intake of foods that are high in K$^+$ would be most important for which client?
   A. A client receiving diuretic therapy
   B. A client with an ileostomy
   C. A client in metabolic acidosis
   D. A client with renal failure

5. Answer: D
Clients with renal disease are predisposed to hyperkalemia due to their inability to excrete K$^+$ along with other substances and fluid, and thus they should decrease their intake of foods high in K$^+$.

6. Hyperkalemia is primarily a disorder of:
   A. Potassium (K$^+$) excess
   B. Lactic acidosis
   C. Calcium depletion
   D. Increased sodium in a person's diet

6. Answer: A
An increase in K$^+$ release from cells or a decrease in K$^+$ excretion brings about total body excess of K$^+$.

7. An expected outcome for a hyperkalemic client would be:
   A. Eosinophil counts will be normal within 24 hours
   B. Serum K$^+$ value will be between 3.5 and 5.0 mEq/L (3.5 to 5.0 mmol/L SI Units)

7. Answer: B
The desired outcome would be that hyperkalemia is controlled, with serum K$^+$ concentrations being within the normal limits of 3.5 to 5.0 mEq/L (3.5 to 5.0 mmol/L SI Units).

C. Pacemaker insertion

D. Weight gain

8. Which nursing intervention should be implemented *first* in a client suspected of having hyperkalemia?
   A. Perform a chest x-ray, lateral field, STAT
   B. Obtain arterial blood gases STAT
   C. Obtain serum K$^+$ specimen STAT
   D. Obtain a 12-lead ECG

8. Answer: C
To make a determination if a client has hyperkalemia, the serum K$^+$ level must be measured.

9. The *first* treatment of choice in a client with hyperkalemia and associated cardiac dysrhythmia would be to:
   A. Dialyze
   B. Administer calcium gluconate IV
   C. Administer a Kayexalate enema
   D. Administer a long-acting insulin infusion over 4 hours IV

9. Answer: B
The administration of calcium gluconate stabilizes the cardiac membrane and increases myocardial contractility to reduce the risk of lethal dysrhythmia and cardiac standstill.

10. The risk of hyperkalemia would be increased *primarily* in the client with:
    A. Lung cancer
    B. Multiple myeloma
    C. Breast cancer
    D. Adrenal metastasis

10. Answer: D
Adrenal metastasis causes decreased adrenal function, which causes a severe increase in serum K$^+$.

REFERENCES

Byers JF, Goshorn J: How to manage diuretic therapy. Am J Nurs 95(2):38–43, 1995.

Chernecky CC, Berger, BJ: Laboratory Tests and Diagnostic Procedures, 2nd ed. Philadelphia: WB Saunders Co, 1997.

Chernecky CC, Ramsey P: Critical Nursing Care of the Client with Cancer. Norwalk, CT: Appleton-Century-Crofts, 1984.

DeFronzo RA, Smith DJ: Hyperkalemia. In Maxwell and Kleeman's Clinical Disorders of Fluid and Electrolyte Metabolism, 5th ed. New York: McGraw-Hill, 1994, pp. 693–754.

Harmon AL: Diagnostics. In Intermed Comunications (ed): Nursing (83 Books). Springhouse, PA: Nurses Reference Library, 1983, pp. 89–92 (Chap 3).

Kelly MA: Chronic renal failure. Am J Nurs 96(1):53–56, 1996.

O'Donnell ME: Assessing fluid and electrolyte balance in elders. Am J Nurs 95(11):40–45, 1995.

Perez A: Hyperkalemia. RN 58(11):32–36, 1995.

Shelton BK, Baker L, Skecher S: Critical care of the patient with hematologic malignancy. AACN Clin Issues Adv Pract Crit Care 7(1):65–78, 1996.

Smith SA: Patient-induced dehydration—Can it ever be therapeutic? Oncol Nurs Forum 22(10):1487–1490, 1995.

Warrell RP Jr: Metabolic emergencies. *In* DeVita V Jr, Hellman S, Rosenberg S (eds): Cancer Principles and Practice in Oncology, 4th ed. Philadelphia: JB Lippincott, 1991, pp. 2128–2140.

Whaley L, Wong D: Balance and imbalance of body fluids. *In* Nursing Care of Infants and Children, 4th ed. St. Louis, MO: Mosby, 1991, pp. 1248–1275.

Whaley L, Wong D: The child with cancer. *In* Nursing Care of Infants and Children, 4th ed. St. Louis, MO: Mosby, 1991, pp. 1656–1710.

CHAPTER 20

HYPERLEUKOCYTOSIS IN CHILDHOOD LEUKEMIA

Wendy Holmes, MSN, RN

CHAPTER OBJECTIVES

At the completion of this chapter, the reader will be able to:

Define hyperleukocytosis in childhood leukemia.

Identify the risk factors for the development of hyperleukocytosis.

Identify the clinical signs of hyperleukocytosis.

Discuss the current management of hyperleukocytosis.

Describe the nursing care as it relates to the client with hyperleukocytosis.

Discuss the outcomes of hyperleukocytosis in relation to remission induction, metabolic complications from cytotoxic therapy, and relapse rate.

Anticipate and prepare the client with hyperleukocytosis for future care needs.

OVERVIEW

HYPERLEUKOCYTOSIS, an elevated peripheral white blood cell (WBC) count exceeding 100,000/μl, is considered a medical emergency in children diagnosed with acute and chronic leukemias. The excessive numbers of leukocytes result in obstruction of the microcirculation, in invasion and damage to vessel walls, and in severe metabolic disturbances in response to rapid destruction following cytotoxic therapy. Clinical sequelae can include intracranial or pulmonary hemorrhage, renal failure, disseminated intravascular coagulation (DIC), and tumor lysis syndrome. Hyperleukocytosis occurs in 9 to 13% of children with acute lymphocytic leukemia (ALL), 5 to 22% of children with acute nonlymphocytic leukemia (ANLL), and 50 to 100% of children with chronic myelogenous leukemia (CML) (Lange, D'Angio, Ross, O'Neil, and Packer, 1993).

DESCRIPTION

The pathogenesis of hyperleukocytosis can be described, based on the following characteristics and properties of leukemic cells: (1) the concentration of leukemic blasts in the peripheral blood, (2) the effect of these cells on blood viscosity, (3) the oxygen consumption of leukemic cells, (4) the invasiveness of leukemic cells through vessel walls, and (5) the metabolic conditions at diagnosis and following cytoreductive therapy (see Fig. 20–1).

The presence of an extremely elevated peripheral WBC count (> 100,000/μl) is associated with fatal hemorrhage resulting from leukostasis, an accumulation of leukocytes in the microvasculature with subsequent ischemia and hemorrhage (Dearth, Fountain, Smithson, Burgert, and Gilchrist, 1978). The lungs and central nervous system (CNS) are most vulnerable. Pulmonary leukostasis is associated with diffuse capillary damage and alveolar hemorrhage. The primary CNS manifestation of hyperleukocytosis is intracranial hemorrhage. The risk for intracranial hemorrhage increases as the WBC count rises and becomes extreme above 200,000/μl. CNS hemorrhage, in fact, is the major cause of early death in children with hyperleukocytosis in childhood leukemias (Allegretta, Weissman, and Altman, 1985).

Blood viscosity is determined by the fraction of cells in a given volume as well as the flow of blood through the vasculature and can be affected by both red blood cells (RBCs) and WBCs. For example, in profound dehydration, in which the volume is greatly reduced, the fraction of RBCs (erythrocrits) is elevated, giving rise to increased viscosity. In leukemic states, as the WBC count

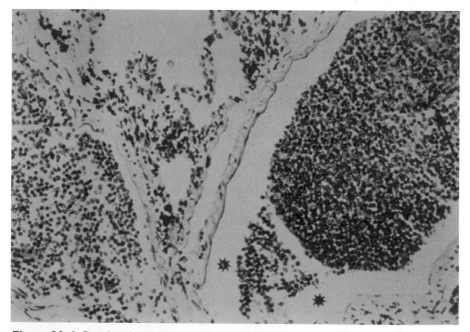

Figure 20–1 Peripheral smear of hyperleukocytosis.

rises, the fractional volume of leukocytes (leukocrit) also rises and may affect blood viscosity, primarily in the microvasculature (Campbell, 1991; Lichtmann and Rowe, 1982). A rise in bulk viscosity of blood is rare in hyperleukocytosis, seen almost exclusively in chronic myelogenous leukemia (Lichtmenn and Rowe, 1982). This development may be due in part to the fact that anemias associated with acute leukemias can be somewhat protective by decreasing RBC numbers and lowering blood viscosity (Dabrow and Wilkins, 1993).

In addition to the number of WBCs present, a second factor affecting blood viscosity relates to the deformability of cells. The size, shape, and function of leukemic leukocytes varies from normal leukocytes, which are small and move easily through the capillaries. Myeloblasts are the largest and most rigid of the leukemic cells and place clients diagnosed with either ANLL or CML in blast crisis (CML-BC) at highest risk for leukostatic complications (Campbell, 1991). That these cells do not circulate easily through small vessels leads to sequestration, vascular damage, and hemorrhage (Bunin and Pui, 1985). Bunin and Pui (1985) found a significantly higher early death rate from intracranial hemorrhage in children with ANLL (11%) as compared with children with ALL (1.2%). Myeloblasts are also sticky and can cause vascular obstruction by leukemic cell aggregates or thrombi (Allegretta et al., 1985).

Clients with ALL are at intermediate risk for the development of leukostatic complications, since lymphoblasts are somewhat smaller than myeloblasts and move through the circulation a bit more easily. Because lymphoblasts are exquisitely sensitive to chemotherapy, complications from hyperleukocytosis in ALL is frequently linked to the metabolic and renal alterations following cytoreductive therapy.

With high numbers of leukocytes, chronically decreased blood flow may decrease oxygen transport to the tissues. Moreover, leukemic cells have an increased oxygen consumption rate and will compete with tissues in areas of obstructed blood flow for available oxygen leading to further damage to vital organs (Campbell, 1991; Lichtmenn and Rowe, 1982).

Local invasion and damage to vessel walls can also be a consequence of hyperleukocytosis. These injured sites can result in the migration of leukemic cells into the surrounding tissues, primarily the lungs and brain (Campbell, 1991).

A final component associated with the pathogenesis of hyperleukocytosis relates to the metabolic and hemorrhagic complications that can occur at the time of diagnosis or once cytoreductive therapy is initiated. At the time of diagnosis coagulopathies may be present, induced by procoagulant substances in the cytoplasm of leukemic cells. The result is activation of thrombin, which leads to DIC, which interferes with the management of acute hemorrhage or thrombosis (Eguiguren, Schell, Crist, Kunkel, and Rivera, 1992). Metabolic alterations at the time of diagnosis are the result of the hypermetabolic states of circulating leukocytes. Presenting metabolic conditions may include pseudo-hypoglycemia and pseudohyperkalemia (Dabrow and Wilkins, 1993).

Once cytoreduction begins, rapid destruction of leukemic cells and increased risk for the development of tumor lysis syndrome ensue. The risk of tumor lysis syndrome is associated with tumor burden and therefore is greater in hyperleukocytosis. This process is characterized by hyperkalemia, hyper-uricemia, hyperphosphatemia and hypocalcemia, and the potential for acute renal failure (see Chapter 42). DIC resulting in both hemorrhage and thrombo-sis has also been reported once therapy has begun. Monocytic leukemia (M4) and acute promyelocytic leukemia (M5) are associated with an increased risk for the development of hemorrhagic complications (Bunin and Pui, 1985).

RISK PROFILE

Cancers: ANLL, CML-BC, ALL.

Conditions: Age < 2 years, WBC count > 100,000/µl, M4 or M5 subtype of ANLL, extramedullary organ involvement at diagnosis.

Environment: None.

Foods: None.

Drugs: None.

PROGNOSIS

Increased morbidity and early mortality have been associated with hyper-leukocytosis in childhood leukemias. Death from the sequelae of hyperleuko-cytosis has been reported in 3 to 6% of children with ALL and 2 to 14% with ANLL (Creutzig, Ritter, Budde, Sutor, and Schellong, 1987). In children with ANLL who present with a WBC count greater than 250,000/µl, the risk increases for a serious intracranial bleed (Basade et al., 1995) and death (Creutzig et al., 1987). In terms of overall prognosis, an increased relapse rate has been reported in children who present with an initial leukocyte count > 100,000/µl (Equiguren et al., 1992).

TREATMENT

Surgery: Placement of indwelling central venous catheter for leukapheresis and/or chemotherapy.

Chemotherapy: Induction chemotherapy for rapid cytoreduction. Protocols will vary based on the type of leukemia. May include agents such as cytosine arabinoside, daunorubicin, idarubicin for ANLL; hydroxyurea for ANLL and CML; adriamycin, vincristine, prednisone, L-asparaginase for ALL.

Radiation: Cranial irradiation (400 to 600 Gy) has been administered to pre-vent cerebral hemorrhage but is not helpful in extraneural cytoreduction (Bunin, Kunkel, and Callihan, 1987).

Medications: Allopurinol to prevent tumor lysis.

Procedures

Leukapheresis to reduce leukemic cell burden. The procedure requires a large-bore catheter and is generally used in children > 30 kg. The goal is to achieve a 30% reduction to initial WBC count. The procedure is done prior to initiation of definitive chemotherapy to decrease the severe metabolic complications (Cuttner et al., 1983).

Exchange transfusion to reduce leukemic cell burden in clients who are less than 30 kg and who are not able to have large-bore catheter placement (Bunin et al., 1987).

Hydration/urine alkalinization to reduce risk of tumor lysis following cytotoxic therapy (Miller and Parnes, 1994).

Administration of blood products to correct coagulation abnormalities (for example, fresh frozen plasma).

Other: Avoid extreme transfusion replacement of RBCs and diuretics that will increase blood viscosity (Allegretta et al., 1985).

ASSESSMENT CRITERIA: HYPERLEUKOCYTOSIS IN CHILDHOOD LEUKEMIA

Vital signs

Temperature	Normal or elevated
Pulse	Tachycardia
Respirations	Tachypnea
O$_2$ saturation	Decreased

History

Symptoms, conditions	Leukemic infiltration in bone marrow, causing increasing WBC count, decreased RBC count, and decreased platelets. Fatigue, weakness (anemia). Increased bruising/bleeding (thrombocytopenia). May present with active infection or history of recurrent infections. Children with ALL may have bone pain in long bones, causing difficulty or inability to walk. Dyspnea on exertion. Progressive respiratory distress. Personality/behavior changes. Increased irritability/unable to comfort child. Headaches or vision disturbances from accumulating leukocytes in CNS.
Hallmark physical signs and symptoms	Tachypnea, respiratory distress, hypoxia, restlessness, ataxia, mental status changes, dizziness, seizures, coma.
Additional physical signs and symptoms	Fever, diminished lung sounds, diffuse pulmonary rales, headache, vomiting, visual blurring, retinal vein distention, papilledema, splenomegaly, hepatomegaly, tinnitus, tachycardia, oliguria/anuria, priapism.

(continued)

ASSESSMENT CRITERIA: HYPERLEUKOCYTOSIS IN CHILDHOOD LEUKEMIA (continued)

Psychosocial signs	Altered personality, anxiety, behavior changes, confusion, disorientation.

Lab values	
WBC count	High, >100,000/µl.
Differential	Blasts—increased.
	Neutrophils—decreased.
RBC count	Normal—CML.
	Decreased—acute leukemia.
Platelet count	Normal or decreased.
BUN and creatinine	Normal or increased (if renal insufficiency).
Coagulation indicators	(If evidence of coagulopathy.)
PT	Increased.
PTT	Increased.
Fibrinogen	Decreased.
Fibrin split product	Increased.
Plasminogen	Decreased.
LDH	Increased (in ALL, CML).
Glucose	Decreased (pseudohypoglycemia).
Potassium	Markedly elevated (if renal failure or tumor lysis).
Phosphate	Markedly elevated (if tumor lysis).
Uric acid	Markedly elevated (if tumor lysis).
Calcium	Decreased (if tumor lysis).

Diagnostic tests	
Chest x-ray	Normal or bilateral pulmonary infiltrates, increased pulmonary vascular markings, pleural effusions, cardiomegaly.
CT scan/MRI	CNS lesions in white matter of brain surrounded by hemorrhage.
Bone marrow biopsy/aspirate	To confirm diagnosis and type of leukemia.

NURSING DIAGNOSIS

The nursing diagnoses will vary, depending on the type of leukemia, the degree of hyperleukocytosis, and the organs affected. Some of the common diagnoses and etiologies are as follows.

(Risk for) injury related to intracranial hemorrhage secondary to hyperleukocytosis.

Potential for ineffective airway clearance related to seizure or coma secondary to intracranial hemorrhage.

Acute confusion secondary to cerebral hemorrhage and/or leukostasis.

Altered tissue perfusion (cerebral, cardiopulmonary, renal) secondary to leukostasis.

Ineffective breathing pattern secondary to pulmonary infiltrates and/or pulmonary hemorrhage.

Knowledge deficit related to new diagnosis of leukemia, sequelae, and treatment of hyperleukocytosis, treatment options, and long-term survival.

(Risk for) injury related to bleeding secondary to coagulopathies following cytoreductive therapy.

(Risk for) injury related to metabolic alterations secondary to tumor lysis following cytoreductive therapy.

Anxiety related to a new cancer diagnosis and unknown outcomes.

NURSING INTERVENTIONS

Immediate nursing interventions

Maintain adequate oxygenation. Assess respirations and oxygen saturation continuously.

Administer oxygen via non-rebreather to maintain oxygen saturation above 90%.

Prepare for emergency endotracheal intubation if acute respiratory failure occurs.

Initiate seizure precautions. Place suction equipment and an oral airway at the bedside.

Assess neurologic status, including level of consciousness, speech pattern, gait, and upper and lower extremity coordination q1h.

Send STAT CBC with differential; platelet count; DIC screen; serum electrolyte panel; complete chemistry panel, including glucose, renal function, uric acid, and lactate dehydrogenase (LDH).

Monitor pulse and blood pressure q1h.

Establish patent IV access and keep vein open.

Measure hourly intake and output (I and O).

Prepare for placement of indwelling central venous access catheter.

Reassure both client and parents and inform them of all activities. Begin preparing client for invasive procedures.

Anticipated physician orders and interventions

Arterial blood gas (ABG) to determine degree of hypoxia. (Arterial O_2 from blood gas may be falsely low because of WBC consumption of O_2 if sample not processed immediately.)

Bone marrow aspirate and biopsy to confirm the diagnosis and the type of leukemia. Educate the client and family about the procedure. Apply EMLA (lidocaine-prilocaine) cream to site to begin anesthetic effect 1 hour prior to the procedure.

Lumbar puncture for diagnosis of CNS involvement. Educate the client and family about the procedure. Apply EMLA cream to site to begin anesthetic effect 1 hour prior to the procedure.

CT scan/MRI of CNS to evaluate for leukostasis and/or hemorrhage. Educate the client and family about the procedure. If the child is very young, he or she may require sedation.

Chest x-ray to evaluate for pulmonary infiltrates.

IV hydration with 5% dextrose 0.45% NaCl at $1\frac{1}{2}$ times maintenance. May add 1 ampule sodium bicarbonate to IV for urine alkalinization.

Begin allopurinol 10 mg/kg by mouth daily.

Insertion of indwelling central venous catheter for leukapheresis and chemotherapy.

Prepare for initiation of cytoreductive therapy, which will vary based on the client's diagnosis, age, and size.

Leukapheresis:
- Explain to the client and parents about leukapheresis.
- Monitor blood pressure q15min × 1 hour, then q30–60min for the duration of leukapheresis.
- Administer albumin if necessary to maintain blood pressure.
- Monitor the client for citrate toxicity, which causes a drop in the serum calcium. Symptoms are manifested by a tingling sensation around the face and lips. Administer Tums or milk.
- Keep the client calm during the procedure. Mild sedation may be required.
- Obtain CBC following leukapheresis.
- Monitor for rapid rebound of leukemic blasts.

Exchange transfusion:
- Administer blood per hospital policy for pediatric clients.
- Monitor vital signs q15min × 1 hour, then q30–60min.
- Observe for signs and symptoms of transfusion reaction.
- Observe for signs of fluid overload.

Cranial irradiation:
- Prepare the client for the procedure.
- Sedation may be required in small children.
- Monitor level of consciousness q shift.

Chemotherapy:
- Hydroxyurea may be administered to certain clients with CML.
- Intrathecal methotrexate/Cytosine Arabinoside (Ara-C) may be administered to certain clients with acute leukemia.
- Administer induction chemotherapy when appropriate.
- Administer antiemetic regimen prior to the start of chemotherapy.

Ongoing nursing assessment, monitoring, and interventions

Assess:
- Level of consciousness q8h and PRN.
- For signs of bleeding (urine, oral mucosa, skin, lungs).
- For signs of infection.
- For signs of congestive heart failure q8h (rales, tachypnea, dyspnea, tachycardia).

- Central venous catheter for patency.
- For signs of tumor lysis (confusion, weakness, renal insufficiency, muscle cramps, lethargy, ECG changes).
- For signs of lactic acidosis (tachypnea, hypotension, nausea, confusion).
- Nutritional status—the client may need total parenteral nutrition.

Measure:
- Blood pressure and pulse q4h and PRN.
- O$_2$ saturation and respirations q4h and PRN.
- I and O qd.
- Weight qd.

Send:
- CBC, differential, platelet count daily.
- Prothrombin time (PT), partial thromboplastin time (PTT), DIC screen qd or PRN.
- Chemistry panel qd.
- 24-hour urine for creatinine clearance prior to or 24 hours after starting chemotherapy.

Implement:
- Seizure precautions until WBC count has decreased.
- Neutropenic precautions if indicated.

TEACHING/EDUCATION

Emergency cytoreduction therapy prior to induction chemotherapy: *Rationale:* Induction chemotherapy will cause most of the leukemic cells to break apart and be destroyed. When the cells die they can release toxic substances. If this occurs when the WBC count is extremely high, the release of these toxic substances could cause severe bleeding or chemical imbalances in the body that could damage your (your child's) major organs or result in potentially fatal cardiac arrythmias.

Central venous access placement: *Rationale:* This catheter lets us take frequent blood samples, as well as give you the chemotherapy, blood products, IV fluids, and IV nutrition that may be needed during your (your child's) therapy. These lines can also be used for leukophoresis and/or exchange transfusion. It will greatly reduce the number of "needle sticks" and pain for your child.

Invasive and noninvasive diagnostic tests: *Rationale:* It is very important to determine the specific type of leukemia you (your child) has, as this will determine the right treatment. These tests will also help us find out what damage has been caused by the high WBC count and what needs to be done to correct that damage.

Chemotherapy administration: *Rationale:* As soon as your (your child's) condition is stable and the WBCs decrease, chemotherapy will begin. With this therapy, called induction therapy, we try to put you (your child) in remission—this means that the leukemia is no longer visible. This therapy will be followed by several more treatments, depending on the type of leukemia.

Breathing or mental status changes: *Rationale:* The lungs and brain are very sensitive when the WBC count is so high. It is very important that you call the nurse if you are (your child is) having trouble breathing, feeling dizzy, or feeling funny in the head or confused.

EVALUATION/DESIRED OUTCOMES

1. The WBC count will be reduced by at least 30% from cytoreductive therapy within 12 to 24 hours.
2. Metabolic alterations will be corrected with hydration and alkalinization.
3. The client's neurologic status will stabilize and is without seizure activity.
4. The client's respiratory status will stabilize, with respirations returning to baseline measurements and $pO_2 > 90$ mmHg.
5. Hematologic abnormalities are corrected with transfusion support.
6. Induction chemotherapy will begin within 24 to 48 hours.
7. Central venous access device will remain patent and free from infection. Teaching the client and/or family about the care of the line will begin.
8. Teaching will begin regarding disease process, ongoing treatment plans, and the side effects of therapy.

DISCHARGE PLANNING

Hyperleukocytosis client may need:

Home nursing visits for care of the central venous catheter, IV hydration, and management of the side effects of chemotherapy.

Referral to community agency for ongoing support, education materials, and financial aid.

FOLLOW-UP CARE

Anticipated care

Office visit to pediatric hematologist within 5 to 7 days.

Regular chemotherapy visits. May need to be rehospitalized, depending on type of leukemia.

Weekly or more frequent laboratory testing of CBC, differential, chemistry profile.

Home nursing visits to monitor status, medication teaching, and central line care.

Referral to support groups for client with leukemia and families of a child with cancer.

Anticipated client/family questions and possible answers

Will this problem of hyperleukocytosis occur again?

"If your (your child's) leukemia were to come out of remission, the WBC count could increase to dangerous levels again, causing some of the same problems. As long as the leukemia is in remission, the WBC count will remain normal or even low following chemotherapy treatments."

"Any breathing problems or changes in your (your child's) ability to think clearly or remember should be reported to your doctor immediately."

What precautions do we have to take at home?

"The chemotherapy treatments will affect the normal blood cells in the bone marrow. It is important to watch for any signs of infection or bleeding. If you (your child) develop fever, cough, sores in the mouth, or difficulty urinating, contact the nurse or doctor right away. Also do so if you notice any abnormal bleeding or bleeding that you cannot stop."

"If your (your child's) blood counts are very low, rehospitalization may be necessary."

"It is important to try and keep as normal a routine as possible during treatment. You (your child) can continue in school and resume regular activities during the time when the blood counts are okay. When the counts are very low, you may need to avoid certain routines for a short period of time."

How long will the chemotherapy treatments continue?

"Even though there is no sign of leukemia cells in your (your child's) blood now, we know there are still many leukemia cells present that we cannot see. It will be necessary to continue therapy for several months or years (based on the type of leukemia) to be sure that you do not come out of remission. Additional therapy such as bone marrow transplantation may be indicated and will be discussed with you by the doctors and nurses who care for you."

CHAPTER SUMMARY

Hyperleukocytosis, an extremely elevated peripheral WBC count, places children with leukemia at high risk for sudden death from massive intracerebral hemorrhage and is one of the established factors indicating a poor response to therapy and higher relapse rate.

The hallmark symptoms of hyperleukocytosis arise from an accumulation of leukocytes in the microvasculature of the lungs and CNS and subsequent pulmonary and cerebral hemorrhage. Attempts to reduce the burden of leukemic cells prior to the initiation of induction chemotherapy are made to reduce the risk for profound metabolic complications when cell lysis occurs.

The focus of nursing care is to assess respiratory and neurologic function, to implement interventions to minimize respiratory distress and increased intracranial pressure, to participate with the medical team to swiftly initiate cytoreductive therapy, followed by chemotherapy to treat the underlying disease, and to provide information and support to the client and family.

TEST QUESTIONS

1. Which two types of childhood leukemia have the highest likelihood to present with hyperleukocytosis?
   A. CLL, ALL
   B. CML (blast crisis), ALL
   C. CML (blast crisis), ANLL
   D. ANLL, ALL

1. Answer: C
The myeloblast that is the cell of origin in both CML and ANLL is the largest and most rigid leukocyte. It is unable to move easily through the microvasculature and has the highest risk for leukostasis and hemorrhage.

2. What metabolic complication is most often associated with rapid leukemic cell destruction in hyperleukocytosis?
   A. Tumor lysis syndrome
   B. Lactic acidosis
   C. Chemical diabetes
   D. Adrenal insufficiency

2. Answer: A
Rapid destruction of leukemic cells can result in tumor lysis syndrome.

3. What factor in addition to total WBC count and type of leukemia influences the type of cytoreduction the client with hyperleukocytosis will undergo?
   A. Prescence of coagulopathy
   B. Degree of hypoxia
   C. Body size
   D. Physician preference

3. Answer: C
A client under 30 kg usually is not able to undergo placement of a large-bore catheter necessary for leukapheresis and therefore would be best treated with exchange transfusion.

4. Which should be the first nursing intervention in a client who is suspected of having hyperleukocytosis and is in no apparent respiratory distress?
   A. Obtain a STAT CBC to confirm a profoundly elevated WBC count.
   B. Sedate the client.
   C. Begin hydration.
   D. Send the client for a STAT chest x-ray.

4. Answer: A
The WBC count must be confirmed serologically as the first step in determining the severity of the problem and appropriate interventions.

5. What intervention would *not* be indicated when a client presents with hyperleukocytosis?
   A. Hydration
   B. RBC transfusion to maintain hemoglobin > 10
   C. Leukapheresis
   D. Allopurinol

5. Answer: B
When the WBC count is profoundly elevated, transfusion of RBCs can increase blood viscosity and increase the risk for intracranial hemorrhage. It is recommended to keep the hemoglobin < 10 until cytoreduction therapy begins.

6. What effect does hyperleukocytosis have on the overall prognosis in children with leukemia?
   A. Better overall prognosis, since aggressive therapy is started early
   B. Harder to achieve a remission but no effect on overall prognosis
   C. Increased relapse rate and poor overall prognosis
   D. Increased complications but no effect on overall prognosis

6. Answer: C
Clients who present with a WBC count > 100,000 have a reported increased relapse rate and poorer overall prognosis.

7. The signs of hyperleukocytosis include:
   A. Tachypnea and mental status changes
   B. Increased urine ouput and hypotension
   C. Increased neutrophils and fever
   D. Visual disturbances and bradycardia

7. Answer: A
The organs most often targeted by hyperleukocytosis are the lungs and CNS; it results in progressive pulmonary distress and intracranial hemorrhage.

8. What would be a desired outcome in clients with hyperleukocytosis at 24 hours following initiation of cytoreduction?
   A. A 10% reduction in the total WBC count
   B. A 30% reduction in the total WBC count
   C. A 50 % reduction in the total WBC count
   D. A 70% reduction in the total WBC count

8. Answer: B
A 30% reduction in the WBC count following cytoreduction is considered to be adequate in reducing the risk for tumor lysis once induction chemotherapy begins.

9. What should the major focus be in terms of discharge teaching for a client who is newly diagnosed with leukemia?
   A. Overall statistics related to survival
   B. Long-term sequelae to chemotherapy
   C. Effect of disease and treatment on bone marrow cells
   D. Available support groups

9. Answer: C
It is most important for the client and family to be knowledgeable about the effects of therapy on the cells in the bone marrow so that they can monitor for signs of early infection and/or bleeding.

10. What would a primary diagnosis be for the clients with hyperleukocytosis?
    A. Diarrhea
    B. Fluid volume deficit
    C. Ineffective breathing pattern
    D. Hyperthermia

10. Answer: C
The client who presents with hyperleukocytosis remains at high risk for leukostasis in the lungs, which causes ischemia and hypoxia and ineffective breathing patterns.

REFERENCES

Allegretta GJ, Weissman ST, Altman A: Oncologic emergencies I: Hematologic and infectious complications of cancer and cancer treatment. Pediatr Clin North Am 32(3):613–624, 1985.

Basade M, Dhar A, Kulkarni SM, Sastry P, Yadav R, Bhavana S, Pai S, Nair C, Kurkure P, Advani S: Rapid cytoreduction in childhood leukemic hyperleukocytosis by conservative therapy. Med Pediatr Oncol 25:204–207, 1995.

Bunin N, Kunkel K, Callihan T: Cytoreductive procedures in the early management in cases of leukemia and hyperleukocytosis in children. Med Pediatr Oncol 15:232–235, 1987.

Bunin N, Pui C: Differing complications of hyperleukocytosis in children with acute lymphoblastic or acute non-lymphoblastic leukemia. J Clin Oncol 3(12):1590–1595, 1985.

Campbell T: Hyperleukocytosis in leukemia. Dimens Oncol Nurs 5(2):11–14, 1991.

Creutzig U, Ritter J, Budde M, Sutor A, Schellong G: Early deaths due to hemorrhage and luekostasis in childhood acute myelogenous leukemia. Cancer 60(12):3071–1079, 1987.

Cutter J, Holland J, Norton L, Ambinder E, Button G, Meyer R: Therapeutic leukapheresis for hyperleukocytosis in acute myelocytic leukemia. Med Pediatr Oncol 11:76–78, 1983.

Dabrow M, Wilkins J: Hematologic emergencies: Management of hyperleukocytic syndrome, DIC, and thrombotic thrombocytopenic purpura. Postgrad Med 93(5):193–202, 1993.

Dearth J, Fountain K, Smithson W, Burgert E, Gilchrist G: Extreme leukemic leukocytosis (blast crisis) in childhood. Mayo Clin Proc 53:207–211, 1978.

Eguiguren J, Schell M, Crist W, Kunkel K, Rivera G: Complications and outcomes in childhood lymphoblastic leukemia with hyperleukocytosis. Blood 79(4):871–875, 1992.

Lange B, D'Angio G, Ross A, O'Neil J, Packer R: Oncologic emergencies. *In* Pizzo PA, Poplack DG (eds): Principles and Practice of Pediatric Oncology, 2nd ed. Philadelphia: JB Lippincott, 1993, pp. 951–972.

Lichtmenn M, Rowe J: Hyperleukocytic leukemias: Rheological, clinical and therapeutic considerations. Blood 60(2):279–283, 1982.

Miller J, Parnes H: Hematologic problems and emergencies. *In* Cameron RB (ed): Practical Oncology. Norwalk, CT: Appleton & Lange, 1994, pp. 77–83.

CHAPTER 21

HYPERNATREMIA

Karen Schulz, RN, MSN

CHAPTER OBJECTIVES

At the completion of this chapter, the reader will be able to:

Define hypernatremia.

State the risks that contribute to hypernatremia in oncology clients.

Describe the nursing care required to prevent and treat
hypernatremic emergencies.

Discuss the nursing assessments most pertinent to the discovery of
hypernatremia.

List the discharge teaching points that will avert hypernatremia in
high-risk clients.

OVERVIEW

HYPERNATREMIA is defined as a laboratory-measured serum sodium >145
mEq/Liter (>145 mmol/L SI Units) (normal value 135 to 145 mEq/L, 135 to
145 mmol/L SI Units). Long, Marin, Bayer, Shetty, and Pathy (1991) found
who the incidence of hypernatremia was only 0.3% in a group of adult inpatients
who included, but was not restricted to, oncology clients. Their study showed that,
although the incidence of hypernatremia is low, there is a high mortality rate (54%)
in clients with hypernatremia. The clients in the Long et al. study were found to
have more than one factor contributing to the hypernatremia, and 60% of the
clients developed hypernatremia after discharge from the hospital. In a study done
by Palevsky, Bhagrath, and Greenberg (1996), it was found that 89% of hospitalized
clients with hypernatremia also had alterations in their urine osmolarity, primarily
due to excessive diuresis. Most (86%) of those in Palevsky's study were unable to
take fluids orally. The Palevsky study also reported a significant mortality rate associated with hypernatremia: 41%. Hypernatremia was found to be a major contributing factor in at least 16% of these deaths.

Even in clients with severe fluid losses, hypernatremia is rare as long as they
obtain sufficient amounts of water. Thus, hypernatremia occurs in clients who can-

not drink, who are very old or very young, or who are very sick (Ellison and Johnson Bia, 1987). Nurses should be alert to the fact that oncology clients may be at risk for hypernatremia under specific conditions, and although rare, hypernatremia has a high mortality. The study by Long et al. (1991) underscores the need for careful discharge planning and teaching of the oncology client and his or her family, because the seriously ill client may be particularly vulnerable to hypernatremia after discharge from the hospital.

DESCRIPTION

Sodium concentration can be elevated in the presence of normal, increased, or decreased body sodium content. The status of total body sodium will depend on the fluid status of the client, the IV and oral sodium intake, and the functioning of the body organs, especially the kidneys and the endocrine system. The oncology clients at highest risk for hypernatremia will most likely fall into three categories, described in Table 21-1.

Normal mechanisms of sodium balance

In the presence of healthy kidneys, an increase in the sodium of the extracellular fluid increases serum osmolarity (the normal range is 280 to 294 mOsm/kg) and stimulates the release of antidiuretic hormone (ADH, also called vasopressin) from the posterior pituitary gland. ADH increases water reabsorption by the distal renal tubules in response to an elevation in serum osmolality (Lancour, 1978). Hypernatremia also suppresses aldosterone secre-

Table 21-1
Causes of Hypernatremia

Type of Hypernatremia	State of Sodium and Body	Water Possible Causes
Euvolemic hypernatremia	Elevated body sodium with normal extracellular fluid volume.	Uncompensated state after high sodium intake in medication, foods, and IV fluids.
Hypervolemic hypernatremia	Total body sodium increased more than extracellular fluid volume increased.	Malfunction of the adrenal glands, which may occur with adenomas. High aldosterone increases sodium and water reabsorption by the kidneys.
Hypovolemic hypernatremia	Normal total body sodium with loss of extracellular fluid volume.	Dehydration due to DI, HHNK, diabetic ketoacidosis, or diuretics. Diarrhea, vomiting, or polyuric renal disease.

tion, increasing the amount of sodium excreted in the urine (Sotis, 1979). This mechanism of ADH secretion and aldosterone inhibition works so well that it is rare to have sodium excesses for which the body cannot compensate.

Euvolemic hypernatremia

An abnormally large ingestion of sodium without water can overwhelm the ADH reabsorption of water and aldosterone inhibition mechanisms. The inability to handle sodium excesses is most common in the elderly, in people with inefficient excretion of body fluids, and in clients with congestive heart failure or renal damage resulting from chronic ingestion of multiple medications (Sonnenblick and Algur, 1993). High-sodium IV fluids and near drowning in salt water are common causes of high-sodium intake (Oh and Carroll, 1992). Occasionally, sodium bicarbonate (used to treat acidosis) or sodium-containing antibiotics such as carbenicillin or ticarcillin may also produce hypernatremia (Flombaum, 1991).

Although less likely, it is possible for sodium ingestion to be so excessive as to rate the diagnosis of hypervolemic hypernatremia. Such clients would be those with concomitant conditions such as congestive heart failure or renal damage severe enough to cause hypervolemia.

Hypervolemic hypernatremia

The most common cause of sodium increase greater than fluid volume increase is excessive adrenocortical secretion of aldosterone. Malfunction of the adrenal glands can be seen with adenomas, administration of steroids, Cushing's syndrome, or the consumption of large quantities of licorice (Cella and Watson, 1989). All of these conditions increase the amount of aldosterone released by the adrenal glands and increase the reabsorption of sodium and water in the distal renal tubules of the kidneys. Aldosterone is a mineralcorticoid normally released by the adrenal cortex in response to hyponatremia or hypovolemia and will cause hypernatremia if released into the bloodstream in abnormally large amounts. Clients with mineralcorticoid excess syndromes usually have a slightly higher serum osmolality with serum sodium concentrations of 145 to 148 mEq/L (145 to 148 mmol/L SI Units) and expansion of the extracellular fluid volume by 1 to 3 L (Narins, Jones, Stom, Rudnick, and Bastl, 1982).

Hypovolemic hypernatremia

Hypovolemic hypernatremia is caused by an inadequate intake of water, which leads to hemoconcentration of the extracellular fluid. Water loss may contribute, but it is never the sole cause of hypernatremia (Kovacs and Robertson, 1992). Hypovolemia with dehydration normally increases the concentration of sodium in the serum and activates the sodium regulatory mechanisms of thirst, ADH release, and aldosterone inhibition. Hypovolemia that exceeds the body's normal compensatory ability will cause symptoms of both hypernatremia and dehydration. The most common causes of dehydration resulting in hypernatremia that cannot be regulated are uncontrolled diabetes mellitus, renal damage or disease, high-protein tube feedings, hyperventilation without humidification, fever, and diabetes insipidus (Cella and Watson, 1989). In addition to these common causes, the critically ill cancer client will most likely compound his or her hypernatremia by chemotherapy side effects of nausea, vomiting, and the inability to drink fluids as a result of mucositis.

HHNK: In uncontrolled diabetes mellitus, the high glucose level in the bloodstream causes a high osmotic pressure that draws water from the interstitial spaces into the intravascular space. The excess glucose and water are excreted into the urine by the kidneys. This osmotic diuresis increases serum sodium concentration. Kahn and Weir (1994) described another condition that can contribute to hypernatremia. Hyperglycemic, hyperosmolar nonketotic state (HHNK), which may or may not be present in conjunction with diabetic ketoacidosis, is defined by an extreme hyperglycemia level >600mg/dl (>31.2 mmol/L SI Units), increased serum osmolarity, and severe dehydration. Hypernatremia results from severe diuresis and the inability to replace fluids orally. HHNK is seen mainly in the elderly, clients with newly diagnosed diabetes, and diabetes mellitus type II. The commonly insidious onset of HHNK often makes it difficult to diagnose. The elderly are further endangered when they are mentally impaired and/or unable to recognize the need for food and fluid. The mortality rate from HHNK ranges from 40 to 70%, as opposed to 1 to 10% for normal diabetic ketoacidosis.

Polyuric hypernatremia can be caused by a variety of renal diseases such as partial urinary tract obstruction or therapy with diuretics, and by prolonged use of renal-dose dopamine (Narins et al., 1982). High-protein tube feedings can also increase osmolarity in the kidney tubules, increasing the excretion of water in the urine. Hyperventilation without humidification may cause dry mucous membranes and dehydration, increasing serum sodium concentration. Fever is a contributing factor for many clients with hypernatremia, as fever increases the body's fluid losses to manage hyperthermia.

Diabetes insipidus (DI) is a problem of fluid imbalance that results from either a deficiency of ADH or a renal insensitivity to the action of ADH (Patterson and Noroian, 1989). Clients with DI lose water through a dilute urine of low osmolality, despite a hyperosmolarity of the serum and extracellular fluid. Hypernatremia and hyperosmolarity of the serum is seen in DI when clients with massive urine outputs are unable to take in adequate fluids orally, or the thirst mechanism fails (Germon, 1987). DI-induced hypernatremia is usually associated with one of the following: (1) tumors in or around the hypothalamus that interfere with the production of ADH and the thirst center, (2) malignant lesions low on the pituitary stalk that result in a partial decrease in ADH release, or (3) primary or metastatic brain cancer causing DI. The reader is referred to Chapter 9 for further details on this condition.

Clinical manifestations of hypernatremia

The clinical symptoms of hypernatremia will be those of dehydration or water excess, depending on the contributing cause(s). In a conscious client, a slight increase in serum sodium concentration (3 to 4 mEq/L, 3 to 4 mmol/L SI Units) above normal will stimulate the thirst mechanism, encouraging an increase in oral fluid intake. If the client is comatose, mentally impaired, or has a defective thirst mechanism due to central nervous system disease and voluntary limited intake of fluids, the ADH mechanism that stimulates water reabsorption may be overwhelmed. If sodium regulation is not achieved, the symptoms of hypernatremia will appear.

The most common sign of hypernatremia is lethargy, brought about by the flow of water from the intracellular tissues of the brain to the vascular spaces in response to an increase in serum osmolarity. The lethargy will progress to coma and convulsions if untreated. Muscular tremor, rigidity, and hyperactive reflexes may also be observed as the cells regulating nerve impulse transmission begin to malfunction due to cellular dehydration. In very acute hypernatremia, the osmotic shift of water from the brain cells can cause shrinkage of the brain that results in tearing of meningeal vessels and intracranial hemorrhage. Slowly developing hypernatremia is less dangerous and better tolerated by most clients. Slow-onset hypernatremia gives the brain a chance to adjust to the change by increasing the intracellular shift of sodium, potassium, chloride, organic solutes, and amino acids to increase the brain's intracellular osmolality and causing water to shift into the brain (Oh and Carroll, 1992).

Symptoms of water excess can be seen with excessive adrenocortical secretion of aldosterone and retention of both sodium and water. Edema, rubbery skin, increased blood pressure, weight gain, dyspnea, and pulmonary congestion may be seen.

RISK PROFILE

Cancers: Hypothalamic, pituitary; other brain tumors involving the supraoptic or paraventricular nuclei. Tumors of the kidney or adrenal glands (adenomas), multiple myeloma, and malignant ascites.

Pediatrics: Accidental salt-tablet ingestion, incorrect preparation of infant feeding formulas. Children with DI caused by Langerhans cell histiocytosis (Ladisch and Jaffe, 1993). Tumors of the pituitary (20% of endocrine tumors). The most common pituitary tumor is craniopharyngioma.

Conditions: Age: infants and the elderly who are unable to voluntarily take oral fluids; congestive heart failure, renal damage, coma, Cushing's syndrome, excessive fluid losses, uncontrolled diabetes, fever, head injury, neurosurgery, chronic hypokalemia or hypercalcemia, pregnancy, central nervous system infections, DI.

Environment: Accidental drowning in salt water.

Foods: Licorice, high-sodium foods, high-protein tube feedings.

Drugs: Catecholamines; ethanol; reserpine; morphine; chlorpromazine; phenytoin; lithium carbonate; demeclocycline; methoxyflurane; cisplatin; sodium bicarbonate; aldomet; apresoline; sodium-containing antibiotics/antifungals, such as carbenicillin, ticarcillin, and amphotericin B (Narins et al., 1982; Flombaum, 1991; Cella and Watson, 1989).

PROGNOSIS

The severity of symptoms of hypernatremia depends on the amount of increase in serum sodium and the length of time over which the hypernatremia occurred. Prognosis is excellent for a hypernatremia that is recognized and treated promptly. Concomitant medical conditions such as HHNK will increase mortality rates significantly.

Symptoms of thirst in a conscious client begin with a slight increase in serum sodium concentration of 3 to 4 mEq/L (3 to 4 mmol/L SI Units). As the concentration increases, the effects become more pronounced, with lethargy proceeding to coma and convulsions. A serum sodium of greater than 160 causes the most life-threatening consequences of coma and death if left untreated.

TREATMENT

To reduce the risk of water intoxication and cerebral edema, it is recommended that serum sodium be lowered by no more than 1 mEq/L (1 mmol/L SI Units) q2h during the first 2 days of treatment.

Surgery: Removal of intracerebral or adrenal tumors.

Chemotherapy: May be indicated as adjuvant treatment for surgically removed tumors or multiple myelomas. The sodium content of chemotherapeutic mixing agents should be minimized whenever possible. Cisplatin may need to be discontinued as a treatment due to its renal toxicity.

Radiation: Might be indicated for treatment of brain tumors affecting pituitary ADH secretion.

Medications
Hypovolemic hypernatremia: isotonic saline replacement followed by hypotonic saline or oral free water.
DI: Clients with complete ADH deficiency may be temporarily or chronically treated with hormones or agents that increase the rate of ADH secretion or renal responsiveness to ADH.

Euvolemic hypernatremia: isotonic or hypotonic saline, depending on urine Na$^+$ level and urine osmolality. Oral free water and diuretics may also be used.

Hypervolemic hypernatremia: diuretics.

Nephrogenic DI: Discontinue drugs that inhibit renal response to ADH, such as catecholamines or phenytoin.

Procedures: Placement of IV access and urinary catheter to provide regulation and accurate measurement of fluid status.

Other: Low-sodium diet.

ASSESSMENT CRITERIA: HYPERNATREMIA

	Hypovolemic State	Euvolemic	Hypervolemic State
Vital signs			
Temperature	Normal or elevated	Normal	Normal
Blood pressure	Decreased	Normal	Increased
Pulse	Elevated	Normal	Elevated
Respirations	Normal	Normal	Tachypneic
CVP	<2 mm Hg	2–6 mm Hg	>6 mm Hg
History	Extremely excessive oral and/or IV intake Fluid losses from GI tract (nausea, vomiting, diarrhea) Mental impairment or coma limiting oral intake Tumors or trauma to the adrenal gland(s), hypothalamus, or pituitary gland Renal trauma or disease. Increased serum osmolality (hyperglycemia, high-protein tube feeding)	Excessive oral and/or IV sodium intake Drug administration (see Risk Profile).	Excessive adrenocortical secretion as seen in adenomas, steroid administration, Cushing's syndrome, or ingestion of large quantities of licorice Congestive heart failure
Hallmark physical signs and symptoms	Thirst, lethargy, dry mucous membranes, decreased skin turgor	Thirst	Weight gain, jugular vein distention
Urine	Diabetes insipidus: high urine output with low specific gravity	Normal to slightly increased urine output	Decreased urine output with normal-to-low specific gravity

ASSESSMENT CRITERIA: HYPERNATREMIA *(continued)*

Additional physical signs and symptoms	Hypercalcemia, malignant ascites, fever	Malignant ascites	Restlessness, dyspnea, agitation, S_3 heart sound, and generalized edema may be present with concomitant congestive heart failure.
Psychosocial signs and symptoms	Confusion, disorientation, apprehension		

Lab values

Sodium, serum	High	High	High
Sodium, urine	Decreased in DI Increased in response to aldosterone in other types of hypernatremia	Increased	Increased or decreased in conditions that cause excessive aldosterone release
Creatinine, urine	Normal or high in renal damage	Normal	Normal
Osmolarity, serum	Increased	Increased	Increased
Osmolarity, urine	Low	Normal or low	High
Specific gravity, urine	High Low in DI	High	High Low in conditions that cause excessive aldosterone release
Potassium, serum	Normal	Normal	Normal or low
Aldosterone, serum	Decreased	Low	High in conditions that increase adrenocortical secretion
ADH, serum	Increased to compensate for fluid volume losses Decreased if fluid volume is low due to diabetes insipidus	Increased	Normal, or may be decreased if fluid volume is high due to condition causing excessive aldosterone release

Diagnostic tests

Deep tendon reflexes	Hyperreactive	Hyperreactive	Hyperreactive
Water deprivation test: To help diagnose DI, a water deprivation test is performed in conjunction with hourly urine osmolality. Fluids are limited for 16–18 hours, followed by administration of vasopressin.	If hypovolemia is due to DI, there will be a twofoldincrease in urine osmolality after the administration of vasopressin (Kopec and Groeger, 1988)	No response to vasopressin	No response to vasopressin

(continued)

ASSESSMENT CRITERIA: HYPERNATREMIA *(continued)*

Other	Assess chemotherapy dosages to limit nausea and vomiting.
	Assess content and rate of IV fluids.
	Assess for medications high in sodium or for those that decrease renal responsiveness to ADH.

NURSING DIAGNOSIS

Potential for ineffective airway clearance related to seizure activity or coma secondary to cerebral dehydration.

Fluid volume deficit related to fluid loss from osmotic diuresis or DI. Compounding factors in oncology clients, such as nausea and vomiting or decreased oral intake of fluids.

Fluid overload secondary to excessive ADH secretion, as seen in adenomas, administration of steroids, and Cushing's syndrome.

Acute confusion secondary to dehydration (serum sodium > 160) or fluid overload.

Potential for injury related to hypernatremia-induced lethargy, coma, or seizures.

NURSING INTERVENTIONS

Immediate nursing interventions

Assess vital signs and neurologic status until stable.

Maintain patent airway. Keep resuscitation and suction equipment at bedside.

Implement seizure precautions. Place oral airway at bedside.

Measure strict intake and output (I and O).

Establish IV access and insert indwelling urinary catheter.

Obtain and carefully monitor electrolyte values.

Encourage oral intake of fluids for dehydration.

Low-salt diet.

Anticipated physician orders and interventions

Calculation of water deficit, if any:

$0.6 \times$ weight $\times$ [serum Na^+ -140/serum Na^+] = Water deficit in liters (Kopec and Groeger, 1988)

Serum osmolality may be calculated from the following formulas:

- If the client's glucose level is normal:

    Serum $Na^+ \times 2$ = Osmolality

- If the client's glucose level is elevated:

    (Serum $Na^+ \times 2$) + (Serum glucose/18) + (BUN/2.4) = Osmolality

Serum electrolytes q2h.

Blood urea nitrogen (BUN) and serum creatinine and osmolality.

Urine electrolytes, osmolality, and specific gravity.

Correct possible cause(s) of hypernatremia:

- Discontinue all medications high in sodium.
- Give insulin if the client has uncontrolled diabetes.
- Discontinue high-protein tube feedings.
- Add humidification to oxygen administration.

Hypovolemic hypernatremia: 0.9% NaCl IV infusion, followed by 0.45% NaCl at rates adjusted to lower serum Na^+ ≤ 1 mEq/L (1 mmol/L SI Units) q2h. Oral free water may also be used.

Euvolemic hypernatremia:

- If urine Na^+ > 20 mEq/L (> 20 mmol/L SI Units) and urine osmolality is < 300 mOsm/kg H_2O): Treat as for hypovolemic hypernatremia above.
- If urine Na^+ > 20 mEq/L (> 20 mmol/L SI Units) and urine osmolality is > 300 mOsm/kg H_2O: Give 0.25% to 0.45% NaCl infusion at rates adjusted to lower serum Na^+ ≤ 1 mEq/L (1 mmol/L SI Units) q2h or give oral free water if symptoms are mild. Diuretics may also be used.

Hypervolemic hypernatremia: Hydrochlorothiazide 50 mg qd (Man and Carroll, 1992).

Nephrogenic DI: Discontinue drugs that inhibit renal response to ADH, such as catecholamines or phenytoin. See also Chapter 9.

Neurogenic DI:

- IV, subcutaneous, or nasal vasopressin for ADH deficiency (diabetes insipidus), as listed below.
- *Desmopressin* (dDAVP)—intranasal spray 0.1 ml twice a day or parenterally 0.5 to 1 ml in two divided doses.
- *Lysine vasopressin*—intranasal spray 1 to 2 sprays four to five times per day.
- *Aqueous pitressin*—2 units IV over 8 hours, 6 units over 24 hours, or 5 units injected subcutaneously every 3 to 4 hours.
- *Pitressin tannate*—5 units subcutaneously every 12 to 24 hours. With the above treatments, salt restriction and thiazide diuretic therapy can help reduce sodium retention.

Ongoing nursing assessment, monitoring, and interventions

Assess:

- Neurologic status q4h and PRN.
- Fluid status (skin turgor, peripheral edema, jugular vein distention, fluid balance) q8h.

Measure:
- Vital signs q4h and PRN.
- Weight qd.
- I and O q1–2h.
- Abdominal girths qd if malignant ascites is present.

Send:
- Blood and urine electrolytes as prescribed.
- Serum sodium q2h until level drops below 150 mEq/L (150 mmol/L SI Units), then q8h × 2 hours.
- Serum and urine osmolarity q8h until serum sodium < 150 mEq/L (150 mmol/L SI Units).

Implement:
- Dietary sodium restriction if applicable.
- Seizure precautions until serum sodium is < 160 mEq/L (< 160 mmol/L SI Units).

TEACHING/EDUCATION

Discontinue all sodium-containing medications and foods: *Rationale:* Certain tumors and medical conditions can cause your body to have trouble getting rid of salt. Until the cause of your salt level can be effectively treated, some of your medicines might be changed to decrease your salt intake. It is also helpful to eliminate salt intake in your diet until your sodium returns to normal.

Fluid administration: *Rationale:* If your high salt level is caused or accompanied by dehydration, you will be asked to drink more fluids. If you are unable to drink enough fluid, the fluids will be given intravenously.

Urinary catheter placement: *Rationale:* If your salt level is dangerously high, a urinary catheter is needed so that your urine can be carefully measured. The amount of urine you make helps us know whether your treatment is working.

Treatment of the cause of hypernatremia: *Rationale:* Correcting your high salt level will most likely require medicine to stop any immediate complications. Following initial treatment, your doctor will order tests to locate the reason your body retains salt. Sometimes surgery, chemotherapy, or radiation is recommended to treat tumors that block the hormones necessary to regulate salt concentration in the body.

Signs and symptoms of hypernatremia: *Rationale:* You and your family will need to be alert for the signs that your high salt level is recurring. Signs of high salt levels can be any of the following: excessive thirst, increase or decrease in urination, weakness, confusion, muscle tremors, convulsions, unconsciousness, and nausea or vomiting.

EVALUATION/DESIRED OUTCOMES

1. Reduction of serum sodium at a maximum rate of 1 mEq every 2 hours, with the goal in acute hypernatremia of reaching a serum sodium level of < 160 mEq/L (< 160 mmol/L SI Units).
2. Prevention of life-threatening complication or injury.
3. Reversal of mental confusion.
4. Permanent return of normal serum sodium level.
5. Return and maintenance of optimum fluid balance.
6. Effective treatment of DI or hyperglycemia.
7. Use of surgery, radiation, or chemotherapy to eliminate tumors that may be blocking the release of ADH.
8. Discharge instructions regarding a low-salt diet, proper fluid intake, and the treatment needs of hypernatremia etiology are to be understood by the client and/or caregiver upon discharge.

DISCHARGE PLANNING/FOLLOW-UP CARE

The hypernatremic client may need:

Medications to treat the condition causing hypernatremia (insulin, vasopressin).

Arrangements for receiving surgery, radiation, or chemotherapy to treat tumors inhibiting ADH release.

IV therapy when experiencing fluid losses as a side effect of chemotherapy or other treatments.

Arrangement for outpatient blood testing.

Education on adequate fluid intake, measurement of I and O, low-salt diet, and medications that may increase sodium level.

Family education on the signs and symptoms of dehydration and hypernatremia.

Possible home care nursing or extended-care-facility placement based on individual needs.

Anticipated client/family questions and possible answers

Can I get high salt/sodium in my blood again?

"Yes, you could develop a high sodium level again. I will teach you the signs of a high sodium level so that we can treat it quickly if it occurs."

"Your cancer treatment should stop the cause of the high sodium, but until the surgery/chemotherapy is effective, we will need to closely monitor your sodium level and treat it when it becomes elevated."

"The medications you are taking might cause high sodium again, so as long as you need your steroids (or other medicines) we will check your blood frequently for sodium elevations."

How long will I have to be on a low-salt diet?

"A low-salt diet will be important for the duration of your cancer treatment. Once the tumor causing your high sodium level is gone, you can return to your normal diet if you have no other medical conditions (like high blood pressure) that might be worsened by the extra salt."

How can I control my sodium level during my cancer treatment before the tumor has fully responded?

"There are several medicines available to replace the hormones that are blocked by your tumor. The type of medicine will depend on the type and location of the tumor. These medicines are generally given in a nose spray or by injection."

Is there anyone who can help me with taking my medicine and monitoring my sodium level at home?

"If you require any special medicines or regular blood tests, we will be able to have a home health nurse stop by to assist you. The nurse will teach you how to give yourself your medication, check your blood for sodium, and look for physical signs that the high sodium level might have returned."

CHAPTER SUMMARY

Hypernatremia is an excess in extracellular sodium concentration that has been reported in one study to occur in about 0.3% of adults who have been hospitalized, with 60% of these cases developing posthospitalization, mainly in elderly clients. Contributing factors for hypernatremia in the oncology client are cancers of the adrenal and endocrine system, dehydration, uncontrolled diabetes, diuretics, steroid use, and other medications high in sodium. Hypernatremia may occur with low, normal, or high levels of extracellular fluid, depending on the cause and serum sodium concentration. In most cases, the signs and symptoms of hypernatremia are related to the fluid status of the client with hypernatremia.

The most common signs of hypernatremia are those seen with dehydration (fluid losses of cancer treatment, malignant ascites, or DI) or fluid overload as seen in excessive adrenocortical secretion (tumors of the kidney or adrenal glands). The onset of symptoms largely depends on the rate of serum sodium elevation, with symptoms such as thirst beginning at 3 to 4 mEq/L (3 to 4 mmol/L SI Units) above normal, or 148 to 149 mEq/L (148 to 149 mmol/L SI Units). Oncologic emergencies occur with a rapid elevation in serum sodium, or a sodium level that exceeds 160 mEq/L (160 mmol/L SI Units). Mortality rates have been reported as high as 54%, regardless of age, and should be largely avoidable with careful monitoring and treatment of clients at risk.

TEST QUESTIONS

1. Hypernatremia is defined as:
   A. An excess in extracellular sodium concentration
   B. High potassium intake
   C. A disorder related strictly to dehydration
   D. An elevated cellular sodium level

1. Answer: A
Hypernatremia is related to high sodium levels in the blood rather than inside the cell. Although high sodium intake and dehydration can cause hypernatremia, these situations do not always cause hypernatremia because of the body's mechanisms for compensation.

2. Sodium concentration can be elevated in the presence of serum sodium that is:
   A. Normal only
   B. Elevated only
   C. Decreased and normal only
   D. Either normal, elevated, or decreased

2. Answer: D
Serum sodium levels do not always depend on the amount of sodium that has been ingested, but on the concentration of this sodium in the blood.

3. Oncology clients at highest risk for hypernatremia are:
   A. Those with malignancies affecting hormones regulating ADH and aldosterone
   B. Tumors of the cervix
   C. Those with excess magnesium losses
   D. Those with hypercalcemia-associated tumor burden

3. Answer: A
Tumors near the hypothalamus may interfere with the production of ADH and cause large fluid volume losses through the kidneys. Large fluid losses increase serum sodium concentration. Clients with tumors of the adrenal gland may have an increased absorption of both sodium and water.

4. Excessive sodium intake puts which of the following clients at the highest risk?
   A. Those taking multivitamins
   B. Those with inefficient excretion of body fluids
   C. Teenagers
   D. Those with multiple sclerosis

4. Answer: B
Normally the body can compensate for abnormally large ingestion of sodium by the release of ADH, which causes reabsorption of more water. Clients with impaired renal function will more quickly demonstrate signs of fluid overload with high sodium intake than will clients with normal renal function.

5. What is the most common cause of hypernatremia?
   A. Excessive fluid loss
   B. High-sodium IV fluid adminis-tration
   C. Deficient water intake
   D. Diabetes mellitus

5. Answer: C
Excessive water losses may con-tribute to hypernatremia but are not sufficient to cause the condition entirely.

6. Tumors centered around the hypothalamus are the most com-mon cause of:
   A. Hypernatremia
   B. Increase in circulating ADH levels
   C. Diabetes insipidus (DI)
   D. Cerebral edema

6. Answer: C
Tumors near the hypothalamus interfere with the release of ADH, causing diabetes insipidus.

7. The clinical symptoms of hyper-natremia include:
   A. Dehydration or water excess
   B. Acidosis
   C. Hyperkalemia
   D. Hypocalcemia

7. Answer: A
Most clients with hypernatremia will have decreased sodium concen-tration from fluid losses (dehydra-tion) or an excessive amount of both sodium and water (excessive adrenocortical secretion).

8. What is the most common clini-cal symptom of hypernatremia?
   A. Increased urine output
   B. Lethargy
   C. Pulmonary congestion
   D. Hypertension

8. Answer: B
Lethargy, the most common sign of hypernatremia, develops as water moves from the intracellular tissues of the brain to the vascular spaces to help compensate for increased osmolarity.

9. Untreated hypernatremia is an oncologic emergency when:
   A. Serum sodium is > 160 mEq/L or > 160 mmol/L.
   B. Hypernatremia causes symp-toms of water excess.
   C. Clients are unable to take oral liquids.
   D. There is a 20 mmHg drop in the systolic blood pressure.

9. Answer: A
A serum sodium of greater than 160 mEq/L or > 160 mmol/L has the most life-threatening consequences of coma and death if left untreated.

10. Surgery is indicated for hypernatremia when there are which of the following:

A. Adrenal tumors
B. Basal cell carcinoma
C. Tearing of the meningeal vessels
D. Diabetes insipidus

10. Answer: A

Surgery is the treatment of choice for endocrine or adrenal tumors. Chemotherapy and radiation may be indicated as adjuvant treatment of surgically removed tumor or those tumors that are nonresectable.

REFERENCES

Cella JH, Watson J: Nurses' Manual of Laboratory Tests. Philadelphia: FA Davis, 1989, pp. 257–258.

Ellison DH, Johnson Bia M: Renal, fluid, and electrolyte disorders in the critically ill immunosuppressed patient. *In* Parrillo JE, Masur H (eds): The Critically Ill Immunosuppressed Patient: Diagnosis and Management. Rockville, MD: Aspen, 1987, pp. 101–103.

Flombaum C: Electrolyte and renal abnormalities. *In* Groeger JS (ed): Critical Care of the Cancer Patient, 2nd ed. St. Louis, MO: Mosby Year Book, 1991, pp. 142–143.

Germon K: Fluid and electrolyte problems associated with diabetes insipidus and syndrome of inappropriate antidiuretic hormone. *In* Chambers JK, Rantz MJ, Maas M (eds): The Nursing Clinics of North America. 22(4). Philadelphia: WB Saunders Co, 1987, pp. 785–796.

Kahn RC, Weir GC: Diabetic ketoacidosis and the hyperglycemic, hyperosmolar nonketotic state. *In* Joslin's Diabetes Mellitus, 13th ed. Philadelphia: Lea and Febiger, 1994, pp. 748–751.

Keen ML: Patients with fluid and electrolyte disturbances. *In* Clochesy JM, Breu C, Cardin S, Rudy EB, Whittaker AA (eds): Critical Care Nursing. Philadelphia: WB Saunders Co, 1993, pp. 863–864.

Kopec ID, Groeger JS: Life-threatening fluid and electrolyte abnormalities. *In* Groeger JS, Carlon GC (guest eds): Critical Care Clinics: Critical Care of the Cancer Patient 4(1):83–84, January 1988.

Kovacs L, Robertson GL: Disorders of water balance—Hyponatraemia and hypernatraemia. Bailliers Clin Endocrinol Metab 6(1):107–127, 1992.

Ladisch S, Jaffe ES: The histriocytosies. *In* Pizzo PA, Poplack DG (eds): Principles and Practice of Pediatric Oncology, 2nd ed. Philadelphia: JB Lippincott, 1993, p. 1787.

Lancour J: ADH and aldosterone: How to recognize their effects. Nursing 8(9):36–38, 1978.

Long C, Marin P, Bayer AJ, Shetty H, Pathy MS: Hypernatraemia in an adult in-patient population. Postgrad Med J 67(789):643–645, 1991.

Narins RG, Jones ER, Stom MC, Rudnick MR, Bastl CP: Diagnostic strategies in disorders of fluid, electrolyte and acid-base homeostasis. Am J Med 72(3):496–519, 1982.

Oh SM, Carroll HJ: Disorders of sodium metabolism: Hypernatremia and hyponatremia. Crit Care Med 20(1):94–103, 1992.

Palevsky PM, Bhagrath R, Greenberg A: Hypernatremia in hospitalized patients. Ann Intern Med 124(2):197–203, 1996.

Patterson LM, Noroian EL: Diabetes insipidus versus syndrome of inappropriate antidiuretic hormone. Dimens Crit Care Nurs 8(4):226–234, 1989.

Sonnenblick M, Algur N: Hypernatremia in the acutely ill elderly patients: Role of impaired arginine-vasopressin secretion. Miner Electrolyte Metab 19(1):32–35, 1993.

Sotis B: Fluid and electrolyte imbalance. *In* Phipps WJ, Long BC, Wood NF (eds): Medical–Surgical Nursing. Concepts and Clinical Practice. St. Louis, MO: CV Mosby, 1979, pp. 306–308.

CHAPTER 22

HYPERURICEMIA

Madeline Heffner, RN, BSN, CPNP

AND

Linda S. Polman, RN, BSN, CPON

CHAPTER OBJECTIVES

At the completion of this chapter, the reader will be able to:

Define hyperuricemia.

Describe the clinical findings associated with hyperuricemia in the client with cancer.

Identify five risk factors associated with the development of hyperuricemia.

List three measures commonly used to prevent renal failure as a complication of hyperuricemia.

Plan appropriate nursing interventions for management of the client who exhibits hyperuricemia associated with cancer or its treatment.

OVERVIEW

HYPERURICEMIA is a potentially fatal disorder of metabolism in which there is an excessive amount of uric acid in the blood resulting either from overproduction, faulty elimination, or a combination of the two (see Table 22–1 for normal levels). As the body attempts to eliminate excessive amounts of uric acid through the kidneys, monosodium urate crystals may precipitate out, obstruct the renal collecting ducts, and result in kidney damage. It is seen most frequently in acute leukemias and high-grade lymphomas. It also occurs in solid tumors and in myeloproliferative disorders. Prior to the institution of prophylactic treatment regimens, hyperuricemia was a common complication of cancer treatment. Even with prophylaxis it has been estimated that approximately 10% of clients with leukemia or lymphoma will experience some degree of renal deterioration as a result of hyperuricemia (Conger, 1990).

Table 22–1
Normal Serum Uric Acid Levels

Adult female	2.4–6.0 mg/dl	143–357 µmol/L
		0.17–0.45 mmol/L
Adult male	3.4–7.0 mg/dl	202–416 µmol/L
		0.21–0.51 mmol/L
Children	2.5–5.5 mg/dl	119–327 µmol/L
		0.15–0.33 mmol/L
Elderly	3.5–8.5 mg/dl	204–550 µmol/L
		0.21–0.51 mmol/L
Panic value	> 12 mg/dl	> 714 µmol/L

Source: From Chernecky CC, Kretch RL, Berger BJ: Laboratory Tests and Diagnostic Procedures. Philadelphia: WB Saunders Co, 1993, p. 343.

DESCRIPTION

Rapid cell breakdown is the most common cause of hyperuricemia in the client with cancer. Uric acid is a normal end product of the breakdown of adenosine triphosphate (ATP) and the nucleic acids that form DNA and RNA (see Fig. 22-1). When cell breakdown occurs, uric acid is released into the bloodstream, where it circulates as sodium urate (also referred to simply as "urate"). Any increase in the rate of cell breakdown is accompanied by a proportional increase in the amount of uric acid released into the blood-

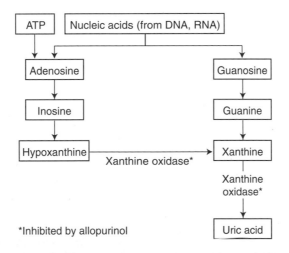

Figure 22–1 Overview of uric acid synthesis. Xanthine oxidase is the critical enzymatic step in the formation of uric acid from the more soluble purine precursors adenosine, inosine, hypoxanthine, and xanthine. Xanthine oxidase actively is inhibited by allopurinol.

stream. Rapid cell breakdown may be related to tumor growth or may be a result of cancer treatments.

Hyperuricemia may be present at the time of diagnosis as a result of tumor growth, if overproduction of cells has been accompanied by an increase in the rate of cell turnover. The disorder is seen most frequently in cancers with a high growth fraction and in clients with large tumor burden. It is a frequent complication of leukemias and lymphomas, especially when there is a high white blood cell (WBC) count, and when lymphadenopathy, hepatomegaly, and splenomegaly are present. It is seen rarely in other solid tumors. When it does occur with other solid tumors, there is usually extensive metastasis present.

Although hyperuricemia may be present at the time of diagnosis, it is more commonly seen after treatment has begun. It is most common in the first 48 hours after initiation of induction chemotherapy, but may be seen up to 7 days after initiation of treatment. This is the time period when the greatest number of tumor cells are likely to undergo rapid breakdown.

Hyperuricemia can occur after chemotherapy, after radiation therapy, or after administration of corticosteroids. It may occur after even a single dose of some drugs, particularly corticosteroids in clients with lymphoma or acute lymphoblastic leukemia. Each of these treatments can bring about rapid tumor cell lysis. The more sensitive a tumor is to treatment, the more rapidly cells will break down and the greater the amount of uric acid released into the bloodstream.

Hyperuricemia may occur as an isolated event or as a part of the tumor lysis syndrome. (The reader is referred to Chapter 43.) It is also associated with diseases (see Table 22–2) and drugs (see Risk Profile) that are unrelated to cancer. Certain disorders of metabolism cause excessive uric acid production and renal disorders that result in decreased uric acid excretion. If one of these metabolic disorders exists in combination with cancer, the risk of complications will be higher.

Elevated levels of uric acid are not directly toxic to the body. However, as

---

Table 22–2
Nonmalignant Causes of Hyperuricemia

Overproduction of Uric Acid	**Underexcretion of Uric Acid**
Acute infectious diseases	Acidic urine
Blood dyscrasias	Alcoholism
Genetic metabolic disorders	Dehydration
High purine diet	Drugs
Hyperparathyroidism	Eclampsia
Rapid tissue breakdown	Hypertension
Severe psoriasis	Lead poisoning
	Renal dysfunction
	Shock

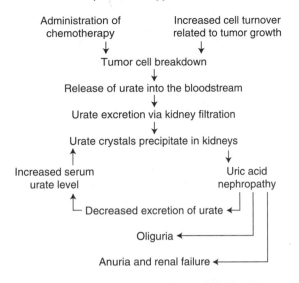

Figure 22–2 Hyperuricemia from cellular breakdown.

serum levels rise, there is a proportional increase in the amount excreted through the kidneys. When serum uric acid levels reach 15 to 20 mg/dl (893 to 1192 μmol/L SI Units), serious renal complications are likely to occur (Thomas and Dodhia, 1991). As serum urate levels rise and the amount excreted by the kidneys increases, maximum solubility in the urine may be exceeded. Urate crystals begin to precipitate out of solution and are deposited in the renal tubules and collecting ducts, where they obstruct urine flow. Obstruction of urine flow results in decreased excretion of uric acid from the body, further elevating serum levels and renal urate deposition. This progressive obstructive uropathy can rapidly lead to complete renal failure (Fig. 22–2).

Measures to prevent uric acid nephropathy are routinely initiated in all clients who have or are at high risk for developing hyperuricemia before the initiation of chemotherapy either at diagnosis or at relapse. These clients include all those with elevated uric acid levels and/or leukemia or lymphoma, especially Burkitt's lymphoma.

The goal of treatment is to prevent the precipitation of urate crystals in the kidney tubules. This can be accomplished by decreasing the amount of uric acid produced, maximizing its solubility in the urine, and ensuring adequate urine flow through the kidneys.

Although a genetically engineered urate oxidase enzyme is currently being tested, at the time of this writing allopurinol is the drug of choice to decrease the formation of uric acid in the client with cancer. It is a xanthine oxidase inhibitor that prevents the formation of uric acid from xanthine during the breakdown of nucleic acids (see Fig. 22–1). Xanthine is more soluble in urine than uric acid and is less likely to precipitate in the renal tubules. Side effects from allopurinol are uncommon. However, an erythematous maculopapular rash can be a sign of hypersensitivity. If a rash develops, allopurinol should be discontinued. In addition, allopurinol interferes with the metabolism of 6-mercaptopurine. To avoid excessive toxicity from 6-mercaptopurine, the dose should be reduced if it is given concomitantly with allopurinol.

Maximum solubility of uric acid occurs at a pH of 7.5. Giving IV fluids containing sodium bicarbonate maximizes the solubility of urate by keeping the urine dilute and at a pH between 7.0 and 7.5. If kidney function deteriorates in spite of the above measures, hemodialysis may be required to remove uric acid from the bloodstream. Progressive oliguria and rising creatinine levels are indications that dialysis should be considered.

The client is often asymptomatic, even in the presence of marked hyperuricemia. When symptoms do occur, they include lethargy, nausea, vomiting, and the presence of uric acid crystals in the urine. Renal colic and hematuria are signs of renal calculi, which are seen infrequently in the client with cancer.

RISK PROFILE

Cancers: Acute leukemias, lymphomas (particularly Burkitt's lymphoma), multiple myeloma, solid tumors other than lymphoma when widespread metastatic disease is present.

Conditions: Tumors with high growth fraction; large tumor burden; tumors that are very sensitive to chemotherapy; first 48 hours following administration of initial chemotherapy, corticosteroids, or irradiation. Compromised renal function, dehydration, acidic urine, elevated serum lactate dehydrogenase (LDH) at diagnosis, elevated pretreatment serum uric acid (see Table 22–2).

Environment: None.

Foods: None.

Drugs: Acetozolamide, alpha interferon, aminothiadiazoles, beta-blockers, chlorthalidone, cimetidine, cisplatin, corticosteroids, cyclosporin, daunorubicin, DDI, diazoxide, dichlorphenamide, ethacrynic acid, ethambutol, filgramstim, furosemide, IV heparin, indapamide, levodopa, lisinopril, 6-mercaptopurine, nicotinic acid, pancreatic enzyme preparations, pyrazinamide, ramipril, ranitidine, low-dose salicylates, tacrolimus, thiazide diuretics, 6-thioguanine, tiazofurin.

PROGNOSIS

Approximately 10% of clients with leukemia or lymphoma will experience some degree of renal deterioration as a result of hyperuricemia (Conger, 1990). Although the incidence of hyperuricemia with other cancers is infrequent, exact statistics regarding morbidity and mortality have not been reported. Prior to 1966, a 47% mortality rate was reported in 30 clients with acute uric acid nephropathy. However, with current prophylactic treatment and early intervention for uric acid nephropathy, permanent renal impairment is extremely rare (Conger, 1990).

TREATMENT

Surgery
> Placement of central venous catheter.
> Placement of Quinton catheter if hemodialysis is required.

Chemotherapy: Decrease dosages of vincristine, cisplatin, daunorubicin, 6-mercaptopurine, 6-thioguanine.

Radiation: Not indicated.

Medications
> Stop medications that may interfere with tubular reabsorption of uric acid: salicylates, probenecid, and thiazide diuretics.
> Administer allopurinol 12 to 24 hours prior to start of chemotherapy.
> IV 5% dextrose in 0.25% NaCl with 50 to 100 mEq sodium bicarbonate.
> Corticosteriods may elevate the uric acid level if given.

Procedures
> Placement of peripheral IV if central venous catheter is not indicated.
> Hemodialysis if uric acid level is > 12 mg/dL (713 µmol/L).
> Leukophoresis or blood exchange transfusion for WBC > 200,000/cu mm.

Other: None.

ASSESSMENT CRITERIA: HYPERURICEMIA

	Without Renal Failure	With Renal Failure
Vital signs		
Temperature	Normal	Normal
Pulse	Normal	Rapid
Respirations	Normal	Tachypneic
Blood pressure	Normal	Increased
History		
Symptoms, conditions	Current medication history	Current medication history
Weight pattern	Stable	Recent weight gain

(continued)

ASSESSMENT CRITERIA: HYPERURICEMIA (continued)

	Without Renal Failure	With Renal Failure
Hallmark physical signs and symptoms	Cloudy urine Crystals in urine	Oliguria, anuria
Additional physical signs and symptoms	Anorexia, diarrhea, lethargy, nausea, vomiting, flank pain, joint pain	CHF, dyspnea, edema, seizure
Psychosocial signs		Confusion, disorientation
Lab values		
Uric acid, serum	<12mg/dl or 714 µmol/L	>15 mg/dl or 892 µmol/L
Creatinine, serum	Normal	High
Urinalysis	Crystals present	Crystals present
Diagnostic tests	None	None
Other	Assess chemotherapy doses.	Stop chemotherapy.

NURSING DIAGNOSIS

Potential nursing diagnoses for the client with hyperuricemia include the following.

Potential for impaired tissue integrity related to:
- Venous access device (peripheral or central venous catheter).
- Skin rash related to allopurinol.

Fluid volume deficit related to:
- Nausea and vomiting associated with the side effects of chemotherapy.
- Inadequate fluid intake.

Fluid volume excess related to:
- Infusion of hydration fluids.
- Oliguria secondary to obstruction of renal tubules with urate crystals.
- Congestive heart failure (CHF) secondary to renal failure.

Altered urinary elimination related to oliguria/urate nephropathy.

Knowledge deficit related to:
- Unfamiliarity with sequelae and treatment for hyperuricemia.
- Unfamiliarity with side effects of allopurinol.

NURSING INTERVENTIONS

Immediate nursing interventions

Assess pulse, respirations, blood pressure qlh × 4, then q4h. Send renal panel, uric acid level, LDH.

Establish patent IV access or prepare for placement of long-line catheter/ access device.

Obtain volumetric infusion pump.

Measure intake and output (I and O) q1h.

Insert indwelling urinary catheter, if necessary.

Strict I and O.

Anticipated physician orders and interventions

Administer allopurinol.

Provide adequate hydration with D5&$\frac{1}{4}$ normal saline with 50 to 100 mEq NaHCO$_3$ per liter to keep urine pH 7.0 to 7.5 with specific gravity ≤ 1.010.

Decrease or discontinue chemotherapy and other medications that cause hyperuricemia.

Check specific gravity and pH of urine with each void or q4h for catheter drainage.

Send uric acid level, renal panel.

Long-line catheter/access device placement for frequent blood sampling.

Possible leukophoresis or exchange transfusion for WBC > 200,000/cu mm.

Ongoing nursing assessment, monitoring, and interventions

Assess:
- Client medication history for medications that would elevate serum urate.
- For nausea and vomiting.
- IV site for redness, edema, pain q4h and PRN.
- For clinical signs of renal failure: oliguria, nausea, vomiting, lethargy, edema, CHF, seizure.

Measure:
- Blood pressure, pulse, and respirations q1h × 4, then q4h.
- Strict I and O q4h × 48 hours, then q8h until hydration fluids are discontinued.
- Weight qd.

Send:
- Repeat urinalysis q24h. (Check pH, specific gravity, crystals in urine.)
- Serum uric acid, renal panel, q8h if elevation in uric acid, and 48 hours after chemotherapy.

Implement:
- Allopurinol administration.
- Medication with antiemetics PRN, as ordered.

- Client and family teaching about hemodialysis as uric acid level rises.

TEACHING/EDUCATION

Decreased/discontinued chemotherapy: *Rationale:* As chemotherapy begins to break down tumor cells, crystals may form in your kidneys and cause kidney damage. Because that might happen, your chemotherapy may need to be decreased or delayed.

IV blood samples and urine samples: *Rationale:* Several blood and urine samples will be taken over the next few days so that we can keep track of how your kidneys are working.

Peripheral IV placement: *Rationale:* You need extra fluid to keep crystals from forming in your kidneys. In addition, some of your medicines need to be given through your IV.

Central venous catheter placement: *Rationale:* The IV line allows us to easily take blood samples and give you fluids and medications.

Strict I and O and use of indwelling urinary catheter: *Rationale:* Accurate urine measurement is very important for you. The urine catheter prevents urine from spilling before it is measured. You will be given extra fluids, so the catheter keeps you from having to get up frequently to go to the bathroom.

IV site symptoms: *Rationale:* Some of the medications you will be given can irritate your vein. This IV may begin to hurt if these medications leak out of the vein and go into the tissue of your hand or arm. A nurse will be checking frequently to see how well the IV is working. However, if it starts to hurt or swell at any time, call the nurse right away.

Signs and symptoms of renal failure: *Rationale:* You and your significant others need to watch for signs of kidney failure. These include any of the following: nausea and vomiting, fatigue, weakness, swelling of feet, hands, or abdomen, cough, difficulty breathing, seizures.

EVALUATION/DESIRED OUTCOMES

1. Urine specific gravity will be ≤ 1.010 from the start of chemotherapy until 48 hours after chemotherapy.
2. Urine pH will be maintained between 7.0 and 7.5.
3. Serum uric acid will be < 8 mg/dl during and 48 hours after chemotherapy.
4. Indwelling urinary catheter will be discontinued within 72 hours.
5. Chemotherapy regimen will continue as prescribed or will be given at reduced dosage within 72 hours.

6. Serum creatinine/blood urea nitrogen (BUN) will be within normal range 48 hours after chemotherapy regimen.
7. The client will be free of any signs of hyperuricemia during and 7 days following chemotherapy.

DISCHARGE PLANNING

The client is hospitalized during the time that he or she is at risk for hyperuricemia. No immediate discharge planning is required.

FOLLOW-UP CARE

Anticipated care

Physician office visit within 1 week.
Discontinue allopurinol, if not done before discharge.
Outpatient lab testing for BUN, creatinine.

Anticipated client/family questions and possible answers

How long do I need to worry about crystals forming in my kidneys?
"It would be very unlikely for this complication to occur later than 7 days after you began your first chemotherapy."

When will my chemotherapy be restarted?
"Your chemotherapy will be restarted when we are sure your kidneys are working well."

CHAPTER SUMMARY

Hyperuricemia is a metabolic disorder that results in some degree of renal compromise in approximately 10% of clients with leukemia or lymphoma, and less frequently in clients with other forms of cancer. Renal compromise occurs when urate crystals precipitate out of the urine and obstruct the kidney tubules. It is seen most frequently during the first 48 hours after initiating chemotherapy, corticosteroids, and/or radiation treatments. The most common cause of hyperuricemia is rapid cell breakdown. The risk is greatest for those clients who have a large tumor burden and/or whose tumor is very sensitive to cytotoxic agents. Serious renal complications are likely to occur when serum uric acid levels exceed 15 to 20 mg/dl. (892 to 1189 µmol/L.) Untreated hyperuricemia in the client with cancer can progress rapidly to complete renal failure. (See Fig. 22–2.)

Treatment modalities include administration of allopurinol to block formation of uric acid, hydration with IV fluids to keep urine dilute, and addition of sodium bicarbonate to IV fluids to alkalinize the urine and thereby maximize urate solubility. In most cases, these measures will effectively prevent or reverse urate nephropathy. Occasionally, urate nephropathy will progress to renal failure in spite of these measures. When this happens, hemodialysis becomes necessary. Permanent kidney damage from hyperuricemia in the client with cancer is rare.

TEST QUESTIONS

1. Untreated hyperuricemia in the client with cancer can result in:
   A. Diarrhea
   B. Renal failure
   C. Hepatic dysfunction
   D. Increased urine production

1. Answer: B
As levels of uric acid in the blood rise, more uric acid is excreted by the kidneys. If levels rise too high, urate crystals precipitate out of the urine, obstruct kidney tubules, and can cause renal failure.

2. Hyperuricemia is most frequently associated with which of the following cancers?
   A. Kaposi's sarcoma
   B. Breast carcinomas
   C. Leukemia and lymphoma
   D. Osteosarcoma

2. Answer: C
Hyperuricemia is seen most frequently in clients with leukemia and lymphoma.

3. When is the client with cancer most likely to develop hyperuricemia?
   A. During the first 48 hours after initial chemotherapy
   B. Following episodes of frequent emesis
   C. During rapid infusion of IV fluids
   D. During transfusion of packed red blood cells

3. Answer: A
Uric acid is an end product of cell breakdown. Levels are most likely to rise during periods of rapid cell breakdown, such as the first 48 hours after initial chemotherapy.

4. Hyperuricemia may be associated with all of the following treatments *except:*
   A. Chemotherapy
   B. Corticosteroids
   C. Radiation therapy
   D. Antiemetics

4. Answer: D
Uric acid is an end product of cell breakdown. All of these treatments can cause cell breakdown, except for the administration of antiemetics.

5. Which of the following is the drug of choice for the treatment of hyperuricemia?
   A. Prednisone
   B. Insulin
   C. Allopurinol
   D. Sulfamethoxazole

5. Answer: C
Allopurinol is a xanthine oxidase inhibitor. It prevents the formation of uric acid from xanthine.

6. The most common cause of renal failure in children with acute leukemia is:
   A. Severe dehydration due to vomiting and diarrhea
   B. Leukemic infiltrate of kidney
   C. Hyperuricemia and uric acid nephropathy
   D. Pyelonephritis

6. Answer: C
Hyperuricemia occurs in acute leukemia at diagnosis or after initiation of therapy as a result of tumor lysis. Uric acid is filtered through the kidneys. Very high levels can result in precipitation of urate crystals, which can block kidney tubules and result in kidney failure.

7. Signs of hyperuricemia include:
   A. Decreased urine osmolarity
   B. Increased serum uric acid
   C. Decreased serum sodium
   D. Confusion

7. Answer: B
Serum uric acid level > 8 mg/dl or > 475 umol/L SI Units.

8. The primary nursing diagnosis for clients with hyperuricemia is:
   A. Knowledge deficit
   B. Fluid volume deficit
   C. Potential for injury
   D. Alteration in nutrition

8. Answer: B
For the client with hyperuricemia, adequate hydration is necessary to help prevent kidney damage as a result of urate crystal formation.

9. Which nursing intervention should be implemented first in a client at risk for hyperuricemia?
   A. Monitor I and O
   B. Obtain a STAT renal panel and serum uric acid level
   C. Insert a urinary catheter
   D. Assess for heart dysrhythmias

9. Answer: B
Serum uric acid levels rise rapidly and can rapidly compromise renal function.

10. Which of the following is an expected outcome for the client with cancer who develops hyperuricemia?
    A. BUN will be within normal limits 1 hour after admission.
    B. Urine will be free of glucose before discharge.
    C. Uric acid level will be within normal limits prior to discharge.
    D. Granulocyte count will be within normal limits in 24 hours.

10. Answer: C
The client will remain in the hospital for IV hydration until hyperuricemia has resolved.

REFERENCES

Allegretta GJ, Weisman SJ, Altman AJ: Oncologic emergencies. Pediatr Clin North Am 32(3):601–605, 1985.

Borgatti RS: Management decisions in hyperuricemia. Patient Care 20(15):93–116, 1986.

Chernecky CC, Kretch RL, Berger BJ: Laboratory Tests and Diagnostic Procedures. Philadelphia: WB Saunders Co, 1993, p. 343.

Conger JD: Acute uric acid nephropathy. Med Clin North Am 74(4):859–871, 1990.

Fernback DJ, Viette TJ: Clinical Pediatric Oncology, 4th ed. St. Louis, MO: Mosby Year Book, 1991, pp. 236–237.

Hande KR, Garrow GC: Acute tumor lysis syndrome in patients with high-grade non-Hodgkin's lymphoma. Am J Med 94(2):133–139, 1993.

Holland P, Holland NH: Prevention and management of acute hyperuricemia in childhood leukemia. J Pediatr 72(3):358–365, 1968.

Kjellstrand CM, Campbell DC, von Hartitzsch B, Buselmeier PJ: Hyperuricemic acute renal failure. Arch Intern Med 133:349–359, 1974.

McCance KL, Huether SE: Pathophysiology: The Biologic Basis for Diseases in Adults and Children, 2nd ed. St. Louis, MO: Mosby Year Book, 1994, p. 1469.

Morris JC, Holland JF: Oncologic emergencies. *In* Holland JF, Frei E III, Bast RC Jr, Kuse DW, Morton DL, Weichselbaum RR (eds): Cancer Medicine, 3rd ed. Philadelphia: Lea and Feibeger, 1993, pp. 2460–2461.

Pizzo PA, Poplack DG: Principles and Practice of Pediatric Oncology, 2nd ed. Philadelphia: JB Lippincott, 1993, pp. 560–561, 966–967.

Plowman PN, McElwain TJ, Meadows AT: Complications of Cancer Management. Oxford: Butterworth-Heinemann, 1990, pp. 62–63.

Porth CM: Pathophysiology: Concepts of Altered Health States, 4th ed. Philadelphia: JB Lippencott, 1994, p. 1263.

Shlafer M: The Nurse, Pharmacology, and Drug Therapy: A Prototype Approach. Redwood City, CA: Addison Wesley, 1993, pp. 1110–1111.

Stucky LA: Acute tumor lysis syndrome: Assessment and nursing implications. Oncol Nurs Forum 20(1):49–59, 1993.

Thomas CR Jr, Dodhia N: Common emergencies in cancer medicine: Metobolic syndromes. J National Med Assoc 83(9):813–815, 1991.

Warell RP, Bockmann RS: Metabolic emergencies. *In* Devita VT, Hellmann S, Rosenberg SA (eds): Cancer: Principles and Practice of Oncology, 3rd ed. Philadelphia: JB Lippincott, 1989, pp. 1995–1996.

CHAPTER 23

HYPOKALEMIA

Bette K. Idemoto, MSN, RN, CS, CCRN

CHAPTER OBJECTIVES

At the completion of this chapter, the reader will be able to:

Define hypokalemia.

Differentiate the etiologies associated with hypokalemia.

State the risk factors associated with hypokalemia in the oncology client.

Describe nursing care as it relates to oncology clients with acute hypokalemia.

Anticipate and prepare the client with hypokalemia for future care needs.

OVERVIEW

HYPOKALEMIA is defined as any condition with a serum potassium (K^+) concentration of <3.5 mEq/L (<3.5 mmol/L SI Units), although signs or symptoms are not always apparent until serum K^+ reaches <3.0 mEq/L (<3.0 mmol/L SI Units). Tight K^+ regulation is maintained by normal homeostatic mechanisms that include aldosterone regulation, kidney excretion or reabsorption, dietary intake, and gastrointestinal (GI) elimination. Regulation is essential to the body because the ratio of extracellular to intracellular K^+ determines cellular resting membrane potential, which is essential for the transmission of electrical impulses. Significant alterations in the ratio can affect neuromuscular excitability, and as the major intracellular cation, K^+ inadequacy can cause muscle weakness. Smooth muscle weakness can cause ileus and flaccid paralysis. Muscle paralysis may become evident with a serum K^+ <2.5 mEq/L (<2.5 mmol/L SI Units). Lower-extremity weakness can progress to upper-extremity and trunk problems, culminating in respiratory failure. Digitalis toxicity, cardiac dysrhythmias, and abnormal electrocardiograms are also seen in hypokalemia. Sinus bradycardia, premature atrial, and ventricular contractions and tachydysrhythmias can be observed as well as T wave depression, prolonged Q-T interval, U waves and depressed S-T segments.

Hypokalemia is noted in approximately 75% of all clients with cancer and can become a potentially life-threatening complication (Mahon and Casperson, 1993).

DESCRIPTION

K^+ is the most abundant exchangeable cation. The majority of the body's K^+ is intracellular, and only the extracellular or serum K^+ can be measured. Only 2% of the total body K^+ is found outside the cell. Serum K^+ levels initially decrease about 1 mEq for each 100 to 200 mEq/L shift or loss. However, in moderate to severe deficits, levels greater than 2 mEq/L will not be accurately reflected in the amount of serum K^+ lost, making diagnosis of the severity of the hypokalemia difficult. The acid-base balance also affects serum K^+ levels due to the complex mechanisms between plasma and K^+. Any change in the balance toward acidemia tends to shift K^+ out of the cells, while alkalemia allows movement of K^+ from extracellular fluid into the cells. The shift of K^+ into the cell can lead to a low serum K^+ level, or hypokalemia.

K^+ has an essential role in many physiologic processes, including cell metabolism and the membrane potential mechanisms of nerve and muscle cells. Cell volume and osmolality of body fluids is determined by K^+. However, with the small percentage of K^+ in the extracellular fluid (ECF), it is the ratio of intracellular to extracellular K^+ that is the principle determinant of cell membrane electrical potential. Small deviations in K^+ concentrations can cause large changes in the ratio, resulting in decreased cell membrane excitability.

Causes of hypokalemia—abnormal intake or metabolism

Decreased K^+ intake: Dietary intake of K^+ does not normally have a major effect on plasma K^+ due to mechanisms related to urinary excretion of K^+. Aldosterone release from the adrenal glands and inhibition of K^+ excretion in the collecting tubules result from the body's response to hypokalemia. However, anorexia and nausea from chemotherapy and radiation can lead to decreased dietary intake and mimic starvation, resulting in hypokalemia.

Increased GI losses: Diarrhea, obstruction, and fistulas can cause loss of K^+ > 10 mEq/L (> 10 mmol/L SI Units). Hypokalemia also can develop with excessive loss of gastric fluid from gastric suction (Wilson, 1992). Excessive diarrhea caused by malignant tumors can worsen pre-existing conditions such as Crohn's disease, cholera, or laxative abuse. Gastrinomas (Zollinger-Ellison syndrome), vipomas, somatostatinoma, corticotropinoma, carcinoid tumors, and calcitoninoma have all demonstrated hypokalemia due to diarrhea. Villous adenoma of the colon can be a direct cause of K^+ loss with stool volumes > 1500 to 3500 ml/day.

Intracellular and extracellular compartmental shifts

Increased entry into cell: Excessive vomiting or nasogastric suction can cause loss of hydrogen ions, which results in exchange of K^+ ions and metabolic alkalosis. K^+ also moves into the intracellular compartment with an increase in insulin, catelcholamines, increased pH, or beta-adrenergic activity.

Disturbances in renal excretion or extrarenal loss

Excessive renal loss and mineralcorticoid excess: Aldosterone and other adrenal corticosteroids cause excretion of chloride and K^+ in exchange for retention of sodium and bicarbonate at the distal renal tubules. Clues that alert the diagnostician to hyperaldosteronism include the combination of hypokalemic metabolic alkalosis and hypertension. Adrenal tumors of the zona glomerulosa cells increase secretion of aldosterone. Aldosterone is also secreted by hyperplastic adrenal cortices, which should normally be secreting cortisol. The additional aldosterone results in hypokalemia, slight hypervolemia, slight hypernatremia, and hypertension. Muscle weakness and occasional periods of muscular paralysis due to hypokalemia can be seen in primary aldosteronism. Nerve fibers are affected by hypokalemia, which depresses the action potential and inhibits transmission of nerve impulses. The diagnosis of primary aldosteronism includes decreased plasma renin and feedback suppression of renin secretion by aldosterone or by excess extracellular volume (Guyton, 1991).

Increased sodium delivery to distal nephron: Diuretics, osmotic diuresis, salt-wasting nephropathies, and Bartter's syndrome are all known to cause K^+ wasting. The symptoms include hypokalemia; metabolic alkalosis; juxtaglomerular hyperplasia; hyperreninemia; hyperaldosteronism; kaliuresis; and sodium bicarbonate retention, without hypertension or edema. These symptoms are also seen in Liddle's syndrome and familial pseudohyperaldosteronism. These electrolyte abnormalities may occur with normal aldosterone levels, causing inhibited sodium reabsorption in proximal tubules to force water excretion. The increased volume of water increases the K^+ excreted.

Other general causes of hypokalemia

Nonreabsorbable anions: K^+ reabsorption decreases in the presence of penicillin, ketoacids, and carbonic acid (metabolic alkalosis). Primary renal tubular acidosis and secondary renal tubular acidosis can result from amphotericin B or toluene abuse.

Intake of large amounts of licorice containing glycyrrhetinic acid blocks the enzyme needed to convert cortisol to cortisone. Cortisol builds in the kidney and triggers high blood pressure and K^+ loss (Long, 1994).

RISK PROFILE

All the risk factors are greater when occurring in an elderly client.

Cancers: Gastrinomas, vipomas, somatostinoma, corticotropinoma, carcinoid and villous adenoma of colon tumors, calcitoninoma, adrenal tumors, serotonin-secreting tumors, acute myeloblastic leukemia.

Pediatrics: Bartter's syndrome.

Conditions: Parasitic infections causing diarrhea, nasogastric tube losses, nausea, vomiting and diarrhea from gastric or colon resection, side effects from chemotherapy and radiation; chemical exposure.

Environment: Radiation therapy.

Foods: Dietary deficiencies from anorexia, nausea, and vomiting. Bile salts (thought to accelerate cancer growth).

Drugs: Chemotherapy, such as vincristine, vinblastin, cisplatin. Diuretics that cause K^+ wasting include loop diuretics (furosemide, ethacrynic acid, bumetanide), thiazides (chlorothiazide, hydrochlorothiazide), or methylxanthines (caffeine, aminophylline). Laxatives, antibiotics.

PROGNOSIS

Severe hypokalemia, while life-threatening and potentially fatal, can be corrected with cautious administration and repletion of K^+.

Serum K^+ < 2.5 mEq/L (< 2.5 mmol/L SI Units)	Acute severe hypokalemia
Serum K^+ < 3.0 mEq/L (< 3.0 mmol/L SI Units)	Symptomatic hypokalemia
Serum K^+ 3.0–3.5 mEq/L (3.0–3.5 mmol/L SI Units)	Asymptomatic hypokalemia

Mortality statistics specific to hypokalemia in the oncology client are not available in the literature.

TREATMENT

Therapy for hypokalemia is determined by the cause of the electrolyte disturbance. For hypokalemia due to alkalosis, the underlying cause of the alkalosis requires correction while supplemental K^+ is administered. For hypokalemia due to depletion of body stores, it is necessary to determine or estimate deficit and replenish K^+. Severe hypokalemia, $K^+ = < 2.5$ mEq/L (< 2.5 mmol/L SI Units), requires hospitalization for IV K^+ replacement and cardiac rhythm monitoring. Other clients require diagnosis and a treatment plan that includes replacement K^+ and continuing follow-up.

Surgery: Surgical removal of the malignant tumor to remove the underlying cause of hypokalemia, such as gastrectomy for gastrinoma, tumor removal of pancreatic tumors, etc.

Chemotherapy: Decrease dosages of chemotherapy that contribute to hypokalemia (vincristine, vinblastin, cisplatin).

Radiation: As indicated for underlying malignancy.

Medications

Decrease dosages of drugs that contribute to hypokalemia, i.e., diuretics. Loop diuretics, thiazides, and methylxanthines (caffeine, aminophylline) all can cause hypokalemia.

Administer K^+ supplements orally or intravenously for hypokalemia due to adrenal tumors or metastasis.

Correct calcium levels (treat hypocalcemia while treating K^+ and treat neuromuscular effects masked by each deficit; treating hypokalemia without treating hypocalcemia can lead to tetany).

Administer antidiarrheal and/or antiemetic medications.

Oral preparations are preferable for slower replacement to prevent hyperkalemia and K^+ rebound. Acute rapid repletion with IV should be given at 10 to 20 mEq/hour. Administration of up to 40 mEq/hour will require central venous access and cardiac monitoring.

With hyperaldosterone states, K^+ loss through the kidneys will continue and may require IV replacement. Glucose solutions should not be used due to insulin's effect on moving K^+ intracellularly, which further decreases serum K^+ level.

Procedures

Related to underlying cause. Therapy may require central line for K^+ administration and nutrition. A soft feeding tube or percutaneous endoscopic gastrostomy (PEG) may be required for adequate nutrition.

Peripheral IV K^+ replacements can cause localized pain and irritation to vein walls, so adequate dilution and rate of administration are essential. Central line administration is often the preferred route.

Other

Correct prolonged gastric suction.

All K^+ replacement therapies must be used with caution due to risk of hyperkalemia in the elderly with potential or actual impaired renal function. Additionally, correction of low magnesium levels is important, due to potential resistance to correction of hypokalemia in the presence of hypomagnesemia. With edematous clients, increasing dietary intake of K$^+$ and giving oral supplements and K$^+$-sparing diuretics can successfully correct hypokalemia when the underlying cause is resolved.

ASSESSMENT CRITERIA: HYPOKALEMIA

Vital signs	
Heart rate	Weak, irregular pulse, bradycardia.
Blood pressure	Hypotension.
Respirations	Weak, shallow.
Temperature	Baseline.
History	Nausea, vomiting, diarrhea from radiation and/or chemotherapy.
Hallmark physical signs and symptoms	Confusion, muscle cramps, bradycardia, depressed T waves on ECG, nausea.
Additional physical signs and symptoms	Drowsiness, apathy, coma, irritability, weakness, paresthesia, muscle pain, tenderness, hyporeflexia, tetany, paralysis, weak pulse, hypoventilation, respiratory weakness, vomiting, anorexia, abdominal distention, cramps, paralytic ileus, polydipsia, polyuria, nocturia.
Psychosocial signs	May have contributing cause of psychologically induced vomiting or laxative abuse.
Lab values	
Potassium	<3.5 mEq/L (<3.5 mmol/L SI Units)
Magnesium	Decreased
Bicarbonate	Increased
pH	Increased or normal
Chloride	<110 mEq/L (<110 mmol/L) (metabolic alkalosis, hypokalemia)
Urine osmolality	Decreased or <500 mOsm/kg
Urine pH	Reflects serum pH.
Urine potassium	Urine K$^+$ will be elevated with a renal cause of hypokalemia; urine K$^+$ will be normal with extrarenal (GI) causes of hypokalemia.
Urine phosphate	Decreased
Diagnostic tests	
Electrocardiogram	12-lead ECGs daily and when changes noted: Hypokalemia is indicated by depressed S-T segment, appearance of U waves, lowering and inversion of the T wave. Rebound hyperkalemia is indicated by tall, peaked T waves, decreasing or disappearing P wave, widening QRS.

ASSESSMENT CRITERIA: HYPOKALEMIA (*continued*)

Other	Assess for medications that affect potassium and electrolyte balance.
	Assess for changes in chemotherapy agents or dosages.

NURSING DIAGNOSIS

The nursing diagnoses will vary depending on the cause of hypokalemia. Following are some of the common diagnoses and etiologies.

Diarrhea, potential for, related to malignancy and/or chemotherapy or radiation therapy.

Nutrition, less than body requirements, related to anorexia, or cachexia.

Decreased cardiac output, potential for, related to cardiac dysrhythmias, hypotension.

Injury, risk for, related to muscle weakness, impaired physical mobility related to parasthesia of extremities, flaccid paralysis.

Activity intolerance, risk for, related to weakness, muscle weakness.

Knowledge deficit related to diagnosis, chemotherapy, K^+ depletion, measures to control nausea and vomiting.

NURSING INTERVENTIONS

Immediate nursing interventions

Assess pulse, respirations, blood pressure, and muscle strength q1h × 4, then q4h.

Send STAT serum electrolyte panel.

Establish patent IV access and obtain volumetric infusion pump.

Measure hourly intake and output (I and O). Insert indwelling urinary catheter if necessary.

Prepare for long-line catheter/access device placement for frequent blood sampling.

Anticipated physician orders and interventions

Decrease/discontinue chemotherapy, radiation therapy, and other medications that may cause hypokalemia.

STAT serum electrolyte panel, serum creatinine, blood urea nitrogen (BUN), aldosterone.

Insert long-line catheter/access device for frequent blood sampling and K^+ replacement therapy.

Administer antiemetic and/or antidiarrheal medication.

Initiate replacement therapy, oral or IV. Oral K^+ supplements and high-

K$^+$ foods are preferred for chronic problems to decrease risk of rebound hyperkalemia.

- Give oral K$^+$ replacement, well diluted to prevent GI irritation.
- Give through the IV route for acute imbalance at a rate of 10 to 20 mEq/hour. *Note:* Give potassium chloride when hypokalemia is associated with alkalemia; give potassium bicarbonate, citrate, acetate, or gluconate when hypokalemia is associated with acidemia.

Monitor cardiac rhythm when serum K$^+$ is < 2.5 mEq/L.

Ongoing nursing assessment, monitoring, and interventions

Assess:
- Blood pressure, heart rate, and respiratory rate q2h with frequent vomiting or diarrhea, or q4h if nausea and vomiting are not present.
- Temperature q4h.
- Skin color, temperature, turgor q8h.
- Level of consciousness (LOC) q8h with mental status assessment for clues that signal rebound hyperkalemia.
- Heart sounds q8h.
- Breath sounds q8h, noting increased respiratory effort or onset of shortness of breath.
- Bowel sounds q4–8h.
- Nausea/amount of emesis.
- ECG monitoring for signs of hypokalemia (sinus bradycardia, premature atrial and ventricular contractions, and tachydysrhythmias can be observed as well as T wave depression, prolonged Q-T interval, U waves, and depressed S-T segments).
- Lab values: Compare client and normal values.
- Muscle strength q4h until K$^+$ > 3.0 mEq/L (> 3.0 mmol/L SI Units).
- Activity tolerance, weakness, and fatigue (client tolerance, organized activities with rest periods, proper body mechanics).
- Elimination pattern, antidiarrheal medications, signs of paralytic ileus; monitor diet.

Measure: Weight every morning; diarrhea/stools for amount, color, consistency.

Send: Serum and urine laboratory tests including electrolyte studies (K$^+$, Mg^{++}, Ca^{++}) q4–6h and PRN.

Implement:
- Promote orientation by providing appropriate stimuli.
- Provide a safe environment and assist with activities of daily living (ADLs) as needed.

- Position the client to facilitate ease of breathing if symptomatic with dysrhythmias.
- If hypokalemia is due to effects of chemotherapy or radiation, review the methods for controlling side effects.
  Topics to review include: mouth sores or dry mouth (soft foods, ice chips); nausea/vomiting (control of odors; eating of small, frequent meals; antiemetic medications); diarrhea (low-fiber foods, bananas, rice, applesauce, toast, mashed potatoes, antidiarrheal medications); muscle aches; weakness or numbness.

TEACHING/EDUCATION

Select from the following items, based on the client's pathophysiology.

Decreased/discontinued chemotherapy and/or radiation therapy: *Rationale:* Nausea or feeling sick to your stomach, vomiting, and diarrhea are side effects from some chemotherapy drugs and some radiation. These side effects will need to be controlled as much as possible. Some of your drugs may be changed and your chemotherapy/radiation plan may be altered or delayed.

IV blood samples and urine samples: *Rationale:* Blood tests will be taken in order to tell us how well your K^+ levels are improving.

IV line placement: *Rationale:* You will need to have an IV line put into one of your veins. The IV helps us give you medicines and fluids and to take some blood samples from you.

Indwelling urinary catheter placement: *Rationale:* Accurate urine measurement is very important to help us know how your kidneys are functioning.

Dietary changes: *Rationale:* Potassium-rich foods will help your potassium levels return to normal. These foods include most meats, beans, broccoli, spinach, lentils, potatoes, milk, bananas, raisins, avocados, and apricots. You may find eating small, frequent meals helpful. (You may also be given medications that will prevent you from feeling as if you will vomit. You may be given medications to prevent or treat stomatitis, mouthwash with lidocaine to help with mouth sores, and you will be encouraged to use good oral hygiene).

IV site symptoms: *Rationale:* It is necessary to give you potassium in your IV instead of (or as well as) your oral supplements. The solution can be strong and may hurt you if it leaks from your vein into your arm or hand tissues. Your nurse will be checking how well your IV is working, but you need to tell your nurse right away if your arm hurts or swells.

Signs and symptoms of hypokalemia: *Rationale:* You (significant others) will need to watch for signs that your potassium is low. Some of the symptoms are the same as other electrolytes, but you should still tell your doctor as soon as you feel any of the following: dizziness, mental confusion, muscle weakness, paralysis (temporary or intermittent), weakness or heaviness of legs, stomach bloating, nausea, vomiting, loss of appetite, irregular heartbeats, generally feeling terrible.

EVALUATION/DESIRED OUTCOMES

1. Serum K$^+$ level increases to >3 mEq/L (>3 mmol/L SI Units) within 48 hours (for acute hypokalemia).
2. Serum K$^+$ level increases to normal values at a rate comparable to the time in which the hypokalemia developed.
3. Urine K$^+$ level returns to normal value within 72 hours.
4. Serum calcium and magnesium levels return to normal.
5. The client is free of the signs of muscle weakness and dysrhythmias.
6. Nausea, vomiting, and diarrhea subside within 48 hours.
7. Chemotherapy/radiation regimen will continue as prescribed within 72 hours.
8. K$^+$ replacement or prophylaxis is understood by client.

DISCHARGE PLANNING

The hypokalemic client may need:

Short-term enteral nutrition and IV fluids when vomiting occurs or nasogastric suctioning is implemented, as these interfere with adequate oral food and fluid intake.

Intermediate care facility, daily home nursing visits, or family caregivers to manage the enteral and parenteral intake.

Training of the client and significant others in I and O measurement and documentation.

Teaching about the signs and symptoms of hypokalemia.

FOLLOW-UP CARE

Anticipated care

Physician office visit within 1 week.

Outpatient laboratory testing for serum electrolytes within 1 week.

Other blood work as appropriate.

Continuation of dietary/fluid regimen.

Daily home nursing visit for clients discharged home with enteral or parenteral fluids.

Home health nursing visit once per week $\times$ 2 weeks for clients discharged home without enteral or parenteral fluids.

Anticipated client/family questions and possible answers

Will this problem with low potassium in my blood happen again?

"It is possible, so it is important that you know the signs of low potassium. You need to know what to do if you have symptoms."

"Whenever you have a lot of vomiting from your chemotherapy, you may lose potassium. You'll need to watch for symptoms and call your doctor."

When can I continue my chemotherapy?

"Your doctor will monitor your lab tests, and when they are more normal, your body will be able to tolerate the side effects of the drugs. This may take a week or so."

What should I do to keep my potassium level normal?

"Knowing what foods are high in potassium is important. Keeping track of what you take in and eliminate is also important."

"Measuring intake should include everything you drink: water, fruit juice, etc., and foods that become liquid at room temperature: ice cream, gelatin. Output is everything that leaves the body as fluid. In measuring intake and output, you may need to convert ounces to milliliters—simply multiply ounces by 30; to convert from milliliters to ounces, divide by 30."

CHAPTER SUMMARY

Hypokalemia is a metabolic complication that occurs in 75% of clients with cancer. The causes include lack of intake and loss of K^+ through GI and metabolic causes. Symptoms occur when the serum K^+ is < 3.0 mEq/L (mmol/L SI Units). Levels < 2.5 mEq/L (mmol/L SI Units) may cause life-threatening cardiac dysrhythmias. Treatment and nursing care depend on the cause(s) of hypokalemia. Chronicity or gradual onset of hypokalemia has a different and slower treatment regimen than does the rapid onset of critical levels of hypokalemia. Understanding electrolyte balances of K^+, magnesium, and calcium will promote definitive care of the person with hypokalemia.

TEST QUESTIONS

1. The diagnosis of hypokalemia is made primarily by which of the following:
   A. Chest x-ray
   B. Laboratory electrolytes
   C. Computed tomography (CT) of the chest
   D. Angiogram

1. Answer: B
Serum electrolytes indicate levels of K^+ < 3.5 mEq/L (< 3.5 mmol/L SI Units).

2. Causes of hypokalemia include:
   A. High intake of K^+, including oranges, tomatoes, potatoes, etc.
   B. Loss through GI tract problems, including nausea, vomiting, or diarrhea
   C. Hypermagnesemia
   D. Hypocalcemia

2. Answer: B
Nausea, vomiting, and diarrhea as side effects of chemotherapy are a major cause of hypokalemia.

3. Symptoms of hypokalemia include:
   A. Muscle rigidity
   B. Cardiac dysrhythmias
   C. Paralytic ileus
   D. Mental alertness

3. Answer: B
Cardiac dysrhythmias are often signs of acute hypokalemia.

4. Which of the following statements is true about hypokalemia?
   A. A slow onset of hypokalemia requires the slow replacement of K^+ as treatment.
   B. Rapid loss of K^+ requires a slow replacement of K^+ as treatment.
   C. IV sodium bicarbonate is often used to treat metabolic alkalosis associated with hypokalemia.
   D. Tetany is the result of a combination of hyperaldosteronism and cardiac dysrhythmia associated with hypokalemia.

4. Answer: A
The body adjustments over time require slow replacement of K^+ to prevent rebound or other complications.

5. K^+ replacement requires:
   A. Cardiac monitoring for severe hypokalemia, < 2.5 mEq/L (< 2.5 mmol/L SI Units)
   B. Chest x-rays every hour
   C. Urine sugar testing hourly
   D. Sedation q4h and PRN

5. Answer: A
Potential and actual dysrhythmias should be monitored to prevent cardiac complications.

6. Follow-up care for clients with hypokalemia should include:
   A. Adjustments in their IV aldosterone dosages
   B. Changes in dietary plans that include frequent, large portions
   C. Monitoring serum laboratory electrolytes
   D. Initial follow-up visit with physician in 1 year

6. Answer: C
Monitoring of serum K^+ is part of a serum electrolyte panel.

7. A potential side effect of K^+ replacement therapy includes all *except:*
   A. Constipation
   B. Rebound hyperkalemia
   C. Alopecia
   D. Decreased deep tendon reflexes

7. Answer: B
Rebound hyperkalemia may occur due to rapid administration of K^+ replacement or renal dysfunction.

8. An appropriate intervention related to the treatment of hypokalemia includes:
   A. Helping the client learn the signs of hypokalemia, such as diarrhea, cramps, irritability, oliguria, and difficulty speaking
   B. Teaching methods to deal with the side effects of chemotherapy, including nausea and vomiting
   C. Helping the client understand how the treatment of the cancer can cause diabetes mellitus, which causes electrolyte imbalance such as hypokalemia
   D. Teaching the client to interpret his or her own ECG changes in order to prevent complications during K^+ replacement

8. Answer: B
Several chemotherapeutic drugs cause nausea and vomiting, which can lead to volume depletion and loss of K^+ in the body.

9. One essential item of client education regarding hypokalemia is the following:
   A. Tell the client not to worry about what foods contain K^+.
   B. Know what signs of hypokalemia to watch for, such as muscle weakness, and when to call the physician.
   C. Chemotherapy medications are never the cause of vomiting related to hypokalemia.
   D. IV K^+ is harmless and painless.

9. Answer: B
Muscle weakness and leg cramping are often an early and reliable sign of hypokalemia.

10. Important laboratory studies associated with the client who has hypokalemia include all of the following *except:*
    A. Serum K^+
    B. Serum Mg^{++}
    C. Serum Ca^{++}
    D. Serum iron

10. Answer: D
Iron is not related to determining K^+ status or hypokalemia. Magnesium and calcium have a related effect on hypokalemia and should therefore be included in monitoring.

REFERENCES

Brimacombe JR, Breen DP: Anesthesia and Bartter's syndrome: A case report and review. AANA J 61(2):193–197, 1993.

Calhoun KA: Serum potassium concentration abnormalities. Crit Care Nurs 13(3):34–38, 1990.

Carlson PA: Antineoplastic agents. Crit Care Nurs Q 18(4):1–15, 1996.

Cheng J, Burke MD: Spurious hypokalemia in a case of acute myeloblastic leukemia. Lab Med 24(11):706–707, 1993.

Chernecky CC, Krech RL, Berger BJ: Laboratory Tests and Diagnostic Procedures. Philadelphia: WB Saunders Co, 1993.

Clochesy JM, Breu C, Cardin S, Rudy EB, Whittaker AA: Critical Care Nursing. Philadelphia: WB Saunders Co, 1993.

DeAngelis R, Lessig ML: Hypokalemia. Crit Care Nurs 11(7):71–72, 1991.

Evans S: Nursing measures in the prevention and treatment of renal cell damage associated with cisplatin administration. Cancer Nurs 14(2):91–97, 1991.

Gordon RD: Mineralocorticoid hypertension. Lancet 34:240–244, 1994.

Guyton AC: Textbook of Medical Physiology, 8th ed. Philadelphia: WB Saunders Co, 1991.

Harvey RA, Champe PC (eds): Pharmacology. Philadelphia: JB Lippincott, 1992.

Held JL: Correcting fluid and electrolyte balances. Nursing 24(4):71, 1995.

Innerarity S: Electrolyte emergencies in the critically ill renal patient. Crit Care Nurs Clin North Am 2(1):89–99, 1990.

Long P: The case of the bone-weary banker. Health 8:100–102, 1994.

Mahon SM, Casperson DS: Pathophysiology of hypokalemia in patients with cancer: Implications for nurses. Oncol Nurs Forum 20(6):937–948, 1993.

Mechanick JI, Morris JC: Clinical case seminar: Hypokalemia in a 52 year old woman with non-small cell lung cancer. J Clin Endocrinol Metab 80(6):1769–1773, 1995.

Moody AM, Ahmed A, Chakrabarty A, Fisher C: Renin-producing leiomyosarcome originating in the uterus. Clin Oncol 7(1):52–53, 1995.

Ramsahoye BH, Davies SV, ElGaylani N, Sandeman D, Scanlon MF: The mineralcorticoid effects of high dose hydrocortisone. Br Med J 310:656–658, 1995.

Santini DL, Lorenzo BJ, Koufis T, Reidenberg MM: Cortisol metabolism in hypertensive patients who do and do not develop hypokalemia from diuretics. Am J Hypertension 8(5):516–519, 1995.

Sica DA: Renal disease, electrolyte abnormalities, and acid-base imbalance in the elderly. Clin Geriatr Med 10(1):197–211, 1994.

Steigerwalt SP: Unraveling the causes of hypertension and hypokalemia. Hosp Pract (Off) 30(7):67–71, 74–75, 79, 1995.

Terry J: The major electrolytes: sodium, potassium, and chloride. J Intravenous Nurs 17(5):240–247, 1994.

von der Ohe MR, Camilleri M, Kvols LK, Thomforde GM: Motor dysfunction of the small bowel and colon in patients with the carcinoid syndrome and diarrhea. New Engl J Med 329(14):1073–1079, 1993.

Williamson JC: Acid-base disorders: Classification and management strategies. Am Fam Physician 52(2):584–590, 1995.

Wilson RF: Critical Care Medicine. Philadelphia: FA Davis, 1992.

CHAPTER 24

HYPOMAGNESEMIA

Eileen M. Glynn-Tucker, RN, MS, AOCN

CHAPTER OBJECTIVES

At the completion of this chapter, the reader will be able to:

Differentiate between hypomagnesemia and magnesium deficiency.

Identify risk factors associated with hypomagnesemia in the oncology client.

State the clinical signs and symptoms of hypomagnesemia.

Describe nursing care as related to clients with hypomagnesemia.

Anticipate and prepare the client with hypomagnesemia for future care needs.

OVERVIEW

HYPOMAGNESEMIA is characterized by serum magnesium levels of <1.5 mEq/L (or <0.8 mmol/L SI Units). The disorder is commonly related to excessive magnesium loss from the gastrointestinal (GI) tract, interference with renal magnesium reabsorption, or inadequate dietary magnesium intake. The incidence of magnesium deficiency ranges from 10% of all clients admitted to urban hospitals to up to 65% of clients in intensive care units (Abbott and Rude, 1993). Clients with hypomagnesemia are most often asymptomatic. When signs and symptoms occur, they are related to neuromuscular hyperirritability, cardiac dysrhythmias, central nervous system dysfunction, and accompanying electrolyte disorders.

DESCRIPTION

Hypomagnesemia and magnesium deficiency

Magnesium is the fourth most abundant cation in the human body and the second most prevalent intracellular cation. More than 99% of magnesium is located intracellularly or in the skeleton. Therefore, serum magnesium measurement does not always reflect the true status of magnesium stores. However, a serum magnesium level < 1.5 mEq/L (< 0.8 mmol/L SI Units) generally indicates some degree of overall magnesium deficiency. A magnesium challenge test is used to explain whether a client's hypomagnesemia actually represents overall body magnesium deficiency. To conduct the test, one measures the 24-hour urine magnesium levels following IV magnesium replacement. Clients with normal renal function and normal body magnesium stores excrete 80% of supplemental magnesium in the urine within 24 hours. In magnesium-deficient clients, the kidneys reduce excretion of magnesium to very low levels (Abbott and Rude, 1993; Arnold, Tovey, Mangat, Penny, and Jacobs, 1994). Thus, a hypomagnesemic client who excretes less than 80% of the IV magnesium supplement is also magnesium deficient.

Physiologic role of magnesium

Magnesium affects the cardiovascular, central nervous and neuromuscular systems, is a necessary cofactor for 300 enzymatic reactions in the body, and is necessary for energy-metabolism processes (see Table 24–1). The clinical signs and symptoms of hypomagnesemia and magnesium deficiency correlate with the physiologic role of magnesium. Although asymptomatic hypomagnesemia is common, asymptomatic magnesium deficiency is rare. Magnesium deficiency has been associated with an increased risk for the occurrence of an ECG abnormality, "torsades de pointes," which can result in death if not treated immediately. Magnesium is necessary for the production of adenosine triphophatase (ATPase), which is necessary to move extracellular potassium ions into the cells during repolarization. It is postulated that a magnesium deficiency leads to prolonged repolarization and increased risk for dysrhythmias during the relative refractory period of cardiac muscle cell repolarization and subsequent "R on T" phenomenon (Fig. 24–1).

Table 24–1
Physiologic Functions of Magnesium

Cofactor for intracellular enzymes necessary for:
    DNA transcription
    Protein synthesis
    Sodium-potassium-ATPase pump regulation
    Anaerobic phosphorylation
Membrane stabilization
Nerve conduction
Calcium channel activity
Ion transport systems

Source: Data from Abbott and Rude, 1993; Whang, Hampton, and Whang, 1994; Toto and Yucha, 1994.

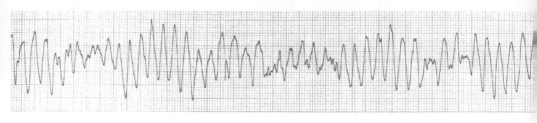

Figure 24–1 Torsades de pointes.
Source: From Phillips RE, Feeney MK: The Cardiac Rhythms: A Systematic Approach to Interpretation, 3rd ed. Philadelphia: WB Saunders Co, 1990, p. 393.

GI magnesium absorption

The oral magnesium intake that a well-rounded diet provides is generally sufficient to meet the U.S. recommended daily allowance (RDA) of magnesium. However, clients with malnutrition, chronic alcoholism, and those receiving enteral or parenteral feedings without magnesium supplementation generally experience hypomagnesemia as a result of inadequate dietary magnesium intake. One-third to one-half of the ingested dietary magnesium is absorbed by the GI tract. The ileum is the primary site of magnesium absorption (Al-Ghamdi, Cameron, and Sutton, 1994; Whang, Hampton, and Whang, 1994). In the absence of adequate oral magnesium intake, the intestines increase their fractional absorption of magnesium (Al-Ghamdi et al., 1994) to compensate. Thus, intestinal magnesium absorption is inversely proportional to the amount ingested.

Disorders affecting the GI absorption of magnesium (including small bowel resection, radiation-therapy-induced intestinal damage, diarrhea, protein-calorie malnutrition, and prolonged nasogastric suctioning or vomiting) often lead to the development of acute and/or chronic hypomagnesemia in the client with cancer. Magnesium located in the salivary, biliary, pancreatic, and intestinal fluids is normally reabsorbed in the large intestine. Clients with cancer who have draining fistulas lose the magnesium in these body fluids.

Renal magnesium handling

The kidney is the principal organ involved in the regulation of magnesium homeostasis. In healthy individuals, approximately 8 mEq is excreted daily in the urine. If excess magnesium is administered parenterally or consumed enterally, the kidneys compensate by excreting unneeded magnesium.

In magnesium-depleted states, the kidneys can normally conserve magnesium, characteristically storing urinary magnesium concentrations of less than 2 mEq per day. When abnormal renal handling of magnesium exists, magnesium excretion exceeds 3 mEq per day, even in the event of marked hypomagnesemia.

Renal tubular injury appears to be the primary factor leading to excess urinary loss of magnesium. Despite the presence of hypomagnesemia, the fractional excretion of magnesium can rise in the presence of renal tubular injury. Chronic parenteral fluid therapy with sodium-containing fluid or use of osmotic diuretics may result in magnesium deficiency, because proximal tubular magnesium reabsorption is proportional to tubular fluid flow and sodium reabsorption. Renal tubular magnesium wasting is thought to be the mechanism of cisplatin-induced hypomagnesemia. A dose-toxicity relationship exists between the total cumulative dose of cisplatin and the degree of hypomagnesemia. A variety of drugs commonly administered to oncology clients cause renal magnesium wasting. (See Risk Profile.)

Associated electrolyte abnormalities

Hypomagnesemia is often accompanied by hyponatremia, hypokalemia, hypophosphatemia, and hypocalcemia. Normally functioning kidneys are unable to conserve potassium in the presence of hypomagnesemia, and this leads to hypokalemia. Hypomagnesemia impairs the secretion of parathyroid hormone, a substance essential for regulation of serum calcium and phosphorus. Correction of hypokalemia and hypocalcemia must be preceded by restoration of a state of normal serum magnesium.

RISK PROFILE

Cancers: Lung (small cell and non-small cell), head and neck, esophagus, testicular, villous adenomas, colon/rectum.

Conditions: Alcoholism, small bowel resection, diarrhea, prolonged nasogastric suction, intestinal biliary fistula, laxative abuse, diuretic phase of acute tubular necrosis, hypertension, metabolic acidosis, insulin-dependent diabetes mellitus, hyperthyroidism, hyperparathyroidism.

Environment: None.

Foods: Low magnesium intake and/or high calcium intake.

Drugs: Cisplatin, amphotericin, parenteral IV fluids or hyperalimentation without magnesium replacement, loop and osmotic diuretics, aminoglycosides, cyclosporine, pentamidine.

PROGNOSIS

The prognosis of clients with cancer and concomitant hypomagnesemia is not documented in the literature. However, the literature indicates that hypomagnesemic clients in intensive care units have higher mortality rates than their normomagnesemic counterparts. The relationship is less clear in nonintensive care units. In one study, the mortality rate of acutely ill medical clients with hypomagnesemia and normal magnesium were measured. In both general medical units and intensive care units, the mortality rate of clients with hypomagnesemia was double the mortality rate of clients with normal serum magnesium values (Rubeiz, Thill-Baharozian, Hardie, and Carlson, 1993).

TREATMENT

Surgery: Not indicated.

Chemotherapy: Add additional magnesium to cisplatin prehydration and posthydration. Possibly decrease cisplatinum dosage.

Radiation: Not indicated.

Medications

    IV magnesium replacement.
    Decreased doses of drugs that may cause hypomagnesemia.
    Potassium replacement is likely when accompanied by hypokalemia.

Procedures: Possible central venous catheter placement for magnesium replacement.

Other: High-magnesium, high-potassium diet to prevent future episodes of hypomagnesemia.

ASSESSMENT CRITERIA: HYPOMAGNESEMIA

Vital signs

Temperature	Normal
Pulse	Tachycardia
Respirations	Normal
Blood pressure	Hypotension or hypertension

History	Loss from the GI tract (emesis, diarrhea, nasogastric suction).
	Loss from the renal system (urine).
	Inadequate oral magnesium intake.

Hallmark physical signs and symptoms	None: Symptoms rarely occur until serum magnesium levels fall below 1.0 mEq/L (0.5 mmol/L SI Units).

Additional physical signs and symptoms	
Gastrointestinal	Anorexia; nausea and/or vomiting.
Central nervous system	Confusion, seizures, vertigo, ataxia, emotional lability or irritability, hallucinations, or psychoses.

ASSESSMENT CRITERIA: HYPOMAGNESEMIA (continued)

Cardiovascular	Tachydysrhythmias, ECG changes (prolonged QT interval, flat broadened T waves, shortened ST segment).
Neuromuscular	Hyperactive deep tendon reflexes; muscle fasciculations, spasticity, tremors, cramping, paresthesias, hyperirritability or weakness of the muscles, dysphagia and/or generalized tremors; positive Chvostek's or Trousseau's sign.

Psychosocial signs	None

Lab values:	
Magnesium, serum	<1.5 mEq/L (<0.8 mmol/L SI Units).
Magnesium, urine	Low (<2 mEq/24 hours).
Potassium	May also be low (<3.5 mEq/L, <3.5 mmol/L SI Units).
Phosphorus, serum	May also be low (<2.8 mg/dl, <0.90 mmol/L SI Units).
Calcium, serum and urine	May also be low.
Sodium, serum	May also be low.

Diagnostic tests	
Magnesium challenge test	Magnesium excretion in 24-hour urine collection is <80% of IV magnesium supplementation in the same 24-hour period.

NURSING DIAGNOSIS

The nursing diagnoses for the client with hypomagnesemia will vary, depending on the cause(s) and treatment(s) of hypomagnesemia. The most common diagnoses and etiologies are described. Because hypomagnesemia is usually asymptomatic, many of the problems will be potential problems unless symptoms develop.

Potential for injury related to central nervous system irritability and neuromuscular hyperirritability.

Potential impaired physical mobility related to tremors, ataxia, muscle weakness, and/or spasms.

Potential decreased cardiac output related to dysrhythmia or hypotension.

Potential alteration in elimination, diarrhea related to oral magnesium supplementation or the disease process.

Denial related to asymptomatic hypomagnesemia.

Knowledge deficit related to unfamiliarity with the sequelae of and treatment for hypomagnesemia.

NURSING INTERVENTIONS

Immediate nursing interventions

Send STAT serum electrolyte panel and magnesium level.

Establish patent IV access and obtain volumetric infusion pump.

If the client exhibits neuromuscular hyperexcitability:

- Initiate seizure precautions. Place suction equipment and an oral airway at the bedside.
- Place the client on bedrest.

Apply telemetry/cardiac monitor.

Assess for neuromuscular irritability and central nervous system changes q1h.

Measure hourly intake and output (I and O).

Assess for rebound hypermagnesemia characterized by loss of deep tendon reflexes q1h during magnesium replacement.

Anticipated physician orders and interventions

STAT serum electrolyte panel and magnesium level.

Magnesium sulfate 4 g IV piggyback over 2 to 6 hours.

0.9% NaCl IV infusion with KCl and $MgSO_4$ at 42 to 125 ml/hour.

Chemotherapy and other medications decreased/discontinued that may cause hypomagnesemia.

High-magnesium, high-potassium diet.

Cardiac telemetry monitor.

12-lead ECG STAT.

Spot urine magnesium and calcium.

Central IV catheter placement for fluid and electrolyte replacement and blood samples.

Ongoing nursing assessment, monitoring, and interventions

Assess:
- Neuromuscular status q8h (tremors, tetany, muscle strength, and movement).
- Presence of Chvostek's or Trousseau's signs.
- Rate, rhythm, and characteristics of pulse.
- ECG waveform for correction of abnormalities as magnesium is replenished.
- Nausea and vomiting, and administer antiemetics as ordered PRN.
- Stool pattern and administer antidiarrheal PRN.
- Level of consciousness q8h and PRN.

Measure:
- I and O q8h × 24 hours.

- VS q4h.
- Weight qd.

Send:
- Serum magnesium, potassium, sodium, and calcium q8–12h × 48 hours or until electrolytes return to normal range.
- Urine magnesium and calcium q48h × 2.
- Blood urea nitrogen (BUN) and creatinine q8–12h × 48 hours or until within normal range.

Implement:
- Bedrest and limited activity as appropriate.
- Comfort measures to relieve nausea and/or vomiting.
- Provide a safe physical environment for the client.
- Provide appropriate stimuli for maintaining orientation.
- Active or passive range-of-motion exercises as appropriate.
- Protect skin integrity from chronic diarrhea.

TEACHING/EDUCATION

Select items, based on the client's pathophysiology.

Oral magnesium supplementation: *Rationale:* Your body needs more of this mineral to work correctly. By taking the pills, you will receive the additional magnesium your body needs. Spacing the pills over the course of each day will make them more likely to be absorbed and less likely to cause diarrhea.

IV blood samples and urine samples: *Rationale:* Blood samples will be taken frequently. They are needed to track the minerals in your blood.

Signs and symptoms of hypomagnesemia: *Rationale:* You and your significant others need to watch for signs of low magnesium levels because early treatment will help you feel better and will prevent other problems. The signs you should watch for are tremors, seizures, muscle weakness, jerky movements, dizziness, confusion, hallucinations, and rapid heartbeats.

Side effects of parenteral magnesium supplementation: *Rationale:* When the magnesium goes in, you might feel burning at the site, sweating, or a warm feeling all over. Tell your nurse so that he or she can slow down the medicine and make the unpleasant feeling go away.

Dietary changes: *Rationale:* Your body will keep the amount of magnesium it needs if you provide enough magnesium in your diet. Foods high in magnesium are nuts, green leafy vegetables, soybeans, cocoa, seafood, peas, dried beans, whole grains, and animal protein.

IV line placement: *Rationale:* The IV line allows us to easily take blood samples and to give you magnesium and other necessary fluids.

Telemetry monitor: *Rationale:* This monitor allows your nurse and doctor to detect any changes in your heart rate or rhythm. If an early problem is detected, it can often be corrected before you develop any symptoms of the problem.

Bedrest/activity restriction: *Rationale:* The low magnesium level can increase the sensitivity of your muscles and nerves. You might develop seizures, weakness, or tremors. For your safety, it is best for you to remain in bed (or to get out of bed only when someone is there to assist you).

EVALUATION/DESIRED OUTCOMES

1. Serum magnesium increases to ≥1.5 mEq/L (≥0.8 mmol/L SI Units) within 24 hours.
2. Any signs and symptoms of hypomagnesemia resolve within 24 hours.
3. The client takes oral magnesium supplements as prescribed without nausea, emesis, or diarrhea within 72 hours.
4. Client remains free of injury resulting from neuromotor excitability and central nervous system hyperactivity.
5. Accompanying serum potassium, phosphorus, sodium, and calcium disorders are corrected within 24 hours.
6. Cancer treatment resumes within 72 hours.
7. Client verbalizes understanding of medication schedule and dietary measures prior to discharge.

DISCHARGE PLANNING

The hypomagnesemic client may need:

IV magnesium and fluid supplementation when client is unable to tolerate oral magnesium supplementation.
Daily home nursing visits or family caregivers to monitor for:
  • Any signs and symptoms of recurrent electrolyte abnormalities.
  • Recurrence or worsening of the factor(s) that led to hypomagnesemia.
Teaching of client and significant others in oral magnesium and electrolyte supplements.

FOLLOW-UP CARE

Anticipated care

Physician office visit within 1 week.
Outpatient lab testing for serum electrolytes within 1 week.
Continuation of high-magnesium, high-potassium diet.
Daily home nursing visits for clients discharged home with IV magnesium supplements.

Home health nursing visits once per week × 2 weeks for clients discharged home with oral magnesium and other electrolyte supplements.

Anticipated client/family questions and possible answers

Will this problem of low magnesium happen again?

"It is possible that the problem of low blood magnesium could happen again. It is very important for you to have your blood checked and to take your magnesium pills as your doctor directs."

"As long as you are taking [insert drug name], the problem of low blood magnesium could return."

"As long as you continue to receive cisplatin chemotherapy, the problem is likely to continue."

"If the [insert condition(s) that led to the development of hypomagnesemia] continues or happens again, the problem of low blood magnesium could return."

When can I stop taking the magnesium pills?

"Cisplatin can cause people's blood magnesium to be low for several months up to many years. It is hard to tell when you can stop taking the pills."

"Once your blood magnesium becomes normal, your doctor will decrease the number of pills you take each day until you can stop completely."

"Once you stop taking the medicine that lowers your magnesium [aminoglycoside, amphotericin B] you will be instructed to stop taking the magnesium pills, too."

Why will a nurse be coming to my home?

"The nurse will come to see whether you are having the low-magnesium symptoms again."

"The nurse will take blood samples from your vein so that your blood magnesium can be checked."

"The nurse will be giving you magnesium into your veins. He or she will start the IV and check on how you are feeling. You or your family members will have to disconnect the IV and flush the IV when the medicine is done."

CHAPTER SUMMARY

Identification of hypomagnesemia in oncology clients using routine serum magnesium monitoring allows for early correction of the disorder. Although the majority of clients with hypomagnesemia are asymptomatic, the signs and symptoms involving the neuromuscular, cardiac, or central nervous system may develop. Assessment of risks factors associated with hypomagnesemia can lead to its early detection and correction. The oncology client should be assessed for accompanying electrolyte disorders of hypokalemia and hypocalcemia. Treatment and nursing care are related to the precipitating factors of hypomagnesemia. Nurses teach asymptomatic clients that oral supplementation and adherence to discharge instructions are essential.

TEST QUESTIONS

1. The primary nursing diagnosis of clients with hypomagnesemia is:
   A. Risk for injury
   B. Impaired physical mobility
   C. Knowledge deficit related to unfamiliarity with sequelae and treatment for hypomagnesemia
   D. Diarrhea

1. Answer: A
Hypomagnesemia is characterized by neuromuscular irritability. Seizures, ataxia, and tremors can result. The client's safety is a priority.

2. The signs of hypomagnesemia include:
   A. Bradycardia and hypertension
   B. Diarrhea
   C. Neuromuscular irritability
   D. Constipation and dehydration

2. Answer: C
Magnesium has a direct effect on the myoneural junction. Magnesium deficiency increases neuromuscular irritability and contractility.

3. Which chemotherapeutic drug may induce hypomagnesemia?
   A. Etoposide
   B. Cisplatin
   C. 5-Fluorouracil
   D. Vincristine

3. Answer: B
Cisplatin's action on the renal tubules can lead to acute and chronic magnesium excretion.

4. Which of the following statements reflects a client's understanding of the signs and symptoms of hypomagnesemia?
   A. "I don't have the diarrhea until I start taking the magnesium pills."
   B. "Even though I don't have any signs or symptoms, my magnesium level can still be low."
   C. "When I feel fatigued and get drowsy easy, I think I need to have my magnesium level checked."
   D. "Low magnesium gives me hot flashes."

4. Answer: B
Hypomagnesemia is often asymptomatic. Symptoms rarely develop until serum magnesium levels fall below 1 mEq/L.

5. Hypomagnesemia is commonly associated with all of the following electrolyte abnormalities *except:*
   A. Hypokalemia
   B. Hypocalcemia
   C. Hyponatremia
   D. Hyperphosphatemia

5. Answer: D
Hypophosphatemia may accompany hypomagnesemia because severe magnesium depletion impairs parathyroid hormone, which is needed to correct the phosphorous abnormality.

6. Oral magnesium supplementation in clients with chronic hypomagnesemia can be complicated by:
   A. The cost of oral magnesium supplements
   B. Supplement-induced diarrhea, which can worsen hypomagnesemia
   C. Intractable nausea
   D. The tendency to easily develop hypermagnesemia

6. Answer: B
Oral magnesium can lead to diarrhea, malabsorption, and severe hypomagnesemia. Clients with chronic hypomagnesemia have difficulty maintaining the low-normal serum magnesium values; subsequent hypermagnesemia would be rare. Magnesium supplements are generally inexpensive and do not cause nausea.

7. Hypomagnesemia is most often associated with which type of cancer?
   A. Breast
   B. Sarcoma
   C. Lung
   D. Multiple myeloma

7. Answer: C
Hypomagnesemia is most common in clients who have lung cancer.

8. A client diagnosed with hypomagnesemia secondary to GI losses (bowel resection) would most likely be taught about:
   A. Management of constipation
   B. Reducing bulk-forming foods in the diet
   C. Adding beans, whole grains, animal protein, and green leafy vegetables to the diet
   D. Restricting activity for 2 hours after meals

8. Answer: C
These foods are high in magnesium and can reduce diarrhea.

9. Hypomagnesemia is most often a result of:
  A. Inadequate dietary intake of magnesium
  B. Chronic renal failure
  C. Excessive losses in the GI tract
  D. Accumulation of ascites

9. Answer: C
Hypomagnesemia is a result of inadequate reabsorption in the ileum. Most Americans consume the RDA of magnesium.

10. Which of the following nursing interventions is most appropriate for the client experiencing severe hypomagnesemia?
  A. Administer opioid analgesia as needed.
  B. Measure central venous pressure every 2 hours.
  C. Institute calorie counts.
  D. Implement seizure precautions.

10. Answer: D
Implementation of seizure precautions can prevent injury associated with neuromuscular irritability and hyperexcitability.

REFERENCES

Abbott LG, Rude RK: Clinical manifestations of magnesium deficiency. Mineral Electrolyte Metab 19:314–322, 1993.

Al-Ghamdi SMG, Cameron EC, Sutton RAL: Magnesium deficiency: Pathophysiologic and clinical overview. Am J Kidney Dis 24(5):737–752, 1994.

Arnold A, Tovey J, Mangat P, Penny W, Jacobs S: Magnesium deficiency in critically ill patients. Anaesthesia 50:203–205, 1994.

Chernecky CC, Krech RL, Berger BJ: Laboratory Tests and Diagnostic Procedures. Philadelphia: WB Saunders Co, 1993.

Evans TRJ, Harper CL, Beveridge IG, Wastnage R, Mansil JL: A randomized study to determine whether routine intravenous magnesium supplements are necessary in patients receiving cisplatinum chemotherapy with continuous infusion 5-Fluorouracil. Eur J Cancer 31A(2):174–178, 1994.

Rubiez GJ, Thill-Baharozian M, Hardie D, Carlson RW: Association of hypomagnesemia and mortality in acutely ill medical patients. Crit Care Med 21(2):203–209, 1993.

Sartori S, Nielsen I, Tassinari D, Rigolin F, Arcudi D, Abbasciano V: Changes in intracellular magnesium concentrations during cisplatin chemotherapy. Oncology 50:230–234, 1993.

Sutton R, Domrongkitchaiporn S: Abnormal renal magnesium handling. Miner Electrolyte Metab 19:232–240, 1993.

Toto KH, Yucha CB: Magnesium: Homeostasis, imbalances and therapeutic uses. Crit Care Nurs Clin North Am 6(4):767–783, 1994.

Whang R, Hampton EM, Whang DD: Magnesium homeostasis and clinical disorders of magnesium deficiency. Ann Pharmacother 28(2):220–226, 1994.

CHAPTER 25

HYPONATREMIA

Cynthia C. Chernecky, PhD, RN, CNS, AOCN
AND
Barbara J. Berger, MSN, RN, CCRN

CHAPTER OBJECTIVES

At the completion of this chapter, the reader will be able to:

Define hyponatremia.

Differentiate hyponatremias that occur with low, normal, and high blood volumes.

State the risk factors associated with hyponatremia in the oncology client.

Describe nursing care as it relates to oncology clients with acute hyponatremia.

Anticipate and prepare the client with hyponatremia for future care needs.

OVERVIEW

HYPONATREMIA is a disorder of hypo-osmolality in which the rate of sodium loss exceeds the rate of water loss (true hyponatremia) or in which the rate of water intake exceeds the ability of the kidneys to excrete free water and maximally dilute the urine (relative hyponatremia). It is a condition characterized by *both* a low serum sodium and a low serum osmolality and occurs in persons with malignancy more frequently than in hospitalized persons in general. Specifically, hyponatremia occurs in approximately 5% of all persons with a malignancy and in 33 to 46% of persons on parenteral nutrition (Batuman, Dreisbach, Maesaka, Rothkopf, and Ross, 1984). Additionally, the elderly are at increased risk for hyponatremia owing to decreased renal function associated with aging and the increased renal burden from the use of multiple medications.

DESCRIPTION

True hyponatremia

Hypovolemic: Fluid and electrolyte loss through the gastrointestinal (GI) tract from the side effects of vomiting and diarrhea associated with chemotherapeutic drugs and from sweating may cause hypovolemic hyponatremia. Clients who develop mucositis after chemotherapy may have a poor oral intake of sodium and fluids and develop hypovolemic hyponatremia. In both cases, serum sodium levels decrease, and there is a depletion of extracellular body fluid from the above symptoms and from an osmotic shift of fluid from the vascular (extracellular) space to the intracellular space. This intravascular fluid volume deficit causes hypotension and can result in neurologic changes caused by brain cell swelling. The symptoms include those typical of dehydration, combined with symptoms of hyponatremia, which may range from vague muscle cramping to coma and respiratory arrest (see Table 25–1). The body's normal response to hypovolemia is to release more arginine vasopressin (AVP, also known as antidiuretic hormone, or ADH), which promotes reabsorption of water by the kidneys. This normal compensatory mechanism may further lower the plasma sodium level owing to a dilutional effect. Adrenal tumors are another common cause of hypovolemic hyponatremia. Aldosterone, a mineralcorticoid, normally helps maintain fluid and sodium balance by promoting reabsorption of sodium, chloride, and water and excretion of potassium and hydrogen at the distal renal tubules and collecting ducts. When adrenal metastasis occurs, reduced levels of aldosterone lead to abnormal urinary sodium and water loss and abnormal serum potassium retention. This type of hyponatremia is associated with urine sodium values > 20 mEq/L, serum potassium levels > 5 mEq/L, increased blood urea nitrogen (BUN) and serum creatinine levels, and metabolic acidosis.

Euvolemic: Ectopic production of AVP by tumors causes euvolemic hyponatremia. The condition, called syndrome of inappropriate antidiuretic hormone secretion (SIADH), results in abnormally high urine sodium excretion and abnormally high water reabsorption by the kidneys (see Chapter 42 for further information on this condition). Another cause of euvolemic hyponatremia is thyroid insufficiency after radiation for head and neck cancer.

Table 25–1
Clinical Manifestations of Acute Hyponatremia

PNa 125 mEq/L*	Nausea, malaise, muscle cramps
PNa 110–120 mEq/L*	Headache, dizziness, lethargy, obtundation
PNa < 110 mEq/L*	Seizures, coma, respiratory arrest

Source: Used with permission, from Clochesy JM, Breu C, Cardin S, Rudy EB, Whittaker AA: Critical Care Nursing. Philadelphia: WB Saunders Co, 1993.

*P = plasma.

Table 25–2
Drugs That May Cause Hyponatremia

Increased ADH or ADH-like Effect	Increased Renal Sodium Loss	Unknown Action	Osmotic Dilution of Serum
Aminoglutethimide	Aminoglycosides	Adenosine	Albumin
Amphotericin-B	Chlorpropamide	Arabinoside	Hypertonic glucose
Barbiturates	Cyclophosphamide	Amitriptyline	
Beta-adrenergics	Diuretics (thiazide > loop)	Antidepressants	
Bromocriptine	Heparin	Antipsychotics	
Carbamazepine	NSAIDs	Cholestyramine	
Carboplatin	Aspirin	Clonidine	
Chlorpropamide	Spironolactone	Indomethacin	
Cisplatin	Tolbutamide	Ketoconazole	
Clofibrate		Lithium	
Cyclophosphamide		Lorcainide	
Desmopressin		MAO inhibitors	
Histamine		Miconazole	
Metoclopramide		Tienilic acid	
Morphine			
Nicotine			
Oxytocin			
Vasopressin			
Vinblastine			
Vincristine			

Source: Adapted from Tietz, 1995; Mulloy and Caruana, 1995; McDonald and Dubose, 1993; Vassal, Rubie, Kalifa, Hartmann, and Lemerle, 1987.

Severe hypothyroidism is associated with sustained nonosmotic AVP release and reduced sodium reabsorption at the distal renal tubules and collecting ducts. Other causes in the oncology population are the neurotoxic, antidiuretic, and renal complications of antineoplastics and other drugs (see Table 25–2).

Relative (hypervolemic) hyponatremia

In relative hyponatremia, total body sodium may be increased or normal, but the plasma or serum value is low because the sodium is diluted by a relatively greater increase in total body water. Postoperative infusions of large volumes of hypotonic solutions are a common cause of relative hyponatremia. Renal dysfunction from chemotherapeutic drugs such as cyclophosphamide can result in oliguria and a relative hyponatremia. Hepatic dysfunction that occurs in liver metastasis and/or cirrhosis and congestive heart failure (CHF) leads to increased total body water, with reduced effective circulating volume, increased venous pressure, and decreased arterial pressure. Reduced arterial filling leads to baroreceptor stimulation of the renin-angiotensin system, as well as inhibition of atrial natriuretic peptide (ANP) release, stimulation of the sympathetic nervous system, and increased AVP release. Thus, even though osmolality may be normal, low arterial volume provides a nonosmotic stimulant for AVP release with subsequent sodium excretion and water retention.

Pseudohyponatremia

"Pseudohyponatremia" may occur when other osmotically active substances such as glucose and proteins become elevated in the blood, a condition that may occur in clients on steroidal drugs or with increased tissue catabolism, as in cancer cellular exponential growth. These substances draw fluid from the intracellular space into the intravascular space, which dilutes the serum sodium value. Serum glucose, protein, BUN, osmolality, and electrolytes should all be measured in a client exhibiting signs of hyponatremia.

RISK PROFILE

All the factors below are greater risks when occurring in an elderly client.

Cancers: Lung (commonly small cell), pancreas, duodenum, larynx, leukemia, brain, esophagus, colon, ovary, prostate, Hodgkin's disease, lymphosarcoma, nasopharynx, and multiple myeloma.

Pediatrics: Suprasellar tumors.

Conditions: Renal failure, renal tubular acidosis, CHF, hepatic failure or cirrhosis, hyperglycemia; adrenal insufficiency or adrenal metastasis from lung, breast, colon, melanoma, renal cell, or lymphoma cancers; clients receiving chemotherapy (causing anorexia, nausea, vomiting) or irradiation (causing mucositis, diarrhea, or hypothyroidism), hypothyroidism, malnutrition.

Pediatrics: Diabetes insipidus in children with Langerhans histiocytosis.

Environment: None.

Foods: Low salt intake. Foods with diuretic properties, which include asparagus, artichokes, cabbage, caffeine-containing foods, corn, cucumbers, grapes, herbal tea, spinach, and watermelon.

Drugs: Cyclophosphamide (high dose), vincristine, vinblastine, cisplatin, amphotericin B, ifosfamide, parenteral nutrition; also see Table 25–2 for other medications (Tietz, 1995).

PROGNOSIS

The severity of the symptoms of hyponatremia depends on the serum sodium level and the length of time over which the hyponatremia developed. "Acute" and "chronic" hyponatremia are differentiated by whether the hyponatremia developed over less than or more than 48 hours (McDonald and Dubose, 1993). Clients who have developed hyponatremia over a long period of time may exhibit lower-severity symptoms than those in whom the condition developed quickly. Those at risk for high mortality rates require intensive medical and nursing intervention.

Prognosis	*Mortality*
Acute hyponatremia with serum or plasma sodium < 120 mEq/L (< 120 mmol/L SI Units)	50%
Symptomatic hyponatremia with serum or plasma sodium 120 to 135 mEq/L (120 to 135 mmol/L SI Units)	15%
Asymptomatic hyponatremia	0%
Asymptomatic hyponatremia with serum sodium levels < 110 mEq/L (< 110 mmol/L SI Units)	Possible permanent neurologic change.

TREATMENT

Surgery: LeVeen shunt for hyponatremia due to cirrhosis.

Chemotherapy: Decrease dosages of cyclophosphamide, vincristine, vinblastine, cisplatin.

Radiation: Not indicated.

Medications

Decrease dosages of drugs that may cause hyponatremia (see Table 25–2).

Administer:
- IV normal saline (NS) with potassium and/or mineralcorticoids for hypovolemic hyponatremia secondary to adrenal tumor or metastasis.
- Thyroid hormone replacement for head and neck cancer clients with hyponatremia due to thyroid damage from irradiation.
- Drugs that interfere with the action of AVP for clients with SIADH.
- IV NS at 1.4 to 2.0 mEq/L/hour for acute symptoms.
- IV NS at the rate of $1/2$ mEq/hour × 24 hours for chronic hyponatremia.
- IV loop diuretic therapy for hypervolemic hyponatremia.
- IV vasodilator therapy and/or angiotensin-converting enzyme (ACE) inhibitors for CHF.
- Antidiarrheal and/or antiemetic medications.

Procedures: Placement of IV long-line catheter/access device for frequent blood draws and regulation of IV intake.

Other

Fluid intake restriction with renal failure or asymptomatic hyponatremia. Fluid and sodium restriction for hypervolemic hyponatremia.

Most cases of hyponatremia are successfully treated and have a positive outcome. However, it is thought that either severe hyponatremia causing hypoxic damage or rapid administration of IV sodium may result in cerebral brain cell osmotic dehydration known as osmotic demyelinating syndrome (central pontine myelinolysis). In this condition, there is disruption of the myelin in the pons, causing behavioral disturbances, movement disorders, akinetic mutism, and seizures. For this reason, hyponatremia requires close airway monitoring and extreme caution when determining the rate of sodium replacement.

ASSESSMENT CRITERIA: HYPONATREMIA

	True Hyponatremia		Relative Hyponatremia
	Hypovolemic State	Euvolemic State	Hypervolemic State
Vital signs			
Temperature	Elevated	At or below baseline	At or below baseline
Pulse	Rapid and weak	Normal	Rapid
Respirations	Tachypneic	Normal	Tachypneic, dyspneic on exertion

ASSESSMENT CRITERIA: HYPONATREMIA *(continued)*

	True Hyponatremia		Relative Hyponatremia
	Hypovolemic State	**Euvolemic State**	**Hypervolemic State**
Blood pressure	Systolic BP <90 mmHg or 20 mmHg below baseline	Normal	Increased
Central venous pressure	<2 mmHg	2–6 mmHg	>6 mmHg
History			
Symptoms, conditions	Decreased oral intake; volume and electrolyte loss from GI tract (nausea, vomiting), integumentary system (sweating), and renal system (urine); adrenal disease or metastasis; mucositis after chemotherapy.	Radiation-induced hypothyroidism, SIADH, drug therapy (see Table 25–2).	Increased hypotonic fluid intake (oral, nasogastric, IV); renal disease or dysfunction (especially elderly on multiple prescriptions); hepatic dysfunction; CHF; uncontrolled diabetes (pseudohyponatremia).
Weight pattern	Decrease of 1–2kg/day.	Stable or increasing.	Increase of 1–2 kg/day.
Hallmark physical signs and symptoms	Malaise, lethargy, weakness, muscle cramps, hyperreflexia, muscle twitching, seizures, coma, vomiting.		
Additional physical signs and symptoms	Abdominal cramps, anorexia, dry mucous membranes, decreased saliva, swollen and red tongue, nausea, oliguria, postural hypotension, diminished skin turgor, decreased urine output.	Decreased urine output.	Dyspnea; tachypnea; tachycardia; S_3; JVD; restlessness; watery diarrhea; increased salivation; arterial hypotension or hypertension; decreased or increased urine output, depending on cause of the hypervolemic state.
Psychosocial signs	Apprehension, confusion, disorientation.		

(continued)

ASSESSMENT CRITERIA: HYPONATREMIA *(continued)*

	True Hyponatremia		Relative Hyponatremia
	Hypovolemic State	Euvolemic State	Hypervolemic State
Lab values			
Sodium, serum	Low	Low	Low
Sodium, urine	Low (GI fluid and electrolyte losses) or high (deficiency of mineralcorticoid).	High	Low (renal dysfunction) or high (reduced effective arterial volume).
Creatinine, urine	Normal	Normal	High (renal problems).
Osmolarity, urine	Low or high (>800 mOsm/kg H_2O).	High	Low (<100 mOsm/kg H_2O) or high (>300 mOsm/Kg H_2O).
Potassium, serum	High (in adrenal metastasis).	Normal	High (in renal dysfunction); otherwise normal.
Aldosterone, serum	Low (in adrenal metastasis).	N/A	N/A
AVP (ADH), serum	Decreased	Increased (in SIADH, thyroid insufficiency, and drug side effects).	Increased (in reduced effective circulating volume); otherwise normal.
Diagnostic tests			
Deep tendon reflexes	Diminished	Diminished	Diminished
Other	Assess chemotherapy dosages. Assess content and rate of IV fluids.		

NURSING DIAGNOSIS

The nursing diagnosis will vary, depending on the cause(s) of hyponatremia. Some of the common diagnoses and etiologies are as follows.

> *(Potential for) ineffective airway clearance* related to seizure activity or coma secondary to cerebral edema.
> *Acute confusion* related to cerebral edema associated with hyponatremia.
> *Fluid volume deficit* related to:
> - Nausea and vomiting associated with the side effects of chemotherapeutic drugs.
> - Decreased oral intake secondary to mucositis.
> - Abnormal fluid loss, secondary to reduced adrenal production of aldosterone.

Fluid volume excess related to:
- Infusion of hypotonic fluids or tube feeding associated with post-operative treatments.
- Hepatic dysfunction secondary to liver metastasis.
- CHF secondary to hepatic dysfunction.
- Oliguria secondary to renal side effects of chemotherapeutic medications.

Potential for injury related to motor deficits associated with hyponatremia.

Altered oral mucous membranes related to mucositis associated with chemotherapy side effects.

Impaired physical mobility related to muscle weakness, twitching, and/or cramping associated with hyponatremia.

Knowledge deficit related to unfamiliarity with sequelae and treatment for hyponatremia.

NURSING INTERVENTIONS

Immediate nursing interventions

Assess pulse, respirations, blood pressure, and deep tendon reflexes q1h × 4, then q6h.

Initiate seizure precautions. Place suction equipment and an oral airway at the bedside.

Send STAT serum electrolyte panel.

Establish patent IV access and obtain volumetric infusion pump.

Measure hourly intake and output (I and O). Insert indwelling urinary catheter, if necessary.

Prepare for long-line catheter/access device placement for frequent blood sampling.

Anticipated physician orders and interventions

Spot urine electrolytes and urine osmolality.

24-hour urine collection for urine sodium measurement.

Chemotherapy and other medications decreased/discontinued that may cause hyponatremia.

STAT serum electrolyte panel, serum creatinine, BUN, aldosterone, and AVP.

Long-line catheter/access device placement for frequent blood sampling.

Antidiarrheal and/or antiemetic medication administration.

Hypovolemic hyponatremia
- Give high-sodium foods (beef, ham, green olives, salted pretzels, soups).
- Initiate sodium replacement for severe hypo-osmolality, Na^+ < 120 mEq/L (< 120 mmol/L SI Units), or with severe neurologic symptoms:

Administer 3% or 5% saline IV at a rate that increases the plasma or serum Na⁺ level no more than 1 mEq/L/hour (McDonald and Dubose, 1993). Discontinue infusion when Na⁺ level reaches 120 to 125 mEq/L (120 to 125 mmol/L SI Units). May add potassium and/or mineralcorticoid, depending on the cause of the hyponatremia.

Euvolemic hyponatremia
- Fluid restriction of 1500 ml/day for Na⁺ 125 to 135 mEq/L (125 to 135 mmol/L SI Units).
- 0.9% NaCl IV infusion at 60 to 120 ml/hour.
- Demeclocycline for SIADH (see also Chapter 42).

Hypervolemic hyponatremia
- Fluid restriction and/or dietary sodium restriction.
- Loop diuretic IV push (usually furosemide), combined with hypertonic saline infusion.
- For symptoms of acute hyponatremia, administer 3% saline IV at a rate adjusted hourly based on hourly urine sodium output.
- Vasodilator or ACE inhibitor IV for CHF.

Ongoing nursing assessment, monitoring, and interventions

Assess:
- Level of consciousness q8h and PRN.
- Skin turgor qd.
- For nausea and vomiting and medicate with antiemetics as prescribed PRN.
- For signs of CHF q8h (rales, tachypnea, dyspnea, S₃, tachycardia, jugular vein distention [JVD], peripheral edema, bounding pulses).
- IV site for redness, edema, pain, q4h and PRN. Increase observations to q1h for 3% and 5% saline infusions.

Measure:
- Blood pressure (BP), pulse, and respirations q1h × 4, then q2h × 4, then q4h × 3.
- I and O q1h × 24 hours.
- Weight qd.

Send:
- Repeat urine electrolytes and urine osmolality in 24 hours.
- Serum creatinine and BUN in 24 hours and PRN.
- *For severe symptoms of hyponatremia, during sodium replacement:* electrolytes q1h × 4, then q2h × 8, then q4h × 2 (for Na⁺ and K⁺).

Implement:
- Water and/or sodium intake restriction PRN, as prescribed.
- Seizure precautions until serum Na⁺ level is > 120 mEq/L (> 120 mmol/L SI Units).

TEACHING/EDUCATION

Select items, based on the client's pathophysiology.

Decreased/discontinued chemotherapy: *Rationale:* Certain chemotherapy drugs can make your kidneys have trouble getting rid of water from your body. Some of your drugs may be changed or alternated with other drugs. There may be a delay in your chemotherapy treatment regimen.

IV blood samples and urine samples: *Rationale:* Several blood and urine samples will be taken during the next day. They are needed to track the amount of salt and water in your body.

IV line placement: *Rationale:* The IV line allows us to easily take blood samples and to give you necessary treatments with fluids.

Indwelling urinary catheter placement: *Rationale:* Accurate urine measurement is very important for people with low salt levels. The catheter prevents any urine from spilling before it is measured. We may also give you medicine that will make your kidneys make more urine, so the catheter keeps you from having to get up frequently to go to the bathroom.

Fluid restriction: *Rationale:* Limiting how much water you can drink is needed to keep the fluid from building up in your body while your kidneys aren't able to get rid of extra fluid. If too much water builds up, it can make it too hard for your heart to pump.

Dietary changes: *Rationale:* Adding high-salt foods to your diet for a few days is necessary to bring your body's salt level back to normal (*Note:* This measure is necessary only for hypovolemic hyponatremia).

IV site symptoms: *Rationale:* Your body's salt level is so low that we have to give you a very strong salt solution through the IV in your vein. This IV may hurt you if it starts to leak out into the tissues of your hand (arm, etc.). Your nurse will be checking how well this IV is working every hour, but if it starts hurting you or swelling at any time, call your nurse right away.

Signs and symptoms of hyponatremia: *Rationale:* You and your significant others need to watch for signs of low salt levels because early treatment helps you feel better and live a higher quality of life. The signs include any of the following: fatigue, weakness, confusion, muscle cramps, muscle twitching, convulsions, nausea, vomiting. (Also signs of hypo-/hypervolemia, as appropriate).

EVALUATION/DESIRED OUTCOMES

1. Serum Na^+ increases to ≥ 120 mEq/L (≥ 120 mmol/L SI Units) within 48 hours (for acute hyponatremia).
2. Serum Na^+ increases to normal values at a rate comparable to the time over which the hyponatremia developed.
3. Urine Na^+ and urine osmolality return to normal values within 72 hours.

4. Serum K^+ decreases to normal values (3.5 to 5.0 mEq/L, 3.5 to 5.0 mmol/L) within 24 hours.
5. Systolic BP returns to baseline within 72 hours.
6. The client is free of signs of osmotic demyelinating syndrome at 48 hours after saline infusion.
7. The lungs are clear to auscultation within 48 hours.
8. Indwelling urinary catheter is discontinued within 72 hours.
9. Nausea, vomiting, and diarrhea subside within 48 hours.
10. Chemotherapy regimen will continue as prescribed within 72 hours.
11. High-salt diet and fluid restrictions are understood by the client and/or caregiver prior to discharge.

DISCHARGE PLANNING

The hyponatremic client may need:

Short-term enteral nutrition and IV fluids when vomiting or mucositis interfere with adequate food and fluid oral intake.
Intermediate care facility, daily home nursing visits, or family caregivers to manage the enteral and parenteral intake.
Training of the client and significant others in I and O measurement and documentation.
Short-term intermediate care facility for IV fluid and diuretic regimen for SIADH.

FOLLOW-UP CARE

Anticipated care

Physician office visit within 1 week.
Outpatient lab testing for serum electrolytes within the next week.
Other blood work as appropriate (thyroid hormone, AVP, K^+, BUN/creatinine, etc.).
Continuation of dietary/fluid restrictions or regimen.
Daily home nursing visit for clients discharged home with enteral or parenteral fluids.
Home health nursing visit once per week × 2 weeks for clients discharged home without parenteral or enteral fluids.

Anticipated client/family questions and possible answers

Will this problem with low salt/sodium in my blood happen again?
"It is possible that this problem will happen again. It is very important for you to know the signs of hyponatremia and what to do when you recognize these signs."

"Whenever you have a lot of vomiting after chemotherapy, there is a chance that you will lose salt/sodium again. This is when you have to be especially watchful for the signs of hyponatremia and call the doctor."

"As long as you are taking [replacement mineralcorticoids (insert drug name)], and the blood level of this drug is where it should be, you probably won't have this problem again. However, hyponatremia could return when you have a lot of vomiting or don't eat food or drink fluids, or from certain chemotherapy drugs. Because of this, you must know the signs of low blood sodium and call your doctor or nurse if you notice them."

When can I continue my chemotherapy?

"When your lab values are back to normal and your body can tolerate the side effects of the drug again. This is usually within a week's time."

Why will a nurse be coming to my home?

"The nurse will come to see whether any low-sodium problems are happening again. The nurse will take blood samples from your vein; listen to your lungs with a stethoscope; weigh you; ask about any recent nausea, vomiting, or diarrhea; see if you understand your fluid restriction; take your blood pressure, heart, and breathing rate; check your reflexes with a small rubber hammer; check your legs for swelling; check your mouth and skin to see if they are dry; and talk with you to see how alert you are. All of these checks can help show whether or not your problem with low sodium in your blood is happening again."

Should I eat extra salt to make sure my blood levels don't drop again?

(For hypovolemic hyponatremia) "You may be able to eat higher-salt foods, close to your chemotherapy, if it normally causes loss of sodium through vomiting. Check with your doctor to see if this is advisable for your situation."

(For euvolemic or hypervolemic hyponatremia) "No. Eating extra salt can cause your body to keep too much water in your bloodstream. This can add extra work for your heart and body, which would be bad for you."

CHAPTER SUMMARY

Hyponatremia is a metabolic complication that occurs in 5% of people with cancer and in up to 46% of people receiving parenteral nutrition. It may occur with normal, low, or high blood sodium content because the serum sodium value is a reflection of fluid balance. Hyponatremia may be caused by the tumor itself, by the effect of metastasis on the body, or by the side effects or actions of chemotherapeutic drugs. Symptoms generally appear when sodium levels drop below 120 mEq/L (120 mmol/L SI Units), and permanent neurologic damage may occur if levels reach ≤110 mEq/L (≤110 mmol/L SI Units). Serum sodium levels that drop quickly or cause neurologic symptoms constitute an acute oncologic emergency. Treatment and nursing care are related to the cause(s) of hyponatremia and the rapidity of development of the problem. A definitive understanding of water and sodium homeostasis is essential to underlying treatment and care.

TEST QUESTIONS

1. Hyponatremia is primarily a disorder of:
   A. Excess cerebrospinal fluid
   B. Lactic acidosis
   C. Hypo-osmolality
   D. Chloride depletion

   1. Answer: C
   Hypo-osmolality occurs when the rate of sodium loss exceeds the rate of water loss (true hyponatremia) or when the rate of water intake exceeds the ability of the kidneys to excrete free water and maximally dilute the urine (relative hyponatremia).

2. The primary nursing diagnosis of a client with hyponatremia is:
   A. Alteration in coping mechanisms
   B. Potential for infection
   C. Alteration in tissue perfusion
   D. Fluid volume deficit (or excess)

   2. Answer: D
   Hyponatremia is a disorder of body fluid osmolality characterized by either a fluid volume excess (hypotonic hyponatremia) or by a fluid volume deficit, caused by depletion of extracellular fluid.

3. Which chemotherapeutic drug may induce hyponatremia?
   A. Procarbazine
   B. Vincristine
   C. Methotrexate
   D. 5-Fluorouracil

   3. Answer: B
   Plant alkaloids have the potential to cause hyponatremia as well as SIADH. Vincristine is a plant alkaloid.

4. A common cause of hyponatremia in persons with cancer is a deficiency in mineralcorticoids that is caused by tumors in the:
   A. Pons of the brain
   B. Adrenal gland
   C. Loop of Henle in the kidney
   D. Pancreas

   4. Answer: B
   The adrenal gland is associated with mineralcorticoid production. Both primary adrenal tumors and metastasis of other tumors to the adrenal gland(s) may result in underproduction of aldosterone. This results in decreased reabsorption of sodium by the kidneys.

5. Hyponatremia is most often associated with which type of cancer?
   A. Cervical
   B. Testicular
   C. Rhabdomyosarcoma
   D. Lung

   5. Answer: D
   Hyponatremia is most common in persons who have small cell carcinoma of the lung.

6. The signs of hyponatremia include:
   A. Decreased serum sodium and decreased deep tendon reflexes
   B. Increased serum sodium and increased blood pressure
   C. Increased urine osmolality and decreased confusion
   D. Decreased serum creatinine and lymphocytes

6. Answer: A
Serum sodium is less than 135 mEq/L. Deep tendon reflexes are decreased owing to intracellular edema that occurs as a result of an osmotic shift of fluid out of the vascular system to the intercellular spaces.

7. Which nursing intervention should be implemented first in a client suspected of having hyponatremia?
   A. Insert urinary catheter STAT.
   B. Assess deep tendon reflexes.
   C. Obtain serum electrolytes STAT.
   D. Initiate seizure precautions.

7. Answer: C
To determine if a client is hyponatremic, a serum sodium level needs to be drawn, which is part of a serum electrolyte panel.

8. A client diagnosed with hyponatremia secondary to renal, hepatic, or cardiac dysfunction would most likely be taught about:
   A. Alopecia
   B. Hypertension
   C. Low-fat diet
   D. Restriction of water intake

8. Answer: D
Water restriction as part of dietary changes is necessary to avoid excess water retention by the body, thereby decreasing the potential for CHF.

9. A diuretic would *not* be indicated for which type of hyponatremia?
   A. Hypovolemic hyponatremia
   B. Euvolemic hyponatremia
   C. Hypernatremic hyponatremia
   D. Pseudohyperkalemia.

9. Answer: A
Clients with hypovolemic hyponatremia have experienced a sodium *and* water loss. Both sodium and fluid replacement are indicated for neurologic symptoms and Na^+ < 110 mEq/L (< 110 mmol/L SI Units).

10. A desired outcome when treating a person who has hyponatremia would be that his or her:
   A. Cardiac enzymes would be within normal limits within 1 hour of admission.
   B. Chest tubes would be removed within 72 hours of admission.
   C. Chemotherapy regimen would continue as prescribed within 72 hours after admission.
   D. Thrombocyte count would be within normal limits 24 hours after admission.

10. Answer: C
Chemotherapy, especially regimens containing plant alkaloids, cyclophosphamide, and/or cisplatin, will be changed or discontinued because these agents increase ADH release, thereby adding to water retention and hypo-osmolality. A desired outcome would be that within 72 hours hyponatremia is controlled and chemotherapy may be restarted.

REFERENCES

Batuman V, Dreisbach A, Maesaka JE, Rothkopf M, Ross E: Renal and electrolyte effects of total parenteral nutrition. J Patenter Enter Nutr 8(5):546–551, 1984.

Cain JW, Bender CM: Ifosfamide-induced neurotoxicity: Associated symptoms and nursing implications. Oncol Nurs Forum 22(4):659–666, 1995.

Chernecky CC, Berger BJ: Laboratory Tests and Diagnostic Procedures, 2nd ed. Philadelphia: WB Saunders Co., 1997.

Clochesy JM, Breu C, Cardin S, Rudy EB, Whitteker AA: Critical Care Nursing. Philadelphia: WB Saunders Co, 1993.

Kokatsu T, Tsukuka M: Hypopituitarism and hyponatremia in a case with nasopharyngeal carcinoma. Otorhinolaryngol Related Specialties 456(6):347–351, 1994.

Lange B, D'Angio G, Ross AJ III, O'Neill JA Jr, Packer RJ: Oncologic emergencies. In Pizzo PA, Poplack DG (eds): Principles and Practice of Pediatric Oncology, 2nd ed. Philadelphia: JB Lippincott, 1993, pp. 951–972.

McDonald GA, Dubose TD: Hyponatremia in the cancer patient. Oncology 7(9):55–64, 1993.

Mulloy AL, Caruana RJ: Hyponatremic emergencies. Med Clin North Am 79(1):155–168, 1995.

Reeves WB, Andreoli TE: The posterior pituitary and water metabolism. In Wilson JD, Foster DW (eds): Williams Textbook of Endocrinology, 8th ed. Philadelphia: WB Saunders Co, 1992, pp. 342–356.

Roth Y, Lightman SL, Kronenberg J: Hyponatremia associated with laryngeal squamous cell carcinoma. Euro Arch Otorhinolaryngol 251(3):183–185, 1994.

Sane T, Rantakari K, Poranen A, Tahtela R, Valimaki M, Pelkonen R: Hyponatremia after transsphenoidal surgery for pituitary tumors. J Clin Endocrinol Metab 79(5):1395–1398, 1994.

Tietz NW: Clinical Guide to Laboratory Tests. Philadelphia: WB Saunders Co, 1995.

Tscherning C, Rubie H, Chancholle A, Claeyssens S, Robert A, Fabre J, Bouissou F: Recurrent renal salt wasting in a child treated with carboplatin and etoposide. Cancer 73(6):1761–1763, 1994.

Vassal G, Rubie H, Kalifa C, Hartmann O, Lemerle J: Hyponatremia and renal sodium wasting in patients receiving cisplatinum. Pediatr Hematol Oncol 4(4):337–344, 1987.

CHAPTER 26

INCREASED
INTRACRANIAL PRESSURE

Janice L. Hickman, MSN, RN, CS

CHAPTER OBJECTIVES

At the completion of this chapter, the reader will be able to:

Define increased intracranial pressure (ICP).

State the risk factors associated with increased ICP in the oncology client.

Describe nursing care as it relates to clients with increased ICP.

OVERVIEW

ICP is the term used to describe the pressure exerted within the skull and meninges by brain tissue, cerebrospinal fluid (CSF), and cerebral blood volume (Hickey, 1992). Any growth within the cranial vault can cause symptoms of increased ICP by compressing the brain against the bony calvarium. Because of the rigid, bony encasement of the brain, even a benign tumor can produce significant symptoms and, if not treated, death. Increased ICP can occur with little or no warning and is a common life-threatening complication of cerebral metastasis.

Intracranial tumors may lead to a generalized disturbance of cerebral functions and to signs and symptoms of increased ICP. Lesions that gradually enlarge over days to months often cause no symptoms until the lesions or the tissue in the surrounding area of reactive edema are large enough to distort or compress functionally important regions of the brain and induce increased ICP. Intracranial tumors behave in this fashion.

DESCRIPTION

Normal state of ICP

The intracranial space is comprised of three components: brain tissue, CSF, and blood. The intracranial volume is essentially constant within the rigid cranial vault known as the skull. According to the Monro-Kellie hypothesis

(Hickey, 1992), the expansion of the volume of one of these three components must be compensated for by a decrease in the volume of one or more of the other compartments in order for the ICP to remain normal.

ICP is not a constant. It is a continuously fluctuating phenomenon within a normal range of 0 to 15 mmHg. Transient increases in ICP are benign, but sustained increases in ICP can be life-threatening. Brain tumors account for approximately 20% of all cancers. Primary brain tumors account for nearly 2% of all cancer deaths, with rates varying with age, sex, and race. The American Cancer Society statistics show that brain tumors occur most commonly in adults over the age of 45, in Caucasians more than blacks, and slightly more often in women than in men. In children, primary brain tumors are the second most common cancer. Although some tumors are classified as congenital or hereditary, the etiology of the majority of primary brain tumors is unknown (Lord and Coleman, 1991).

Pathologic causes of increased ICP

Most malignant central nervous system (CNS) tumors are metastatic from a distant site. The most common primary sites include the breast, lung, and colon along with the kidney, thyroid, and prostate. Increased ICP is caused by rapidly increasing tumor mass; associated edema; and, less commonly, hemorrhagic or infarction within the tumor. A rapid increase in the tumor mass or associated edema can cause early symptoms such as headache, nausea, vomiting, and later depression of the level of consciousness (LOC). In contrast, slow-growing tumors, such as low-grade gliomas or meningiomas, may be present for years and become large before symptoms are caused by increased ICP within the skull. Tumors that cause obstructions of CSF flow through the ventricles can also cause a rapid and severe rise in ICP (Fig. 26–1).

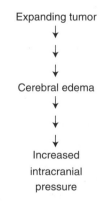

Figure 26–1   Progression of ICP with tumor mass.

Clinical manifestations of increased ICP

The clinical manifestations of generalized increased ICP include mental changes, papilledema, headache, vomiting, and changes in vital signs.

Change in Mental Status

Changes in mental status include alterations in the LOC, confusion, short-term memory loss, and personality changes. Each client may exhibit a wide variety of mental changes. Frequently, these changes are gradual in onset and evident only to the client's family. In the early stages of increased ICP, clients may complain of decreased attention span, drowsiness, and memory loss. Families may observe personality and behavior changes, poor judgment, mood changes, or decreasing intellectual functioning.

Papilledema

Papilledema is considered a major sign of increased ICP. An increase in CSF pressure around the optic nerve impairs the outflow of venous blood, causing edema and swelling of the optic disk. Papilledema may be an early or late sign related to the location and type of the brain tumor.

Headaches

Approximately one-third of clients with a brain tumor report headaches. These headaches, if caused by increased ICP, are usually bilateral and are generally located in the frontal or occipital regions. Clients may give a history of early-morning headache, which subsides on arising. They also may report that bending over, coughing, or performing the Valsalva maneuver may increase or cause a headache. The pain may be described as dull, sharp, or throbbing. Headaches will increase in severity, frequency, and duration over time (Wegmann and Hakiner, 1990).

Vomiting

Another symptom of increased ICP is vomiting, which appears unrelated to food ingestion. It may be preceded by nausea and is often sudden and projectile. Increased pressure on the medulla's vomiting center is thought to cause the symptom.

Altered Vital Signs

Late findings of increased ICP are changes in vital signs. This results from increased pressure on the vasomotor centers of the medulla. As ICP increases, circulatory and respiratory responses in intracranial hypertension occur.

The systolic blood pressure rises, diastolic pressure drops, and the pulse pressure widens. Bradycardia and slow irregular respirations are exhibited (Cushing's triad). This response is a late finding, and the client is usually comatose.

A growing tumor mass and the edema associated with it cause increased ICP. If not treated, increased ICP can lead to brain herniation. Herniation is a neurologic emergency. Shifting brain tissue causes compression, cerebral edema, and ischemia, and if the condition is not treated, death will occur.

> **Pediatrics:** The clinical signs of increased ICP include those of the adult, along with macrocephaly, excessive rate of head growth.

RISK PROFILE

Cancers: *Brain tumors:* Cerebellar, midbrain, pineal, ventricular (related to obstruction of CSF flow). Intrinsic brain stem tumors (late in course). Tumors most likely to cause increased ICP without conspicuous focal or lateralizing signs are medullo-blastoma, ependymoma of the fourth ventricle, hemangioblastoma of the cerebellum, pineodoma, colloid cyst of the third ventricle, and craniopharyngioma.

> **Pediatrics:** Cerebellar tumors.

Conditions: Primary and metastatic brain or skull tumors; tumor growth; bleeding diatheses; CNS infection, increased $PaCO_2$, decreased PaO_2, syndrome of inappropriate antidiuretic hormone secretion (SIADH), or acute sodium depletion; alteration in internal jugular vein flow by head/neck tumors; obstruction of CSF circulation resulting in hydrocephalus; failure of autoregulation.

Environment: None.

Foods: None.

Drugs: ≥6,000 rads of whole-brain irradiation with or without methotrexate, radiosurgery (symptoms may occur months after treatment).

PROGNOSIS

Brain tumors become space-occupying lesions at the expense of the space available for the brain's normal contents. The tumor becomes the fourth component of the cerebral contents and eventually displaces the brain tissue, blood, and CSF. The extent to which a tumor produces symptoms of increased ICP is a reflection of three factors: (1) the rapidity of tumor growth, (2) the ability of the brain to compensate for the expanding lesion, and (3) the tumor location. Intracerebral lesions can produce signs and symptoms of increased ICP in four ways (the so-called four Ds): destruction, distortion, displacement, and dissemination. Initially, built-in compensatory mechanisms resist elevations in ICP. Eventually, decompensation follows, and ICP increases. Failure to identify a client's early and often subtle signs and symptoms of increased ICP places the client at great risk. If treatment is delayed, brain herniation will occur, and the client can die from cardiac or respiratory arrest related to compression of the brain stem.

TREATMENT

In the past, surgical intervention was the only option for managing increased ICP. Today, there are a variety of medical approaches that reduce the need for acute surgical measures. The management plan selected is determined partially by the severity of the condition and the status of the client.

Surgery

The emergency intervention involves making a small burr hole into the skull and inserting a ventriculostomy catheter into the anterior horn of the lateral ventricle. This procedure allows for controlled drainage of CSF and results in immediate decrease in ICP.

Tumor resection and debulking.

Chemotherapy: Depends on tumor type.

Radiation: In many cases of increased ICP resulting from intracranial tumor, the primary treatment is radiation therapy, particularly when the increased ICP is caused by multiple metastatic lesions. It is also used when surgery is contraindicated because of the client's condition, treatment preferences, or tumor location.

Medications

Treatment focuses on diagnosing the cause and intervening with the appropriate pharmacologic, medical, and/or surgical interventions (see Table 26–1).

Osmotic diuretics have a high osmotic concentration that causes water to be drawn from the edematous brain tissue into the vascular system.

Glucosteroids are effective in reducing focal cerebral edema.

Barbiturate therapy is used in instances of severe, uncontrolled increased ICP unresponsive to usual treatment modalities. Barbiturate therapy reduces cerebral blood flow and cerebral blood volume by causing cerebral vasoconstriction.

Antiseizure drugs: Although anticonvulsants do not specifically treat

Table 26–1
Medications That Decrease ICP or Control Symptoms

Osmotic diuretics	Mannitol (Osmitrol)
Glucocorticoids	Dexamethasone (Decadron)
Loop diuretics	Furosemide (Lasix)
	Bumetanide (Buprex)
	Ethacrynate sodium (Sodium Edecrin)
Barbiturates	Pentobarbital
	Nembutal
Antiseizure drugs	Phenytoin (Dilantin)
Neuromuscular blocking agents	Atacurium (Tracrium)
	Pancuronium (Pavulon)
	Vecuronium (Norcuron)

cerebral edema, they control seizure activity of the brain (see Chapter 37 for further information on seizure control).

Procedures: Placement of arterial line for arterial blood gases (ABGs), blood sampling, and for monitoring blood pressure.

ASSESSMENT CRITERIA: INCREASED INTRACRANIAL PRESSURE

Baseline neurologic assessment

A baseline neurologic assessment is essential in detecting changes indicating increased ICP and should include assessment for the following:

Alteration in LOC: subtle behavior changes, restlessness, irritability, drowsiness, confusion, or apathy.

Orientation:
- To person, place, time.
- Difficulties in verbalization.

Muscle strength: motor strength, bilateral equality, extremity drift, flexion/dorsiflexion.

Vital signs: widening pulse pressure, bradycardia, irregular breathing patterns.

Pupillary response: size and shape, equality, and reaction to light.

History   History of confusion, restlessness, and lethargy. Disorientation to time, then to place and to person.

ASSESSMENT CRITERIA:
INCREASED INTRACRANIAL PRESSURE (continued)

Hallmark physical signs and symptoms	Headache, nausea, and projectile vomiting progressing to depression of LOC.
	Pediatrics: macrocephaly.

	Early Signs of Increased ICP	Late Signs of Increased ICP
LOC	Restlessness Disorientation Lethargy	Somnolence Stupor Coma
Headache	Present	Increase in intensity
Motor function	Contralateral hemiparesis	Decorticate/decerebrate posturing
Vital signs	Normal	Cushing's triad: Increased blood pressure Decreased pulse Widening pulse pressure
Pupils	Dilated ipsilaterally Sluggish reaction	Dilated bilaterally and fixed
Visual disturbances	Blurring Decreased visual acuity Diplopia	Unable to assess due to decreased LOC
Papilledema	Not present Note: In some clients this may be the first sign observed if an increase in ICP has developed gradually.	Present

Additional physical signs and symptoms	Decreased attention span, drowsiness, memory loss.

Psychosocial signs	Personality and behavior changes, poor judgment, mood changes, decreased intellectual functioning.

Diagnostic tests	CT scan, MRI of brain.

Other	ICP monitoring.

NURSING DIAGNOSIS

The nursing management of the client with increased ICP is directed toward principles implemented within the context of the nursing process. Following are the nursing diagnoses and related outcomes most commonly applicable to a client with increased ICP.

Tissue perfusion, altered cerebral, related to increased ICP secondary to tumor.

Fluid volume deficit, risk for, related to osmotic diuretic therapy.

(Potential for) ineffective breathing pattern related to alteration in LOC.

Skin integrity, potential for, impaired, related to immobility and/or hypothermia therapy.

Family processes, altered, related to loss of client's well-being.

NURSING INTERVENTIONS

Immediate nursing interventions

Assess client for baseline neurologic status and reassess q1h and PRN for neurologic changes. (See Assessment Criteria section.)

Elevate head of bed (HOB) 30 to 45 degrees.

Maintain head and neck in neutral position.

Avoid extreme hip flexion.

Maintain patent airway and adequate ventilation.

Avoid "clustering" client care activities.

Anticipated physician orders and interventions

Drain CSF, as prescribed, if ventriculostomy is inserted.

ABGs.

Intake and output (I and O) and urinary specific gravity q1h.

Serum electrolytes, osmolality, and creatinine qd.

Administration of steroids, osmotic agents, and diuretics. (Dosages and frequencies will vary with the client's clinical presentation.)

Maintenance of normothermia with antipyretic medications and hypothermia blanket.

Control of seizures with prophylactic and with anticonvulsant(s) PRN.

Insert indwelling urinary catheter.

Use of sedatives, barbiturates, or paralyzing agents for severe increased ICP unresponsive to other treatment.

Stool softeners qd.

Maintenance of blood pressure within the client's norm by using volume expanders, vasopressors, or antihypertensives.

Ongoing nursing assessment, monitoring, and interventions

Assess:
- Neurologic status q1h and PRN.
- Peripheral circulation, color, temperature of skin every 2 to 3 hours (if hypothermia used).

- For signs of hypovolemia (if diuresis is ordered): serum osmolality > 300 mOsm/kg H_2O, tachycardia, hypotension.
- For Cheyne-Stokes respirations, which indicate increasing ICP.
- For signs of seizure activity and infection.
- Family's ability to cope with client's altered neurologic status.
- For signs of brain herniation (Cushing's response, Cushing's triad).

Measure:

- Temperature, pulse, respirations, and neurologic status q1h.
- I and O q1h and specific gravity q4h.
- CSF drainage q1h (if applicable).

Send:

- Serum electrolytes and osmolality q24h.
- ABGs qd and PRN.
- Blood for levels of antiseizure drugs every other day.

Implement:

- Organization of nursing care to allow for optimal rest periods.
- Seizure precautions.
- Turning client q2h.
- A bowel program.
- Control of environment to avoid noxious stimulation (i.e., limit visitors, provide dark, quiet environment, avoid clustering of nursing activities).
- Maintenance of patency of airway.
- Passive range of motion schedule.
- Maintenance of bedrest and HOB elevation of 30 to 45 degrees.
- Explanation of all procedures to family, client.
- Referrals to other disciplines, i.e., clergy, physical therapy.

TEACHING/EDUCATION

Neurologic examination: *Rationale:* It is an important part of your care to have your awareness of yourself and your environment checked often so that we will know if it is changing and choose the proper treatment if it does change.

Limitation of noxious stimulation: *Rationale:* Speaking softly to the client and avoiding discussion of disturbing topics will help keep the ICP from increasing.

Instruct each client (if able) to exhale when being turned and to avoid pushing feet against footboard: *Rationale:* When you exert pressure using your chest and stomach muscles, you increase ICP, so you must avoid such action.

Application of hypothermia blanket: *Rationale:* When the body temperature rises, your body metabolism increases, and this can cause your ICP to rise.

EVALUATION/DESIRED OUTCOMES

1. Stable ICP, within normal limits, within 24 hours.
2. Stable vital signs and baseline neurologic status.
3. Absence of cardiovascular or pulmonary complications.
4. Normal fluid and electrolyte balance.
5. Skin integrity intact.
6. Family acceptance of actual or potential altered abilities of client within 24 hours.

DISCHARGE PLANNING

The client at risk for ICP may need:

Training of family members to recognize signs and symptoms of increased ICP.

Intermediate short-term rehabilitation, home nursing visits, or family member caregivers to assist in self-care.

Home evaluation of physical environment for changes to promote optimal safety.

Physical therapy for activity and use of assistive devices.

Social service for placement, financial evaluation, and community services.

Information about local support groups.

Referral, if appropriate, to a hospice setting to allow for increased control over environmental factors.

FOLLOW-UP CARE

Anticipated care

Physician office visit within 1 week.

Home care visits for re-evaluation and ongoing client/family teaching and support.

Anticipated client/family questions and possible answers

Will this problem happen again?

"It is possible that the problem will happen again. It is important for you to know the symptoms of increased ICP and notify the doctor."

"Whenever you have a brain tumor, there is a chance of tumor regrowth. That is why you have to be watchful of the symptoms and notify the doctor."

CHAPTER SUMMARY

Increased ICP is a complication that can occur in a person with brain tumor. Elevated ICP can be produced when a mass lesion reaches critical size, obstructs the intracranial venous system, or obstructs the CSF pathways. Accurate assessments can play a significant role in selection of the treatment to be instituted for increased ICP and in the client's recovery potential. Nursing interventions, including ongoing assessment and documentation, combined with aggressive treatment of increased ICP when it occurs help to prevent neurologic damage and to identify progress or deterioration in the client's condition. Effective assessment and interaction are based on knowledge of the dynamics of ICP and the factors associated with its increase.

TEST QUESTIONS

1. The normal range of ICP is:
   A. 0 to 15 mmHg
   B. 10 to 20 mmHg
   C. 20 to 30 mmHg
   D. 25 to 35 mmHg

1. Answer: A
Normal ICP is 0 to 15 mmHg under normal physiologic conditions.

2. A *major* sign of increased ICP is:
   A. Anorexia
   B. Thrombocytopenia
   C. Papilledema
   D. Behavior changes

2. Answer: C
Papilledema is considered a major sign of increased ICP. An increase in CSF pressure around the optic nerve impairs the outflow of venous blood, causing edema and swelling of the optic disc.

3. If not treated, prolonged increased ICP can lead to:
   A. Headache
   B. Tumor growth
   C. Vomiting
   D. Brain herniation

3. Answer: D
Herniation is a neurologic emergency. Shifting brain tissue causes compression, cerebral edema, and ischemia, and if the condition is not treated, death will occur.

4. *Early* signs of increased ICP in the client's level of consciousness are:
   A. Restlessness, disorientation, and lethargy
   B. Stupor
   C. Somnolence
   D. Coma

4. Answer: A
Early signs of increased ICP are restlessness, disorientation, and lethargy.

5. The primary nursing diagnosis of clients with increased ICP is:
   A. Ineffective breathing pattern
   B. Altered cerebral perfusion
   C. Altered family processes
   D. Impaired skin integrity

5. Answer: B
Increased ICP alters cerebral perfusion to brain tissue. With increased pressure, brain tissue is compressed and lacks blood and oxygen.

6. Which of the following nursing interventions should be implemented *first* in a client with increased ICP?
   A. Maintain head in neutral position.
   B. Initiate baseline neurologic assessment.
   C. Insert indwelling urinary catheter.
   D. Send blood for STAT lab.

6. Answer: B
A baseline neurologic exam is essential in determining changes as ICP increases.

7. Position of the bed in a client with increased ICP should be:
   A. Flat
   B. Trendelenburg
   C. 90-degree angle head of bed (HOB)
   D. 30- to 45-degree angle HOB

7. Answer: D
Maintenance of the HOB at a 30- to 45-degree angle promotes venous return and decreases cerebral blood volume.

8. A ventriculostomy drain insertion is performed to:
   A. Decrease client's respiratory rate
   B. Decrease client's temperature
   C. Allow for drainage of CSF and immediately reduce increased ICP
   D. Remove brain tissue to reduce increased ICP

8. Answer: C
A ventriculostomy is an emergency intervention in which a burr hole is made in the skull and a catheter is inserted in the anterior horn of the lateral ventricle. This procedure allows for controlled drainage of CSF and decreases ICP.

9. The etiology of the *majority* of brain tumors is:
   A. Sex
   B. Age
   C. Race
   D. Unknown

9. Answer: D
Although some tumors are classified as congenital or hereditary, the etiology of the majority of brain tumors is unknown.

10. The symptoms of Cushing's triad, a late sign of increased ICP, are:
    A. Increased pulse, decreased systolic blood pressure, narrow pulse pressure
    B. Rising systolic blood pressure, dropping diastolic blood pressure, abnormal respirations, bradycardia
    C. Normal blood pressure, rapid pulse, narrow pulse pressure
    D. Normal pulse, low systolic pressure, high diastolic pressure

10. Answer: B
Cushing's triad is a late finding, and the client is usually comatose. The symptoms include a widening of the pulse pressure (an increased systolic and a decreased diastolic blood pressure), bradycardia, and abnormal respirations.

REFERENCES

Adam RD, Victor M: Neurology, 4th ed. New York: McGraw-Hill, 1989.

Barker E: Neuroscience Nursing. St. Louis, MO: CV Mosby, 1994.

Bendal BA, Sowaya R, Leavens ME, Lee JJ: Surgical treatment of multiple brain metastases. J Neurosurg 79:210–216, 1993.

Betz CL, Hunsberger M, Wright S: Family Centered Nursing Care of Children, 2nd ed. Philadelphia: WB Saunders Co, 1994.

Gross J, Johnson BL: Handbook of Oncology Nursing. Boston: Jones and Bartlett, 1994.

Hickey JV: The Clinical Practice of Neurological and Neurosurgical Nursing, 3rd ed. Philadelphia: JB Lippincott, 1992.

Lord J, Coleman EA: Chemotherapy for glioblastoma multiforme. J Neurosci Nurs 230(1):68–70, 1991.

Otto SE: Oncology Nursing, 2nd ed. St. Louis, MO: CV Mosby, 1994.

Rising CJ: The relationship of selected nursing activities to ICP. J Neurosci Nurs 25(5):302–307, 1993.

Tierney LM, McPhee SJ, Papadaleis MA: Current Medical Diagnoses and Treatment. Norwalk, CT: Appleton and Lange, 1995.

Wegmann JA, Hakiner P: Central Nervous System Cancers in Cancer Nursing: Principles and Practice, 2nd ed. Boston: Jones and Bartlett, 1990.

Werner WJ, Goetz CG: Neurology for the Non-Neurologist. Philadelphia: JB Lippincott, 1994.

CHAPTER 27

LACTIC ACIDOSIS—Type B

Anna M. Pignanelli, BSN, RN, C

AND

Michelle Budzinski-Braunscheidel, BSN, RN, C

CHAPTER OBJECTIVES

At the completion of this chapter, the reader will be able to:

Differentiate between type A and type B lactic acidosis.

Review the possible etiologies of type B lactic acidosis associated with malignancy.

Describe nursing care, including the initial and ongoing nursing assessments, of oncology clients experiencing type B lactic acidosis secondary to malignancy.

Review the rationale for the medical treatments of type B lactic acidosis associated with malignancy.

Discuss the prognosis of oncology clients with type B lactic acidosis secondary to malignancy and relate it to future care needs.

OVERVIEW

TYPE B lactic acidosis is a very rare metabolic complication that occurs in both adult and pediatric clients with malignancies. Unlike type A lactic acidosis, type B lactic acidosis is not associated with tissue hypoperfusion or hypoxia as occurs with shock or cardiac arrest but is rather the result of anaerobic glycolysis. Type B lactic acidosis is characterized by a pH ≤ 7.35 and an arterial blood lactate level of ≥ 5 mEq/L (≥ 5 mmol/L SI Units). Blood gases are reflective of a metabolic acidosis. Typically the presenting symptoms include changes in mental status and hyperventilation. Type B lactic acidosis is generally a complication of advanced oncologic disease, but it has also occurred as the presenting symptom, and this should be noted. The prognosis is based on the client's response to treatment of the underlying disease. A review of the case studies in the literature, for both adult and pediatric clients, indicate that treatment using combination chemotherapy yields the best prognosis for clients with type B lactic acidosis secondary to malignancy.

DESCRIPTION

Lactic acidosis was first defined in 1961 by Huckabee, and in 1976, Cohen and Woods further defined lactic acidosis into two classifications, type A and type B (as cited in Stacpoole, 1993). Type B lactic acidosis is a very rare finding and a rare metabolic complication in the oncology client. Although generally associated with advanced disease, type B lactic acidosis has been reported to occur as the presenting symptom of malignancy. Therefore, it is imperative for the practitioner to understand the difference between type A and type B lactic acidosis, although most certainly either of these conditions and their related etiologies may affect the oncology client. This chapter will focus on type B lactic acidosis secondary to the malignancy.

Type A versus type B

Lactic acidosis is defined as a pH ≤ 7.35 and an arterial blood lactate level ≥ 5 mEq/L (≥ 5 mmol/L SI Units). An increased anion gap is present, and blood gases will reflect a metabolic acidosis. In addition to the pH being ≤ 7.35, the bicarbonate level will be below normal (< 24 mEq/dl, < 24 mmol/L SI Units), and the $PaCO_2$ will be within normal range unless the lungs are compensating by hyperventilation (normal $PaCO_2$ is 35 to 45 mmHg, 4.7 to 5.0 kPa SI Units). Type A lactic acidosis is caused by tissue hypoxia or poor tissue perfusion. The etiologies of type A lactic acidosis include shock (cardiogenic, septic), cardiac arrest, severe anemia, congestive heart failure, carbon monoxide poisoning, pheochromocytoma, and catecholamines. Type B lactic acidosis has a variety of causes or etiologies; however, none of them are associated with inadequate tissue oxygenation. Examples of these are diabetic ketoacidosis, renal failure, liver failure, infections, drugs (i.e., theophylline or cocaine), exercise, and malignancies. Diarrhea can also result in lactic acidosis as a result of loss of bicarbonate from the gastrointestinal (GI) tract. In clients with insulin-dependent diabetes mellitus (IDDM), type B lactic acidosis is caused by insulin deficiency, in liver disease by decreased lactate clearance by the liver, and in renal failure by accumulation of volatile acids. Type B lactic acidosis has unclear etiologies when associated with malignancy in clients without perfusion problems. In malignancy, type B lactic acidosis is postulated to be associated with lactate production by malignant cells, but the association is not clear. Nonetheless, when oncology clients are being assessed for type B lactic acidosis secondary to malignancy, other etiologies should be ruled out.

Lactate production

Lactate is produced by the skin, muscles, brain, erythrocytes, leukocytes, and platelets and is the end product of anaerobic glycolysis. The serum lactate level reflects the balance between production and elimination of lactate. Both the kidneys and liver eliminate lactate. The liver has a huge physiologic reserve for eliminating lactate and is responsible for about 70% of the elimination of daily lactate production, while the kidney handles the rest (Thomas and Dodhia, 1991). Lactate is taken up by the kidney and liver and transformed into glucose via gluconeogenesis. The normal rate of lactate production is in the estimated range of 1290 mEq/L/day.

Etiologies of type B lactic acidosis secondary to malignancy

The etiologies of type B lactic acidosis secondary to malignancy remain obscure and difficult to elucidate. One suggestion is that type B lactic acidosis occurs from an overproduction of and an underutilization of lactate. Many clients with type B lactic acidosis have hematologic malignancies, while others have solid tumors with or without liver metastasis. Following are some explanations that have been offered for type B lactic acidosis in the oncology client, but all remain theoretical.

1. When there is a large tumor mass, or tightly packed bone marrow, anaerobic glycolysis occurs because of decreased oxygenation to the area producing lactate (Ellis, 1985).
2. Microvascular aggregates of leukocytes and leukostasis result in decreased blood flow, causing local tissue hypoxia and anaerobic metabolism (Ellis, 1985).
3. Liver metastasis may result in the accumulation of lactate due to decreased uptake by the liver (Ellis, 1985).
4. In the laboratory under hypoxic conditions, leukemic and lymphomatous cells can produce lactate. Interestingly, acute leukemic cells produce more lactate than chronic myelogenous leukemic cells. This phenomenon may explain why type B lactic acidosis is more common in acute leukemias (Sculier, Nicaise, and Klastersky, 1983). It, however, does not explain the rarity of tumor-induced type B lactic acidosis (Rose, 1994). It is important to note that not all clients with type B lactic acidosis have a heavy tumor burden or liver metastasis.

Pediatrics: Type B lactic acidosis secondary to malignancy has been reported in pediatric clients but is very rare. A case of type B lactic acidosis has occurred secondary to thiamine deficiency from total parenteral nutrition (TPN) (Oriot, Wood, Gottesman, and Huault, 1991), and this should be considered. Acute lymphocytic leukemia in children has been associated with type B lactic acidosis (Field, Block, Levin, and Rall, 1966) as well as Burkitt's lymphoma (Révész, Obeid, and Mpofu, 1995).

RISK PROFILE

This risk profile is specific to type B lactic acidosis secondary to malignancy.

Cancers: Acute myelogenous leukemia, breast, colon, small and large cell lung, Hodgkin's and non-Hodgkin's lymphoma, multiple myeloma, osteogenic sarcomas, oat cell cancer of the lung, acute lymphocytic leukemia, all malignancies.

Pediatrics: ALL, lymphosarcoma, Burkitt's lymphoma.

Conditions: Liver metastasis.

Pediatrics: Thiamine deficiency while on TPN.

Environment: None.

Foods: None.

Drugs: None.

PROGNOSIS

The prognosis for clients experiencing type B lactic acidosis secondary to malignancy is varied and depends on the rapid identification of the cause of lactic acidosis and subsequent cytoreductive therapy. Treatment should not be directed toward the acidosis but, rather, at the underlying cause, which is the malignancy. The symptomatic treatment of acidemia has proved unsuccessful. If there is a poor response to cytoreductive therapy, the acidemia will continue, and the outcome will be poor. Conversely, if the tumor mass is decreased, then the prognosis can be favorable. Many clients with type B lactic acidosis from malignancy require prompt intensive medical and nursing interventions. Type B lactic acidosis can result in a comatose and ventilatory-dependent client. Type B lactic acidosis can also recur if the client has a relapse. The prognosis remains the same for clients experiencing recurrence of their malignancy and lactic acidosis. Clients can have a regression of type B lactic acidosis if there is a positive response to cytoreductive therapy.

Pediatrics: The prognosis is the same as for adult clients.

TREATMENT

The overall goal when treating type B lactic acidosis secondary to malignancy is to treat the underlying cause, which is the cancer.

Surgery: For removal of tumor mass if indicated.

Chemotherapy: Combination chemotherapy for the specific malignancy.

Radiation: As an adjunct to chemotherapy or surgery.

Medications: The use of IV sodium bicarbonate as a treatment remains controversial. If the underlying cause of the lactic acidosis is not found and treated, bicarbonate therapy results in only a transient, if any, improvement, and may actually make the condition worse. In addition, IV sodium bicarbonate has been found not to improve the hemodynamics of critically ill clients with metabolic acidosis and increased blood lactate levels (Cooper, Walley, Wiggs, and Russell, 1990). Treatment toward a positive outcome must be directed toward the malignancy and not the acidosis. Nonetheless, the use of sodium bicarbonate as a therapy is felt, by some, to buy time to treat the underlying cause (Mizock, 1987), and the need should be evaluated on an individual basis.

Procedures

Placement of a central line or long-line catheter for chemotherapy, IV fluids, and blood transfusions.

Arterial line placement for intensive care unit (ICU) clients for arterial blood gases (ABGs) and other laboratory tests.

Other: For severe acidosis and for clients who are compensating via hyperventilation, be alert for respiratory fatigue and the need for subsequent ventilatory support.

ASSESSMENT CRITERIA: LACTIC ACIDOSIS

Vital signs

Temperature	Normal, but assess elevations due to infections or sepsis, which can cause type A lactic acidosis.
Pulse	Tachycardia
Respirations	Shortness of breath, dyspnea, or tachypnea can progress to compensatory hyperventilation, Kussmaul's breathing, or respiratory muscle fatigue.
Blood pressure	Hypotension systolic blood pressure <90 mmHg
Pulmonary artery catheter	Normal cardiac function
Pulse oximetry	Normal

History

Symptoms, conditions	Changes in respiratory rate/patterns, dyspnea, hyperventilation.
	Changes in mental status, lethargy, confusion, disorientation, somnolence, coma.
	Hematologic malignancies, solid tumors with or without liver metastasis.
	Advanced disease.
	History of previous episodes of type B lactic acidosis secondary to malignancy.
	Recurrence of the malignancy.

Hallmark physical signs and symptoms	Changes in mental status, hyperventilation, lethargy.

Additional physical signs and symptoms	Headache, disturbed perception, mental dullness, loss of coordination, myalgia, hepatomegaly.

ASSESSMENT CRITERIA: LACTIC ACIDOSIS (continued)

Psychosocial signs	Disorientation, confusion, anxiety, due to respiratory distress.

Lab values	
ABGs	Reflective of a metabolic acidosis pH ≤7.35.
PaO$_2$	Normal
PaCO$_2$	Normal, but may be decreased if lungs are compensating.
Bicarbonate	Low <22 mEq/L (<22 mmol/L SI Units).
Blood lactate	Hyperlactemia ≥5 mEq/L (≥5 mmol/L SI Units).
Liver function tests	May or may not be normal. If liver metastasis is present:
Alkaline phosphatase	Increased
Acid phosphatase	Increased
Alanine aminotransferase (ALT) (serum glutamic pyruvic transaminase) (SGPT)	Increased
Aspartate aminotransferase (AST) (serum glutamic-oxaloacetic transaminase) (SGOT)	Increased
Lactate dehydrogenase (LD), total, LD$_4$, LD$_5$	Increased
Aldolase	Increased
Gamma glutamyl transpeptidase (GGTP)	Increased
5′ Nucleotidase	Increased
Leucine aminopeptidase	Increased
Renal function tests (urea nitrogen, blood, serum creatinine)	Normal
Anion gap	Increased
Blood cultures	Negative
Thiamine	Normal

Diagnostic tests	
Abdominal CT scan	May or may not show liver metastasis.

Other	
Abdominal assessment	May or may not reveal hepatomegaly.

NURSING DIAGNOSIS

The following are potential nursing diagnoses for clients experiencing type B lactic acidosis secondary to malignancy.

Breathing pattern, ineffective, related to respiratory compensation for metabolic acidosis.

Confusion, acute, related to cerebral lactic acidosis buildup causing increased intracranial pressure (ICP). A buildup of lactate acid in the brain causes a localized acidosis. An increase in hydrogen ion concentration increases vasodilation and increases ICP (by a process of metabolic autoregulation).

Injury, risk for, related to changes in mental status associated with metabolic acidosis.

Physical mobility, impaired, related to cognitive impairment, impaired coordination, and changes in mental status/level of consciousness (LOC).

Nutrition, altered, less than body requirements related to inability to eat associated with changes in mental status and altered breathing pattern.

Knowledge deficit related to unfamiliarity with complication and prognosis.

Grieving anticipatory, related to perceived potential loss of physical well-being.

NURSING INTERVENTIONS

Nursing and medical interventions are based on the treatment of the malignancy primarily, and supportive therapy is based on the condition of the client.

Immediate nursing interventions

Assess neurologic status q1h.
Assess respiratory rate, rhythm, depth q1h.
Assess blood pressure, pulse, temperature q1h × 4, then q4h, if stable.
Auscultate lung sounds.
Establish IV access and obtain volumetric infusion pump.
Prepare for central line or long-line catheter access for chemotherapy.
Monitor for respiratory muscle fatigue.
Elevate head of bed 30 degrees.
Insert indwelling catheter, measure intake and output (I and O) q1h × 4, then q4h.
Continuous pulse oximetry.
Initiate safety precautions, with frequent monitoring.
Place suction equipment at bedside.
Send STAT ABGs, electrolyte panel, serum lactate levels.

Anticipated physician orders and interventions

Diagnostic studies for malignancy workup.
Combination chemotherapy particular to the tumor, malignancy involved.
Initiate surgery or radiation therapy, if necessary, to reduce tumor mass.
Assess cardiac function to rule out type A lactic acidosis.
Lab work: renal function tests; liver function tests; glucose; blood cultures to rule out sepsis; urine cultures, sputum cultures, and toxicology screen (salicylates, methanol, ethanol, cocaine).

Thiamine level for clients on TPN without thiamine.

Calculation of anion gap (Chernecky and Berger, 1997):

$$\text{Anion Gap} = (Na^+) - (Cl^- + HCO_3^-)$$

$$OR$$

$$= (Na^+ + K^+) - (Cl^- + HCO_3^-)$$

Insertion of arterial line (possibly) for ABGs.

Chest x-ray.

Oxygen therapy—possible intubation.

IV sodium bicarbonate therapy.

Ongoing nursing assessment, monitoring, and interventions

Assess:
- Neurologic status plus LOC q4h and PRN.
- Respirations for rate, rhythm, depth.
- Lung sounds q4h.
- IV site/central line site for redness.
- Monitor client for side effects of chemotherapy.
- Blood gases and lactate level for improvement of metabolic acidosis.

Measure:
- Temperature, pulse, blood pressure, respirations q4h.
- I and O q4–8h.

Send:
- Blood sample for lactate level and ABGs.
- Blood sample for electrolyte levels for use in calculating the client's anion gap.

Implement:
- Safety precautions.
- Nutritional support.

TEACHING/EDUCATION

Depending on the condition of the client, teaching may need to be directed to a family member or significant other.

Changes in mental status or level of consciousness: *Rationale:* The brain is very sensitive to any increase in body acids. When these acids are increased, persons can become confused. They may not know their name, where they are, or the date or time. In addition, they may not be able to do normal daily activities or become tired, sleepy, or difficult to wake.

Changes in respiratory pattern: *Rationale:* The level of acid in your body has affected how fast and how deep you breathe. Your lungs are helping your body to change the amount of acid in it. When you breathe faster and deeper, more carbon dioxide (CO_2) is eliminated from the body, helping to decrease the level of acid.

Chemotherapy/surgery/radiation: *Rationale:* In order to bring your body back to a normal, nonacid environment, the cause has to be treated. The cause is the cancer. Chemotherapy will help to shrink your tumor (or cause remission of the leukemia). Generally, once the amount of tumor is decreased (or the leukemia is in remission), the acid environment will resolve, your breathing will return to normal, and you won't be sleepy, tired, or forgetful. In addition, your doctor may also recommend surgery or radiation to help bring your body back to a normal, nonacid state.

Blood sampling: *Rationale:* Several blood samples will be taken daily to monitor the amount of lactate in the body. Your body continues to produce blood at a regular rate to replace the samples.

IV line/central line/arterial line: *Rationale:* The IV lines allow us to draw blood samples as well as provide fluids to you. If the doctor orders chemotherapy, it can be given through these lines, also.

Frequent respiratory assessments/oxygen therapy: *Rationale:* It is necessary for us to evaluate your breathing frequently and listen to your lungs. The oxygen was prescribed by your doctor to help make you comfortable.

Ventilator: *Rationale:* Owing to the acid state of the body and the rapid breathing of your loved one, his or her respiratory muscles become tired or weak, and the ventilator is helping him or her to breathe.

Prognosis: The nurse will be part of the team working with the family, physician, social worker, and chaplain in supporting the client. *Rationale:* If the tumor/leukemia responds well to treatment, there can be a good outcome. If the tumor or leukemia does not respond well to treatment, the outcome can be poor.

Signs and symptoms of lactic acidosis type B secondary to malignancy: *Rationale:* This acid state can recur, so it is important for you and your significant others to watch for any signs and symptoms. These include changes in how you breathe, such as shortness of breath, difficulty in breathing, or breathing too quickly. Other symptoms include confusion, being sleepy, feeling disoriented, or not waking up. If any of these symptoms occur, your doctor should be called.

EVALUATION/DESIRED OUTCOMES

The time frames for the desired outcomes depend on the type of malignancy and how responsive it is to cytoreductive treatment, as well as on the client's condition.

1. The solid tumor is decreased, or remission of hematologic malignancy occurs.

2. Blood gases:
   pH returns to between 7.35 to 7.45.
   PaO_2 within normal limits.
   $PaCO_2$ within normal limits.
   Bicarbonate, serum level, within normal limits.
3. Blood lactate < 5 mEq/L (< 5 mmol/L SI Units).
4. Anion gap is within normal limits.
5. Client's mental status returns to baseline.
6. Respiratory rate is 12 to 20/minute with normal breathing pattern.
7. Lung sounds are clear to auscultation.
8. The client is free of injury.
9. The client is able to ingest oral nutrition and meet nutritional needs.
10. The signs and symptoms of type B lactic acidosis secondary to malignancy are understood by the client and family (significant others).
11. If a long-line catheter or central line or IV remains in the client, the client and/or significant other verbalize and demonstrate care.

DISCHARGE PLANNING

The client with type B lactic acidosis secondary to malignancy may need:

Home care or hospice, based on the severity of the malignancy and general condition of the client.
Short-term home nursing visits for line care.
Training of the client and/or significant others in line care.
Education about the signs and symptoms of type B lactic acidosis.
Education about the signs and symptoms of chemotherapy or radiation treatment side effects.
If surgery is performed, care for the incisional wound.

FOLLOW-UP CARE

Anticipated care

Physician office visit within 1 to 2 weeks.
Outpatient blood work as indicated, i.e., blood gas analysis and lactate level.
Possible continued chemotherapy treatments and/or radiation therapy.
For clients discharged home, home nursing visits for line care and further instructions about line care as needed.

Anticipated client/family question and possible answer:

Will this problem with acid in my body occur again?
"It is possible that you can experience this problem again. Sometimes when

cancer recurs the acid can build up in your body. This is why it is important for you and your significant others to know the signs and symptoms of acid accumulation in your body."

CHAPTER SUMMARY

Type B lactic acidosis is a rare metabolic complication of malignancy that occurs in both the adult and pediatric populations. This oncologic emergency, unless recognized and treated, will be fatal. It is generally a complication of advanced disease but can occur as the presenting symptom of malignancy. Unlike type A lactic acidosis, type B lactic acidosis is not the result of tissue hypoxia or hypoperfusion, but rather the result of a malignancy. It is generally accepted that lactic acidosis is present when the pH is ≤7.35 and the blood lactate is ≥5 mEq/L (≥5 mmol/L SI Units). Treatment for this oncologic complication is always directed toward the underlying cause of the lactic acidosis. Because of the rarity of the complication, it is important for the clinician to recognize the hallmark signs and symptoms of lactic acidosis, which are changes in mental status and changes in respiratory pattern. In addition, other causes of lactic acidosis, either type A or type B, should be ruled out, and prompt treatment of the malignancy and supportive care of the client begun. The prognosis and follow-up care are based on the severity of the malignancy and the client's response to cytoreductive therapy.

TEST QUESTIONS

1. Type A lactic acidosis can be the result of:
   A. Diabetic ketoacidosis
   B. Liver failure
   C. Shock
   D. Exercise

1. Answer: C
Type A lactic acidosis has as its etiology tissue hypoxia or hypoperfusion that are the result of shock. Type B lactic acidosis has multiple etiologies, but none of them are due to hypoperfusion. Malignancy is one etiology for type B lactic acidosis.

2. Signs and symptoms of type B lactic acidosis secondary to malignancy include:
   A. Shallow, slow respirations and a pH ≥7.35
   B. Positive blood cultures
   C. An increased blood lactate level ≥5 mEq/L and hyperactivity
   D. Hyperventilation and lethargy

2. Answer: D
Hyperventilation occurs as the lungs attempt to compensate for the metabolic acidosis, and mental status is altered owing to the acidic environment of the brain.

3. The prognosis of the oncologic emergency of type B lactic acidosis secondary to malignancy is:
   A. Based on the client's response to cytoreductive therapy
   B. Always fatal
   C. 25% if the acidosis is treated within 1 hour
   D. More favorable if liver metastasis is not present

3. Answer: A
Treatment is always aimed at the malignancy, and the prognosis is based on the client's response to cytoreductive treatment.

4. Treatment of type B lactic acidosis secondary to malignancy should always include:
   A. Radiation therapy to the chest wall
   B. Chemotherapy
   C. Ventilatory support
   D. Antibiotics

4. Answer: B
A review of the case studies of the literature for both adult and pediatric clients indicate that treatment using combination chemotherapy yields the best prognosis for clients with type B lactic acidosis secondary to malignancy.

5. Type B lactic acidosis can be the result of:
   A. Shock
   B. Congestive heart failure
   C. Severe anemia
   D. Malignancy

5. Answer: D
Shock, congestive heart failure, and severe anemia result in tissue hypoxia or hypoperfusion, causing type A lactic acidosis. Type B lactic acidosis is not associated with perfusion problems. In the case of malignancy, it is postulated that the malignant cells are the cause of increased lactate production.

6. The primary nursing diagnosis for clients experiencing type B lactic acidosis secondary to malignancy is:
   A. Potential for infection
   B. Fluid volume deficit
   C. Breathing pattern ineffective
   D. Grieving, anticipatory

6. Answer C
In an attempt to compensate for metabolic acidosis, clients will hyperventilate and can become ventilatory dependent from respiratory muscle fatigue.

7. Lactate is:
   A. The end product of anaerobic glycolysis
   B. An enzyme produced by the liver
   C. A colony stimulating factor produced by the kidney
   D. A metabolic end product of angiogenesis

7. Answer: A
Lactate is produced by the skin, brain, muscles, and blood cells and is the end product of anaerobic glycolysis.

8. Type B lactic acidosis secondary to malignancy:
   A. Occurs only in clients with liver metastasis
   B. Can occur with any malignancy
   C. Commonly occurs in solid tumor sarcomas
   D. Occurs only in clients with elevated serum creatinine levels

8. Answer: B
Type B lactic acidosis secondary to malignancy can occur with any cancer, although a review of the literature suggests that it occurs most commonly with hematologic malignancies.

9. An arterial line may be placed in the client with lactic acidosis to:
   A. Instill chemotherapy
   B. Administer IV fluids
   C. Obtain blood gas specimens
   D. Prevent potential pneumothorax

9. Answer: C
An arterial line is placed in the client for purposes of monitoring as well as obtaining blood gases and other arterial (not venous) laboratory blood samples that may be necessary.

10. An immediate nursing intervention for a client with lactic acidosis associated with malignancy would be to assess:
    A. I and O output daily
    B. Serum sodium values q4h
    C. Urine pH q2h
    D. Neurologic status q1h

10. Answer: D
Assessment of neurologic status is important to determine the client's condition and the success of the associated treatment.

REFERENCES

Afshan AA, Flombaum CD, Brochstein JA, Gillio AP, Brussel JB, Boulad F: Lactic acidosis and renal enlargement at diagnosis and relapse of acute lymphoblastic leukemia. J Pediatr 125:584–586, 1994.

Brambilla McFarland M, Moeller Grant M: Nursing Implications of Laboratory Tests, 3rd ed. New York: Delmar Publishers, 1994.

Casper CB, Oelz O: Lactic acidosis in malignant lymphoma. Am J Med 91:197–198, 1991.

Chernecky CC, Berger B (eds): Laboratory Tests and Diagnostic Procedures, 2nd ed. Philadelphia: WB Saunders Co, 1997.

Cooper DJ, Walley KR, Wiggs BR, Russell JA: Bicarbonate does not improve hemodynamics in critically ill patients who have lactic acidosis: A prospective, controlled clinical study. Ann Intern Med 112(7):492–498, 1990.

Doolittle GC, Wurster MW, Rosenfeld CS, Bodensteiner DC: Malignancy induced lactic acidosis. South Med J 81(4):533–536, 1988.

Ellis RW: Breast cancer and lactic acidosis: An unusual metabolic complication. Minn Med 68:441–442, 1985.

Evans JR, Stein RC, Ford HT, Gazet JC, Chamberlain GV, Coombs RC: Lactic acidosis: A presentation of metastatic breast cancer arising in pregnancy. Cancer 69(2):453–456, 1992.

Field M, Block JB, Levin R, Rall DP: Significance of blood lactate elevations among patients with acute leukemia and other neoplastic proliferative disorders. Am J Med 40:528–547, 1966.

Fraley DS, Adler S, Bruns FJ, Zett B: Stimulation of lactate production by administration of bicarbonate in a patient with a solid neoplasm and lactic acidosis. New Engl J Med 303(19):1100–1102, 1980.

Mizock BA: Controversies in lactic acidosis: Implications in critically ill patients. J Am Med Assoc 258(4):497–501, 1987.

Mizock BA, Glass J: Lactic acidosis in a patient with multiple myeloma. West J Med 161(4):417–418, 1994.

Nadiminti Y, Wang JC, Chou S, Pineles E, Tobin M: Lactic acidosis associated with Hodgkin's disease: Response to chemotherapy. New Engl J Med 303(1):15–17, 1980.

Oriot D, Wood C, Gottesman R, Huault G: Severe lactic acidosis related to acute thiamine deficiency. J Parenter Enter Nutr 15:105–109, 1991.

Raju R, Kardinal CG: Lactic acidosis in lung cancer. South Med J 76(3):397–398, 1983.

Révész T, Obeid K, Mpofu C: Severe lactic acidosis and renal involvement in a patient with relapsed Burkitt's lymphoma. Pediatr Hematol Oncol 12:283–288, 1995.

Rice K, Schwartz SH: Lactic acidosis with small cell carcinoma: Rapid response to chemotherapy. Am J Med 79:501–503, 1985.

Rose DB: Clinical Physiology of Acid-Base and Electrolyte Disorders, 4th ed. New York: McGraw-Hill, 1994.

Sculier JP, Nicaise C, Klastersky J: Lactic acidosis: A metabolic complication of extensive metastastic cancer. Eur J Clin Oncol 19:597–601, 1983.

Sing RF, Branas CA, Sing RF: Bicarbonate therapy in the treatment of lactic acidosis: Medicine or toxin? J Am Osteopath Assoc 95(1):52–57, 1995.

Stacpoole PW: Lactic acidosis. Endocrinol Metabol Clin North Am 22(2):221–245, 1993.

Thomas CR, Dodhia N: Common emergencies in cancer medicine: Metabolic syndromes. J Natl Med Assoc 83(9):809–818, 1991.

Vincent Corbett J: Laboratory Tests and Diagnostic Procedures with Nursing Diagnosis, 3rd ed. Norwalk, CT: Appleton and Lange, 1992.

CHAPTER 28

LAMBERT-EATON MYASTHENIC SYNDROME

Carol S. Potter, RN, MS, AOCN

CHAPTER OBJECTIVES

At the completion of this chapter, the reader will be able to:

Explain the pathophysiology of the Lambert-Eaton myasthenic syndrome (LEMS).

Describe the major signs and symptoms of LEMS in relation to its pathophysiology.

Anticipate the diagnostic procedures that identify LEMS and prepare the client.

Describe the nursing care of the client with LEMS.

Plan for ongoing care of the client with LEMS.

OVERVIEW

LEMS occurs as the result of an autoimmune attack against the voltage gated calcium channels at the neuromuscular junction, causing proximal muscle weakness, hyporeflexia, and autonomic dysfunction. Clinically, the syndrome may resemble myasthenia gravis. This rare syndrome was first reported by Anderson, Churchill-Davidson, and Richardson in 1953 as an abnormal neuromuscular transmission occurring concomitantly in a 47-year-old man with oat cell carcinoma of the lung (cited in Sanders, 1994). Three years later, Lambert, Eaton, and Rooke (1956) reported three clients with neuromuscular transmission defects and lung cancer. The syndrome thereafter was referred to as the Lambert-Eaton (or Eaton-Lambert) myasthenic syndrome.

Approximately 3 to 6% of clients with small cell lung cancer (SCLC) will be diagnosed with LEMS. O'Neill and his colleagues reported a series of 50 clients with LEMS in which 21 of the 25 with cancer had SCLC (O'Neill, Murray, and Newsom-Davis, 1988). Of all clients with LEMS 60% have SCLC (Darnell, 1996). Malignant tumors never develop in about 30% of clients. Most tumors are evident within 2 years of the diagnosis of LEMS, with a latency period of 3.8 years reported. Among those who are tumor-free, there is an increased frequency of organ-specific antibodies and autoimmune diseases such as thyroiditis, pernicious anemia, systemic lupus erythematosus, and antibody-positive myasthenia gravis (Scully, Mark, McNeely, and McNeely, 1994). The average age at diagnosis is 60 years, but the syndrome does occur rarely in children and all other adult age groups. The paraneoplastic form more typically develops in middle-aged to elderly clients (McEvoy, 1994). Recently showing less predominance due to the increased number of female smokers, men with LEMS still outnumber women 2 to 1. There tends to be a female predominance among LEMS clients with primary autoimmune disorders (Sanders, 1994).

DESCRIPTION

LEMS is a disorder of the neuromuscular junction. It can be paraneoplastic or a primary autoimmune disorder. The neuromuscular junction (NMJ) is the area of contact between nerve and muscle fibers. It is a chemical synapse (connection) that consists of an axon (the terminal end of the nerve fiber that conducts an impulse away from the nerve cell body to another tissue), a muscle cell endplate with a folded postsynaptic membrane, and a synaptic cleft (the space between the nerve and muscle cells). It is through this space, or synapse, that an impulse is sent from one cell to another. This impulse is called an action potential. This action potential stimulates calcium entry into the axon, causing acetylcholine (Ach), a neurotransmitter substance, to be released from vesicles in the presynaptic nerve fiber. The vesicles are clustered under active zones that consist of double parallel rows of large intramembrane particles. These particles form the voltage gated calcium channels that mediate the release of Ach. Ach then diffuses across the synaptic cleft and binds to the Ach receptors in the junctional folds of the muscle cell endplate. This process concludes with muscle contraction (Scully et al., 1994; Maselli, 1994; Sanders, 1993).

The pathophysiologic mechanism of LEMS is an autoimmune antibody-mediated destruction of the presynaptic voltage gated calcium channels (VGCCs) (Scully et al., 1994). In the case of a malignancy, the tumor antibodies cross-react with the VGCCs of the NMJ. The mechanism in nonmalignant cases is unclear, but the physiologic behavior is the same (Scully et al., 1994). Antibodies bind to the active zone particles that form the VGCCs, causing clumping and disorganization of the particles. This clumping and disorganization causes a decrease in the amount of calcium allowed through the channels as well as a decrease in the number of Ach particles available to be released (Maselli, 1994). Because the probability of Ach release is primarily dependent on the amount of available intracellular calcium, decreased calcium availability causes decreased Ach to be released (Scully et al., 1994). In addition, anatomically the NMJ exhibits an increased number of postsynaptic junctional folds (Fukuhara, Takamori, Gutmann, and Chou, 1972). This increases the surface area that Ach must stimulate before an action potential can be initiated. Both the decreased amount of Ach and the increased surface area of the postsynaptic junctional folds contribute to muscle weakness by inhibiting the propagation of the action potential in the muscle fiber.

RISK PROFILE

Cancers: Lung (commonly small cell), non-Hodgkin's lymphoma, mixed parotid tumors, systemic mastocytosis, renal cell (McEvoy, 1994).

Conditions: Genetic tendency to organ-specific autoimmune diseases (e.g., thyroid disease, pernicious anemia, vitiligo, celiac disease, type I diabetes), rheumatoid arthritis, psoriasis, asthma, ulcerative colitis, scleroderma, multiple sclerosis.

Environment: Tobacco use.

Foods: None.

Drugs: None.

PROGNOSIS

Prognosis in those cases of LEMS with an underlying malignancy is related to the success with which that malignancy is treated. Clients responsive to antineoplastic therapy may experience resolution of the syndrome as the activity of the cancer decreases. Chemotherapy produces tumor regression and effective symptom relief in 70 to 90% of clients with SCLC. The median survival for clients with limited disease (confined to the hemithorax, including the ipsilateral supraclavicular lymph nodes) is 12 to 15 months. Clients with extensive disease (metastatic spread) have a median survival of 6 to 9 months. These survival rates refer to clients receiving treatment. For clients without treatment, the median survival is 2 to 3 months from the time of diagnosis (Eisen, Hickish, Sloane, Eccles, and Smith, 1995).

Data regarding prognosis for clients without a malignancy are scarce. In O'Neill's series of 50 clients with LEMS, 25 never developed a malignancy. At the time of his publication, 3 were dead from unrelated causes, 21 were alive at a median time of 6.9 years from the onset of LEMS, and data were unavailable on the twenty-fifth client (O'Neill et al., 1988).

TREATMENT

Surgery: Generally not indicated with a diagnosis of SCLC, as SCLC is characterized by rapid local and metastatic spread (Eisen et al., 1995). If diagnosis of breast, stomach, prostate, or rectal cancer is made, surgery may be indicated to remove the primary tumor and to determine the extent of local disease. In cases without an identified malignancy, there is no role for surgery.

Chemotherapy: Chemotherapy regimens containing one or more of the following drugs: doxorubicin, cisplatin, cyclophosphamide, etoposide, carboplatin, vincristine. In cases without a malignant cause, chemotherapy is not indicated.

Radiation: Rarely indicated except in the case of superior vena cava syndrome or another obstructive malignant pulmonary emergency in SCLC. Radiation therapy is not indicated in cases without an underlying malignancy.

Medications

> Pyridostigmine, guanine hydrochloride, aminopyridines, prednisone, azathioprine, cyclosporine, IV immunoglobulin (IVIG).
>
> Medications to avoid: drugs that compromise neuromuscular transmission, including competitive neuromuscular blocking agents (succinylcholine, d-tubocurarine), nondepolarizing neuromuscular blocking agents (atracurium, cisatracurium, pancuronium, vecuronium), antidysrhythmics (quinine, quinidine, procainamide), antibiotics (aminoglycosides), beta-blockers (propranolol), calcium channel blockers (Sanders, 1994).
>
> (See Counsell, McLeod, and Grant, 1994; Eisen et al., 1995; McEvoy, 1994; Sanders, 1994; Sanders, Howard, and Massey, 1993.)

Procedures: Plasma exchange every day or every other day for 1 to 2 weeks (McEvoy, 1994; Sanders, 1994).

Other: Physical and/or occupational therapy.

ASSESSMENT CRITERIA:
LAMBERT-EATON MYASTHENIC SYNDROME

The signs and symptoms for clients with and without a malignancy are the same.

Vital signs	
Pulse	Normal
Blood pressure	Normal
Respirations	May have decrease in rate and depth if muscles involved in ventilation are affected.
Temperature	Normal

History	
Onset	Slow and insidious over years. Rapid onset over weeks to months is associated with an increased incidence of malignancy.
Strength	Lower extremity weakness with increased weakness in the morning, improving throughout the day; presents with difficulty climbing stairs or rising from a chair; may increase on hot days or after a hot bath or shower. Upper extremity weakness may manifest in activities such as opening jars. Aching, stiff muscles exacerbated by activity or muscle cramping.

(continued)

ASSESSMENT CRITERIA:
LAMBERT-EATON MYASTHENIC SYNDROME (continued)

Gait	Altered gait, beginning as impaired balance and progressing to a waddling gait.
Fatigue	Generalized fatigue: prominent, occurs after protracted exercise but characterized by increased strength after mild exercise.
Other	Dry mouth (80% of clients), constipation, abnormal sweating, blurred vision. Vaginal dryness, erectile failure. Difficulty regaining spontaneous respiratory function after anesthesia (rare presenting symptom).
Hallmark physical signs and symptom	Dry mouth, fatigability, hyporeflexia, muscle weakness (lower >upper extremity, proximal >distal).
Additional physical signs and symptoms	Blurred vision; chewing difficulty; constipation; diplopia; drooping eyelids; head lolling; muscle aches, pain, and stiffness; muscle wasting; numbness/paresthesias of extremities; pain: low back; ptosis; pupillary light reflexes: sluggish; respiratory distress requiring ventilatory support; slurred speech; dysphagia; weakness: jaw, facial muscles, neck, voice.
Psychosocial signs	Anxiety, depression.
Lab values	
Antibody assay	Positive for anti-P/Q-type calcium channel antibodies or organ-specific autoantibodies.
Diagnostic tests	
Repetitive nerve stimulation	Decremental response at low frequencies; incremental response at higher frequencies; amplitude increase of 400% with voluntary contraction compared with resting amplitude characteristic and diagnostic of LEMS.
Single-fiber electromyography	Increased neuromuscular jitter with frequent blocking out of proportion to the severity of weakness.
Conventional EMG	Markedly unstable motor unit action potentials varying in shape with voluntary activation (a manifestation of increased neuromuscular jitter, can be quantified with single-fiber EMG).
Deep tendon reflexes	Decreased or absent.
Chest CT, abdomen/pelvis CT, chest x-ray, MRI of brain	If positive for malignancy, indicates probable cause of LEMS.
Other	Bronchoscopy with endobronchial biopsies and bronchoalveolar washings. Mediastinoscopy for biopsy.
	Assess client's drugs to identify receipt of drugs that interfere with neuromuscular transmission (see list under Treatment section).

NURSING DIAGNOSIS

The following are potential nursing diagnoses for clients with LEMS.

(Potential for) injury related to muscle weakness and impaired balance.

Activity intolerance related to muscle weakness and fatigability.

(Potential for) ineffective individual coping related to loss of function and new diagnosis of malignancy.

Knowledge deficit related to diagnosis of malignancy and neuromuscular disorder.

Inability to sustain spontaneous ventilation related to weakness affecting the muscles of ventilatory support.

Altered oral mucous membrane related to autonomic dysfunction: dry mouth.

NURSING INTERVENTIONS

Immediate nursing interventions

Assess client's ability to maintain effective ventilation.

Perform baseline neuromuscular and neurologic function assessment.

Assess the client's ability to safely perform ambulation and the activities of daily living.

Assess the client's environment for safety.

Assess autonomic function, specifically, dry mouth, bowel status, and sexual function.

Assess the client's medications to identify any that interfere with neuromuscular transmission (see list under Treatment section). Notify the physician of any such drugs the client has received.

Anticipated physician orders and interventions

Chest x-ray.

Computed tomography (CT) scans of the chest, abdomen, and pelvis: may require oral and/or IV contrast.

Magnetic resonance imaging (MRI) of the brain.

Bronchoscopy/mediastinoscopy.

Electrodiagnostic testing: repetitive nerve stimulation, conventional electromyogram (EMG), single-fiber EMG.

Antibody assays.

Pyridostigmine 30 or 60 mg by mouth (PO) every 4 to 6 hours.

Guanidine hydrochloride 5 to 10 mg/kg/day PO to a maximum dose of 30 mg/kg/day in divided doses.

Aminopyridines (3,4-diaminopyridine) 5 to 25 mg PO 3 to 4 times/day.

Prednisone 60 to 80 mg/day until symptoms improve, then 100 to 120 mg every other day, tapered over weeks to months.

Azathioprine 50 mg/day, increased by 50 mg/day q 3 days to a total of 150 to 200 mg/day.

Cyclosporine 5 to 6 mg/kg/day, divided into 2 doses q12h initially, increased to produce blood levels of 100 to 150 ng/L until maximum response achieved, then tapered.

IVIG: total dose of 2 g/kg over a 2- to 5-day course.

Plasma exchange.

Ongoing nursing assessment, monitoring, and interventions

Assess:
- Patency of airway.
- Neuromuscular and neurologic function.
- Safety factors.
- Emotional coping.
- Side effects of chemotherapy or other medications.
- Response to treatment based on improvement or lack of improvement of symptoms.
- Oral mucous membranes for signs of infection.
- Bowel status for constipation.

Measure:
- I and O if receiving nephrotoxic or bladder-toxic chemotherapy.
- Respiratory rate, rhythm, depth.

Send:
- Repeat antibody assay for calcium channel antibodies or organ-specific autoantibodies.
- Complete blood count (CBC) and electrolytes to monitor effects of chemotherapy.

Implement:
- Steps for MRI of the brain: Prepare the client for the procedure, and if the client is claustrophobic, obtain an order for and administer a sedative.
- Steps for bronchoscopy or mediastinoscopy: Prepare the client for the procedure, and prepare for the administration and monitoring of procedural sedation.
- Steps for electrodiagnostic testing: Prepare the client for potential discomfort during the procedure.
- Administration of chemotherapy: Administer antineoplastics, and instruct the client regarding side effects and self-care management strategies.
- Administration of cholinergics and/or immunosuppressants: Instruct the client on their use and side effects.
- Preparation of the client for the plasma exchange procedure: assure adequate venous access.
- Initiation of safety precautions: provide assistance with the activities of daily living and ambulation.

TEACHING/EDUCATION

Safety precautions/activity assistance: *Rationale:* Because your muscles are weak, you could fall and hurt yourself or even break a bone. Having somebody help you or using this walker or cane will keep you from hurting yourself.

Mouth care: *Rationale:* When your mouth is dry, it is easier for you to get an infection. You need to keep your mouth clean and moist.

Ventilator: *Rationale:* Your muscles are too weak to allow you to breathe on your own. This machine will help you breathe.

Chemotherapy side effects: *Rationale:* Chemotherapy affects cancer cells and normal cells. Because it harms normal cells, you may have hair loss. It is best to shop for a wig or hairpiece before you lose your hair. You can also wear turbans or hats, but it is important to protect your scalp. You may also have fewer white blood cells, the ones that help you to fight infection; fewer red blood cells, so you may have less energy; and fewer platelets, so you may have a higher chance of bleeding. These drugs can also cause harm to your kidneys. You will get a lot of fluid through the IV line to protect your kidneys and your bladder. You will also need to drink a lot of fluid. We will measure how much urine you make to make sure everything is okay. You could also have numbness or tingling in your hands or feet and a change in your hearing. We will ask you about these sensations, because they may determine the amount of drugs we give you.

Chemotherapy initiation: *Rationale:* The symptoms you are having are the result of the cancer. Chemotherapy will treat the cancer, so the symptoms will go away.

Medication initiation (if no malignant source found): *Rationale:* We are not sure why you are having these symptoms. These medications will help make the symptoms better and may help them go away.

Blood tests: *Rationale:* We will take blood to see if there is a substance called an antibody that may tell us why you are having these symptoms. The blood tests will also help us see if you are having side effects from the chemotherapy or other medications.

Plasma exchange: *Rationale:* Two IV lines will be put in. One line allows blood to be removed. This blood goes through a machine that takes away the harmful antibodies that we talked about. The blood without the antibodies then comes back to you through the other IV.

IVIG: *Rationale:* This IV immunoglobulin is being given to you to help your body fight the substances that are causing your symptoms. The nurse will take your blood pressure, pulse, and temperature every 15 minutes to every hour to make sure your body is handling the drug properly.

EVALUATION/DESIRED OUTCOMES

1. The client demonstrates return of spontaneous ventilation.
2. Initiation of chemotherapy regimen within 48 hours of confirmation of SCLC.
3. The client and family or significant others demonstrate knowledge of self-care management of the side effects of chemotherapy or other medications before discharge to home.
4. The home environment is safe for the client at the time of discharge.
5. The client returns to an independent level of functioning in regard to the activities of daily living and ambulation.
6. Coping mechanisms are developed, allowing the client and his or her family to live with the syndrome and underlying malignancy or with the uncertainty of the symptoms if no malignancy is found.
7. The client regains normal bowel and sexual function.
8. The client demonstrates the ability to perform good oral hygiene.

DISCHARGE PLANNING

The LEMS client may need:

Home physical therapy for safety evaluation and strengthening therapy.

Home occupational therapy to maximize the client's ability to function independently.

A visiting nurse to evaluate symptoms, draw lab samples, and evaluate client/family coping.

An intermediate care facility if care cannot be safely managed at home.

Discussion of resuscitation status with focus and immediacy, dependent on the client's disease status and ventilatory function.

Advance Directives and a "Do Not Resuscitate" order.

FOLLOW-UP CARE

Anticipated care

Physician office visit initially in 1 to 2 weeks, then monthly.

Blood work with CBC and electrolytes every 1 to 2 weeks.

Repeat scans after two cycles of chemotherapy if malignancy is present or every 3 to 6 months if no malignancy is found on the initial scans.

Continued physical and occupational therapy as well as visiting nurses until the client's level of functioning is independent.

Anticipated client/family questions and possible answers

Will these symptoms go away?

"If the problem causing these symptoms responds to the treatment, your symptoms should gradually go away over the next couple of months."

Why does physical and occupational therapy have to come to my home?

"We need to make sure your home environment is safe. Physical therapy can help you learn how to move around in your home if the health care team knows how it is set up. Occupational therapy can help you learn to take care of yourself in your own home if the health care team knows how it is set up."

How are these symptoms related to my cancer?

"The cancer makes a substance that attacks the area where your muscles and nerves talk to each other to make your muscles move or contract. Your muscles then get weak. Your muscles control a lot of activities, and that is why you have the other symptoms."

What is causing these symptoms (if a malignancy has not been identified)?

"For some reason, your body is attacking itself in the area where your nerves and muscles talk to each other. This is called an autoimmune attack. When the nerves and the muscles can't talk to each other, you get weak and get the other symptoms you are having."

Why is this syndrome affecting my ability to breathe?

"Breathing is partly controlled by muscles. If the muscles are weak, it is more difficult for you to take a deep breath."

How long will I be on this treatment?

Malignancy present: "You will stay on the chemotherapy until there are no more signs of the cancer and then perhaps undergo a couple of cycles more."

Malignancy not present: "You will be on this treatment as long as it keeps your symptoms away. If your symptoms get worse, a different treatment may be tried."

CHAPTER SUMMARY

LEMS is a disorder of the neuromuscular junction that occurs as a result of a malignancy or an autoimmune disorder. The severity of the symptoms ranges from mild muscular weakness and dry mouth to an inability to breathe independently and perform the activities of daily living. The origin of the disorder in 60% of cases is SCLC and is therefore classified as a paraneoplastic syndrome. In this situation, treatment is successful with chemotherapy, and resolution of the symptoms occurs in a majority of cases. In the other 40% of cases in which an autoimmune disorder is confirmed or suspected, treatment is not so straightforward. The symptoms may be slow to resolve or not resolve at all, and several treatments may need to be attempted.

The effect of this syndrome on the client's quality of life and the overall functioning of the family can be profound. The syndrome often develops quickly over weeks to months, not allowing the client and his or her family to adapt to the changes it causes in lifestyle and function. The client with both LEMS and a malignancy requires much emotional and nursing support to maintain effective coping mechanisms and good quality of life.

TEST QUESTIONS

1. LEMS is paraneoplastic in what percentage of clients?
   A. 10%
   B. 30%
   C. 40%
   D. 60–70%

1. Answer: D
60% present with small cell lung cancer (SCLC); another 10% develop a malignancy later; 30% are unrelated to cancer.

2. Lambert-Eaton myasthenic syndrome can be briefly defined as:
   A. A form of myasthenia gravis
   B. A disorder of the neuromuscular junction
   C. A degenerating muscle syndrome
   D. A disorder of nerve fibers only

2. Answer: B
The symptoms of LEMS mimic those of myasthenia gravis. There is no muscle degeneration, and both the nerve and muscle are involved.

3. LEMS is most commonly seen in which malignancy?
   A. SCLC
   B. Ovarian cancer
   C. Thyroid cancer
   D. Non-SCLC

3. Answer: A
60% of LEMS is seen in SCLC.

4. What is the pathophysiologic mechanism of LEMS?
   A. Destruction of postsynaptic junctional folds
   B. Antibody-mediated destruction of the presynaptic voltage gated calcium channels
   C. Destruction of calcium needed to cause acetylcholine release
   D. Decreased surface area of the postsynaptic junctional folds

4. Answer: B
The surface area of the postsynaptic junctional folds increases, but it is not destroyed. Because there is not enough Ach to cover the increased surface area, an ineffective action potential develops, with a subsequent decrease in muscle contraction. In this process, calcium is not destroyed but depleted, which leads to decreased Ach release.

5. What is the most common environmental factor associated with LEMS?
   A. Asbestos
   B. Tobacco use
   C. Air pollution
   D. Paint fumes

5. Answer: B
Tobacco use is associated with 90% of SCLC.

6. The treatment of choice for a client diagnosed with LEMS and SCLC is:
   A. Surgery
   B. Radiation therapy
   C. Chemotherapy
   D. Biotherapy

6. Answer: C
SCLC responds to chemotherapy in approximately 70 to 90% of clients. SCLC is usually a diffuse tumor for which radiation and surgery are not effective. An exception to this would be limited stage disease.

7. The triad of symptoms in LEMS is:
   A. Hyporeflexia, autonomic dysfunction, muscle weakness
   B. Neuropathy, autonomic dysfunction, muscle weakness
   C. Hyperreflexia, muscle spasm, autonomic dysfunction
   D. Hyperreflexia, autonomic dysfunction, muscle weakness

7. Answer: A
Clients rarely experience neuropathies; reflexes are decreased, and muscles are weak because of inadequate stimulation; muscle spasm is not present.

8. Which electrodiagnostic test is most likely to result in a diagnosis of LEMS?
   A. Electroencephalogram (EEG)
   B. Conventional EMG
   C. Single-fiber EMG
   D. Repetitive nerve stimulation

8. Answer: D
Facilitation > 400% is conclusive evidence for the presence of LEMS. The single-fiber EMG quantifies results better than the conventional EMG, but the single-fiber EMG is not sensitive enough to be conclusive for LEMS. The EEG is not a useful diagnostic test.

9. Which nursing intervention is most important for the chronic care of the client with LEMS?
   A. Performing plasma exchange
   B. Administering chemotherapy
   C. Assistance with options to maximize independent function
   D. Preparing the client for radiation therapy

9. Answer: C
Assistance with options to maximize independence with the activities of daily living and ambulation will provide safety and foster self-esteem. Assistive efforts may include utilizing physical and occupational therapy. The other options are short-term medical interventions.

10. Which baseline nursing assessment will allow definition of treatment response?
    A. Neurologic and neuromuscular assessment
    B. Vital signs
    C. I and O
    D. Results of follow-up CT scans

10. Answer: A
As the client responds to treatment, neurologic and neuromuscular function improve. Vital signs and I and O are assessments related to the treatment itself. CT scan evaluation is a medical interpretation.

REFERENCES

Counsell CE, McLeod M, Grant R: Reversal of subacute paraneoplastic cerebellar syndrome with intravenous immunoglobulin. Neurology 44:1184–1185, 1994.

Darnell RB: Onconeural antigens and the paraneoplastic neurologic disorders: At the intersection of cancer, immunity, and the brain. Proc Natl Acad Sci 93:4529–4536, 1996.

Eisen T, Hickish T, Sloane J, Eccles S, Smith IE: Small cell lung cancer: Grand rounds. Lancet 345:1285–1289, 1995.

Fukuhara N, Takamori M, Gutmann L, Chou S: Eaton-Lambert syndrome: Ultrastructural study of the motor end-plates. Arch Neurol 27:67–78, 1972.

Howard JF, Sanders DB, Massey JM: The electrodiagnosis of myasthenia gravis and the Lambert-Eaton myasthenic syndrome. Neurol Clin North Am 12(2):305–330, 1994.

Lambert EH, Eaton LM, Rooke ED: Defect of neuromuscular conduction associated with malignant neoplasms. Am J Physiol 187(3):612–613, 1956.

Maselli RA: Pathophysiology of myasthenia gravis and Lambert-Eaton syndrome. Neurol Clin North Am 12(2):285–303, 1994.

McEvoy KM: Diagnosis and treatment of Lambert-Eaton myasthenic syndrome. Neurol Clin North Am 12(2):387–399, 1994.

O'Neill JH, Murray NMF, Newsom-Davis J: The Lambert-Eaton myasthenic syndrome: A review of 50 cases. Brain 111:577–596, 1988.

Pelucchi A, Ciceri E, Clementi F, Marazzini L, Foresi A, Sher E: Calcium channel autoantibodies in myasthenic syndrome and small cell lung cancer. Am Rev Respir Dis 147:1229–1232, 1993.

Sanders DB: Lambert-Eaton myasthenic syndrome: Pathogenesis and treatment. Semin Neurol 14(2):111–117, 1994.

Sanders DB: Clinical neurophysiology of disorders of the neuromuscular junction. J Clin Neurophysiol 10(2):167–180, 1993.

Sanders DB, Howard JF, Massey JM: 3,4-Diaminopyridine in Lambert-Eaton myasthenic syndrome and myasthenia gravis. Ann New York Acad Sci 681:588–590, 1993.

Scully RE, Mark EJ, McNeely WF, McNeely BU: Case records of the Massachusetts General Hospital: Case 32-1994. New Engl J Med 331(8):528–535, 1994.

Struthers CS: Lambert-Eaton myasthenic syndrome in small cell lung cancer: Nursing implications. Oncol Nurs Forum 21(4):677–685, 1994.

CHAPTER 29

MALIGNANT ASCITES

Gail Wych Davidson, RN, BSN

AND

Beth Griebel, MSN, RN

CHAPTER OBJECTIVES

At the completion of this chapter, the reader will be able to:

Define malignant ascites.

Describe the signs and symptoms associated with the diagnosis of malignant ascites.

Identify methods of treatment for malignant ascites.

Describe nursing care in the treatment of malignant ascites.

Identify nursing assessments and interventions for the complications of malignant ascites.

OVERVIEW

CLIENTS with end-stage colorectal, gastric, liver, breast, and gynecologic cancer are at risk for developing malignant ascites. Malignant ascites, caused by compromised drainage or hydrodynamic disequilibrium, is a prognostically poor symptom in the cancer trajectory. Treatment options are limited, and none of the therapies available completely resolve the ascites. Comfort and relief of the symptoms are the goals of treatment. Nursing assessment and interventions should emphasize alleviation of physical discomfort and the provision of emotional support for the client and his or her family or significant others. Nursing care should be focused on anticipation of client needs, teaching related to medical treatment options, and facilitation of home health care or hospice referral.

DESCRIPTION

Malignant ascites is a serious prognostic event in the progression of several tumors. These tumors include breast, colorectal, gastric, pancreatic, hepatocellular, and gynecologic cancers (Kehoe, 1991; Baker and Weber, 1993; Fraught,

Kirkpatrick, Krepart, Heywood, and Lotocki, 1995). Metastatic disease to the liver, peritoneal lining, or lung; testicular cancer; or, less frequently, melanoma also lead to malignant ascites (Kehoe, 1991). The pathophysiology of malignant ascites is multifactorial. Invasion of the subdiaphragmatic lymphatic channels and plexuses compromises the drainage of the peritoneal cavity (Feldman and Knapp, 1974). While ascites from cirrhosis of the liver is usually related to excessive fluid formation, some tumors, particularly ovarian, alter humoral factors, which increases capillary leakage of proteins and fluids into the peritoneum (Garrison, Kaelin, Heusser, and Galloway, 1986; Groenwald, Frogge, Goodman, and Yarbro, 1993). When the liver has been extensively replaced by metastatic disease, hydrodynamic disequilibrium occurs due to hypoalbuminemia, portal venous obstruction, or hepatic venous obstruction, and this disequilibrium leads to ascites (Baker and Weber, 1993). Runyon (1994) cites multiple mechanisms for the cause of malignant ascites, including (1) liver metastases and hepatocellular carcinoma occluding the portal venous flow, (2) peritoneal carcinomatosis, (3) combination of peritoneal carcinomatosis and extensive liver metastases, (4) malignant lymph node obstruction with lymph overflow into the peritoneal cavity, and (5) Budd-Chiari syndrome from tumor occluding the hepatic veins.

RISK PROFILE

Cancers: Those at risk for developing malignant ascites include diagnosis of lymphoma, breast, ovarian, colorectal, gastric, pancreatic, hepatobiliary, and uterine cancers (Baker and Weber, 1993; Kehoe, 1991).

Conditions: Extensive liver involvement from metastatic disease; cirrhosis; congestive heart failure; nephrosis with protein wasting; and, infrequently, complications of radiation. Pancreatic disease, hepatic encephalopathy, infectious peritonitis, and gut lymphatic or thoracic duct injury can be etiologies of ascites (Baker and Weber, 1993; Arroyo, Gines, and Planas, 1992).

Environment: Exposure to hepatitis has been speculated to be an environmental risk (Elcheroth, Vons, and Franco, 1994).

Foods: Long-term alcohol abuse, high-sodium diet, or increased water intake with liver or renal disease have been linked to the formation of ascites (Elcheroth et al., 1994).

Medications: Noncompliance with drug regimen in chronic renal or liver disease (Elcheroth et al., 1994); complications of chemotherapy can lead to ascites (Baker and Weber, 1993; Arroyo et al., 1992).

PROGNOSIS

Malignant ascites is an indicator of end-stage disease, and treatment is guided toward palliation of symptoms, although effective palliation of the symptoms causing ascites is difficult to achieve (Fraught et al., 1995). Baker and Weber (1993) did a meta-analysis of client survival after peritoneovenous shunt placement, with reports of 5 to 33 weeks survival. The median survival for a diagnosis with malignant ascites is approximately 2 months (Labovich, 1994; Baker and Weber, 1993; Scholmerich, 1991).

TREATMENT

Determination of the cause of ascites should be based on the client's history and a physical examination. An abdominal paracentesis is performed to determine the etiology of the ascites. Bloody or serosanguinous fluid characterizes malignant ascites. Cirrhotic, nephrotic, pancreatic, or cardiac disease results in serous fluid, and cloudy fluid is characteristic of infectious peritonitis. Ascitic fluid cytology should be ordered only in clients with (1) a history of cancer, (2) no physical findings suggestive of liver disease, or (3) an initial ascitic fluid sample with a high lymphocyte count and low number of neutrophils (Runyon, 1994).

A limited amount of literature is available about well-controlled studies that compare alternative treatments for management of malignant ascites. Since the prognosis is usually poor, once a diagnosis of malignant ascites has been made, most therapy is directed toward palliation of symptoms rather than long-term remission. Generally, the medical approach is initiated with noninvasive options and proceeds to more invasive treatments as the malignant ascites becomes more refractory (Baker and Weber, 1993; Runyon, 1993).

Surgery

Sugarbaker (1991) studied responses from clients with colorectal and gastric cancers undergoing aggressive tumor debulking and intraperitoneal chemotherapy, or occasionally abdominal radiation. His results were impressive, considering the seriousness of the gastrointestinal malignancies, but further research follow-up is needed.

Use of a silastic catheter, such as the LeVeen or Denver shunt, for peritoneovenous shunting has been evolving over the last several decades and has been used with some success (Fraught et al., 1995; Baker and Weber, 1993). The shunts have been associated with several risk factors, and current medical recommendations are to use shunts only when the ascites have proven to be refractory to other treatments. This is especially true when the client has ovarian cancer, since, in this case, ascites appears in the early stages and can be controlled with a hysterectomy-salpingo-oophorectomy (Runyon, 1993). Surgical placement of a silastic catheter into the peritoneal space may relieve symptoms, but multiple complications can occur, predisposing the shunt to infection and/or occlusion of flow. Tube kinking or tip malposition are immediate technical failures. Later failure of the shunt can occur from fibrin clot formation and debris accumulation at the valve. Leakage of ascitic fluid at the peritoneal insertion site increases the client's risk of infection (Sonnenfeld and Tyden, 1986). Removal of approximately 50% of the fluid during catheter placement decreases the potential for fluid overload after shunt placement (Baker and Weber, 1993).

Recent research by Fraught et al. (1995) indicates an improved efficacy in the use of peritoneovenous shunts for clients with gynecologic malignancies. Shunts were placed in 25 women with refractory ascites. Placement, done for palliation only, provided relief of gastrointestinal discomfort and dyspnea, and decreased abdominal girth. This study also examined quality of life, but despite symptom relief, no change in Karnofsky scores were found. As quality of life is a primary objective in palliative care, the benefits of peritoneovenous shunts for palliation should be further explored.

Chemotherapy

Use of chemotherapy agents intraperitoneally, such as doxorubicin, 5-fluorouracil, mitoxantrone, or cisplatin, have demonstrated a decrease in the amount of ascitic fluid present in clients with ascites (Alberts, Young, Mason, and Salmon, 1985). There is a risk of bleeding, infection, or chemical peritonitis that can carry significant morbidity (Piccart et al., 1985).

Education should include the risks of chemotherapy, although due to the limited systemic exposure, there are few toxicity symptoms.

Biologic response modifiers like interferon alpha and interleukin 2 have been used with some success in decreasing the amount of ascitic fluid. The risks with the use of biologic response modifiers include peritoneal fibrosis and abdominal pain (Berek et al., 1985).

Radiation: Not indicated, other than its use in the treatment regimen for the causative type of cancer.

Medications: Loop diuretics and aldosterone-inhibiting diuretics may be ordered, although efficacy is poor in malignant ascites as compared to ascites secondary to cirrhosis. A study by Greenway, Johnson, and Williams (1982) found that high doses of spironolactone (150 to 450 mg/day) decreased the malignant peritoneal effusions in 13 of 15 clients. Research may be needed to further explore high-dose drug therapy.

Procedures: Repeat paracentesis may be offered, but complications from frequent abdominal taps can include protein depletion, postural hypotension, and electrolyte abnormalities. Repeated insertion of the catheter into the peritoneal space is painful and inconvenient and can lead to bleeding and infection (Fraught et al., 1995; Belfort, Stevens, DeHaek, Soeters, and Krige, 1990).

Other: Low-sodium diet and water restriction, although efficacy is poor.

ASSESSMENT CRITERIA: MALIGNANT ASCITES

Vital signs

Temperature	Unchanged unless infectious peritonitis present.
Pulse	Unchanged unless infectious peritonitis is present.
Blood pressure	Unchanged unless infectious peritonitis is present.
Respiratory rate	Increased. Client may exhibit shortness of breath, tachypnea, or orthopnea.

History

Symptoms, conditions — Increased abdominal girth, shortness of breath, respiratory compromise, anorexia, early satiety, gastric reflux, swollen ankles, fatigue, constipation, decreased bladder capacity.

Hallmark physical signs and symptoms — Weight gain, increased abdominal girth, respiratory compromise.

Additional physical signs and symptoms — Abdomen: distended abdomen with ability to elicit a fluid wave, shifting dullness upon percussion; everted umbilicus.

Other: difficulty with ambulation, lower extremity edema, stretched skin.

Psychosocial signs — No signs directly related to the disease process; however, the client may need emotional support when ascites occurs, due to its grim prognosis.

Lab values

Ascitic fluid

Gross appearance	Bloody or serosanguinous.
Cell count and differential	>300–500/mm^2 with primarily polymorphonuclear cells in malignant ascites.
Total protein	High
Lactate dehydrogenase (LD)	High
Carcinoembryonic antigen (CEA)	High
Cytology	Positive only when malignant cells line the peritoneal cavity.
Microbiology	Gram stain and culture (positive in infection).
Serum-ascites albumin gradient	High

Diagnostic tests

Abdominal flat plate	Air-filled loops of small bowel separated by fluid between loops.
Ultrasound of the abdomen	Obtain if a small amount of ascites is suspected and to monitor the complications of ascites.
CT scan of the abdomen	Obtain if a small amount of ascites is suspected and to monitor the complications of ascites.

Source: Data from Labovich, 1994; Runyon, 1994; Baker and Weber, 1993; Groenwald et al., 1993; Kehoe, 1991.

NURSING DIAGNOSIS

The nursing diagnosis will vary, depending on the severity (extent of accumulation) of the malignant ascites. Suggested nursing diagnoses include the following:

Impaired gas exchange related to the accumulation of ascites with diaphragmatic displacement.

Fluid volume deficit related to:
- Draining or shunting of ascites.
- Osmotic shift with hypoalbuminemia.
- Diuresis with spironolactone or furosemide.
- Increased antidiuretic hormone (ADH).

Activity intolerance related to:
- Respiratory compromise.
- Weakness secondary to anorexia.

Anxiety related to:
- Respiratory compromise, physical deterioration.
- Poor prognosis, end-stage disease.

NURSING INTERVENTIONS

Immediate nursing interventions

Elevate head of bed to decrease respiratory compromise and alleviate discomfort.

Assess pulse, respirations, blood pressure, and temperature.

Monitor for fluid shifts and signs of bacterial peritonitis.

Monitor fluid balance through intake and output (I and O) measurements.

Assess abdomen, and measure girth.

Weigh the client.

Assess for gastroenteral and urologic distress due to increased abdominal pressure.

Monitor function of ascitic drains or shunts, if in place.

Anticipated physician orders and interventions

Bedrest.

Low-sodium, fluid-restricted diet.

Diuretic therapy.

Serum electrolytes, complete blood count (CBC) qd.

I and O monitoring.

Antacids for indigestion as needed.

Following paracentesis, monitor for:
- Hypotension related to hypovolemia or fluid shift.
- Infection/peritonitis.

Following peritoneovenous shunting, monitor for:
- Heart failure/pulmonary edema due to rapid infusion of peritoneal fluid intravascularly.
- Disseminated intravascular coagulation due to procoagulants in ascitic fluid.
- Shunt malfunction due to malposition.
- Potential fluid volume deficit and potential electrolyte imbalance due to increased diuresis.
- Infection due to contamination of the intravascular or intraperitoneal systems.

Ongoing nursing assessment, monitoring, and interventions

Assess:
- Pulmonary status (breath sounds, labor of respirations, oxygen saturation) q4h.
- For abdominal rigidity.
- For gastrointestinal/genitourinary (GI/GU) compromise.
- Paracentesis site or shunt placement incision for signs of infection qd.
- Client comfort q4h.
- Weight pattern to evaluate the effectiveness of interventions.
- Client/family coping qd.

Measure:
- Temperature, respirations, pulse, blood pressure q4h.
- I and O q8h.
- Weight qd.
- Abdominal girth qd.
- Urine specific gravity qd.

Send:
- CBC, serum electrolytes qd.
- Ascitic fluid for specific gravity, protein count, cell count, bacteriology, amylase, carcinoembryonic antigen (CEA) when drained (Kehoe, 1991).

Implement:
- Activity restriction.
- Low-sodium, fluid-restricted diet.

TEACHING/EDUCATION

The client should be instructed on the rationales for the nursing interventions related to ascites.

Ascites: *Rationale:* Your doctors have told you that your cancer is causing excess fluid to build up in your belly. This fluid is called *ascites*. Your doctor may try to control the fluid by a number of different ways, including limiting your activity, changing your diet, limiting the amount of fluid you drink, ordering special medications, draining the fluid through a needle, or possibly surgery. Although you may be able to get rid of the extra water through these methods, you may also find that none of these treatments works well. Remember, these treatments are to help you be more comfortable.

Limit Activity: *Rationale:* Resting in bed with your head propped up will give your lungs more room to expand. This will help you breathe easier. More rest will also help your body get rid of extra water.

Diet changes: *Rationale:* Drinking less fluids and eating food without salt may help your body to keep from adding any more fluid. Eating small meals many times each day will help with your indigestion and help you not to feel so full.

Blood sampling: *Rationale:* Blood samples may be taken as often as every day to watch for changes in the minerals in your body. If changes are found, you may need some medicine to make you feel better.

Monitoring I and O: *Rationale:* It is important that we measure what you drink and measure your urine to keep your body in balance and to see if the treatments are working.

Abdominal girth, weight: *Rationale:* By measuring around your gut and weighing you, we can see how well the extra fluid (ascites) is coming off.

Your doctor has decided to use the following treatment to help your body get rid of the extra fluid:

Paracentesis: *Rationale:* A paracentesis is done to take out some of the fluid (ascites) that is causing you discomfort and making it hard to breathe. After a spot on your stomach is numbed, a needle is put in to drain the fluid.

Intracavitary chemotherapy or radiation: *Rationale:* Chemotherapy drugs or radiation can be placed directly inside your gut during surgery or by a small tube to try to kill the cancer cells that may be causing the fluid buildup.

Shunt: *Rationale:* In surgery, a tube can be put inside you that will drain or "shunt" the fluid inside your gut into a vein. This procedure will help your body to control the fluid better and may help you feel more comfortable. The tube placed in you may have a pump on it. You will need to push the pump to drain the fluid. Ask your nurse or doctor if this is the kind of tube you will have. They will show you how to pump the tube.

EVALUATION/DESIRED OUTCOMES

1. Decreased abdominal girth.
2. Improved respiratory status, less-labored breathing.

3. Decreased anorexia, indigestion.
4. Activity, dietary, and fluid restrictions are understood by the client and caregivers.
5. Effective coping skills, related to prognosis, exhibited by the client and significant others.

DISCHARGE PLANNING

The client with malignant ascites may need:

Long-term assistance with the activities of daily living, depending on the severity of the remaining symptoms.

A hospice referral, since the prognosis of a client with this complication is often poor. Under this care, the client and significant others will receive the attention that will help meet their needs during an anxious and stressful time.

Caregiver teaching about comfort measures, signs of infection, and severe respiratory compromise, all of which may require medical intervention.

Discussion of advance directives and wishes for life support should be addressed early in the course of the disease. However, if life support decisions have not been addressed before the client reaches the terminal stage, the health care provider must initiate and facilitate this discussion. The client's wishes should be respected and will guide the nurse in giving caregivers appropriate information about comfort measures and when to seek medical intervention. Should the client not choose further medical intervention, the client and caregivers must be taught about what to expect at the end of life.

FOLLOW-UP CARE

Anticipated care

Physician office visit as needed.
Continuation of dietary/fluid recommendations.
Continuation of activity restrictions.
Hospice or home health referral.

Anticipated client/family questions and possible answers

What can I do to feel better?
"It is important to continue to eat a diet low in salty foods and continue to restrict the amount of fluid you drink. You need to continue to rest, and save your energy to help you breathe better. Placing pillows behind your

back to support you will make it easier for your to breathe and decrease the pressure on the lungs caused by your abdomen. You might find a reclining chair to be more comfortable for resting. Also, using a hospital bed for positioning may help you stay in a comfortable position. Limiting your activity and eating smaller but more frequent meals may also help you to be more comfortable."

What can I do so the fluid does not come back?

"By following instructions, you may be able to decrease fluid buildup, but malignant ascites is due to your disease, and you may not be able to control it yourself. We will continue to help you feel the best you can."

When should I call the doctor?

You should call the doctor if you have a fever, or if it gets harder to breathe, or if you become uncomfortable.

CHAPTER SUMMARY

Malignant ascites, a prognostically poor symptom of breast, ovarian, colorectal, gastric, pancreatic, hepatocellular, and uterine cancers, has a multifactorial pathophysiology. The risk profile includes injury or disease to the liver, renal disease, infectious peritonitis, or alcohol abuse, to list a few of the most common causes. Treatment should be directed toward palliation of symptoms. Diet and medication are the most conservative and least successful of the medical therapies. Repeat paracentesis is a more invasive approach, and it carries a higher risk of problems. It cannot be used as a solution for long-term management of ascites. Silastic catheters, such as the LeVeen or Denver shunts, have been used for years with limited success in controlling ascitic fluid. As research further investigates this arena, it may become a more desirable option. Intraperitoneal chemotherapy and biologic response modifiers have also demonstrated success in decreasing the amount of ascitic fluid, although further research in these areas is needed. The nursing diagnoses are related to management of symptoms and comfort measures. Assessment of the client is crucial in identifying the nursing interventions needed. Knowledge of symptoms and treatment of malignant ascites are necessary in order to anticipate physician orders, interventions, and potential complications from the disease process and medical treatment. Nurses caring for clients with malignant ascites need to be sensitive to the emotional needs of the client and caregivers. As malignant ascites usually carries a poor prognosis, facilitation of comfort measures and hospice referral need to be offered.

TEST QUESTIONS

1. Malignant ascites is the result of:
   A. Pulmonary edema
   B. Cardiac insufficiency
   C. Compromised drainage of peritoneal lymphatics
   D. Chemotherapy toxicity

1. Answer: C
Malignant ascites is the result of compromised drainage of the peritoneal lymphatics that occurs when the formed lymph fluid accumulates faster than the thoracic duct can drain the abdomen.

2. Median survival for a client diagnosed with malignant ascites is:
   A. 2 months
   B. 6 months
   C. 1 year
   D. 5 years

2. Answer: A
Based on a study by Baker and Weber (1993), the median survival for a client with malignant ascites was found to be 2 months, despite moderately aggressive treatment.

3. The goal of treatment of malignant ascites is:
   A. Restoration of previous status/Karnofsky score
   B. Palliation of symptoms
   C. Absence of micro metastases within the ascitic fluid
   D. Decreased potential for liver failure

3. Answer: B
Because malignant ascites is indicative of end-stage disease, palliation of symptoms is the goal.

4. The most common treatment options for malignant ascites include diuretics, dietary management, paracentesis, and:
   A. Peritoneovenous shunting
   B. Intraperitoneal chemotherapy
   C. Intracavitary radiation
   D. Metered-dose inhalers

4. Answer: A
One of the most common treatment options for malignant ascites, depending on the status of the client, is peritoneovenous shunting, whereby a catheter is placed to drain ascites into the venous system. Intraperitoneal chemotherapy and radiation can be treatment options but are much less common.

5. Nursing assessment of the client with malignant ascites should include:
   A. Neurologic integrity
   B. Evaluation of generalized edema
   C. Pulmonary assessment
   D. Sensory deficits

5. Answer: C
The nursing assessment of a client with ascites should include a pulmonary assessment to assess the extent of respiratory compromise related to diaphragmatic displacement.

6. Nursing diagnoses that could be utilized with the client with malignant ascites include:
   A. Fluid volume deficit
   B. Confusion, acute
   C. Functional incontinence
   D. Impaired swallowing

6. Answer: A
One of the nursing diagnoses that would be appropriate is fluid volume deficit. As the treatment of ascites typically includes diuresis of some type, intravascular fluid volume deficit must be closely monitored.

7. Nursing interventions for a client with malignant ascites should include:
   A. Abdominal assessment, girth
   B. Oxygen therapy
   C. Postural drainage
   D. Urinary catheter placement

7. Answer: A
As GI/GU compromise is a concern, as is the potential for umbilical rupture, abdominal assessment is critical.

8. Client education regarding malignant ascites should include:
   A. Elevation of edematous extremities
   B. Valsalva maneuvers
   C. Dietary and activity restrictions
   D. Use of metered-dose inhalers

8. Answer: C
The client and significant other should be taught about activity restrictions that are important when fatigue and respiratory compromise can be limiting factors. Dietary recommendations, including small, frequent low-sodium meals, should be discussed to aid symptom management of indigestion, anorexia, and necessary sodium restrictions to prevent increased water gain.

9. Peritoneovenous shunting:
   A. Is a successful method of managing ascites
   B. Should be the first line of treatment after malignant ascites is diagnosed
   C. May provide relief of discomfort from ascites if other medical treatments fail
   D. Has few problems after insertion

9. Answer: C
Ascites may be relieved by use of a peritoneovenous shunt, but it should only be used if other medical treatments fail to offer relief of symptoms. There are numerous problems associated with the shunts.

10. Formation of malignant ascitic fluid is caused by all of the following *except:*
   A. Invasion of the subdiaphragmatic lymphatic channels inhibiting fluid drainage
   B. Excessive fluid formation
   C. Increased capillary leakage
   D. Hydrodynamic disequilibrium

10. Answer: B
   Excessive fluid formation is usually related to cirrhosis of the liver rather than a metastatic disease process.

REFERENCES

Alberts DS, Young L, Mason N, Salmon SE: In vitro evaluation of anticancer drugs against ovarian cancer at concentrations achievable by intraperitoneal administration. Oncology 12(Suppl 4):38–42, 1985.

Arroyo V, Gines P, Planas R: Treatment of ascites in cirrhosis: Diuretics, peritoneovenous shunt, and large-volume paracentesis. Gastroenterol Clin North Am 21(1):237–256, 1992.

Baker AR, Weber JS: Treatment of malignant ascites. *In* DeVita VT, Hellman S, Rosenberg SA (eds): Cancer: Principles and Practice of Oncology, 4th ed. Philadelphia: JB Lippincott, 1993.

Belfort MA, Stevens RJ, DeHaek K, Soeters R, Krige JE: A new approach to the management of malignant ascites, a permanently implanted abdominal drain. Eur J Surg Oncol 16(1):47–53, 1990.

Berek JS, Hacker HF, Lichtenstein A, Jung T, Spina C, Knox RM, Brady J, Greene T, Ettinger LM, et al.: Intraperitoneal recombinant for "salvage" immunotherapy in stage III epithelial ovarian cancer. Cancer Treat Rev 12(Suppl. B):23–32, 1985.

Elcheroth J, Vons C, Franco D: Role of surgical therapy in management of intractable ascites. World J Surg 18(2):240–245, 1994.

Feldman GB, Knapp RC: Lymphatic drainage of the peritoneal cavity and its significance in ovarian cancer. Am J Obstet Gynecol 119(7):991–994, 1974.

Fraught W, Kirkpatrick JR, Krepart GV, Heywood MS, Lotocki RJ: Peritoneovenous shunt for palliation of gynecologic malignant ascites. J Am Coll Surg 180:427–474, 1995.

Garrison RN, Kaelin LD, Heusser LS, Galloway RH: Malignant ascites. Ann Surg 203(6):644–651, 1986.

Greenway B, Johnson PJ, Williams R: Control of malignant ascites with spironolactone. Br J Surg 69(8):441–442, 1982.

Groenwald SL, Frogge MH, Goodman M, Yarbro CH: Cancer Nursing: Principles and Practice, 3rd ed. Boston: Jones and Bartlett, 1993.

Howell SB, Pfiefle CE, Wang WE, Oshen RA, Lucas WE, Von JL, Green M: Intraperitoneal cisplatin with systemic thiosulfate protection. Ann Intern Med 97(6):845–851, 1982.

Kehoe C: Malignant ascites: Etiology, diagnosis, and treatment. Oncol Nurs Forum 18(3):523–530, 1991.

Labovich TM: Selected complications in the patient with cancer: Spinal cord compression, malignant bowel obstruction, malignant ascites, and gastrointestinal bleeding. Semin Oncol Nurs 10(3):189–197, 1994.

Ozols RF, Speyer JL, Markman M, Myers CE: Phase II trial of 5-FU administration with refractory ovarian cancer. Cancer Treat Rep 68(10):1229–1232, 1984.

Piccart MJ, Speyer IL, Markman M, ten Bokkel Huinink WW, Albert D, Jenkins J, Muggia F: Intraperitoneal chemotherapy experience at five institutions. Semin Oncol 12(3, Suppl. 4):90–96, 1985.

Runyon BA: Refractory ascites. Semin Liver Dis 13(4):343–351, 1993.

Runyon BA: Editorial: Malignancy-related ascites and ascitic fluid "humoral tests of malignancy." J Clin Gastroenterol 18(2):948, 1994.

Scholmerich J: Strategies in the treatment of ascites. Hepato-gastroenterology 38(5):365–370, 1991.

Sonnenfeld T, Tyden G: Peritoneovenous shunts for malignant ascites. Acta Chir Scand 152:117–121, 1986.

Straus AK, Roseman DL, Shapiro RM: Peritovenous shunting in the management of malignant ascites. Arch Surg 114(4):489–491, 1979.

Sugarbaker PH: Mechanisms of relapse for colorectal cancer: Implications for peritoneal therapy. J Surg Oncol 52(Suppl 2):36–41, 1991.

CHAPTER 30

MALIGNANT PERICARDIAL EFFUSION AND CARDIAC TAMPONADE

Peggy Dragonette, MS, RN, CCRN

CHAPTER OBJECTIVES

At the completion of this chapter, the reader will be able to:

Describe the pathophysiology of malignant pericardial effusion and cardiac tamponade.

Identify risk factors that contribute to the development of malignant pericardial effusion.

Describe the presenting symptoms of cardiac tamponade.

Discuss the treatment options for the client with malignant pericardial effusion, as well as the emergency treatment of cardiac tamponade.

Describe how to prepare the client for future care needs.

OVERVIEW

PERICARDIAL effusion is an accumulation of fluid in the pericardial sac and can be caused by infection, radiation-induced pericarditis, and malignancy. In the cancer client, about half of the pericardial effusions are malignant. Malignant pericardial effusion can result from metastasis, most often from lung, breast, or other cancers, and, less commonly, from primary tumors of the heart. Because the effusion often develops gradually, the client may be asymptomatic. Autopsy reports have found that 8 to 20% of clients who die from cancer have pericardial disease (Kilbride, 1994; Maxwell, 1993; Olopade and Ultmann, 1991) and of those who have symptomatic malignant pericardial effusion, the effusion itself contributed to the cause of death in 86% of cases (Thurber, Edwards, and Achor, 1962).

Cardiac tamponade is an emergency that can occur when the pericardial effusion compresses the heart, resulting in low cardiac output. It is likely to develop

425

when the effusion accumulates rapidly or becomes so large that compensatory mechanisms fail. It is estimated that 10 to 30% of clients who have a malignancy involving the heart develop cardiac tamponade (Maxwell, 1993; Schafer, 1991).

DESCRIPTION

Malignant pericardial effusion

The pericardial sac encases the heart and consists of two layers: the visceral and parietal pericardium (Fig. 30–1). The visceral pericardium is a serous membrane that is contiguous with the outer surface of the heart. The parietal pericardium is a dense fibrous membrane separated from the visceral layer by the pericardial space. This space normally contains no more than 50 ml of fluid, which serves to prevent friction between the two layers of the pericardium as the heart contracts and relaxes.

Pericardial fluid is maintained in equilibrium by a balance of four processes: capillary filtration, hydrostatic pressure, osmotic pressure, and lymphatic drainage (Mangan, 1992; Maxwell, 1993). Capillary filtration is the movement of fluid and particles between the capillaries and interstitium. Hydrostatic pressure, within the capillary, is the result of arterial and venous pressure. Osmotic pressure refers to the concentration of osmotically active

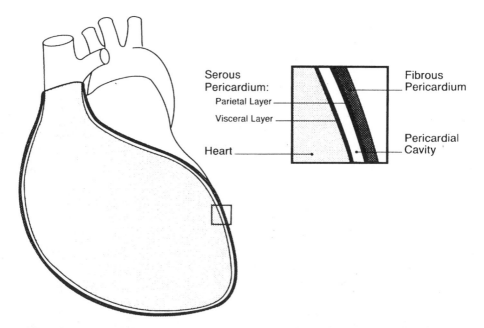

Figure 30–1 Layers of the pericardium (From Mangan CM: Malignant pericardial effusions: Pathophysiology and clinical correlates. Oncol Nurs Forum 19(8):1215–1221, 1992.)

particles, such as protein, that serve to hold fluid within the capillary, interstitium, or intracellular space. Finally, the lymph system drains excess fluid and protein from the interstitium and returns it to the vasculature.

Neoplastic disease of the pericardium interferes with these processes. Malignant pericardial effusions develop because of obstruction of venous and lymphatic drainage. When venous flow is obstructed, capillary hydrostatic pressure is increased. As a result, fluid leaks from the vessel into the interstitium and, ultimately, into the pericardial space. When lymphatic flow is obstructed, less interstitial fluid and protein are reabsorbed. Therefore, interstitial osmotic pressure rises and contributes to fluid seeping into the pericardial space. Fluid dynamics can also be altered by hypoproteinemia, which is not uncommon for the client with cancer owing to poor nutritional intake. Hypoproteinemia results in a decrease of osmotically active particles required to hold fluid in the vascular space and, as a result, can lead to an increased loss of fluid from the capillaries into the pericardial space.

The tumor itself can also contribute to an effusion because of irritation to the pericardial membranes (Kilbride, 1994; Mangan, 1992). This irritation triggers an inflammatory response, which brings leukocytes, fibrin, platelets, and fluid to the area. During this process, capillaries become more permeable, and additional fluid can leak into the interstitium and pericardial space.

Many clients with malignant pericardial effusion are asymptomatic because the effusion tends to develop slowly and because the pericardium is capable of stretching to accommodate up to 4 liters of fluid. However, when the effusion becomes so large that it compresses the heart, the client can develop signs and symptoms of cardiac tamponade. This scenario is even more likely to occur if the client has poor ventricular function, a decreased blood volume, or a noncompliant pericardial sac. In the latter case, the sac is stiff and unable to stretch, as a result of bacterial or viral pericarditis, radiation therapy, uremia, or collagen-vascular disease such as rheumatoid arthritis. In addition, when effusions develop rapidly, even 150 to 200 ml may be enough to compress the heart and cause cardiac tamponade.

Cardiac tamponade

Cardiac tamponade is an emergency that is caused when fluid in the pericardial space compresses the heart and decreases the cardiac output (Fig. 30–2). Normally, intrapericardial pressure is 3 to 5 mmHg less than the pressure in the central veins and right atrium, and central venous pressure (CVP) is 3 to 5 mmHg less than pressure in the peripheral veins. This pressure gradient maintains continuous blood flow from the systemic veins to the right atrium.

With cardiac tamponade, as fluid accumulates in the pericardial space, intrapericardial pressure rises and equilibrates with central venous and right atrial pressure, which is normally 0 to 8 mmHg. This process impairs right ventricular filling and may even cause the thin-walled right ventricle to collapse during diastole. Therefore less blood is delivered to the lungs and, ulti-

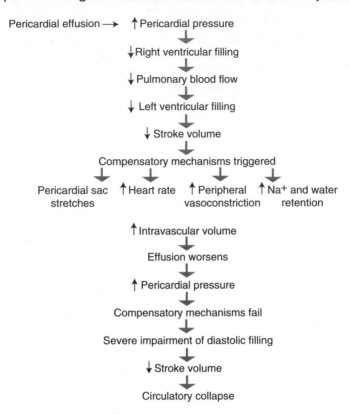

Figure 30–2   Pathophysiology of pericardial effusion and cardiac tamponade.

mately, to the left ventricle, which results in a decreased stroke volume. In response to the decreased stroke volume, the pericardial sac stretches to accommodate the increased fluid, and compensatory mechanisms are triggered. These compensatory mechanisms include an increased heart rate and constriction of peripheral blood vessels, which decrease venous pooling and boost venous return to the heart. The decrease in renal blood flow stimulates the renin-angiotensin-aldosterone system, causing sodium and water retention and vasoconstriction.

These compensatory mechanisms initially increase intravascular volume but ultimately fail as the effusion worsens. Intrapericardial pressure continues to rise, along with the central venous and right atrial pressure, to the level of the left atrial and left ventricular end-diastolic pressure, which is normally 4 to 12 mmHg. As the effusion worsens, all pressures continue to rise together, severely impairing diastolic filling. The stroke volume, which is normally 60 to 120 ml, progressively falls, causing arterial hypotension. Concurrently, the vasoconstriction that has occurred to attempt to boost venous return to the heart causes systemic venous hypertension. The arterial hypotension and venous hypertension result in a critical reduction in the pressure gradient necessary to maintain blood flow. Hypoperfusion of all organ systems ensues.

RISK PROFILE

Cancers: Any malignancy has the potential for spread to the pericardium via metastasis or direct tumor extension. However, most cases result from metastasis, especially from lung (36.5%) or breast cancer (22.3%), as well as from lymphoma and leukemia (17.2%), sarcoma (3.5%), and melanoma (2.7%) (Maxwell, 1993; Olopade and Ultmann, 1991; Schafer, 1991; Thurber et al., 1962).

Conditions: Neoplastic constrictive pericarditis, radiation pericarditis, uremia, collagen-vascular disease, and viral or bacterial pericarditis.

Environment: None.

Foods: None.

Drugs: Anthracyclines (doxorubicin, daunorubicin), anticoagulants, apresoline, procainamide (Schafer, 1991).

PROGNOSIS

The prognosis for clients with a malignant pericardial effusion is grave. Regardless of the treatment option, several studies have found that clients usually survive only 1 to 13 months (Moores et al., 1995; Okamoto, Shinkai, Yamakido, and Saijo, 1993; Vaitkus, Herrmann, and LeWinter, 1994; Wang, Feikes, Morgensen, Vyhmeister, and Bailey, 1994).

TREATMENT

Surgery

Pericardial window or pericardiectomy: Pericardial window involves resecting a piece of the pericardium that is a few square centimeters in size so that fluid can drain. Pericardiectomy involves removal of the pericardium. Because it is a more extensive surgery than pericardial window, it is usually not well tolerated by the client with cancer and is not as common.

Pericardioperitoneal shunt: This intervention involves placing a conduit between the pericardial space and peritoneum. The conduit, which is tunneled subcutaneously, contains a pumping chamber that is manually compressed several times a day so that fluid continues to drain. A more recently developed procedure, it has only been performed on a few clients but is showing some promise (Wang et al., 1994).

Chemotherapy: May be given systemically to treat the primary disease or may be instilled into the pericardial space.

Radiation: External beam radiation may be given to clients with a radiosensitive tumor. Treatment administered over 3 to 4 weeks can help control the effusion. Internal radiation therapy is less common.

Medications: Less severe cases of neoplastic cardiac tamponade may be treated with a corticosteroid and a diuretic. A common prescription is prednisone (40 to 60 mg/day) and furosemide (40 mg/day) or aldactazide (25 to 200 mg/day) (Kilbride, 1994; Schafer, 1991).

Procedures

Pericardiocentesis is performed to tap the effusion and is the treatment of choice for cardiac tamponade. It is performed through a needle inserted into the pericardial sac. A catheter for continuous drainage may be left in place.

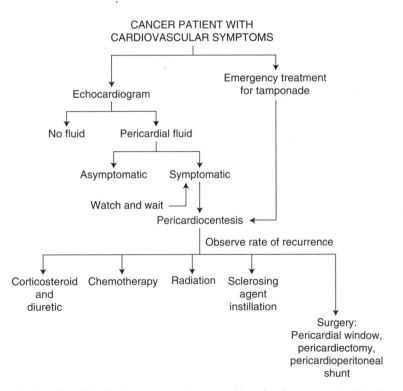

Figure 30–3 Algorithm for diagnosis and management of malignant pericardial effusion. (Adapted from Maxwell MB: Malignant effusions and edemas. *In* Groenwald SL, Frogge MH, Goodman M, Yarbro CH [eds]: Cancer Nursing: Principles and Practice, 3rd ed.. Boston: Jones and Bartlett, 1993.)

A sclerosing agent, such as bleomycin, cisplatin, or tetracycline, may be
instilled into the pericardial space. These agents produce an inflammatory response that ultimately obliterates the space.

The choice of treatment for malignant pericardial effusion depends on
the physiologic impairment that it causes (see Fig. 30–3). On one end of the
continuum, the client may be asymptomatic, and no intervention may be
necessary except for routine physician office visits. On the other end of the
continuum, the client may present with cardiac tamponade, a life-threatening emergency that requires an immediate pericardiocentesis. In another scenario, the client could present with symptoms of decompensation that are
not life-threatening. In that case, treatment options, such as a pericardial
window or sclerosis, may be effective in alleviating symptoms.

ASSESSMENT CRITERIA: MALIGNANT PERICARDIAL EFFUSION AND CARDIAC TAMPONADE

The assessment criteria for cardiac tamponade are listed in the table at the
end of this section. Elevated CVP, distant heart sounds, and arterial hypotension have been considered the hallmark signs, but these may not appear in
all clients and may not be present until the advanced stages (Mangan, 1992;
Schafer, 1991). Dyspnea and tachycardia are the symptoms that have been
found to occur with the most frequency (Maxwell, 1993). Other classic signs
of cardiac tamponade are pulsus paradoxus, hepatojugular reflux, and electrical alternans (Kilbride, 1994; Mangan, 1992; Schafer, 1991). In addition,
for the client with a pulmonary artery catheter, some characteristic changes
in hemodynamic parameters occur.

Pulsus paradoxus

Pulsus paradoxus is an abnormal finding in which the pulse becomes weaker
during inspiration because of a greater than normal decrease in the systolic
blood pressure. The arterial pressure typically decreases during inspiration
because the increased negative pressure in the thoracic cavity causes blood
pooling in the pleural vasculature. This decreases venous return to the heart
and therefore decreases the stroke volume, resulting in a weaker pulse and a
lower systolic blood pressure. Cardiac tamponade exaggerates this process
because the increase in intrapericardial pressure also impairs ventricular filling
and decreases the stroke volume. Pulsus paradoxus is present when the pulse is
weaker or even absent during inspiration or when the systolic blood pressure is
more than 10 mmHg lower during inspiration as compared to expiration.

There are three ways to assess pulsus paradoxus: palpation, cuff sphyg-
momanometry, and arterial waveform analysis (Sultzbach, 1989). In the first
method, the carotid or femoral pulse is palpated, and the pulse is noted to be
weaker or absent during inspiration. In the second method, the blood pres-

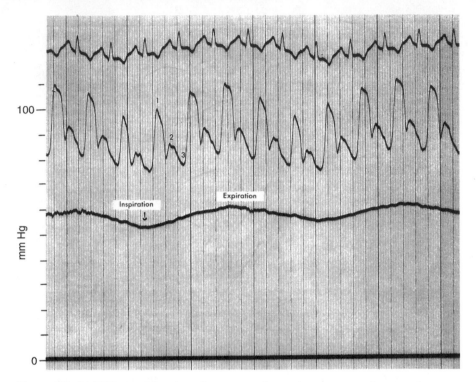

Figure 30–4   ECG, arterial, and respiratory waveforms demonstrate pulsus paradoxus. (From Daily EK, Schroeder JS: Hemodynamic Waveforms: Exercises in Identification and Analysis. St Louis, MO: CV Mosby Co.)

sure cuff is inflated above the client's systolic blood pressure and then is deflated slowly until the first Korotkoff sound is heard. This reading is noted because, with pulsus paradoxus, the Korotkoff sounds are initially auscultated during expiration only. The cuff is further deflated until sounds can be auscultated during both inspiration and expiration. That reading is noted and compared to the previous one. If the difference is greater that 10 mmHg, pulsus paradoxus is present.

The third method requires an indwelling arterial line and a simultaneous paper recording of the arterial and respiratory waveforms. In this method, the height of the arterial waveform is measured during expiration and compared to the height of the waveform during inspiration (see Fig. 30–4). Again, if the difference is greater than 10 mmHg, pulsus paradoxus is present.

Hepatojugular reflux

Hepatojugular reflux is the result of venous engorgement of the liver. It occurs because the pericardial effusion compresses the heart and eventually collapses the thin-walled right ventricle. This process results in an increased

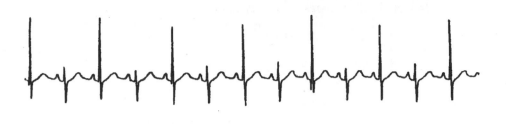

Figure 30–5 ECG tracing that demonstrates electrical alternans. (From Mangan CM: Malignant pericardial effusions: Pathophysiology and clinical correlates. Oncol Nurs Forum 19(8):1215–1221, 1992.)

systemic venous pressure, which ultimately congests the liver. Reflux can be assessed by having the client lie down with the head of the bed elevated to a level at which jugular venous pulsations are visible. Then pressure is exerted continuously over the periumbilical area of the abdomen for 30 to 60 seconds. Reflux is present when there is a sustained rise of > 1 cm in jugular venous pulsations while pressure is exerted.

Electrical alternans

Electrical alternans is an ECG finding in which the height of the QRS complex changes with each successive beat so that it is alternately increased and decreased (Fig. 30–5). It represents the swinging movement of the heart within the effusion, which results in changes in the electrical axis with each beat.

For the client with a pulmonary artery catheter, the CVP (normal 0 to 8 mmHg), pulmonary artery diastolic pressure (PAD, normal 6 to 12 mmHg), and pulmonary capillary wedge pressure (PCWP, normal 4 to 12 mmHg) typically equalize and may be > 15 mmHg. This equalization occurs because the effusion compresses the heart uniformly during the later stage of cardiac tamponade. Because of the impaired filling, the cardiac output (CO) decreases below 4 to 8 L/minute. Concurrently, the systemic vascular resistance (SVR, normal 770 to 1500) increases in proportion to the decreased stroke volume.

Vital signs

Blood pressure	Decreased systolic blood pressure <90 mmHg
Pulse	Increased heart rate >120 bpm
Respiratory rate	Increased >26/min; dyspnea

Hemodynamic measurements

Central venous pressure (CVP)	>0–8 mmHg

(continued)

ASSESSMENT CRITERIA: MALIGNANT PERICARDIAL EFFUSION AND CARDIAC TAMPONADE *(continued)*

Pulmonary capillary wedge pressure (PCWP)	>4–12 mmHg
Pulmonary artery diastolic pressure (PAD)	>6–12 mmHg
Cardiac output (CO)	<4 L/min
Cardiac index (CI)	<2.5 L/min/m^2
Systemic vascular resistance (SVR)	>770–1500 dynes/sec/cm^{-5}
History	Malignancy, especially lung cancer, breast cancer, leukemia, lymphoma, sarcoma, melanoma; previous radiation therapy to the chest.
Hallmark physical signs and symptoms	*Early:* weakness, fatigue, secondary to decreased CO from pericardial effusion.
	Later, signs of cardiac tamponade appear: narrowed pulse pressure secondary to impaired diastolic filling of the ventricles.
	Arterial hypotension secondary to low CO, muffled (distant) heart sounds and elevated CVP, dyspnea, tachycardia, pulsus paradoxus.
Additional physical signs and symptoms	Ascites, chest pain: initially, fullness and heaviness; later, retrosternal pain, cool, clammy extremities, cough, cyanosis, diaphoresis, dyspnea, dysphagia, fatigue, hepatojugular reflux, hepatomegaly, hiccoughs, hoarseness, JVD, nausea and vomiting, normal breath sounds (rales in severe cardiac tamponade), oliguria, pericardial friction rub, peripheral edema, and weak, thready pulse.
Psychosocial signs	Anxiety, altered mental status (i.e., diminished level of consciousness).
Lab values	
Pericardial fluid	Usually serosanguinous; usually contains malignant cells; protein >3 gm/dl; specific gravity >1.015; hematocrit and fibrinogen lower than that of circulating blood.
Hematocrit, potassium, calcium, ABGs	Not conclusive for cardiac tamponade, but assists with differential diagnosis.
Diagnostic tests	
Echocardiography	Presence of fluid between the heart and pericardium. (Normally, the visceral and parietal layers are contiguous.)
Chest x-ray	Cardiomegaly, hilar adenopathy, mediastinal widening.

ASSESSMENT CRITERIA: MALIGNANT PERICARDIAL EFFUSION AND CARDIAC TAMPONADE (continued)

ECG	Elevated ST segments, depressed T waves, diminished QRS voltage, electrical alternans.
Cardiac catheterization	Determination of the size and exact location of the effusion; increased intracardiac pressures and an equalization of diastolic pressures in all chambers.
Computed tomography (CT), magnetic resonance imaging (MRI)	Pericardial effusion vs. pericardial thickness, as from radiation fibrosis.

NURSING DIAGNOSIS

Decreased CO related to impaired diastolic filling.

Activity intolerance related to decreased CO.

Anxiety related to the illness and fear of the unknown.

Knowledge deficit related to unfamiliarity with the disease process and treatment options.

Potential for injury secondary to trauma related to invasive procedures and surgery.

NURSING INTERVENTIONS

Immediate nursing interventions

Assess vital signs at least q15min until the systolic blood pressure is > 100 and then q1h.

Assess for increased CVP via a central venous line or pulmonary artery catheter, if placed, or assess jugular venous distention (JVD).

Auscultate heart sounds with assessment of vital signs.

Assess for signs of respiratory distress such as dyspnea and use of accessory muscles, and auscultate lungs with assessment of vital signs.

Position the client to assist with chest expansion.

Assess for pulsus paradoxus with assessment of vital signs.

Assess extremities for color, temperature, and pulses q1h.

Monitor ECG for elevated ST segments, inverted T waves, decreased QRS voltage, and electrical alternans q1h.

Monitor urine output q1h.

Establish patent IV access.

Prepare for a pericardiocentesis.
- Explain the procedure to the client.
- Premedicate the client to decrease anxiety and pain.
- Obtain a pericardiocentesis tray.
- Have a 12-lead ECG machine available. Some physicians attach the pericardiocentesis needle to the V lead. During the procedure, if

the needle is advanced too far and touches the epicardium, acute elevation of the ST segment or premature atrial or ventricular contractions will be apparent on the ECG tracing, and the needle can be withdrawn into the pericardial space.
- Other physicians use echocardiogram to identify the size and location of the effusion.
- Have emergency equipment available.
- Position the client in semi-Fowler's position.

Assist with the procedure.

Continue to monitor vital signs and cardiovascular status.

Assess for potential complications of pericardiocentesis: puncture of the myocardium or coronary artery, dysrhythmia, laceration of lung tissue, and air embolus.

Anticipated physician orders and interventions

Rapidly infuse a volume expander, such as saline, fresh frozen plasma, blood, or dextran. A fluid bolus can be administered as rapidly as 300 to 500 ml over 10 to 15 minutes.

Administer oxygen therapy.

Administer isuprel, dopamine, dobutamine, or amrinone to increase the CO.

Obtain echocardiography.

Ongoing nursing assessment and interventions

Since the effusion can recur, nursing assessment is similar to the assessment for cardiac tamponade.

Assess q8h unless otherwise indicated:
- For cardiac signs that the effusion is worsening, such as, JVD, distant heart sounds, and fatigue.
- For symptoms of respiratory distress.
- For symptoms of decreased tissue perfusion such as pale or cyanotic skin color, cool skin temperature, and weak peripheral pulses.
- For pulsus paradoxus.
- For deteriorating level of consciousness (LOC).
- For ECG changes that may be indicative of cardiac tamponade, such as elevated ST segments, depressed T waves, decreased QRS voltage, and electrical alternans.
- Abdomen for tenderness and ascites, and assess for nausea and vomiting.
- For hepatojugular reflux.

For client with pericardial catheter in place, assess:
- Pericardial catheter site q4h for erythema and edema, and obtain client's temperature.
- White blood cell count qd.

- For symptoms of infective pericarditis, such as pericardial friction rub and new onset of chest pain, described as sharp and increasing with respirations.
- That catheter is patent by assessing for clots and debris in drainage and noting any abrupt decrease in drainage.
- Color of catheter drainage. Pericardial fluid is normally clear and straw-colored, whereas malignant drainage is often serosanguinous.

Measure:
- Blood pressure, pulse, and respirations q4h.
- CVP q4h.
- Intake and output (I and O) q4–8h.
- Weight qd.
- Abdominal girth q8h.
- Pericardial catheter drainage.

Send:
- Pericardial drainage for hematocrit, fibrinogen, specific gravity, protein, cell count, stains, cultures, and cytologic analysis × 1. The hematocrit and fibrinogen are useful in distinguishing between a bloody effusion and puncture of the myocardium during pericardiocentesis. Bloody effusions have a lower hematocrit and fibrinogen than circulating blood (Schafer, 1991).
- Serum electrolytes, especially calcium and potassium, qd × 2.
- Arterial blood gases (ABGs), if the client develops respiratory distress.

Implement:
- Assistance with activities of daily living (ADL) to reduce cardiac workload.
- Provision of a safe environment for the client with decreased LOC by frequent, close observation and by instructing the client in the use of the call light.
- Provision of emotional support and opportunity to verbalize feelings.
- Aseptic care after insertion of pericardial catheter. Due to the risk of infection, the catheter is usually left in only 24 to 48 hours.
- Care for the client undergoing a pericardial sclerosis:
  Premedicate the patient with an analgesic, since the procedure is painful.
  Evaluate the need for an antiemetic, analgesic, and antipyretic during and after the procedure, since nausea, pain, and fever are potential sequelae.
  Monitor for signs and symptoms of infection.
  Assess client for dysrhythmias.

TEACHING/EDUCATION

Respiratory distress: *Rationale:* We are applying an oxygen mask and rolling the head of your bed up so you can breathe more easily.

Vital signs: *Rationale:* Your blood pressure and pulse will be taken frequently so that any changes that need to be treated will be treated quickly.

IV line placement: *Rationale:* The IV line allows us to give you fluids and medicine. At first, you will be receiving fluids very rapidly so that your heart can pump better.

Urine output: *Rationale:* Measuring your urine tells us how well your heart is pumping blood to your kidneys. When the kidneys don't make enough urine, it may mean the fluid is building up around your heart.

Echocardiography: *Rationale:* An echo is a study of how well your heart is pumping. It involves placing a special microphone on your chest and moving it over the areas of your heart. It doesn't hurt, but the gel used with the microphone feels cool.

Pericardiocentesis: *Rationale:* You are feeling short of breath because fluid has built up in the sac around your heart, and it is preventing your heart from pumping very well. The fluid will be removed from the sac by a needle. The procedure will take only a few minutes, and you will receive medicine to help you relax.

Pericardial catheter: *Rationale:* After the fluid is removed from the sac, a tube will be left in place so that any remaining fluid will drain out into a bag.

Pericardial sclerosis: *Rationale:* Fluid can build up again in the sac around your heart. To prevent this, the doctor will place medicine into the tube near your heart. This medicine will cause an inflammation in the sac and close it off. Your heart can still beat normally with the sac closed off. You will receive pain medicine before the procedure.

Pericardial window: *Rationale:* Because fluid is still building up in the sac around your heart, a small piece of the sac will be removed. This will allow the fluid to drain out.

Symptoms of cardiac tamponade: *Rationale:* You and your family members need to watch for symptoms that the fluid is building up again. These symptoms include shortness of breath, feeling tired all the time, fast heart rate, a lightheaded or dizzy feeling, fullness or heaviness in the chest, stomach or belly pain, and swollen feet. If you have any of these symptoms, call your doctor.

EVALUATION/DESIRED OUTCOMES

The first four outcomes below should be achieved immediately after pericardiocentesis.
1. Blood pressure and pulse are at client's baseline.
2. The symptoms of respiratory distress improve.
3. The CVP is at client's baseline, or JVD is absent.

4. Heart sounds are easily auscultated.
5. Mental status is at client's baseline within 8 hours.
6. Urine output is > 30 ml per hour within 8 hours.
7. The client appears less anxious within 8 hours.
8. The client verbalizes understanding of treatment plans after explanations are given.
9. The pericardial catheter, if placed, is removed within 24–48 hours.
10. Prior to discharge, the client understands which symptoms indicate that the effusion is recurring.

DISCHARGE PLANNING

The client with a history of pericardial effusion may need:

Instruction in energy conservation techniques due to the impaired cardiac output that an effusion causes.
Home nursing visits or an extended-care facility, depending on the debilitation of the client and availability of family caregivers.

FOLLOW-UP CARE

Anticipated care

Physician office visit within 1 week.
Home nursing visits twice a week for detection of recurrent effusion.
Mental health professional or support group for assistance in coping with the illness.

Anticipated client/family questions and possible answers

Can the fluid build up again in the sac around my heart?
"It's possible that it will happen again. However, the fluid tends to build up slowly, and you may not have any symptoms at first. That's why it's important to recognize the symptoms when they first appear, before the amount of fluid gets very large."

Why will a nurse be visiting me at home?
"A nurse can help identify symptoms that the amount of fluid around the heart is increasing, for example, by taking your blood pressure and pulse and by asking you about your symptoms."

Why can't the drainage catheter stay in the sac around my heart?
If the catheter stayed there, you would be at high risk for an infection. The catheter can be inserted again at a later time if you need it. Since the fluid tends to build up slowly, you don't need the catheter all the time.

CHAPTER SUMMARY

Neoplastic pericardial effusion can be caused by any malignancy but is most commonly the result of metastasis, especially from lung or breast cancer. Because the effusion tends to develop slowly, many clients are asymptomatic. However, when the effusion compresses the heart, the client can develop cardiac tamponade—a life-threatening emergency.

The treatment for cardiac tamponade is pericardiocentesis, which allows the fluid to be removed from the pericardial space. A catheter can be left in for continuous drainage but should be left in for only 24 to 48 hours because of the risk of infection.

The client may receive treatment, such as sclerosis or pericardial window, to prevent the recurrence of an effusion. However, there is still a chance the effusion will recur, and the client must be educated in identifying the early symptoms and must receive follow-up care.

TEST QUESTIONS

1. Most malignant pericardial effusions result from:
   A. Tumors of the heart
   B. Metastasis of lung or breast cancer
   C. Leukemia
   D. Metastasis of colon cancer

1. Answer: B
Any malignancy has the potential for spread to the myocardium; however, most cases result from metastasis of lung or breast cancer.

2. Clients with a pericardial effusion may be asymptomatic because:
   A. The effusion may develop slowly and the pericardial sac stretches to accommodate it.
   B. The volume of the effusion is usually small.
   C. The effusion is usually absorbed by the lymph system.
   D. The heart's pumping action is usually not affected.

2. Answer: A
Malignant pericardial effusions tend to develop slowly and can be very large. The pericardium is capable of stretching to accommodate up to 4 liters of fluid.

3. Clients who have cardiac tamponade typically have the following symptoms:
   A. Hypertension, tachycardia, and tachypnea
   B. Rales throughout the lung fields

3. Answer: D
Tachycardia is a compensatory response in tamponade. Then, as the effusion compresses the heart, the thin-walled right ventricle collapses, and the CVP rises. Less

C. A low CVP and decreased urine output

D. Tachycardia, elevated CVP, and hypotension

blood is pumped to the lungs and, therefore, less blood returns to the left side of the heart. This causes decreased cardiac output and resultant hypotension.

4. Electrical alternans is evidenced by:

A. A decreased systolic blood pressure during inspiration

B. Lowered QRS voltage

C. Alternating height of the P wave and QRS complex

D. Nonspecific ST changes

4 Answer: C
Electrical alternans is an alternating height of the ECG complex and is caused by the changing position of the heart as it swings within the pericardial fluid.

5. Besides pericardiocentesis, the emergency treatment of cardiac tamponade includes:

A. Rapid infusion of fluids

B. Diuretics

C. Intermittent positive pressure breathing (IPPB) treatment

D. Calcium channel blockers

5. Answer: A
With cardiac tamponade, the problem is low cardiac output due to impaired diastolic filling. Therefore, fluids are rapidly infused to increase filling pressures.

6. Initially, with cardiac tamponade, the following compensatory mechanisms are triggered:

A. The heart rate increases, and peripheral vessels dilate.

B. The heart rate increases, and the urine output increases.

C. The heart rate decreases, and peripheral vessels constrict.

D. The heart rate increases, and peripheral vessels constrict.

6. Answer: D
When ventricular filling is impaired, the heart rate increases, and peripheral vessels constrict, which serves to decrease venous pooling and boost venous return to the heart.

7. Potential complications of a pericardiocentesis are:

A. Fractured ribs

B. Pneumothorax

C. Aneurysm

D. Lacerated liver

7. Answer: B
The potential exists for lung tissue to be lacerated during a pericardiocentesis. Other potential complications during the procedure are puncture of the myocardium or coronary artery, dysrhythmia, and air embolus.

8. Malignant pericardial fluid is typically:
   A. Bloody and contains no protein
   B. Has the same hematocrit and fibrinogen as the circulating blood volume
   C. Has a specific gravity < 1.015
   D. Contains protein

8. Answer: D
Malignant pericardial effusions usually contain protein. Also, they are usually serosanguinous, have a lower hematocrit and fibrinogen than circulating blood, and have a specific gravity > 1.015.

9. The client undergoing a pericardial sclerosis, is likely to have all of the following except:
   A. Nausea
   B. Pain
   C. Fever
   D. Dyspnea

9. Answer: D
With pericardial sclerosis, an agent, such as tetracycline, is instilled into the pericardial space. This causes an inflammation that serves to obliterate the space. Clients typically have transient nausea, pain, and fever.

10. Before discharge, the client with a pericardial effusion should be taught the following except:
    A. How to care for the pericardial catheter, since it is usually left in for several days
    B. Energy conservation techniques
    C. Symptoms that the effusion is increasing
    D. The purpose, dosage, and potential side effects of medications.

10. Answer: A
The pericardial catheter should only be left in for 24 to 48 hours because of the risk of infection.

REFERENCES

Barbiere CC: Cardiac tamponade: Diagnosis and emergency intervention. Crit Care Nurs 10(4):20–22, 1990.

Clark JC, McGee RF, Preston R: Nursing management of responses to the cancer experience. *In* Clark JC, McGee RF (eds): Core Curriculum for Oncology Nursing, 2nd ed. Philadelphia: WB Saunders Co, 1992, pp. 151–155.

Corey GR, Campbell PT, Van Tright P, Kenney RT, O'Connor CM, Sheikh KH, Kisslo JA, Wall TC: Etiology of large pericardial effusions. Am J Med 95(2):209–213, 1993.

Daily EK, Schroeder JS: Hemodynamic Waveforms: Exercises in Identification and Analysis. St. Louis, MO: CV Mosby, 1983.

Darovic GO: Hemodynamic Monitoring: Invasive and Noninvasive Clinical Applications. Philadelphia: WB Saunders Co, 1995.

Hiller G: Cardiac tamponade in the oncology patient. Focus Crit Care 14(4):19–23, 1987.

Joiner GA, Kolodychuk GR: Neoplastic cardiac tamponade. Crit Care Nurs 11(2):50–58, 1991.

Kilbride SS: Cardiac tamponade. In Gross J, Johnson BL (eds): Handbook of Oncology Nursing, 2nd ed. Boston: Jones and Bartlett, 1994, pp. 658–673.

Mangan CM: Malignant pericardial effusions: Pathophysiology and clinical correlates. Oncol Nurs Forum 19(8):1215–1221, 1992.

Maxwell MB: Malignant effusions and edemas. In Groenwald SL, Frogge MH, Goodman M, Yarbro CH (eds): Cancer Nursing: Principles and Practice, 3rd ed. Boston: Jones and Bartlett, 1993, pp. 677–687.

Moores DW, Allen KB, Faber LP, Dziuban SW, Gillman DJ, Warren WH, Ilves R, Lininger L: Subxiphoid pericardial drainage for pericardial tamponade. J Thorac Cardiovasc Surg 109(3):546–551, 1995.

Okamoto H, Shinkai T, Yamakido M, Saijo N: Cardiac tamponade caused by primary lung cancer and the management of pericardial effusion. Cancer 71(1):93–98, 1993.

Olopade OI, Ultmann JE: Malignant effusions [Review]. CA 41(3):166–179, 1991.

Otto SE (ed): Oncology Nursing. St Louis, MO: Mosby Year Book, 1991.

Schafer SL: Oncologic complications. In Otto SE (ed): Oncology Nursing. St. Louis, MO: Mosby Year Book, 1991, pp. 490–498.

Sultzbach LM: Measurement of pulsus paradoxus. Focus Crit Care 16(2):142–145, 1989.

Thurber DL, Edwards JE, Achor RW: Secondary malignant tumors of the pericardium. Circulation 26(2):228–241, 1962.

Vaitkus PT, Herrmann HC, LeWinter MM: Treatment of malignant pericardial effusion [Review]. J Am Med Assoc 272(1):59–64, 1994.

Wang N, Feikes JR, Mogensen T, Vyhmeister EE, Bailey LL: Pericardioperitoneal shunt: An alternative treatment for malignant pericardial effusion. Ann Thorac Surg 57(2):289–292, 1994.

CHAPTER 31

MALIGNANT PLEURAL EFFUSIONS

Patricia Manda Collins, RN, MSN, OCN

CHAPTER OBJECTIVES

At the completion of this chapter, the reader will be able to:

Discuss the pathophysiology of pleural effusions.

State the risk factors associated with pleural effusion in the oncology client.

Discuss the common signs and symptoms of malignant pleural effusion.

Discuss the advantages and disadvantages of the various treatments for pleural effusion.

Describe nursing care as it relates to oncology clients with pleural effusion.

OVERVIEW

PLEURAL effusion is an accumulation of fluid in the pleural space and is caused by a variety of malignant and nonmalignant conditions. *Malignant* pleural effusion refers to effusions caused by solid tumors or hematologic malignancies. The most common malignancies causing pleural effusion are lung cancer, breast cancer, and lymphoma (Light, 1990). The severity of symptoms depends on how fast the fluid has accumulated and the degree to which the fluid compromises lung function. The presence of a pleural effusion in an individual whose cancer is untreatable indicates a grim prognosis, although symptom relief from the effusion is achievable. Individuals with malignancies responsive to cancer therapies and who have a pleural effusion respond well to the treatment of the malignancy. Many of these individuals will have no further problems with pleural effusions.

DESCRIPTION

Anatomy and physiology of the pleurae

The outer surface of the lungs is covered by a smooth covering, the visceral pleura. The interior surface of the lung cavity is covered by the parietal pleu-

444

ra. These linings join together at the hilar root of the lungs and are lined with a thin layer of mesothelial cells. The pleurae primarily allow movement of the lung in relation to the chest wall, but also provide support and shape for the lungs. There is a gap or "pleural space" between these linings, and approximately 5 to 15 ml of lubricating pleural fluid is present, with as much as 1 to 2 liters passing through the space each day. Pleural fluid flow is determined by Starling's law of transcapillary exchange. Fluid moves through the capillaries in the parietal pleura to the pleural space and exits through the visceral pleura based on a differential in hydrostatic pressure. Other factors that influence the flow of pleural fluid through the pleural space are oncotic pressures, interstitial osmotic pressures, and capillary permeability (Light, 1990).

Pathophysiology of malignant pleural effusion

Malignant pleural effusion results when more fluid enters the pleural space than can exit. Either the rate of entry exceeds the pleura's ability to clear it, or the drainage mechanism of the pleura is defective. Sometimes both conditions occur. The presence of tumor cells irritates the pleura, causing inflammation and subsequent increases in capillary permeability. Plasma oncotic pressure decreases as protein leaks into the pleural space. These events are followed by osmotic movement of capillary fluid into the pleural space to dilute the excess protein. The overabundance of pleural fluid accumulation overwhelms the ability of the visceral pleura to remove it. Excessive entry of protein into the pleural space may be the result of neoplastic involvement of the pleura either by metastasis, direct extension (e.g., lung cancer), or primary growth

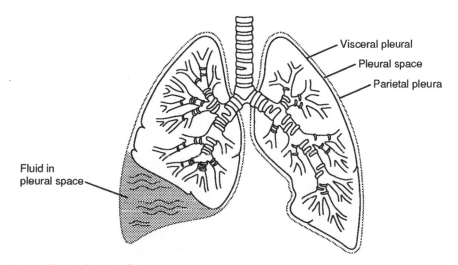

Figure 31–1 Pleural effusion.

(malignant mesothelioma) (Light, 1990). The most common mechanism responsible for the majority of malignant pleural effusions is impaired lymphatic drainage from the pleural space caused by the following: a primary neoplasm of the lymphatic system (e.g., lymphoma); metastasis via the lymphatics from another site; or, rarely, fibrosis of lymph nodes from radiation therapy. Other mechanisms that may cause pleural effusion in the person with cancer are related to various pressure changes in the cardiopulmonary system that impact on the pleural pressures. These mechanisms include: hypoproteinemia, pulmonary emboli, pneumonia, lung infections, pericardial effusions, and superior vena cava syndrome (Light, 1990).

Diagnosis of malignant pleural effusion

The first symptom of a pleural effusion may be the client's report of respiratory difficulties. Otherwise, an asymptomatic pleural effusion may be first diagnosed with a chest x-ray. Further diagnostic testing depends on the individual's symptomatology, medical condition, and pre-existing diseases. In most situations, a thoracentesis will be performed for diagnosis and for relief of symptoms. Analysis of pleural fluid for differentiation of transudative versus exudative qualities and pleural fluid cytology can help guide interventions. If the pleural fluid is not diagnostic, the physician may obtain a pleural needle biopsy. When pleural fluid cytology and needle biopsy are nondiagnostic, thoracoscopy may be indicated. Video-assisted thoracoscopy also can be used to determine the extent of pleural involvement, lyse adhesions, place drainage tubes, and instill a sclerosing agent (Viallat and Boutin, 1994). Other tests, such as ultrasound, CT scan, lung scan, or bronchoscopy may be helpful in diagnosis and staging.

RISK PROFILE

Cancers: Lung, breast, lymphomas (Hodgkin's and non-Hodgkin's), stomach, ovarian, mesothelioma, melanoma, leukemia. All cancers, except intracranial malignancies have been known to cause pleural effusions (Fingar, 1992; Kennedy, Rusch, Strange, Ginsberg, and Sahn, 1994; Light, 1990).

Pediatrics: Leukemia.

Conditions: Congestive heart failure, bacterial pneumonia, pulmonary embolization, viral pneumonia, cirrhosis with ascites, hypoproteinemia, gastrointestinal disease, collagen vascular disease, tuberculosis, and asbestosis are nonmalignant conditions that can cause pleural effusions in the person with cancer. Superior vena cava syndrome can cause pleural effusion.

Environment: History of asbestos exposure.

Drugs: Chemotherapeutic agents such as methotrexate, cyclophosphamide, and procarbazine and the drugs nitrofurantoin, dantrolene, methysergide, or bromoscriptine.

Other: History of chest irradiation.

PROGNOSIS

Malignant pleural effusion is often associated with advanced cancer, and therefore the prognosis is poor. A low pleural fluid pH (< 7.20) and low pleural fluid glucose level (< 60 mg/dl) indicates poor survival (Milanez, Vargas, Filomeno, et al., 1995). Individuals with this distressing complication may live for just a few months after developing pleural effusion, unless their disease (such as breast cancer, lymphoma, small cell lung cancer, ovarian cancer) is responsive to therapy.

TREATMENT

The treatment options for malignant pleural effusion may be grouped into four categories: (1) eliminate the cause, (2) remove the fluid, (3) obliterate the pleural space so there is no room for fluid to collect, and (4) do nothing (for asymptomatic clients). (See Table 31–1.)

Surgery: Thoracotomy, thoracoscopy, or video-assisted thoracoscopy may be used to resect tumor, perform a pleurectomy or pleural abrasion, position chest tubes, and/or place a pleuroperitoneal shunt (Lee, Harvey, Reich, and Beattie, 1994).

Chemotherapy: Systemic chemotherapy for chemosensitive tumors.

Radiation: To affected lymph nodes when lymph node involvement is the cause of effusion; to responsive tumors.

Medications

> Intrapleural sclerotics (talc, doxycycline, bleomycin), analgesics, antianxiety agents.
> Biologic response modifiers: interferon, interleukin 2, and tumor necrosis factor (Viallat and Boutin, 1994).

Procedures: Thoracentesis, pleural biopsy, tube thoracostomy for drainage and instillation of a sclerosant, placement of an external catheter for drainage (Robinson, Fullerton, Albert, Sorensen, and Johnston, 1994).

Other

> Correct/treat nonmalignant causes: hypoproteinemia, infections, pulmonary emboli.
> Intrapleural fibrin "glue" to obliterate the pleural space (Boutin and Rey, 1994).
> Urokinase for loculated effusions (Robinson et al., 1994).

Table 31–1
Treatment Options for Malignant Pleural Effusion

Treatment	Purpose	Advantages	Disadvantages
Chemotherapy and/or radiation therapy	Treat underlying cause of pleural effusion.	If effective, prevent(s) recurrence of effusion.	Side effects associated with therapy.
Thoracentesis	Drain fluid for relief of dyspnea and pain. Pleural fluid analysis.	Bedside or office procedure. Generally easy to perform. Immediate relief of symptoms. Relatively easy method of obtaining material for diagnosing etiology of effusion.	Thoracentesis alone will not prevent fluid reaccumulation if cause for effusion remains. Potential adverse effects: depletion of fluid/protein stores; hypotension from rapid removal of a large volume of fluid; pneumothorax; hemothorax; fever; infection. Repeated thoracentesis carries increased risks.
Chest tube drainage (tube thoracostomy)	Drain fluid. Restore negative pressure in pleural space. Re-expand lung.	Relieves symptoms. Provides access for instilling sclerosing drugs.	Painful procedure. Potential complications: bleeding, infection, lung injury, subcutaneous emphysema.
Chemical pleurodesis	Obliterate pleural space by instilling an agent to produce fibrotic adhesions, causing the pleurae to stick together.	Bedside procedure except for talc pouderage.	Painful. Not always effective. Talc pouderage must be done in surgery.
Mechanical pleurodesis (pleurectomy/pleural abrasion)	Obliterate pleural space.	Permanent, most effective of the procedures.	Must be done in surgery. Long, bloody procedure.
Pleuroperitoneal shunt	Drain pleural space when pleurodesis has failed or lung cannot re-expand, e.g., in the case of trapped lung.	Drainage system is internal. Treatment is client-activated. Treatment spares client from repeated thoracentesis. Fluid/protein is reabsorbed. Extended hospital stay avoided.	Must be inserted in surgery. Client/caregiver must pump valve manually many times a day. Potential complications: pneumothorax; possible clogging of system or malfunctioning of valve; infection; cellulitis; and seeding of cancer cells along tract or into peritoneum.

Source: Data from Boutin and Rey, 1994; Fingar, 1992; Keller, 1993; Lee et al., 1994; Robinson et al., 1994; Ruchdeschel, Moores, Lee, et al., 1991; Walker-Renard et al., 1994.

Table 31–2
Pros and Cons of the Most Commonly Used Sclerosing Agents

Agent		Pro	Con
Talc			
	Pouderage	Most effective of the agents. Painless, since client is anesthetized. Is instilled using thoracoscopy, thus permitting visualization of pleurae and deloculation if needed. Bedside procedure. Least expensive agent.	Requires thoracoscopy to instill. Involves expense of a surgical procedure. Potential adverse effects (especially with doses over 5 g): re-expansion edema, pleuritic chest pain, fever.
	Slurry		May not be as effective as pouderage, owing to uneven application of talc. Pain on instillation. Potential adverse effects: acute respiratory distress syndrome, respiratory failure.
Bleomycin		Bedside procedure. Causes minimal pain on instillation. Usually requires only one instillation to be effective.	Most expensive agent. Potential adverse effects: fever, nausea.
Doxycycline		Bedside procedure. Inexpensive.	May require multiple dosing. Causes pain on instillation. Potential adverse effect: fever.

Source: Data from Aelony, King, and Boutin, 1991; Fingar, 1992; Keller, 1993; Kennedy et al., 1994; Milanez et al., 1995; Robinson et al., 1993; Ruchdeschel et al., 1991; Walker-Renard et al., 1994.

If the pleural effusion persists despite systemic chemotherapy or radiation therapy, and the client is symptomatic, the pleural effusion will be drained. Then, depending on the physician's preference and the client's condition, pleurodesis is attempted with one of several drugs (see Table 31–2). Pleurodesis is achieved after chemical injury produces inflammation and irritation of the pleural linings, producing fibrotic adhesions that cause the two pleurae to stick together. Tetracycline was the drug of choice until the manufacturer could no longer procure sterile tetracycline salt (Heffner and Unruh, 1992). Talc, an old sclerosant and the most effective of the chemical agents, is making a comeback because of its availability in a pure and sterile form. Its drawback is that it is most effective when instilled as a fine, dry powder (pouderage) over all the pleural surfaces. This procedure must be performed in surgery by means of thoracoscopy. Some clinicians instill talc in solution (slurry), using a chest tube (Kennedy et al., 1994). Opponents to this method of application, suggest that the talc may clump and not cover all the surfaces (Kennedy, Harley, Sahn, and Strange, 1995). Bleomycin is an effective sclerosant often after just one instillation via chest tube, but it is expensive

(Walker-Renard, Vaughan, and Sahn, 1994). Doxycycline, a relative of tetracycline, is being used by many clinicians (Robinson, Fleming, and Galbraith, 1993). It is inexpensive initially, but becomes an expensive procedure if it must be instilled two or three times in order to achieve effective pleurodesis (Fingar, 1992). Numerous agents have been used to attempt pleurodesis (nitrogen mustard, fluorouracil, thiotepa, cisplatin, quinacrine, and others) (Robinson et al., 1993), including a fibrin "glue," but the most common agents are talc, bleomycin, and doxycycline. Studies of the biologic agents, interferon, interleukin 2, tumor necrosis factor, and others are in progress. (See Table 31–2.)

Other means of obliterating the pleural space include removing the parietal pleura and abrading the visceral pleura, or abrading both pleurae. Abrasion is accomplished by rubbing the pleura with a gauze or polyethylene pledget. These procedures must be done in surgery, and the client should be in good physical condition because these techniques are risky in clients with advanced disease or concurrent medical problems.

Pleurodesis is not performed when the individual has trapped lung. The pleural surfaces cannot come together because of a thickened pleura. The lung has lost its' elasticity and cannot re-expand; therefore, it is "trapped" (Boutin and Rey, 1994; Weissberg and Ben-Zeev, 1993).

ASSESSMENT CRITERIA:
MALIGNANT PLEURAL EFFUSIONS

Vital signs	
Pulse	Increased
Blood pressure	Increased
Respirations	Increased
Temperature	Normal or increased if infection is present.
History*	History of breathing problems and absence or presence of risk factors.
Hallmark physical signs and symptoms	Cough, dyspnea, heaviness or pain in chest, diminished or absent breath sounds, decreased fremitus, dullness to percussion.
Additional physical signs and symptoms	Anorexia, confusion, cyanosis, fever, malaise, memory loss, must sit upright to breathe, protrusion of abdomen and restricted chest wall expansion on affected side, tachycardia, tachypnea, weight loss.
Psychosocial signs	Distressed, anxious expression.

ASSESSMENT CRITERIA:
MALIGNANT PLEURAL EFFUSION (continued)

Lab values	Abnormal blood gases (PaO_2 <50 mmHg and $PaCO_2$ >50 mmHg)
Pleural fluid analysis	*Transudative effusions* (clear or straw-colored, low specific gravity, lactate dehydrogenase [LD] and protein) usually indicate a problem outside the pulmonary system, e.g., congestive heart failure, hypoproteinemia.
	Exudative effusions (bloody, cloudy or white in the case of thoracic duct obstruction, high specific gravity, LD, and protein) usually indicate a problem within the pulmonary system, e.g., malignancy, parapneumonic problems (tuberculosis, pneumonia, pulmonary emboli, infections). Cytologic studies on exudative effusions may demonstrate malignant cell (Light, 1990).

Diagnostic tests and procedures

Chest x-ray	Reveals increase in pleural fluid (if >300ml of pleural fluid present).**
Thoracentesis	Drains fluid for examination and relief of symptoms.
Pleural fluid examination	Assesses color and specific gravity, protein content, protein ratios, LD levels and LD ratios, depending on whether transudate or exudate.*** May or may not contain malignant cells.
Ultrasound	Reveals location of loculated effusions, if present.
CT scan	May reveal neoplastic involvement of mediastinal lymph nodes.
Pleural biopsy	May reveal cause of pleural effusion when analysis of fluid is inconclusive.
Bronchoscopy	May reveal obstructive bronchial lesion as cause of pleural effusion.
Lung scan	May reveal pulmonary emboli as cause for pleural effusion.
Video-assisted thoracoscopy	May reveal extent of disease, presence of adhesions/loculations.

* Malignant pleural effusions often occur over time; therefore, clients may have a pleural effusion and be asymptomatic.

** Areas of increased density, blunted costophrenic angle, horizontal or meniscus-shaped fluid level, fluid in interlobar fissure.

*** Transudate is clear or straw-colored, specific gravity < 0.016, protein < 3 g/100 ml, protein/serum ratio < 0.5, LDH l < 200 IU, LDH/serum ratio < 0.6. Exudate-color cloudy, bloody, or purulent, specific gravity > 0.016, protein > 3 g/100 ml, protein/serum ratio > 0.5, LDH > 200 IU, LDH/serum ratio > 0.6.

Source: Data from Keller, 1993; Light, 1990; Viallat and Boutin, 1994.

NURSING DIAGNOSIS

The nursing diagnoses will vary, depending on the severity and onset of pleural effusion. Some of the common diagnoses and etiologies are as follows.

Ineffective breathing pattern related to:
- Partial or total collapse of the lung.
- A change in intrathoracic pressure as a result of the application of suction to the chest tube.
- Pain.
- Anxiety.

Impaired gas exchange related to partial or total collapse of the lung owing to effusion.

Pain caused by compression of bronchial walls; as a result of procedures and/or surgery.

Anxiety related to dyspnea, pain, implications and lack of knowledge of the illness, procedures, and/or surgery.

Risk for infection related to thoracentesis needle, chest tube, thoracotomy, or thoracoscopy.

NURSING INTERVENTIONS

Immediate nursing interventions

Assess respiratory status: inspection, palpation, percussion, and auscultation; pulse oximetry or arterial blood gas (ABG) analysis.

Perform mental status assessment.

Promote comfort: positioning, analgesics, sedatives, information, quiet environment, orientation, emotional support.

Prepare supplies and client/family for anticipated pleural fluid removal (thoracentesis or chest tube insertion).

Assess other body systems.

Anticipated physician orders and interventions

STAT ABGs.

Continuous pulse oximetry.

Oxygen as needed to maintain oxygen saturation ≥90%.

Stat chest x-ray (decubitus and upright).

Analgesic PRN.

Thoracentesis (guided by ultrasound if pleural fluid is loculated).

Chest tube.

Ongoing nursing assessment, monitoring, and interventions

Assess:
- Breath sounds as lung re-expands after drainage procedure.
- Respiratory status q15min × 2, then q30min × 2, then q1h × 4, then q4h after thoracentesis.

- Effectiveness of analgesia.
- For relief of dyspnea and hypoxia after thoracentesis or chest tube insertion.
- For side effects after drainage procedures (pneumothorax, hemothorax, pain, hypotension, mediastinal shift).
- For patency and placement of chest tube, amount and character of drainage, drainage system function (e.g., presence or absence of air leaks).
- Mental status.
- Incision sites for signs of infection.
- Nutritional status.
- Psychological, social, and spiritual well-being.
- Educational needs.

Measure:
- Vital signs as indicated.
- Intake and output.

Send:
- Pleural fluid to laboratory for analysis, as ordered.
- Arterial blood for blood gas analysis, as ordered.

Implement:
- Turning, coughing, and deep breathing after drainage procedure to aid in lung re-expansion and in ventilation and to prevent atelectasis.
- Semi-Fowler's position to promote adequate gas exchange and comfort.
- Strict aseptic techniques when caring for drains, wounds, tubes, and invasive lines.
- Measures to promote comfort, particularly prior to coughing.
- Measures to facilitate chest tube drainage:
  Position client so as to prevent kinking.
  Milk tubing, but do *not* strip it if drainage is thick (Robinson, 1993).
  Avoid dependent loops when positioning chest drainage system.
  Change positioning after instillation of sclerosing agent, if ordered.
  Measures to increase activity as tolerated.

TEACHING/EDUCATION

Select items, based on the client's situation.

Pleural effusion: *Rationale:* Our lungs have two thin coverings around them. Between these two linings is a space that has a small amount of liquid our body makes to help the linings move more easily as we breathe. Your type of cancer has cells that leave the main tumor and travel to this lining. These tumor cells cause the body to make extra liquid. This liquid is made faster than the body can get rid of it. This extra liquid presses on the lung, making it hard for the lung to work. That is why you might be having a hard time breathing. Some types of cancer (e.g., lymphoma) cause the liquid to be trapped in the space between the two linings because the tumor cells block the drainage glands, called lymph nodes. Some people have extra liquid, which can be seen on an x-ray, but they don't have any breathing problems. This usually happens when the liquid collects slowly over several weeks or months. If this extra liquid makes it hard to breathe, your doctor can remove it.

Thoracentesis: *Rationale:* This procedure can be done in the hospital or the doctor's office. The purpose is to remove the extra liquid from between the two linings that cover your lung. To begin, you will sit on the side of the bed or examination table and lean on a bedside table. This position makes the procedure more comfortable for you and easier for the doctor or specialized nurse to perform it. He or she will numb a little spot on your side or back and then put a needle into the space where the liquid is located. The liquid will be drained into a special bottle or bottles. It is important not to move or cough during the procedure. After the liquid is removed, some people feel the need to cough because the lung has been able to spread out again after being pushed on by the liquid. Coughing at this time is okay and helps your lung to work better. The liquid is usually sent to the laboratory for tests so your doctor can learn more about why this extra liquid has accumulated.

Chest tube insertion: *Rationale:* This procedure is done in the hospital, usually in your room. The purpose is to drain the extra liquid from the space between the two linings that cover your lung. You will be given medicine beforehand to help relax you and to lessen any discomfort you might have with the procedure. The doctor numbs your side or back and after making a small hole, puts a small tube about as thick as a finger in the space between the two linings. This tube is attached to a container for the liquid to drain. It is important that the tube stay straight so the liquid will drain. Sometimes another tube will be attached to a suction device, which may cause a bubbling sound. Usually, after a day or two, most of the liquid has been drained, and the tube can be removed. After the liquid has been drained, the doctor will sometimes put medicine into the space to help keep liquid from reaccumulating (see pleurodesis).

Pleurodesis: *Rationale:* This procedure is done either in your hospital room or in the operating room after most of the liquid has been drained from the space. The purpose is to put medicine into the space between the two linings that cover the lung. This medicine causes the two linings to stick together so there is no room for liquid to collect. There are several different medicines, including a form of talc, that are known to make the linings stick together. Your doctor will discuss which medicine is best for you. If talc is used, it can be given in a liquid form or a dry form. If the liquid form is used, the procedure is usually done in your hospital room. If dry talc is used, the procedure is done in the operating room, where the talc is "puffed" into the space with a small device. When the procedure is done in your hospital room, the medicine is put into the space by using the same tube that drained the liquid. The tube is then clamped for several hours. Your doctor may want you to change position periodically so that the medicine will spread all around the space. After several hours, the tube is unclamped and allowed to drain again, because the medicine has caused more liquid to form and will continue to do so for a day or two. After the drainage stops, your doctor will remove the tube. For most people, the linings stick together, and no more liquid is formed. You might wonder how your lungs can work if you no longer have this space, but people who have had this procedure have no difficulty breathing without the space (Weissberg and Ben-Zeev, 1993).

Oxygen: *Rationale:* Sometimes, the liquid presses on your lung and your lung can't work as well to help you breathe. If this happens, you may need extra oxygen.

ABGs/pulse oximeter: *Rationale:* This test measures the amount of oxygen in your blood and carried by your red blood cells.

Chest x-ray: *Rationale:* This x-ray is used to see the extra liquid in the space between the two linings of the lung and to check the lung after drainage to see if the lung has spread out to its proper place.

Turning, coughing, and deep breathing after drainage procedure: *Rationale:* These activities will help your lung to spread out to its proper place and help you to breathe better.

Signs and symptoms of pleural effusion: *Rationale:* Call your doctor if you have breathing problems, coughing, or chest pain, because these are signs that liquid may have collected again in the space between the two linings of the lung.

EVALUATION/DESIRED OUTCOMES

1. The client reports relief of symptoms (dyspnea, cough, chest pain, anxiety).
2. Chest x-ray demonstrates fully expanded lungs and absence of pleural effusion.
3. Blood gases and blood chemistries are normal.
4. Symptoms of recurrent pleural effusion are understood by the client and/or caregiver.

DISCHARGE PLANNING

The client with malignant pleural effusion may need:

Reinforcement of previous teaching about the signs and symptoms to report and about activities to promote health (nutrition, exercise, energy conservation techniques, relaxation techniques).

A long-term drainage system if pleural effusion persists—external catheter/Heimlich-flutter valve (Shuey, 1994) or pleuroperitoneal shunt.

Home nursing visits, depending on the status of the underlying disease and symptoms.

FOLLOW-UP CARE

Anticipated care

Physician office visit within 1 week.

Home nursing visits, depending on the client's condition and whether a drainage system is in place.

Periodic chest x-rays to assess lungs for recurrent effusion.

Anticipated client/family questions and possible answers

Will this problem of too much liquid in the space between the linings of my lung happen again?

"It is possible that this problem will happen again. It is very important for you to call your doctor if you have problems with breathing, coughing, or chest pain."

"In some individuals, the liquid collects but doesn't cause breathing problems. Your doctor will probably have you get chest x-rays periodically in order to see how your lungs are doing."

"You are receiving treatment for your cancer, so the liquid shouldn't become a problem again. If the liquid collects again and causes breathing problems, your doctor can remove it."

"If the liquid keeps collecting, your doctor might put a permanent, 'portable' tube in the space, and then the liquid will drain out as it collects. There are several different types of drainage tubes. Some drain into the body and some outside the body. A lot of detail about these now may not be helpful, especially if you won't ever need one of them."

How will I know if the fluid is building up again?

"You might have a cough, trouble breathing, or chest discomfort. Often, people have none of these problems, but the doctor can see the fluid on a chest x-ray."

CHAPTER SUMMARY

Although malignant pleural effusion is often associated with end-stage disease, effective treatment is available. Because various treatment options exist as well as different opinions about which option to choose, treatment decisions should be based on the goal of improving quality of life. Nursing interventions focus on symptom relief, education, and psychosocial support and on facilitating home care.

TEST QUESTIONS

1. The three areas of malignancy that cause the majority of malignant pleural effusions are:
   A. Lung, sarcoma, and breast
   B. Breast, lung, and brain
   C. Bone, lymphomas, and stomach
   D. Lung, breast, and lymphomas

1 Answer: D
Lung, breast, and lymphomas are the most common malignancies causing malignant pleural effusions.

2. The primary nursing diagnosis of clients with pleural effusion is:
   A. Altered tissue perfusion
   B. Impaired gas exchange
   C. Infection
   D. Fluid volume deficit

2. Answer: B
Frequently, because the lung is partially or totally collapsed from the effusion, lung ventilation is impaired.

3. A client should be scheduled for an ultrasound-guided thoracentesis in which of the following situations?
   A. Fluid cannot be seen on x-ray.
   B. Fluid is free-flowing.
   C. Fluid is bloody.
   D. Fluid is trapped in pockets.

3. Answer: D
Ultrasound is helpful in identifying fluid that is trapped in pockets within the pleural space.

4. What is the definition of pleurodesis?
   A. Removal of excess pleural fluid
   B. Removal of the parietal pleural lining
   C. Production of adhesions between the parietal and visceral pleurae
   D. Injection of medications into the pleural space

4. Answer: C
Production of adhesions between the parietal and visceral pleurae is accomplished by several methods. Injection of medications is one method.

5. Which of the following methods has not been used to achieve pleurodesis?
   A. Rubbing the pleural surfaces with a gauze sponge
   B. Bleomycin pouderage
   C. Fibrin glue
   D. Talc pouderage

5. Answer: B
Pouderage is the application of a powder to the pleural space in order to produce pleurodesis. Bleomycin is instilled in a liquid form.

6. The most common symptoms of pleural effusion include:
   A. Cough, chest pain, and dyspnea
   B. Increased fremitus, dyspnea, and cough
   C. Dyspnea, diminished breath sounds, and pain
   D. Cough, increased breath sounds, and dyspnea

6. Answer: A
Cough, chest pain, and dyspnea are the most common complaints reported by clients experiencing pleural effusion.

7. Pleurodesis cannot be attained when:
   A. The effusion quickly reaccumulates.
   B. The client has a trapped lung.
   C. Chemotherapy is ineffective.
   D. The platelet count is > 50,000/µl.

7. Answer: B
Trapped lung maintains the pleurae in opposition, owing to adhesions; therefore, pleurodesis cannot be attained.

8. A client treated for pleural effusion would most likely be taught about:
   A. Fluid restrictions
   B. Low-protein diet
   C. Weight loss strategies
   D. Symptoms of recurrent pleural effusion

8. Answer: D
Some individuals will experience recurrent effusions.

9. An expected outcome for a client treated with thoracentesis alone is:
   A. Immediate relief of symptoms
   B. No relief of symptoms
   C. Prevention of further effusions
   D. Achievement of pleurodesis

9. Answer: A
The client can expect immediate relief of symptoms. Thoracentesis alone will not prevent further effusions, nor will it obliterate the pleural space.

10. A sclerosing drug has been instilled into the pleural space, and the client says, "I shouldn't have any more fluid come out of the chest tube now." What is your response?
    A. "That's right; the medicine will stop the liquid from forming."
    B. "The medicine will cause more liquid to form over the next day or two; then we expect it to stop."
    C. "Ask your doctor."
    D. "Yes, the sclerosant acts just as a huge plug, like a cork in a bottle."

10. Answer: B
    The sclerosant is an irritant and will cause an increase in fluid formation for a few days.

REFERENCES

Aelony Y, King R, Boutin C: Thoracoscopic talc pouderage pleurodesis for chronic recurrent pleural effusions. Ann Intern Med 115(10):778–782, 1991.

Boutin C, Rey F: Complications of thoracoscopy and preventive measures. *In* Brown WT (ed): Atlas of Video-Assisted Thoracic Surgery. Philadelphia: WB Saunders Co, 1994, pp. 138–152.

Fingar B: Sclerosing agents used to control malignant pleural effusions. Hosp Pharm 27:622–628, 1992.

Heffner J, Unruh I: Tetracycline pleurodesis: Adios, farewell, adieu. Chest 101(1):5–6, 1992.

Jewell D, Olak J: Postoperative management. *In* Brown WT (ed): Atlas of Video-Assisted Thoracic Surgery. Philadelphia: WB Saunders Co, 1994, pp. 134–137.

Keller S: Current and future therapy for malignant pleural effusion. Chest 103(1, Suppl):63–67, 1993.

Kennedy L, Harley R, Sahn S, Strange C: Talc slurry pleurodesis. Chest 107(6):1707–1712, 1995.

Kennedy L, Rusch V, Strange C, Ginsberg R, Sahn S: Pleurodesis using talc slurry. Chest 106(2):342–346, 1994.

Lee KA, Harvey JC, Reich H, Beattie E: Management of malignant pleural effusions with pleuroperitoneal shunting. J Am Col Surg 198: 586–588, 1994.

Light RW: Pleural Diseases, 2nd ed. Philadelphia: Lea and Febiger, 1990.

Milanez R, Vargas F, Filomeno L, Teixeira L, Fernandez A, Jatene F, Light P: Intrapleural talc for the treatment of malignant pleural effusions secondary to breast cancer. Cancer 75(11):2688–2692, 1995.

Robinson C: Thoracic cavity management. *In* Boggs RL, Wooldridge-King M (eds): AACN Procedure Manual for Critical Care. Philadelphia: WB Saunders Co, 1993, pp. 165–198.

Robinson LA, Fleming WH, Galbraith TA: Intrapleural doxycycline control of malignant pleural effusions. Ann Thorac Surg 55:1115–1122, 1993.

Robinson RD, Fullerton DA, Albert JD, Sorensen J, Johnston M: Use of pleural Tenckhoff catheter to palliate malignant pleural effusion. Ann Thorac Surg 57:286–288, 1994.

Ruchdeschel J, Moores D, Lee J, Einhorn L, Mandelbaum I, Koeller J, Weiss G, Losada M,

Keller J: Intrapleural therapy for malignant pleural effusions. Chest 100(6):1528–1535, 1991.

Shuey K: Heart, lung, and endocrine complications of solid tumors. Semin Oncol Nurs 10(3):177–188, 1994.

Viallat J, Boutin C: Diagnostic and therapeutic thoracoscopy in pleural effusion. *In* Brown WT (ed): Atlas of Video-Assisted Thoracic Surgery. Philadelphia: WB Saunders Co, 1994, pp. 159–170.

Walker-Renard PB, Vaughan L, Sahn S: Chemical pleurodesis for malignant pleural effusions. Ann Intern Med 120(1):56–64, 1994.

Weissberg D, Ben-Zeev H: Talc pleurodesis. J Thorac Cardiovasc Surg 106(4):689–695, 1993.

CHAPTER 32

MALNUTRITION/CACHEXIA

Eileen M. Glynn-Tucker, RN, MS, AOCN

CHAPTER OBJECTIVES

At the completion of this chapter, the reader will be able to:

Define malnutrition and cachexia.

Describe the pathophysiology of cancer cachexia.

Describe the interdisciplinary and nursing care of clients with malnutrition and cancer cachexia.

Help prepare the client with malnutrition and cancer cachexia for the future.

OVERVIEW

MALNUTRITION is the most common secondary diagnosis in clients with cancer. Malnutrition in the client with cancer is described as an inadequate supply of nutrients to a cell as a result of inadequate intake, impaired absorption, or hypermetabolic processes. Cancer cachexia, the most severe form of malnutrition, is experienced by 40 to 60% of all oncology clients (Ottery, 1995; Skipper, Szeluga, and Groenwald, 1993; Ovesen, Allingstrup, Hannibal, Mortensen, and Hansen, 1993). Cancer cachexia is a syndrome of progressive, profound loss of body weight, fat, and muscle accompanied by anorexia, weight loss, and altered metabolism. Weight loss with accompanying malnutrition and cachexia is one of the most common presenting signs of cancer, affecting up to 50% of patients at the time of diagnosis. Malnutrition and cachexia are most often seen in patients with gastric, lung, head and neck, pancreatic, and other carcinomas of the gastrointestinal (GI) tract. The elderly are at higher risk for the development of malnutrition and cachexia because of the physiologic changes associated with aging, diminishing oral intake, depletion of protein stores, and increased sensitivity to the side effects of cancer treatment.

DESCRIPTION

Malnutrition and cancer cachexia occur when the client's physiologic requirement of protein and calories exceeds the client's dietary consumption of protein and calories, creating a situation in which the body's reserves are used to meet energy and protein needs. Both visceral adipose tissue and protein stores are markedly depleted in cachectic patients (Ogiwara et al., 1994). Malnutrition and cancer cachexia can be caused by a variety of factors, including metabolic effects of the tumor, mechanical effects of the tumor, and effects of cancer treatment.

Metabolic effects of the tumor

It has been repeatedly observed that the degree of cachexia bears no simple correlation to tumor burden, tumor cell type, or anatomic site of involvement. Metabolic effects produced by tumors and independent of anatomic aberrations or insufficient delivery of nutrients must be considered (Daly et al., 1990; Heber, Byerley, and Tchekmedyian, 1992). Such effects are of substantial importance, as they imply secretion of peptides by the tumor cells (Table 32–1). Thus, cancer cachexia is a paraneoplastic syndrome that involves more than simply a negative balance between calorie intake and expenditure of energy. Table 32–1 identifies specific metabolic effects of the tumor, at least partly caused by the release of tumor necrosis factor (cachectin) and other cytokines.

Table 32–1
Metabolic Effects of the Tumor

Increased basal metabolic rate
Altered carbohydrate metabolism:
    Anaerobic glycolysis replaces oxidative phosphorylation.
    Rate of gluconeogenesis increases.
    Glucose intolerance develops with marked resistance to peripheral insulin.
Altered protein metabolism:
    Muscle mass decreases.
    Protein breakdown increases.
    Protein synthesis diminishes, possibly due to decreased albumin synthesis.
    Protein stores are depleted via fistulas, skin ulcerations, etc.
Altered fat metabolism:
    Lipid stores are utilized for energy.
    Hyperlipidemia develops.
Malabsorption of nutrients
Fluid and electrolyte abnormalities
Taste changes
Anorexia
Immunosuppression:
    Lymphoid tissue mass decreases.
    Circulating lymphocytes decrease in number.

Source: Data from Heber, Byerley, and Tchekmedyian, 1992; Skipper, Szeluga, and Groenwald, 1993.

Mechanical effects of the tumor

Mechanical interference of tumors of the GI tract can lead to impaired chewing with dysphagia, early satiety, obstructive symptoms, nausea and vomiting, diarrhea, constipation, pain, and/or a sensation of food becoming "stuck" after swallowing. Cancer treatment modalities are aimed at reducing tumor burden and consequently decreasing these mechanical effects of the tumor. However, cancer treatment creates further malnutrition and cachexia.

Effects of cancer treatment

Surgery

Surgery is often associated with a prolonged period of malnutrition, which can include the prediagnostic workup, perioperative period, and the often complicated recovery period. Malnutrition is often the result of radical dissection of the head, neck, or GI tract, as these resections impair the ability to ingest, digest, or absorb nutrients. In these malignancies, the tumor burden has often interfered with ingestion and digestion long before diagnosis. Malnutrition and cachexia are magnified in surgical patients as a result of increased catabolism and accelerated metabolic demands.

Abdominal surgery affects nutritional status, as ascites, gas, constriction, early satiety, and pain may contribute to postsurgical anorexia. Two critical factors in resuming normal bowel function are the extent and location of the resection and the adaptive ability of the remaining bowel. These factors influence the absorption of fat, protein, fat-soluble vitamins, calcium, and magnesium, creating a significant impact on nutrition.

Chemotherapy

The side effects of chemotherapy include nausea and vomiting, anorexia, fatigue, diarrhea, mucositis (including stomatitis and esophagitis), and taste changes. Each of these side effects can decrease a client's appetite and physical activity, further resulting in weight and muscle loss. Myelosuppression places the client at risk for infection. Infection accompanied by fever, chills, anorexia, and increased metabolism can lead to further deterioration in the nutritional state of the patient. The GI tract is a very sensitive target for cytotoxic drugs, because of the rapid turnover of cells in the mucosa. Toxic effects on the mucosal lining include oral ulcerations, esophagitis, pharyngitis, and generalized mucositis. Mucositis can result in dysphagia, diarrhea, and bleeding; consequently, dehydration, electrolyte imbalances, and malnutrition may ensue. Nausea and vomiting result in decreased oral intake, fluid and electrolyte imbalances, general weakness, and weight loss. Thus, the side effects of chemotherapy can contribute to malnutrition and cachexia in multiple ways.

Radiation Therapy

The nutritional deficits are related to the location of the tumor and the area being irradiated. Mucositis resulting from irradiation of the upper GI tract leads to diminished oral intake. Radiation injury to the taste buds greatly affects the client's appetite. Xerostomia makes chewing and swallowing difficult and diminishes the taste of foods. Taste changes lead to different dietary habits and disinterest in food, which often result in further malnutrition. Diarrhea, nausea and vomiting, and flatus production can result from radiation therapy to the abdominal region. Each of these factors leads to diminished oral intake, contributing to the negative energy balance.

RISK PROFILE

Cancers: Gastric, head and neck primaries, pancreatic, lung, colon, duodenum, rectum, esophageal, liver, ovary, prostate, myeloma, acute leukemia, brain, and lymphoma.

> **Pediatrics:** Acute leukemia.

Conditions: Inability to chew, swallow or feed self, anorexia, early satiety, malabsorption syndromes, GI tract obstruction, fluid and electrolyte abnormalities, alcoholism, hormonal abnormalities, changes in taste and smell, smoking.

> **Pediatrics:** Clients requiring emergent oncologic surgery for cessation of bleeding, spinal cord compression, relief of superior vena cava syndrome, and palliative relief of pain.

Environment: Living alone or having to prepare meals for one's self.

Foods: None.

Drugs: Any medication that places the client at risk for nausea and vomiting, anorexia, taste changes, fullness/bloating, or diarrhea.

PROGNOSIS

The presence of malnutrition in a client with cancer indicates a poor prognosis in both children and adults. Weight loss at the time of cancer diagnosis is an independent predictor of survival (Ovesen et al., 1993). Cachexia has been implicated as the most common immediate cause of death in the cancer patient. There is no evidence that cancer cachexia syndrome can be

Table 32–2
Measures to Promote Nutritional Intake

Cause of Reduced Intake	Measures to Promote Intake
Anorexia	Eat six small frequent meals daily. Avoid foods with strong odors. Snack on high-calorie, high-protein foods. Avoid empty calories. Eat meals in a clean, unhurried atmosphere. Drink wine or fruit juice before a meal.
Taste changes	Sample foods to determine what tastes best. Add mild seasonings, sauces, or sugar to enhance palatability. If beef and pork taste bitter, obtain protein from fish, poultry, eggs, and cheese. Rinse mouth before meals and snacks.
Xerostomia	Carry a squirt bottle of water or juice. Use artificial saliva preparations, if effective for client. Chew sugarless gum or suck on sugarless candy. Moisten foods with gravies or sauces.
Dysphagia	Soft, pureed, or liquid foods are easiest to swallow. Adding creams and grains can facilitate swallowing. Experiment with food temperature to determine which foods are easiest to swallow.
Diarrhea	Drink liberal fluids to prevent dehydration. Avoid caffeine and cold foods, which stimulate GI motility. Administer antidiarrheals. Consume foods at room temperature.
Nausea, vomiting	Administer antiemetics 30 minutes before meals. Take small, frequent meals. Consume foods at room temperature. Avoid foods with strong odors.
Stomatitis	Avoid irritating foods. Consume nonacidic, bland foods with a soft consistency. Consume cold foods and beverages. Use topical/systemic anesthetics as needed.
Early satiety	Drink beverages between meals (not with meals). Eat six small meals a day. Eat light foods that "slide down" easily. Eat slowly; avoid hurrying.

reversed or cured. The longer cancer cachexia remains untreated, the more susceptible the client becomes to the continued muscle wasting, fat mobilization, organ dysfunction, and hypermetabolic state (Nelson, Walsh, and Sheehan, 1994).

TREATMENT

Surgery

> Gastrostomy or jejunostomy tube placement for long-term enteral nutrition.
> Central venous access device placement for parenteral nutrition.
> Removal or bypass of tumor if obstruction interferes with nutrition.

Chemotherapy: Chemotherapy is indicated when a chemoresponsive tumor burden leads to malnutrition or cachexia.

Radiation: To area of partial obstruction of alimentary tract.

Medications

> Megestrol acetate 800 mg orally (PO) qd.
> Corticosteroids to stimulate appetite and improve sense of well-being.
> Metoclopramide 10 mg PO 4 times a day for treatment of early satiety and postprandial fullness related to delayed gastric emptying.
> Dronabinol to increase food intake, promote weight gain.

Procedures: Placement of nasogastric, nasojejunal, or nasoduodenal feeding tube for short-term feeding.

Other

> Increase of oral intake. Use measures described in Table 32–2 to counteract the cause of diminished appetite.
> Enteral tube feeding to meet caloric, protein, and carbohydrate needs that are not met with oral intake.
> Combined enteral and parenteral feeding when enteral feeding alone does not meet client's needs.
> Parenteral nutrition when enteral nutrition is contraindicated.

ASSESSMENT CRITERIA: MALNUTRITION/CACHEXIA

Vital signs	
Temperature	No anticipated deviation from normal.
Pulse	Tachycardia if dehydrated.
Respiration	Tachypnea or normal.
Blood pressure	Decreased systolic and diastolic values.
History:	
Symptoms, conditions	GI symptoms (anorexia, taste changes, nausea and vomiting, dysphagia, stomatitis, xerostomia, diarrhea, malabsorption), GI obstruction (by tumor, or treatment-related), GI surgery, cancer treatment, other medical illnesses.
Weight pattern	Decreased by 10% or more from baseline in 6 months, or 5% in the past 1 month, unintentional weight loss.

ASSESSMENT CRITERIA: MALNUTRITION/CACHEXIA *(continued)*

Hallmark physical signs and symptoms	Loss of muscle mass, depletion of fat stores, poor muscle tone, cachectic, fatigued appearance.
Additional physical signs and symptoms	Skin dry with poor turgor; evidence of gum disease; stomatitis; broken or missing teeth; ill-fitting dentures; dry or pale oral mucosa; dull, brittle hair; brittle nails; possibly swollen abdomen.
Psychosocial signs	Anxiety, depression, difficulty preparing or purchasing foods/meals, living alone, social isolation.

Lab values

Serum albumin	Decreased
Serum transferrin	Decreased
Total lymphocyte count	Decreased
Hemoglobin and hematocrit	Decreased
	Increased in the process of dehydration
Glucose	Decreased
Blood urea nitrogen (BUN)/ creatinine ratio	Decreased
Sodium	Increased
Total iron binding capacity (TIBC)	Decreased
Folate	Decreased

Diagnostic tests

Anthropometric measurements	Weight for height is low. Midarm muscle circumference, triceps skin fold thickness, and subscapular skin fold thickness are low compared to age-specific and sex-specific reference values.
Skin testing/anergy panel	Client is anergic and exhibits delayed hypersensitivity response.

Other	Assess nutritional history and dietary intake (weight loss; pattern of weight loss; 24-hour recall of foods consumed; vitamins, minerals, or other supplements; food allergies or intolerances; food preferences).
	Assess performance status in activities of daily living.

NURSING DIAGNOSIS

The nursing diagnosis will vary depending on the cause(s) of malnutrition and cachexia. The most common diagnoses and etiologies are as follows.

Altered nutrition, less than body requirements, related to inability to ingest or digest food or absorb nutrients because of biologic or psychological factors, tumor location, and side effects of cancer treatments.

Fluid volume deficit related to inadequate intake or inability to absorb fluids.

Social isolation as a result of decreased oral intake or alternative methods of nutritional supplementation.

Knowledge deficit related to manifestations and treatment of malnutrition and cachexia.

Impaired swallowing related to side effects of cancer treatment or obstruction by tumor.

Diarrhea related to inability to ingest or digest foods or absorb nutrients.

NURSING INTERVENTIONS

Immediate nursing interventions

Assess for signs and symptoms of hypoglycemia, dehydration, and critical electrolyte disorders.

Send STAT complete blood count (CBC) and electrolyte panel with albumin, protein, folate, and glucose levels.

Establish patent IV access and obtain volumetric infusion pump.

Monitor intake and output (I and O).

Anticipated physician orders and interventions

STAT serum electrolyte panel.

IV isotonic crystalloid hydration to correct electrolyte abnormalities.

Placement of nasogastric, nasojejunal, or nasoduodenal feeding tube.

Begin enteral feedings and water boluses.

If enteral route is unavailable or inadequate, establish central venous access for parenteral hyperalimentation.

Diagnostic workup to determine causes(s) of malnutrition/cachexia.

CBC, complete electrolyte panel, folic acid, zinc, iron studies (serum iron and total iron-binding capacity [TIBC], serum prealbumin, protein, and serum and urine osmolality.

Nutritional consultation for anthropometric measurements (baseline) after acute dehydration is resolved.

Ongoing nursing assessment, monitoring, and interventions

Assess:
- IV sites for erythema, edema, pain q4h and PRN.
- For signs and symptoms of fluid and electrolyte imbalance q8h.
- Skin turgor qd.
- Extensive dietary history, including dietary habits, responses to food intake, methods of food storage and preparation, sociocultural influences, events leading to current cachexia/malnutrition.

- Bowel status.
- Tolerance to oral, enteral, and parenteral feedings.

Measure:
- I and O q8h × 48 hours.
- Weight twice a day.
- Oral intake for calorie count.
- Gastric residual for the client receiving enteral feedings.
- Baseline height.
- Urine specific gravity q8h.

Send:
- Blood glucose q6h.
- Electrolytes qd (from line other than the one used for parenteral nutrition if applicable).

Implement:
- Calorie count.
- Enteral and/or parenteral feedings as prescribed.
- Measures to promote intake (see Table 32–2).
- Patient/family teaching programs.
- Oral care regimen q4–6h.

TEACHING/EDUCATION

Enteral feedings: *Rationale:* The tube feedings provide the nutrients you need to meet your body's energy needs.

Calorie count: *Rationale:* By measuring the amount of calories, protein, and nutrients you eat, we can determine the amount of extra nutrition you need.

IV line placement: *Rationale:* The IV line allows us to give you necessary fluids and nutrients. In some cases, we can take blood samples from the IV.

Dietary changes: *Rationale:* By making the changes in your diet, you might be able to eat and drink more of what your body needs. The more you can eat, the stronger your body will become.

Parenteral feedings: *Rationale:* Nutrition in your IV gives you the calories, protein, vitamins, minerals, and other nutrients your body needs to do its work. When you are able to eat more, we will decrease or stop the IV feedings.

Blood specimen collection: *Rationale:* Several blood specimens will be taken each day. They are needed to check the sugars, vitamins, and other nutrient levels in your blood.

Signs and symptoms of dehydration and/or hypoglycemia: *Rationale:* You and your significant others need to watch for signs of low fluid or low blood sugar because early treatment helps you feel better and prevents other problems. Signs include feeling light-headed, dizzy, or tired, headaches, trembling, confusion, dry mouth, weight loss, or rapid heart rate.

EVALUATION/DESIRED OUTCOMES

The goal for patients is to plan a diet that meets nutritional needs and minimizes GI disturbances. The primary goal in this population remains nutritional support; thus, replacing fluid and electrolytes, maintaining or regaining weight, and improving functional status and quality of life are important outcomes.

1. Euvolemic state is restored.
2. Weight is stable or increasing.
3. Electrolyte abnormalities are corrected.
4. Serum protein, albumin, and folic acid are stable or improving.
5. Oral, enteral, and/or parenteral supplements are meeting the client's requirements.
6. Additional IV fluids are discontinued.
7. Mechanical effects of tumor are resolved or bypassed.
8. The client or caregiver verbalizes understanding of interventions to maximize oral intake.
9. The client or caregiver demonstrates measures necessary to manage malnutrition/cachexia, including administration of enteral or parenteral feedings and care of feeding tube and access site.

DISCHARGE PLANNING

The malnourished/cachectic client may need:

Oral nutrition supplements, enteral feedings, and/or parenteral nutrition when oral intake alone does not meet client's nutrient requirements.

Intermediate care facility, daily nursing visits, or family caregivers to manage enteral and/or parenteral intake.

Training of the client and significant other in measuring and documenting food/supplement log, daily weights, blood glucose levels via fingerstick, and enteral feeding residuals.

The client with prolonged, severe cancer cachexia may need referral for hospice care and preparation for end-of-life decision making.

FOLLOW-UP CARE

Anticipated care

Nurse or physician office visit within 1 week.

Outpatient lab testing for complete serum electrolyte panel, albumin, CBC, and other blood work as appropriate, within the next week.

Continuation of measures/interventions to promote oral intake.

Weekly home health nursing visits with laboratory testing for clients discharged home with enteral tube feedings.

Three times weekly high-tech home nursing visits with laboratory testing for clients discharged home with parenteral nutrition.

Ongoing specialized nutrition intervention with anthropometric measurements and laboratory testing (prealbumin, folate, TIBC, trace elements) monthly.

Anticipated client/family questions and possible answers

Will I always need IV nutrition?

"It is very unlikely that you will need it for longer than 1 to 2 months. Once we can feed you through your GI tract, we will stop the IV nutrition."

"Once we are able to give you all your nutrients through the feeding tube, we will be able to decrease and eventually stop the IV nutrition."

Will I always need the tube feedings?

"Because you are unlikely to be able to swallow, you will always need the tube feedings to get enough food to meet your body's requirements."

"Once you are able to eat and drink all the nutrition your body needs, we will stop the tube feedings."

"Once your cancer treatment is completed, we might be able to stop the feedings."

Will the nausea and vomiting (or dry mouth, anorexia, taste changes, dysphagia, early satiety, stomatitis) go away?

"Yes, the symptom(s) you describe is (are) an acute effect of the cancer treatment that start(s) to go away a few weeks after your treatment ends."

"Some of the symptoms can last for up to 6 months or a year after treatment. However, they will get better in time."

"No, the xerostomia and taste changes can continue forever. As you begin to feel better in other ways, they might not be so bothersome to you."

Will the tube feeding continue every day and night?

"Once you are receiving the total amount your body requires, we can try to increase the rate so that you can be off the feedings during the day or night. You can decide which hours you prefer not to receive the feedings."

How come I'm not gaining weight? Shouldn't I regain the weight I lost?

"Our goal is to help you maintain your present weight. After the cancer treatment ends, you might begin to gain the weight you lost."

"Cancer causes changes in your body's energy patterns that make you particularly likely to lose weight. When the cancer growth slows, it will be easier for you to regain the weight."

CHAPTER SUMMARY

Weight loss with accompanying malnutrition and cachexia is one of the most common presenting signs of cancer. Up to 60% of all oncology clients experience cancer cachexia, a condition associated with a poor prognosis. Early nutritional support is critical because attempts to reverse cancer cachexia are generally unsuccessful. The goals of nutritional support in the client with cancer are to prevent further nutritional deterioration, support body composition and functional status, and to maintain quality of life. Treatment and nursing care for the client experiencing malnutrition/cachexia are designed to resolve the cause(s) of the problem and support the client with the least invasive and most effective interventions.

TEST QUESTIONS

1. Which of the following laboratory findings would be found in the patient experiencing cachexia?
   A. Decreased serum albumin
   B. Increased protein
   C. Normal hemoglobin
   D. Increased serum folate

1 Answer: A
Albumin is a plasma protein that is low in clients who experience malnutrition lasting a few weeks or more.

2. The goal of nutritional interventions in clients experiencing malnutrition/cachexia is to:
   A. Prevent further nutritional deterioration
   B. Provide double the number of calories the client requires
   C. Provide protein and calories to rebuild and correct the malnutrition
   D. Use the parenteral route first

2. Answer: A
Reversing the malnutrition/cachexia process so that the client maintains current status is a reasonable goal. Correcting nutritional deficits is generally an unattainable goal. Hyperfeeding is generally discouraged.

3. Cachexia is defined as:
   A. Profound loss of weight, fat, and muscle
   B. Loss of appetite
   C. The presenting sign of most cancers
   D. A metabolic effect of tumors

3. Answer: A
Cachexia is a syndrome of progressive profound loss of body weight, fat, and muscle, accompanied by anorexia, weight loss, and altered metabolism.

4. Cancer can alter the metabolism and utilization of:
   A. Protein
   B. Glucose and carbohydrates
   C. Fat
   D. All of the above

4. Answer: D
Metabolic effects of the tumor include changes in protein, glucose, carbohydrate, and fat metabolism and utilization.

5. Surgery can compound malnutrition and cachexia by all of the following *except:*
   A. Interfering with absorption of nutrients
   B. Creating a loss of digestive enzymes
   C. Resecting a large portion of the colon
   D. Removing a tumor that was obstructing the esophagus

5. Answer: D
Removing an obstructive tumor should allow the client to swallow and eat more effectively.

6. An expected outcome for a malnourished/cachectic client would be:
   A. Restoring albumin and protein levels to normal
   B. Maintaining current weight and euvolemic state
   C. Gaining 1% of body weight weekly
   D. Return to ideal body weight

6. Answer: B
Preventing further cachexia by maintaining weight and euvolemic state is reasonable. Resolving cancer cachexia is usually impossible.

7. A common cause of malnutrition/cachexia in the client with cancer is:
   A. Tumor obstruction of the GI tract
   B. Side effects of treatment
   C. Metabolic alterations
   D. All of the above

7. Answer: D
Malnutrition and cachexia can be attributed to metabolic alterations, mechanical effects of the tumor, and side effects of cancer treatment.

8. A client experiencing anorexia would most likely be taught to:
   A. Eat three meals daily
   B. Cook foods with strong odors
   C. Snack on high-calorie, high-protein foods
   D. Drink two glasses of water with meals

8. Answer: C
High-calorie, high-protein foods provide maximal nutrient benefit.

9. Which of the following malignancies is associated with the highest incidence of malnutrition and cachexia?
   A. Gastric carcinoma
   B. Breast cancer
   C. Lymphoma
   D. Acute leukemia

9. Answer: A
Gastric carcinoma and other malignancies of the GI system are associated with high incidence of malnutrition and cachexia.

10. Because many activities in our society revolve around food, clients experiencing anorexia may experience:
    A. Diarrhea
    B. Social isolation
    C. Self-care deficit
    D. Depression

10. Answer: B
Social isolation results as the client withdraws from activities involving eating and drinking. The social isolation can contribute to further malnutrition/cachexia.

REFERENCES

Brown JK: Gender, age, usual weight and tobacco use as predictors of weight loss in patients with lung cancer. Oncol Nurs Forum 20:466–472, 1993.

Daly JM, Hoffman K, Lieberman M, Leon P, Redmond HP, Shou J, Torosian MH: Nutritional support in the cancer patient. J Parenter Enter Nutr 14:(Suppl):244S–248S, 1990.

Heber D, Byerley LO, Tchekmedyian NS: Hormonal and metabolic abnormalities in the malnourished cancer patient: Effects on host-tumor interaction. J Parenter Enter Nutr 16(Suppl):60S–64S, 1992.

Nelson KA, Walsh D, Sheehan FA: The cancer anorexia-cachexia syndrome. J Clin Oncol 12:213–215, 1994.

Ogiwara H, Takahashi S, Kato Y, Uyama I, Takahara T, Kikuchi K, Iida S: Diminished visceral adipose tissue in cancer cachexia. J Surg Oncol 57:129–133, 1994.

Ottery FD: Cancer cachexia: Prevention, early diagnosis, and management. Cancer Practice 2:123–131, 1994.

Ottery FD: Supportive nutrition to prevent cachexia and improve quality of life. Semin Oncol 22(Suppl 3):98–111, 1995.

Ovesen L, Allingstrup L, Hannibal J, Mortensen EL, Hansen OP: Effect of dietary counseling on food intake, body weight, response rate, survival, and quality of life in cancer patients undergoing chemotherapy: A prospective randomized study. J Clin Oncol 11:2043–2049, 1993.

Sarna L, Lindsey AM, Dean H, Brecht M, McCorkle R: Nutritional intake, weight change, symptom distress, and functional status over time in adults with lung cancer. Oncol Nurs Forum 20:481–489, 1993.

Skipper A, Szeluga DJ, Groenwald SL: Nutritional disturbances. *In* Groenwald SL, Frogge MH, Goodman M, Yarbro CH (eds): Cancer Nursing: Principles and Practice. Boston: Jones and Bartlett, 1993, pp. 620–643.

CHAPTER 33

PAIN MANAGEMENT: SOMATIC, VISCERAL, AND NEUROPATHIC

Christine Miaskowski, PhD, RN, FAAN

CHAPTER OBJECTIVES

At the completion of this chapter, the reader will be able to:

Differentiate among the etiologies of somatic, visceral, and neuropathic pain in the oncology client.

Develop a pain management plan for somatic, visceral, and neuropathic pain problems.

Anticipate and prepare the client for the side effects associated with the pharmacologic management of somatic, visceral, and neuropathic pain problems.

OVERVIEW

ONCOLOGY clients can experience acute or chronic pain from their cancer, diagnostic procedures, treatments, or pre-existing conditions. Approximately 30 to 50% of oncology clients experience moderate to severe pain at the time of their cancer diagnosis and at the intermediate stages of their disease (Daut and Cleeland, 1982). During the advanced stages of the disease, 75 to 90% of oncology clients will experience moderate to severe pain (Bonica, 1990). Effective management of cancer-related pain requires that the etiology of the pain be determined and that appropriate treatment be initiated. Pain related to cancer can be categorized based on its pathophysiologic mechanisms into somatic, visceral, or neuropathic pain. Each type of pain has unique etiologies and distinct clinical features, and each responds to different types of therapeutic interventions. Careful assessment of the oncology client experiencing cancer-related pain will result in an accurate diagnosis of the underlying cause of the pain and the initiation of an effective treatment plan.

DESCRIPTION

Somatic pain

Somatic pain results from the activation of nociceptors in cutaneous and deep tissues. Thermal (e.g., excessive heat), mechanical (e.g., surgical incision), and chemical (e.g., stomatotoxic chemotherapy) stimuli activate A-delta and C-fiber primary afferent nociceptors. Activation of primary afferent nociceptors results in the transmission of electrical impulses from the peripheral nervous system into the dorsal horn of the spinal cord. Pain signals are transmitted through the dorsal horn of the spinal cord to the thalamus and cerebral cortex, where pain perception occurs. The most common causes of somatic pain complaints in oncology clients are listed in Table 33–1. Somatic pain is typically described as constant and well localized. Somatic pain descriptors include such words as "aching," "throbbing," "sharp," or "gnawing." Somatic pain responds well to nonsteroidal anti-inflammatory drugs (NSAIDs) or opioid analgesics.

Visceral pain

Visceral pain results from damage to organs innervated by the sympathetic nervous system. The character of the pain can vary, depending on the underlying cause. For example, acute visceral pain may occur in waves (i.e., paroxysmal) and be described as cramping. Acute visceral pain is often associated with nausea, vomiting, diaphoresis, and changes in heart rate and blood pressure. Oncology clients may experience visceral pain as a result of a lesion in the abdomen or pelvis. Abdominal or pelvic pain is often described as vague in distribution and quality. Clients may use words like "deep," "dull," "aching," "squeezing," or "pressure-like" to describe their pain. The major mechanisms for visceral pain in oncology clients include abnormal distention or contraction of a hollow viscera (e.g., intestine); rapid capsular stretch (e.g., liver capsule); ischemia of a visceral muscle (e.g., tumor emboli); and necrosis. The most common causes of visceral pain in oncology clients are listed in Table 33–1.

Neuropathic pain

Neuropathic pain refers to pain that is initiated or caused by a primary lesion or dysfunction in the nervous system. The pain is usually localized to the area of neural injury. Neuropathic pain is typically described as dysesthetic in nature. Dysesthesia refers to discomfort and altered sensations, distinct from the ordinary, familiar sensations of pain. Clients experiencing a dysesthetic, neuropathic type pain will use words like "burning," "tingling," "numbing," or "pressing" to describe their pain. Neuropathic pain may be constant and steady in nature. Some clients report that in addition to a con-

Table 33–1
Common Causes of Cancer-Related Pain

Somatic pain
  Bone metastasis
  Mucositis
  Pathologic fractures
  Spinal cord compression
  Surgery
  Tissue inflammation/necrosis

Visceral pain
  Acute ischemia
  Chemical irritation
  Distention of the capsule of a solid viscus
  GI malignancies
  Hepatic metastasis
  Infectious peritonitis
  Inflammation of the parietal peritoneum
  Invasion or compression of splenic and renal veins
  Obstruction of a hollow viscus
  Omental metastasis
  Thrombosis or engorgement of splenic and renal veins

Neuropathic pain
  Base of the skull metastases
  Chemotherapy (e.g., vincristine, cisplatin, taxol)
  Leptomeningeal disease
  Postherpetic neuralgia
  Radiation-induced damage to peripheral nerves
  Surgery (e.g., limb amputation, mastectomy, nephrectomy, radical head and neck, thoracotomy)

stant, steady, dysesthetic pain, they may experience a shocklike pain (e.g., shooting, electrical, jolting) superimposed on the steady pain. The most common causes of neuropathic type pain in oncology clients are listed in Table 33–1. Neuropathic pain tends to respond to treatment with tricyclic antidepressants, anticonvulsants, or oral local anesthetics.

RISK PROFILE

Cancers

> *For somatic pain problems:* breast, kidney, lung, multiple myeloma, prostate, thyroid.
>
> *For visceral pain problems:* GI cancers, ovarian cancer.
>
> *For neuropathic pain problems:* myeloma, metastases to the base of the skull; brachial plexopathy from breast, lung, and lymphoma; cervical plexopathy from head and neck tumors; and lumbosacral plexopathy from colorectal, endometrial, renal, sarcoma, and lymphoma.

Conditions

For somatic pain problems: surgery, administration of somatotoxic chemotherapy, infectious processes in soft tissues, radiation-induced skin desquamation, and extravasation of chemotherapy.

For visceral pain problems: intraperitoneal chemotherapy, intestinal obstruction, hepatic metastasis, abdominal radiation (diarrhea), and pelvic radiation (cystitis).

For neuropathic pain problems: surgical procedures that damage peripheral nerves (i.e., limb amputation, mastectomy, nephrectomy, radical head and neck, thoracotomy), herpes zoster infection, and radiation-induced damage to peripheral nerves.

Environment: None.

Foods: None.

Drugs

For somatic pain problems: administration of stomatotoxic chemotherapy (e.g., methotrexate, 5-fluorouracil, doxorubicin, bleomycin, dactinomycin, daunorubicin, vinblastine) and administration of chemotherapy that can produce extravasation (e.g., actinomycin D, daunomycin, doxorubicin, mechlorethamine, mithramycin, mitomycin C, streptozotocin, vinblastine, vincristine).

For visceral pain problems: administration of intraperitoneal chemotherapy.

For neuropathic pain problems: cisplatin, taxol, and the vinca alkaloids.

PROGNOSIS

Ninety percent of all cancer pain can be effectively managed by means of noninvasive pharmacologic and nonpharmacologic interventions (Jacox, Carr, Payne, et al., 1994). The use of nonopioid and opioid analgesics in combination with adjuvant medications, which are administered by the oral, transdermal, or rectal routes, provide cost-effective pain control for the majority of oncology clients experiencing cancer-related pain.

TREATMENT

Surgery: Orthopedic procedures are used to treat the pain associated with pathologic fractures; surgery may be performed to debulk tumors or relieve obstructions caused by tumors; neurosurgical procedures (e.g., peripheral neurectomy, dorsal rhizotomy, anterolateral cordotomy, hypophysectomy) are appropriate in approximately 10% of oncology clients when more conservative pain treatment is no longer tolerated or effective and when adequate expertise and follow-up care are available.

Table 33–2
Nonopioid Analgesics

Drug	Usual dose for adults ≥50 kg body weight	Usual dose for adults <50 kg body weight
Acetaminophen	650 mg q4h 975 mg q6h	10–15 mg/kg q4h 15–20 mg/kg q6h (rectal)
Aspirin	650 mg q4h 975 mg q6h	10–15 mg/kg q4h 15–20 mg/kg q6h (rectal)
Choline magnesium trisalicylate	1000–1500 mg TID*	25 mg/kg TID*
Ibuprofen	400–600 mg q6h	10 mg/kg q6–8h
Naproxen	250–275 mg q6–8h	5 mg/kg q8h

* TID = three times a day.

Source: Adapted from Jacox A, Carr DB, Payne R, et al.: Management of Cancer Pain. Clinical Practice Guideline No. 9. (AHCPR Publication No. 94-0592). Rockville, MD: Agency for Health Care Policy and Research, U.S. Department of Health and Human Services, Public Health Service, 1994.

Table 33–3
Opioid analgesics

Drug	Approximate Equianalgesic Dose	
	Usual dose for adults ≥50 kg body weight	Usual dose for adults <50 kg body weight
Morphine	30 mg q3–4h (repeated around-the-clock dosing)	10 mg q3–4h
Morphine (controlled release)	90–120 mg q12h	N/A
Fentanyl (transdermal delivery system)	0.1 mg q48–72h	N/A
Hydromorphone	7.5 mg q3–4h	1.5 mg q3–4h
Levo-Dromoran	4 mg q6–8h	2 mg q6–8h
Meperidine	300 mg q2–3h	100 mg q3h
Methadone	20 mg q6–8h	10 mg q6–8h

Source: Adapted from Jacox A, Carr DB, Payne R, et al.: Management of Cancer Pain. Clinical Practice Guideline No. 9. (AHCPR Publication No. 94-0592). Rockville, MD: Agency for Health Care Policy and Research, U.S. Department of Health and Human Services, Public Health Service, 1994.

Table 33–4
Adjuvant Analgesics

Drug	Approximate Adult Daily Dose Range
Antidepressants	
Amitriptyline	10–150 mg
Doxepin	25–150 mg
Imipramine	20–100 mg
Trazodone	75–225 mg
Anticonvulsants	
Carbamazepine	200–1600 mg
Clonazepam	2–8 mg
Phenytoin	300–500 mg
Valproic acid	1500–3000 mg
Oral Local Anesthetics	
Mexiletine	600–900 mg
Tocainide	600–1200 mg

Source: Adapted from Jacox A, Carr DB, Payne R, et al.: Management of Cancer Pain. Clinical Practice Guideline No. 9. (AHCPR Publication No. 94-0592). Rockville, MD: Agency for Health Care Policy and Research, U.S. Department of Health and Human Services, Public Health Service, 1994.

Chemotherapy: Chemotherapeutic agents and hormonal therapies may produce analgesia if they cause significant tumor shrinkage.

Radiation: Radiation therapy can relieve metastatic pain as well as pain associated with local extension of primary disease. In addition, radiopharmaceuticals (e.g., iodine-131, phosphorus-32, strontium-89) are used to treat the pain associated with bone metastasis.

Medications: The major groups of drugs used to treat cancer-related pain are nonopioids, opioids, and adjuvant analgesics. The most common analgesics in each class with their recommended dosing regimens are listed in Tables 33–2 (nonopioids), 33–3 (opioids) and 33–4 (adjuvants).

Procedures: Anesthetic nerve blocks using a local anesthetic or neurolytic agent are useful in some patients with cancer-related pain.

Other: A variety of nonpharmacologic interventions can be used as adjuvant therapies in the management of cancer-related pain. Nonpharmacologic strategies that can be used to supplement the pharmacologic management plan include application of heat or cold, transelectrical nerve stimulation (TENS), acupuncture, relaxation therapy, guided imagery, distraction, hypnosis, peer support groups, and pastoral counseling.

ASSESSMENT CRITERIA: CANCER-RELATED PAIN

	Somatic	Visceral	Neuropathic
Vital signs			
Pulse	Normal or increased.	Normal or increased.	Normal or increased.
Respirations	Normal or increased.	Normal or increased.	Normal or increased.
Blood pressure	Normal or increased.	Normal or increased.	Normal or increased.
History			
Description	Aching, throbbing, sharp, gnawing.	Paroxysmal cramping pain or deep, dull, aching, squeezing, pressurelike.	Burning, tingling, numbing, pressing with a shooting electrical, jolting component.
Location	Usually well localized to the site.	Usually more diffuse; may be referred to other sites.	Usually well localized to the site of neural injury.
Severity	Use a 0-to-10 numeric rating scale (0 = no pain to 10 = worst pain you can imagine) to assess patient's self-report of pain intensity.		
Aggravating factors	May include movement; increased activity; stress.	May include food or fluid intake.	May include clothing rubbing against the site, water or wind hitting the site.
Relieving factors	May include application of heat and cold, splinting the affected site.	May include abdominal decompression.	May include gentle rubbing of the affected site.
Additional physical signs and symptoms	Muscle spasms.	Diaphoresis; distention; feelings of fullness; nausea and vomiting.	Allodynia; atrophy; hair loss; hyperalgesia; loss of reflexes; loss of normal sensations; dysesthesias; smooth, fine skin.
Psychosocial signs	Depression, anxiety, fear.		
Diagnostic tests	Bone scan, MRI, skeletal x-rays.	CT scan, abdominal x-rays, workup of the GI tract.	Electromyography, somatosensory testing.

NURSING DIAGNOSIS

The nursing diagnosis will vary, depending on the cause of the pain, the pain management plan, and the condition of the client. Some of the common diagnoses and etiologies are as follows.

Acute pain related to:
- Diagnostic procedures.
- Surgery.
- Stomatotoxic chemotherapy.
- Skin desquamation from radiation therapy.

Chronic pain related to:
- Somatic etiology.
- Visceral etiology.
- Neuropathic etiology.

Constipation related to:
- Intake of opioid analgesics.
- Intake of tricyclic antidepressants.

Fatigue related to chronic pain.

Sleep pattern disturbance related to chronic pain.

NURSING INTERVENTIONS

Immediate nursing interventions

Assess description, location, severity, aggravating and relieving factors, and previous treatments related to the pain problem.

Position patient to enhance comfort.

Establish patent IV access (if pain is uncontrolled and excruciating).

Anticipated physician orders and interventions

Diagnostic workup to evaluate the cause of the pain may include a bone scan, magnetic resonance imaging (MRI), diagnostic x-rays, electromyography, somatosensory testing, or a computed tomography (CT) scan.

Somatic pain:
- Nonopioid analgesics (see Table 33–2).
- Opioid analgesics (see Table 33–3).

Visceral pain:
- Nasogastric tube or long intestinal tube to relieve obstruction.
- Nonopioid analgesics (see Table 33–2).
- Opioid analgesics (see Table 33–3).
- Antiemetic medication administration.
- Antispasmodic medication administration.

Neuropathic pain:
- Tricyclic antidepressants (see Table 33–4).
- Anticonvulsants (see Table 33–4).
- Oral local anesthetics (see Table 33–4).

Ongoing nursing assessment, monitoring, and interventions

Assess:
- Pain intensity twice a day (BID) and PRN.
- Effectiveness of analgesics at a suitable time after administering each dose.
- For bowel movement qd.
- For signs of tolerance (i.e., duration of analgesia shortens) qd.
- For side effects of nonopioid analgesics, including abdominal pain, bleeding, renal failure, central nervous system toxicity, and hepatotoxicity (with acetaminophen) qd.
- For side effects of opioid analgesics, including constipation, sedation, nausea, pruritus, urinary retention, and respiratory depression qd.
- For side effects of the tricyclic antidepressants, including sedation, orthostatic hypotension, constipation, dry mouth, dizziness, precipitation of acute-angle glaucoma, constipation, urinary retention, and cardiac dysrhythmias, qd.
- For side effects of anticonvulsants qd, including dizziness, ataxia, sedation, diplopia, and nausea and vomiting with carbamazepine; dizziness, sedation, and fatigue with clonazepam; gingival hyperplasia and acne with phenytoin; and hepatocellular toxicity, pancreatitis, nausea and vomiting, insomnia, and headache with valproic acid.
- For side effects of the oral local anesthetics qd, including cardiac dysrhythmia, confusion, dysarthria, nystagmus, tremor, nausea, vomiting, and constipation.

Measure: Blood pressure, pulse, and respirations BID.

Send: Blood for anticonvulsant drug levels, monthly.

Implement:
- Around-the-clock administration of analgesic regimen.
- A bowel protocol (senna and docusate).
- A nonpharmacologic pain management plan based on client preferences.

TEACHING/EDUCATION

Around-the clock administration of pain medication: *Rationale:* Pain medicine will work best if the medicine is taken on a regular schedule. *Do not* skip a dose of medicine or wait for your pain to become very bad before taking your pain medicine.

Cause of the pain: *Rationale:* The pain you have is caused by [explain the specific cause of the pain]. The pain can be well controlled by using pain medicines and other types of treatments.

Side effects of pain medicines: *Rationale:* All pain medicines have side effects. One of the most common side effects of pain medicine is constipation (not being able to have a bowel movement). The best way to prevent constipation is to drink lots of liquids and eat more fruits and vegetables. You may need to take a stool softener or a laxative for the constipation. Nausea and vomiting are another side effect of pain medicine that usually goes away 1 to 2 days after starting the pain medicine. Sleepiness is another side effect of pain medicine that often goes away after a couple of days. Tell your doctor or nurse if you have any of these problems.

Development of tolerance: *Rationale:* Sometimes your body gets used to the pain medicine. This effect is called tolerance. Tolerance is not a problem, because the amount of pain medicine can be changed to keep your pain under control.

Development of addiction: *Rationale:* You will not "get hooked" or become addicted to pain medicine. You need to take your pain medicine to treat your pain just as you would take antibiotics to treat an infection.

EVALUATION/DESIRED OUTCOMES

1. Pain is controlled to tolerable levels.
2. Bowel elimination pattern is normal.
3. The client is free of side effects of the analgesic regimen.
4. The client uses preferred nonpharmacologic pain management strategies on a routine basis.

DISCHARGE PLANNING

The oncology client experiencing cancer-related pain may need:

A referral to a pain specialist when pain is not controlled by conventional means and more specialized pain management strategies are required.

A referral to hospice care during the terminal stages of the illness to manage escalating doses of pain medication and additional symptoms of the disease and treatments.

A referral for psychological counseling and support in order to manage some of the psychosocial issues associated with a chronic illness and chronic pain.

Training of the client and family members in pain assessment and how to communicate about unrelieved pain to health care professionals.

FOLLOW-UP CARE

Anticipated care

Escalate the dose of pain medication as tolerance develops.

Watch for increases in pain intensity if tolerance to pain medication develops or the client's disease progresses.

Make weekly evaluations of the efficacy of the pain management plan.

Through education, address the fear on the part of the client and family members about taking opioid analgesics.

Develop a plan to manage the side effects of pain medications should they occur.

Anticipated client/family questions and possible answers

Will my pain get worse?

"It is possible that your pain may increase. You need to tell your doctor or nurses if your pain increases in intensity or changes in any way. Your doctor will be able to adjust your pain medicine to maintain your level of comfort."

Will I become addicted to the pain medication?

"Studies have shown that only a very small number of clients become addicted or 'get hooked' on pain medicine. You need to take your pain medicine to treat the pain associated with your cancer just as you need to take antibiotics to treat an infection. You are taking your pain medicine to help relieve your pain and make you more comfortable."

Will the pain medicine stop working?

"The pain medicine will not stop working. However, sometimes your body will get used to the pain medicine. This effect is called tolerance. If your body does get used to the pain medicine, the doctor can change the dose or give you a different pain medicine to help control your pain."

CHAPTER SUMMARY

The pain associated with cancer or cancer treatment is a significant problem for oncology clients. Approximately 30 to 50% of clients undergoing active treatment and 75 to 90% of clients during the terminal stages of the disease experience moderate to severe pain. The pain associated with cancer or cancer treatment can be classified as three types: somatic, visceral, and neuropathic. Each type of pain has unique etiologies and distinct clinical features and responds to different types of therapeutic interventions. Effective pain management involves a detailed pain assessment, the use of pharmacologic and nonpharmacologic interventions, and ongoing evaluation of the effectiveness of the pain management plan. Ninety percent of all pain that occurs in oncology clients can be managed by noninvasive therapies (i.e., oral, transdermal, or rectal routes of administration). Clients who have pain problems that are not responsive to noninvasive approaches require evaluation by a pain specialist.

TEST QUESTIONS

1. What percentage of oncology clients will have pain during the terminal stages of their illness?
   A. 10%
   B. 25%
   C. 50%
   D. >75%

1. Answer: D
Approximately 75 to 90% of oncology clients will experience moderate to severe pain during the terminal stages of their illness.

2. The major types of cancer-related pain include all of the following *except:*
   A. Somatic
   B. Idiopathic
   C. Neuropathic
   D. Visceral

2. Answer: B
Pain related to cancer can be categorized based on its pathophysiologic mechanism as somatic, visceral, or neuropathic pain. Each type of pain has unique etiologies and distinct clinical features and responds to different types of therapeutic interventions.

3. The type of pain that results from activation of nociceptors in cutaneous and deep tissues is called:
   A. Somatic
   B. Idiopathic
   C. Neuropathic
   D. Visceral

3. Answer: A
Somatic pain results from activation of nociceptors in cutaneous and deep tissues by thermal, mechanical, or chemical stimuli.

4. The type of pain that can be described as paroxysmal and cramping is called:
   A. Somatic
   B. Idiopathic
   C. Neuropathic
   D. Visceral

4. Answer: D
Visceral pain that occurs acutely is often described as occurring in waves (paroxysms) and having a crampy quality. Acute visceral pain is often associated with nausea, vomiting, and diaphoresis.

5. All of the following chemothera-
peutic agents can cause neuro-
pathic pain problems *except:*
A. Adriamycin
B. Cisplatin
C. Taxol
D. Vincristine

5. Answer: A
The vinca alkaloids (i.e., vincristine, vinblastine, vindesine),
taxol, and cisplatin can produce
neuropathic pain.

6. The percentage of cancer-related
pain that can be effectively
relieved by noninvasive means is:
A. 25%
B. 50%
C. 75%
D. 90%

6. Answer: D
Approximately 90% of all cancer
pain can be effectively managed
using noninvasive pharmacologic
and nonpharmacologic interventions. The use of nonopioid and
opioid analgesics in combination
with adjuvant medications provide
cost-effective pain control for the
majority of oncology clients.

7. One of the most effective medica-
tions for neuropathic pain is:
A. Acetaminophen
B. Morphine
C. Amitriptyline
D. Ibuprofen

7. Answer: C
The tricyclic antidepressants are
one of the most effective classes of
medications for the management of
neuropathic pain problems.

8. One of the most troublesome side
effects of opioid analgesics that
needs to be treated prophylacti-
cally is:
A. Pruritus
B. Constipation
C. Respiratory depression
D. Dry mouth

8. Answer: B
Clients taking opioid analgesics will
develop tolerance to all of the side
effects except constipation. These
clients need to be placed on a
bowel regimen.

9. The equivalent dose of hydromor-
phone that one would need to give
a client who was taking 30 mg of
morphine q4h, orally, is:
A. 1.5 mg q3–4h
B. 3.5 mg q3–4h
C. 7.5 mg q3–4h
D. 10.5 mg q3–4h

9. Answer: C
The equianalgesic dose of hydromorphone is 7.5 mg, orally, q3–4h.

10. In developing a teaching plan for a client with cancer-related pain, all of the following information needs to be included *except:*
    A. How to reverse respiratory depression
    B. An explanation of tolerance
    C. The problem of addiction
    D. How to measure pain intensity

10. Answer: A

Respiratory depression is not a problem with the chronic administration of opioid analgesics. This information does not need to be included in the teaching plan for a client with cancer-related pain.

REFERENCES

Bonica JJ: Cancer pain. *In* Bonica JJ (ed): The Management of Pain, 2nd ed. Philadelphia: Lea and Febiger, 1990, pp. 400–460.

Daut RL, Cleeland CS: The prevalence and severity of pain in cancer. Cancer 50(9):1913–1918, 1982.

Jacox A, Carr DB, Payne R, et al: Management of Cancer Pain. Clinical Practice Guideline No. 9. (AHCPR Publication No. 94–0592). Rockville, MD: Agency for Health Care Policy and Research, U.S. Department of Health and Human Services, Public Health Service, 1994.

McGuire DB, Yarbro CH, Ferrell BR: Cancer Pain Management, 2nd ed. Boston: Jones and Bartlett, 1995.

Miaskowski C: Current concepts in the assessment and management of cancer-related pain. MEDSURG Nurs 2(1):113–118, 1993.

Patt RB: Cancer Pain. Philadelphia: JB Lippincott Co, 1993.

CHAPTER 34

PATHOLOGIC FRACTURE

Roberta Anne Strohl, RN, MN, AOCN

CHAPTER OBJECTIVES

At the completion of this chapter, the reader will be able to:

Define pathologic fracture.

State the risk factors for pathologic fracture in the client with cancer.

Describe treatment modalities for pathologic fracture.

Describe nursing care for the oncology client with potential or actual fracture.

Prepare the client with pathologic fracture and his or her family for future care needs.

OVERVIEW

PATHOLOGIC fracture is a fracture that occurs in a bone weakened by bone disease. While cancers account for a significant number of these fractures, they are not the only etiology of this problem. Pathologic fractures occur in Paget's disease, fibrous dysplasia, senile osteoporosis, tuberculosis, infections such as pyogenic osteomyelitis, and in association with benign cysts (Harrington, 1977). In one study, about 54% of pathologic fractures were found to be related to metastatic cancer, 13% to primary malignant tumors of the bone, and 41% to benign conditions (Harrington, 1977). The management of pathologic fracture in the client with cancer is predicated on the extent of the underlying disease.

DESCRIPTION

When bone is diseased, even trivial trauma may result in severe compression or fracture of bone. It is estimated that 30 to 70% of clients newly diagnosed with cancer will develop bone metastases and that 9 to 10% will experience pathologic fracture requiring surgical intervention. Untreated fractures result in immobility and all of its associated sequelae (Townsend, Rosenthal, Smalley, Cozad, and Hassanein, 1994).

Bone metastases are frequently associated with severe and debilitating pain. The cellular mechanism by which cancer cells metastasize to bone is not well understood. Tumor cells become lodged adjacent to the bone surface and develop the ability to influence bone cells. The cells of the bone are able to produce growth factors and angiogenic factors that support tumor growth. Some tumor cells may be responsive to the local ambient concentration of calcium in the extracellular fluid of bone. Most tumors cause osteolytic destruction of bone, producing lytic lesions (see Fig. 34–1). Some tumors stimulate new bone formation, though this new bone may have a destructive component. Tumors are able to cause mineral release from bone and stimulate matrix resorption. Humoral mediation by tumor cells also activates osteoclasts to further destroy bone. Tumors also release osteoclastic stimulating factors including parathyroid-hormone-related protein, transforming growth factor-alpha and -beta, prostaglandins, and cytokines. Tumor cells can also produce factors that activate immune cells, which, in turn, release powerful osteoclastic-stimulating cytokines such as tumor necrosis factor and interleukin 1. These factors produce weakened bone that is highly susceptible to fracture, particularly in weight-bearing areas (Garrett, 1993).

The repair of bone is a unique healing process in that new bone is regenerated. When fractures occur during malignant disease, aggressive management is often appropriate. Even clients with widely metastatic disease are considered for surgical interventions, as up to 70% may survive 6 months postfracture and 50% survive as long as a year (Harrington, 1977, Connnolly, 1995).

Two processes contribute to fracture repair: intramembranous and endochondral ossification. Intramembranous ossification begins in the areas of loose mesenchyme. Ingrowth of capillaries is associated with differentiation of mesenchymal cells into osteoblasts to lay down organic matrix. This matrix mineralizes into new bony trabeculae on the old fracture fragments. The early fracture callus is formed by this appositional growth. In endochondral ossification bone formation occurs in the primary and secondary growth centers of bone. Such formation occurs in fractures in which the fragments are displaced or unstable, such as the ribs (Connolly, 1995).

There are four overlapping stages of fracture repair, which are described in Table 34–1.

RISK PROFILE

Cancers: Any cancer that involves the bone either as a primary or metastatic site. Involvement of the distal femur accounts for over half of all pathologic long-bone fractures. Cancers causing the most pathologic fractures include those of the breast, lung, kidney, prostate, bowel, and thyroid; myeloma; and lymphoma. The most common sites for pathologic fracture include the femoral neck, trochanteric, subtrochanteric, femoral shaft, supracondylar, acetabulum, tibia, humerus, and ulna. Compression fractures of vertebral bodies, which most commonly occur in breast cancer and in cancer of the

Table 34–1
Stages of Fracture Repair

Stage	Time Frame	Characteristics
Inflammation	Begins after the initial injury and lasts until cartilage and bone begin to form a few days to several months later.	Swelling and pain.
Soft callus	Begins when pain and swelling decrease. May last 3 weeks to 3 months.	Bone fragments are united by fibro-cartilage or fiberbone, and a soft callus is formed. This is the point of clinical stability.
Hard callus	Begins after a soft callus is formed and lasts 3 to 6 months after fracture.	After the soft callus is initially stable, it is converted to bone. This corresponds to clinical and radiologic union.
Remodeling	Begins after clinical and radiologic union and may last years.	Bone structure, including medullary canal, is restored to normal. Primary cortical healing is an extremely slow process, estimated to progress 1 mm each 3 weeks.

Source: Data from Connolly J: Fractures and Dislocations: Closed Management. Philadelphia: WB Saunders Co, 1995.

thoracic spine, can also occur in lung cancer, lymphoma, and myeloma. Total collapse of greater than 50% of the vertebral body is almost always associated with malignant disease (Connolly, 1995; Harrington, 1977).

Conditions: Bone disease, particularly in weight-bearing areas; clients who are at risk for falls because of confusion; conditions that complicate the healing of fractures (diabetes, infection, malnutrition, and alcoholism). Circulation to the bone is the most significant factor in facilitating healing (Connolly, 1995).

Environment: Unsafe environments, increasing the chance of the client's falling (e.g., cluttered floors, throw rugs in pathway, loose edges on floor tiles, uneven floors, icy pavement); lifting of the client by caregivers without enough assistance to minimize trauma.

Pediatrics: Children with metastatic or primary bone lesions are vulnerable to falls when running or playing.

Foods: None.

Drugs: Medications or drugs that may result in confusion, increased risk of falling, and associated bone fracture.

PROGNOSIS

The prognosis for the client with a pathologic fracture is related to the underlying disease process. The degree of bone destruction determines the prognosis for the fracture itself. It has also been found that fractures secondary to breast cancer, prostate cancer, myeloma, and lymphoma unite more frequently than those related to cancers of the lung, kidney, or gastrointestinal tract. If extensive destruction of bone has occurred, secure immobilization of the fracture may not be possible, and the client may not be able to bear weight. If the cancer is uncontrolled and continues to grow within the bone, stability may never be achieved.

The quality of the bone proximal and distal to the fracture site must be adequate to support metallic fixation. An acrylic cement, methylmethacrylate, has been used to fill in fractures, either supplementing fixation or improving prognosis when fixation devices cannot be used (Harrington, 1977). Prophylactic fixation is the treatment of choice for clients at risk for pathologic fracture, particularly when lytic lesions are present in weight-bearing bones.

The effect of radiation on fracture healing also influences prognosis. Without internal fixation, chondrogenesis is a necessary precursor of osteogenesis. Because of the radiosensitivity of chondrogenesis, radiation may prevent bone union in nonfixed fractures. This is the rationale for internally fixing fractures prophylactically. If fixation cannot be achieved, healing cannot be expected when the fracture is radiated (Bonarigo and Rubin, 1967).

Perez, Bradfield, and Morgan (1972) identified internal fixation and postoperative radiation as affording the best prognosis in terms of pain relief and functional status with good function in 70% of subjects, and pain relief in 80%, compared with radiation alone, which yielded good function in 30% of subjects and relief of pain in 44%. Harrington (1981) found that 80% of clients receiving hip replacement and radiation were ambulatory 6 months postoperatively, and 45% were still ambulatory at 2 years. The ability of the client to ambulate facilitates healing by increasing circulation to the fracture site (Fig. 34–1).

TREATMENT

Surgery: Internal fixation of fracture or bone at risk for fracture. Methylmethacrylate is added to fixation for increased stability or used when fixation is not possible to stabilize bone. Figure 34–2 shows stabilization of impending fractures in preparation for radiation.

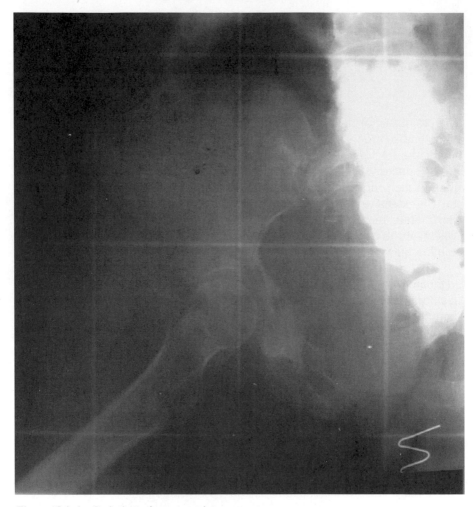

Figure 34–1   Pathologic fracture, pelvis.

Chemotherapy: Depends on the underlying malignancy.

Radiation: Three thousand rad (3000 cGy) given over 10 treatment days, 10 to 14 days, postoperatively. The same dose may also be given to palliate pain if surgery is not indicated.

Medications: Pain medications as needed.

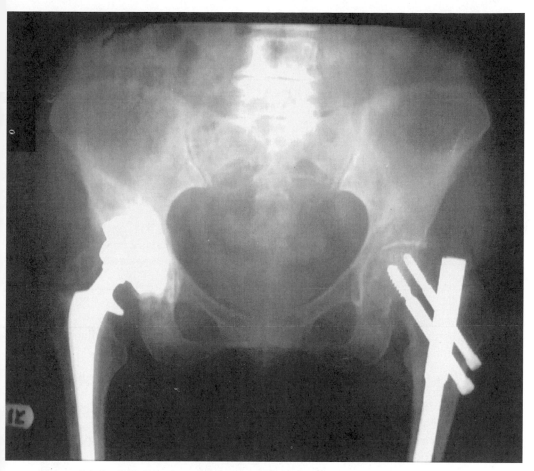

Figure 34–2 Pathologic fracture, with stabilization device.

ASSESSMENT CRITERIA: PATHOLOGIC FRACTURE

Vital signs	Normal or changes typical with pain (i.e., increased heart rate, blood pressure, and respiratory rate). Fever accompanying inflammatory process.

History	
Symptoms, conditions	Bone metastasis or primary tumor.
	Dull, aching, steady pain that increases during the daytime.
	Sharp pain, tenderness, swelling, redness, reduced range of motion.

(continued)

ASSESSMENT CRITERIA: PATHOLOGIC FRACTURE *(continued)*

Hallmark physical signs and symptoms	Sharp pain initially, then dull pain that increases with movement; limited range of motion.
Psychosocial signs	Anxiety, apprehension.
Lab values	
Calcium, serum	Increased in extensive bone disease.
Diagnostic tests	
Radiograph	Variable results, depending on the nature of the fracture, hairline to complete break. Bone exhibits decreased density.
Bone scan	Increased uptake in healing bone. Metastatic disease will light up on a bone scan.

NURSING DIAGNOSIS

The nursing diagnosis will vary, depending on the site and severity of the fracture and the underlying disease process. Some of the common diagnoses and etiologies are as follows.

> *Pain* related to actual fracture or to destruction of bone from malignant disease.
>
> *Risk for injury* related to increased risk for falls from instability of weight-bearing bone.
>
> *Knowledge deficit* related to unfamiliarity of risk factors and sequelae of pathologic fractures.
>
> *Impaired physical mobility* related to actual or potential immobility from instability of bone as healing process continues.

NURSING INTERVENTIONS

Immediate nursing interventions

If client has fallen, assess pulse, respirations, and blood pressure.
Inspect injured area.
Provide comfort measures and measures to prevent further injury.
Summon medical assessment.
Obtain assistance prior to any attempts to move client.

Anticipated physician orders and interventions

X-ray or bone scan of suspected fracture.

Surgical procedure for internal fixation.
Analgesics.

Ongoing nursing assessment, monitoring, and interventions

Assess:
- Site of fracture q4h.
- Wound site q8h.
- Radiation portal.
- Pain characteristics q2h PRN.
- Color, motion, temperature, and sensation distal to fracture if extremity is involved.

Measure: N/A.

Send: N/A.

Implement:
- Weight bearing as directed.
- A safe environment. Lifting and moving the client should be accomplished with enough assistance to minimize trauma. Clients should not be left alone if unable to ambulate.
- Administration of analgesic for pain.

TEACHING/EDUCATION

Select items, based on client's fracture site and treatment.

Ambulation: *Rationale:* The ability to bear weight and to walk will increase the blood supply to the area of the fracture and help it to heal more quickly.

Safety: *Rationale:* The cancer you have has spread to the bones. You are at risk for fractures and need to be careful not to fall, so you must make your environment as safe as possible. Even movements like turning in bed or coughing can cause a fracture if there is a lot of bone destruction. Even if you are very careful, you may not be able to prevent a fracture, so you should not feel guilty if it happens.

Signs and symptoms of bone disease: *Rationale:* You need to let your doctor or nurse know if you have dull aching pain in your bones, because early diagnosis of bone metastases can prevent fractures.

EVALUATION/DESIRED OUTCOMES

1. Timing will depend on the site of the fracture and on treatment.
2. The client is able to ambulate.
3. The client is able to decrease pain medications as fracture heals.
4. The client is able to identify new sites of disease.

DISCHARGE PLANNING

The client with pathologic fracture may need:

Short-term or long-term intermediate care facility if weight bearing is delayed or not possible.

Training of the client and significant other(s) in progressive weight bearing.

Training of the client and significant other(s) in wound care.

FOLLOW-UP CARE

Anticipated care

Physician office visit within 2 weeks.

Follow-up x-rays, scans to monitor bone regeneration.

Home health nursing visit once per week for clients who are not ambulatory.

Anticipated client/family questions and possible answers

Will this problem with my bones happen again?

"It is possible that this problem will happen again. Cancers like yours tend to spread to the bones, and anytime that happens, the inside of the bone gets weak, and fractures may occur."

How can I help to prevent another broken bone?

"You should try to avoid falls and to make your environment as safe as possible. Some ways to do this are to get rid of throw rugs in your walking path, make sure your floors are uncluttered, and avoid walking on uneven surfaces. Use a cane or walker to help you walk. Get someone to help you walk if you feel weak. Move slowly, and turn over in bed very gently."

How will I know if I get another fracture?

"Your doctor will see you often and repeat the x-rays and scans to be sure that new areas are not involved. Anytime you feel a consistent dull and aching pain or a new sharp pain you may have another fracture. If this happens, you should avoid moving as much as possible and call the doctor."

CHAPTER SUMMARY

Pathologic fracture occurs as a result of bone destruction from malignant disease. Cancers that spread to the bone, particularly long bones, place clients at the highest risk for pathologic fracture. Surgical intervention with internal fixation and radiation provides the best prognosis in terms of mobility and relief of pain. Nurses caring for these clients need to identify those at highest risk and must help them to provide safe home environments and to recognize the signs and symptoms of fracture.

TEST QUESTIONS

1. Pathologic fractures occur commonly in all of the following cancers *except?*
   A. Breast cancer
   B. Lung cancer
   C. Kidney cancer
   D. Brain cancer

   1. Answer: D
   Brain tumors do not cause bone metastases.

2. The first phase of bone healing after fracture is:
   A. Soft callus
   B. Inflammation
   C. Hard callus
   D. Remodeling

   2. Answer: B
   After the initial injury, inflammation is the initial phase of healing, lasting until cartilage and bone begin to form.

3. The treatment of choice for pathologic fracture is:
   A. Chemotherapy
   B. Internal fixation and radiation
   C. Radiation alone
   D. Surgery alone

   3. Answer: B
   Internal fixation provides stability to the bone. Radiation prevents tumor growth. The combination allows union, stability, and control of disease.

4. New bone is formed by:
   A. Osteoclasts
   B. Osteoblasts
   C. Mesenchyme
   D. Trabeculae

   4. Answer: B
   Osteoblastic activity results in the formation of new bone.

5. All of the following are characteristic of metastatic bone pain *except:*
   A. Dull
   B. Aching
   C. Gets better during the day
   D. Increases during the day

   5. Answer: C
   Pain from metastatic disease tends to increase during the day, in contrast to arthritic pain, which tends to lessen.

6. The most significant factor facilitating the healing of a fracture is:
   A. Location of fracture
   B. Type of cancer
   C. Circulation to bone
   D. Stage of disease

   6. Answer: C
   Circulation to bone facilitates healing.

7. Which type of cancer produces the fracture least likely to unite?
   A. Breast
   B. Prostate
   C. Lymphoma
   D. Kidney

7. Answer: D
For reasons that are unclear, fractures related to kidney, lung, and gastrointestinal malignancies are less likely to unite than those related to breast cancer, prostate cancer, myeloma, and lymphoma.

8. Most tumors cause destruction in bone, resulting in:
   A. Lytic lesions
   B. Blastic lesions
   C. Mesenchymal lesions
   D. Trabecular lesions

8. Answer: A
Osteolytic destruction results in lytic lesions.

9. The hallmark change in pain at the actual time of fracture is:
   A. Dull pain
   B. Sharp pain
   C. No pain
   D. Aching pain

9. Answer: B
Sharp pain, tenderness, redness, swelling, and limited range of motion occur at the time of actual fracture.

10. The last stage of fracture repair is:
    A. Soft callus
    B. Hard callus
    C. Inflammation
    D. Remodeling

10. Answer: D
Remodeling is the phase when bone structure including the medullary canal is returned to normal.

REFERENCES

Bonarigo BC, Rubin P: Non-union of pathologic fractures after radiation therapy. Radiology 88(5):889–898, 1967.

Connolly J: Fractures and Dislocations: Closed Management. Philadelphia: WB Saunders Co, 1995.

Garrett IR: Bone destruction in cancer. Semin Oncol 20(3):4–10, 1993.

Harrington KD: The management of acetabular insufficiency secondary to metastatic malignant disease. J Bone Joint Surg (Am) 63(4):653–664, 1981.

Harrington KD: The role of surgery in the management of pathologic fractures. Orthoped Clin North Am 8(4):841–859, 1977.

Perez CA, Bradfield JS, Morgan HC: Management of pathologic fractures. Cancer 29(3):684–693, 1972.

Piaseck P: Bone tumors. In Groenwald S, Hansen-Frogge M, Goodman M, Yarbro C (eds): Cancer Nursing: Principles and Practice, 2nd ed. Boston: Jones and Bartlett, 1990, pp. 702–722.

Townsend PW, Rosenthal HG, Smalley SR, Cozad SC, Hassanein RE: Impact of postoperative radiation therapy and other perioperative factors on outcome after orthopedic stabilization of impending or pathologic fractures due to metastatic disease. J Clin Oncol 12(11):2345–2350, 1994.

CHAPTER 35

PERIRECTAL INFECTION

Deborah A. Liedtke, MSN, RN, OCN

CHAPTER OBJECTIVES

At the completion of this chapter, the reader will be able to:

Define perirectal infection.

State the risk factors associated with perirectal infection in the oncology client.

Describe nursing care as it relates to oncology clients with perirectal infection.

Anticipate and prepare the oncology client for future care needs.

OVERVIEW

INFECTION poses the greatest risk to the neutropenic cancer client. It is the proximate cause of death in 50% of clients with solid tumors and lymphomas and in 75% of clients with acute leukemia (Bodey, 1975). Improvements in the supportive care of neutropenic cancer clients has resulted in a reduction in infection-related morbidity and mortality. However, tissue infections such as pneumonitis, colitis, and perianal/perirectal infections are still associated with substantial morbidity and mortality, particularly when caused by aerobic, gram-negative bacilli.

The gastrointestinal (GI) tract serves as an important focus for bacterial and fungal infections. Clients receiving antineoplastic therapy experience the GI side effects of mucosal erosion and diarrhea. Disruption of normal anatomical barriers from surgery, combined with the myelosuppresive effect of chemotherapy, puts clients at significant risk for infections that originate from the GI tract (Rolston and Bodey, 1993).

Perirectal infections remain relatively uncommon, and proper management remains controversial. This complication is an urgent problem, however, requiring prompt therapy. Most of the controversy regarding the management of this sort of infection centers around the necessity for surgical intervention.

DESCRIPTION

The majority of clients with cancer who develop perirectal infections have underlying hematologic malignancies, although these infections are being observed with increasing frequency in clients with solid tumors (Schimpff, Wiernik, and Block, 1972). They have been estimated to occur in 10% of clients with leukemia at the time of autopsy examination and up to 23% of clients with acute leukemia undergoing chemotherapy (Rolston and Bodey, 1993). Perirectal infections have been observed to be particularly common in clients with acute monocytic leukemia and acute myelomonocytic leukemia, suggesting infiltration of rectal tissue by leukemic cells.

The vast majority of perirectal infections occur during relapse of leukemia (Glenn, Cotten, Wesley, and Pizzo, 1988). They may also occur in newly diagnosed clients with leukemia or during initial remission induction chemotherapy. On occasion, perirectal infections may be the presenting sign of acute leukemia (Kott and Urca, 1969). They may also be seen in clients with lymphoma or disseminated solid tumors but are almost never seen during periods of remission for these diseases.

The most common predisposing factor is neutropenia, which is found in over 90% of clients who develop perirectal infections (Glenn et al., 1988). The severity of the neutropenia also appears to be important. Among clients with hematologic malignancies, perirectal infection developed in 11% who had severe neutropenia, defined as < 500 neutrophils/mm^3 (Vanheuverzwyn, Delannoy, Michaux, and Dive, 1980).

The predominant presenting symptom is rectal pain that is aggravated by the act of defecation. Most clients (> 95%) are febrile, often with a hectic or septic temperature pattern. Hypotension or septic shock may occur in up to 10% of clients, particularly those with gram-negative bacteremia (Rolston and Bodey, 1993). The perirectal lesion is usually discrete, erythematous, and indurated. Fluctuation may be elicited as infection progresses. True abscess formation is rare, most likely because of severe neutropenia (Bodey and McKenna, 1986).

RISK PROFILE

Cancers: Acute myelogenous leukemia, acute lymphocytic leukemia, chronic myelogenous leukemia, chronic lymphocytic leukemia, lymphoma, sarcoma, lung carcinoma, and anal carcinoma.

Conditions: Prolonged and severe neutropenia (< 500 neutrophils/mm^3), chemotherapy, radiation therapy to perirectal area, pre-existing fissure or fistula, hemorrhoids, prior intestinal dysfunction (diarrhea, constipation).

Environment: None.

Foods: Foods that are not well digested may irritate the rectal canal and should be avoided. These include corn, nuts, and whole berries.

Drugs: None.

PROGNOSIS

The incidence, severity, and signs of perirectal infection in immunosuppressed clients are inversely related to the peripheral granulocyte count. Infection usually starts at a time of profound neutropenia following chemotherapy and radiation. Because of this, signs of systemic involvement with fever and septicemia predominate (Schimpff et al., 1972). Resolving neutropenia later permits abscess formation with pain or tenderness and, in a lesser degree, erythema and swelling as the only signs of local infection. Typical abscess formation is seen when an increase in granulocytes permits formation of pus (Sickles, Greene, and Wiernik, 1975).

Morbidity and mortality are closely tied to the primary disease, response to chemotherapy and radiation, depth and length of the neutropenic period, and systemic involvement of the infectious process. The overall mortality associated with perirectal infection is in the range of 15 to 35%, with many deaths occurring in clients with bacteremia and septic shock (Rolston and Bodey, 1993).

TREATMENT

Surgery

When used, surgery may consist of incision, digital exploration and destruction of septa, and evacuation.

Needle aspiration to relieve pain and specimen collection.

Diverting colostomy.

Hemorrhoidectomy, if remission of disease permits.

Fissurectomy, if remission of disease permits.

Chemotherapy: Not indicated.

Radiation: Not indicated.

Medications

Various antimicrobial combinations have been used to provide coverage against enteric gram-negative bacilli, gram-positive cocci, and anaerobes. Combinations of aminoglycosides (tobramycin, amikacin) with an antipsuedomonal penicillin (mezlocillin, piperacillin) or an extended-spectrum cephalosporin with activity against *Pseudomonas aeruginosa* (ceftazidime, cefoperazone) are commonly used. B-lactam agents with broad antimicrobial activity (imipenem, ticarcillan/clavulanate) are useful. Vancomycin, clindamycin, and metronidazole are used to provide specific gram-positive and anaerobic coverage. Antifungal therapy (amphotericin B, fluconazole, 5-flucytosine) or antiviral therapy (acyclovir) might be necessary.

Gut-sterilizing oral antibiotic regimens may have some value in reducing contamination of ulcerated lesions by fecal flora.

Stool softeners.

Analgesics for pain.

Reduction of neutropenic days with granulocyte colony-stimulating factors.

Procedures: Sitz baths, warm compresses.

Other: Not indicated.

ASSESSMENT CRITERIA: PERIRECTAL INFECTION

Vital signs	
Temperature	Normal or may be elevated if the client is not immunosuppressed.
Pulse	Normal or increased if infection has produced septicemia.
Respirations	Normal or increased if infection has produced septicemia.
Blood pressure	Normal or may be hypotensive if infection has produced septicemia.
History	History of hemorrhoids, fissures, diarrhea, or constipation; acute myelogenous leukemia, acute lymphocytic leukemia, chronic myelogenous leukemia, chronic lymphocytic leukemia, lymphoma, sarcoma, lung carcinoma, or anal carcinoma; prolonged and severe neutropenia (<500 neutrophils/mm^3), chemotherapy, or radiation therapy.
Hallmark physical signs and symptoms	Rectal pain aggravated by defecation.
	Perirectal lesion that is edematous and indurated and that demonstrates fluctuation or drainage.
	Local necrosis or tissue sloughing.
	True abscess formation.
Additional physical signs and symptoms	None
Psychosocial signs	None
Lab values	
CBC with differential	Neutropenia.
Electrolytes	Possibly reflective of dehydration and imbalance secondary to large volume fluid loss through abscess.
Blood culture and sensitivity	May indicate bacteremia, depending on the extent and duration of the infection.
Culture and sensitivity of abscess drainage or aspirate	Aerobic gram-negative bacilli, anaerobes, and enterococci.

Diagnostic tests	None.

Other	None.

NURSING DIAGNOSIS

The nursing diagnoses associated with perirectal infection include:

Risk for activity intolerance related to pain.

Body image disturbance related to involved perirectal area.

Constipation related to chemotherapeutic agents utilized, pain on defecation.

Diarrhea related to chemotherapeutic agents and antibiotic therapies utilized.

Risk for infection related to depth and duration of neutropenic phase.

Pain related to tissue injury, inflammation, and tissue infiltration.

Impaired tissue integrity related to tissue infiltration, inflammation, hemorrhoids, fissure, and true abscess formation.

NURSING INTERVENTIONS

Immediate nursing interventions

Assess and trend temperature. Avoid use of rectal thermometers, rectal route medications, and rectal manipulation.

Assess pulse, respirations, and blood pressure.

Establish client IV access if client is experiencing septicemia.

Assess area for pain, erythema, fluctuance, and drainage. Culture initial drainage.

Assess for allergies to antibiotic, antifungal, and antiviral medications.

Anticipated physician orders and interventions

CBC qd to monitor neutropenia.

Electrolyte panel qd to monitor for imbalance related to large volume drainage, poor oral intake, or severe diarrhea.

IV crystalloid and electrolyte replacement.

Needle aspiration of abscess formation.

Culture of aspirate.

Broad-spectrum antimicrobial regimens directed against aerobic gram-negative bacilli, anaerobes, and enterococci.

Colony-stimulating factors such as G-CSF and GM-CSF.

Neomycin 50 mg/kg/day orally (PO) in divided doses to sterilize the gut and reduce the number of organisms passing over the wound.

Acetaminophen 650 mg orally q4–6h for temperature >38.5° C or 101° F.

Analgesic PRN.

Docusate sodium 100 mg PO twice a day or other stool softener to relieve constipation.

Antidiarrheal agent to relieve diarrhea.

Ongoing nursing assessment, monitoring, and interventions

Assess:
- Vital signs for return to normal.
- White blood cell (WBC) count to monitor neutropenia.
- Electrolyte panel qd.
- For signs of diarrhea or constipation q8h.
- Need for analgesics q4h.
- Need for antipyretic agent q4h.

Measure:
- Intake and output (I and O) closely owing to risk for high-volume fluid loss through abscess drainage.
- Pulse, blood pressure, and temperature q4h.

Send:
- Blood samples for complete blood count (CBC) and electrolytes as prescribed.
- Cultures from site as prescribed.

Implement:
- Comfort measures such as warm normal saline compresses and sitz baths.
- Administration of antibiotics and gut-sterilizing medication as prescribed.
- Administration of colony-stimulating factors such as G-CSF and GM-CSF.
- Analgesic for perirectal pain.
- Antipyretic for fever.
- Provision of stool softeners if the client is constipated, and caution him or her to avoid straining to pass stool.

TEACHING/EDUCATION

Select items as appropriate to the severity of perirectal infection.

Intravenous blood sampling: *Rationale:* Many blood samples will be taken throughout your neutropenic and fever phase to find out which organisms are causing your infection and to monitor your white blood cell count.

Culture of perirectal area: *Rationale:* Cultures of the affected area will be taken to find out which organisms are causing your infection.

IV line placement and monitoring: *Rationale:* IV fluids and antibiotics may be needed to prevent dehydration and treat the organisms causing the infection.

Dietary changes: *Rationale:* If you have diarrhea or constipation, changes in food may help cut down on this problem.

Frequent monitoring of vital signs: *Rationale:* To check for signs of a total blood system infection, your pulse, blood pressure, and temperature will be checked often.

Inspection of the affected perirectal area: *Rationale:* Looking at and measuring the infected area helps us know how severe the infection is and how well it is healing.

Use of sitz bath: *Rationale:* Sitz baths are needed to relieve your pain and help the tissue heal.

EVALUATION/DESIRED OUTCOMES

1. Resolution of pain and discomfort through use of analgesics and comfort measures within 24 hours.
2. Resolution of infection, with local tissue healing within 72 hours.
3. Resolution of fever and stabilization of pulse, respiration, and blood pressure if signs of septicemia are present within 48 hours.
4. Relief of constipation if present within 24 hours.
5. Resolution of diarrhea if present within 48 hours.

DISCHARGE PLANNING

The client with perirectal infection may need:

Teaching about the signs and symptoms of perirectal infection and abscess formation, use of antibiotics at home, growth-stimulating factors, and analgesics if appropriate.

Discussion of measures to maintain adequate elimination patterns (avoidance of constipation and diarrhea), and measures to promote skin integrity and wound healing.

Home nursing visits every week to assess wound healing and client/family understanding of instructions upon discharge.

Discussion of the possible need to return for surgical intervention if client has a history of hemorrhoids, fissures, or diversion of drainage or if drainage of abscess is present.

FOLLOW-UP CARE

The need for follow-up care will vary with the extent of the perirectal
   infection.
Consult with enterostomal nurse for ostomy and/or wound care.

Anticipated care

Surgical intervention for wound drainage, removal of necrotic tissue, and
   repair of hemorrhoids or fissures will require additional outpatient
   monitoring by the surgical team.
Home nursing visits for dressing changes.
Home nursing visits for clients discharged on colony-stimulating factors
   such as G-CSF and GM-CSF.
The neutropenic client will require lab sampling on an outpatient basis
   as well, every day to every other day.

Anticipated client/family questions and possible answers

Will my infection return?

"It is possible that your infection will return, so it is important that you learn
the signs of early infection and be able to notify your doctor or nurse about
them. It is easier to treat an infection if it is caught early."

Will I ever be able to take suppositories again?

"Once your abscess has healed and your white blood cell count is normal,
you may use suppository medicine again."

When can I stop taking sitz baths?

"When your abscess has healed and you no longer have any discomfort."

CHAPTER SUMMARY

Perirectal infection is an uncommon but serious complication in the neutropenic
cancer client. Medical management consists of antibiotic therapy and supportive
care measures for a large number of affected clients. Broad-spectrum antimicrobial regimens directed against aerobic gram-negative bacilli, anaerobes, and
enterococci is the basis for most treatment. Management of pain and discomfort,
constipation, diarrhea, and fever provides supportive care. Oral, gut-sterilizing
antimicrobial regimens may be of some use to reduce local fecal contamination.
Surgical intervention for drainage may be beneficial for those clients not
responding to conservative medical management. Resolution of the neutropenic
phase of therapy for the underlying disease is paramount to fight infection.

TEST QUESTIONS

1. Which malignancy is most associated with the development of perirectal infection?
   A. Acute lymphocytic leukemia
   B. Lung carinoma
   C. Lymphoma
   D. Sarcoma

1. Answer: A
The majority of clients who develop perirectal infection have underlying hematologic malignancies; among these, acute lymphocytic leukemia carries the most at risk. Leukemic infiltration of tissue is thought to play a role in pathogenesis.

2. The following predisposing signs and symptoms are often seen in the development of perirectal infection *except:*
   A. Diarrhea
   B. Hemorrhoids
   C. Fissures
   D. Nausea and vomiting

2. Answer: D
Infection often arises from the site of a pre-existing fissure or hemorrhoid. Diarrhea may facilitate contamination and infection; therefore, nausea and vomiting are the exception.

3. Controversy over the management of perirectal infections surrounds which of the treatment options available?
   A. Combination antibiotics to treat a broad range of microbes
   B. Surgical intervention
   C. Symptom control of pain and fever
   D. Gut sterilization with oral antibiotics

3. Answer: B
Surgical intervention in the neutropenic, thrombocytopenic client remains controversial because of the possibility of hemorrhage, sloughing, extension of infection, or possible poor wound healing.

4. Lab culture and sensitivity from drainage or aspirate often reveal the cause of a perirectal infection in a person with cancer to be:
   A. *E. coli* only
   B. Gram-negative bacilli only
   C. Polymicrobial, consisting of gram-positive enterococci, gram-negative bacilli, and anaerobes
   D. Aerobic and viral, particularly pseudomonas in origin

4. Answer: C
The majority of infections are polymicrobial, consisting of gram-positive enterococci, gram-negative bacilli, and anaerobes.

5. True abscess formation may not occur in cancer clients with perirectal abscess primarily because the client:
   A. Is hypertensive
   B. Lacks granulocytes
   C. Has a history of hemorrhoids
   D. Has enlarged lymph nodes that block the passage of waste out of the abscess

5. Answer: B
   True abscess formation occurs in 10% or less of clients experiencing perirectal infection because of lack of granulocytes.

6. Which body system is a focal point for bacterial and fungal infections in the person who has cancer?
   A. Reticuloendothelial system
   B. Lymphatic system
   C. GI system
   D. Central nervous system

6. Answer: C
   The GI tract serves as an important focus of bacterial and fungal infections.

7. Severe neutropenia is defined as:
   A. Greater than 100,000 total WBCs
   B. Greater than 10,000 lymphocytes
   C. Less than 2,000 thrombocytes
   D. Less than 500 neutrophils

7. Answer: D
   Less than 500 neutrophils/mm^3 is considered severe neutropenia, which places a client at risk for perirectal abscess.

8. The best way to resolve neutropenia in a client with cancer is to implement which intervention?
   A. Administer G-CSF.
   B. Administer packed red blood cells.
   C. Administer hyperalimentation that consists of high doses of vitamin C, iron, and albumin.
   D. Administer acetaminophen every 4 hours.

8. Answer: A
   Colony-stimulating factors assist in increasing the WBC count, which helps decrease the potential for infection.

9. Which vital sign is most likely to be decreased in a neutropenic client with perirectal infection?
   A. Temperature
   B. Blood pressure
   C. Pulse
   D. Respirations

9. Answer: B
Hypotension is a sign of perirectal abscess with subsequent septicemia in the neutropenic client.

10. To help relieve perirectal pain, a nurse may administer a prescribed:
   A. Antibiotic
   B. Antipyretic
   C. Analgesic
   D. Colony-stimulating factor

10. Answer: C
Analgesics are often prescribed for perirectal pain.

REFERENCES

Bodey JP: Infections in cancer patients. Cancer Treat Rev 2:89–128, 1975.

Bodey JP, McKenna RJ Jr: Surgical considerations in the immunocompromised cancer patient. *In* McKenna RJ Jr, Murphy GP (Eds): Fundamentals of Surgical Oncology. New York: Macmillan, 1986, pp. 114–140.

Corfitsen M, Hansen C, Christensen T, Kane H: Anorectal abscesses in immunosuppressed patients. Eur J Surg 158:51–53, 1992.

Glenn J, Cotton D, Wesley R, Pizzo R: Anecdotal infections in patients with malignant diseases. Rev Infect Dis 10:42–52, 1988.

Kott I, Urca I: Perianal abscess as a presenting sign of leukemia. Dis Colon Rectum 12:338–339, 1969.

McNally J, Star J, Somerville E: Guidelines for Cancer Nursing Practice. Orlando, FL: Grune and Stratton, 1985, pp. 262–266.

Nelson RL, Prased L, Abcarian H: Anal carcinoma presenting as a peri-rectal abscess or fistula. Arch Surg 120(5):632–635, 1985.

North American Nursing Diagnosis Association: Nursing Diagnoses: Definitions and Classifications 1995–1996. St Louis, MO: NANDA, 1995.

Rolston KV, Bodey JP: Diagnosis and management of perianal and peri-rectal infection in the granulocytic patient. Curr Clin Topics Infect Dis 13:164–171, 1993.

Schimpff SC, Wiernik PH, Block JB: Rectal abscess in cancer patients. Lancet 2:844–847, 1972.

Sickles AE, Greene WH, Wiernik PH: Clinical presentations of infection in granulocytopenic patients. Arch Intern Med 135:715–719, 1975.

Vanheuverzwyn R, Delannoy A, Michaux JL, Dive C: Anal lesions in hematologic diseases. Dis Colon Rectum 23:310–312, 1980.

CHAPTER 36

PULMONARY FIBROSIS

Paula Timmerman, RN, MSN, AOCN

CHAPTER OBJECTIVES

At the completion of this chapter, the reader will be able to:

Define pulmonary fibrosis (PF).

Identify oncology clients at risk for developing PF.

Describe the pathogenesis of PF.

List physical signs and symptoms pertinent to the detection of PF.

Anticipate and prepare the client for diagnostic tests performed in the detection of PF.

Describe nursing interventions and teaching strategies for the client with PF.

OVERVIEW

PF is a complication of cancer treatment that can have a devastating effect on a person's quality of life. It is a potentially fatal complication of oncologic therapy in which inflammatory changes lead to progressive fibrosis of the alveoli. The alveoli collapse and become obliterated by connective tissue, leading to restrictive lung disease (McDonald, Rubin, Phillips, and Marks, 1995), which is characterized by decreased lung compliance or elasticity. This impairs the ability of the lung to expand and increases the work of breathing (Thelan, Daire, and Urden, 1990). PF can occur after treatment with numerous chemotherapeutic agents, radiation therapy to the thorax, or following bone marrow transplantation. It can also occur following pulmonary infections, especially in immunocompromised clients. PF is characterized by cough, fatigue, increasing dyspnea, and restrictive ventilatory function (Fischer, Tish Knobf, and Durivage, 1993; Snyder, 1986). Symptoms may appear during active treatment for cancer or not be apparent until months or years after treatment has been completed.

DESCRIPTION

PF is the end result of an inflammatory response to lung tissue damage. The damage may occur to epithelial cells of the alveoli and/or the endothelium of the alveolar capillaries (McDonald et al., 1995; Fulmer, 1994). Exudation of serum protein and cellular debris into the alveolar spaces occurs, resulting in impaired gas exchange. Capillary endothelial damage leads to decreased perfusion of the alveolar surfaces. Cellular breakdown products, resulting from alveolar ischemia, initiate the release of cytokines, causing an inflammatory response (alveolitis). The alveolitis promotes the recruitment of repair cells and fibroblasts. The lung damage may be successfully repaired or lead to permanent scarring of the damaged area. If the lung injury is chronic, such as that which occurs in PF, proliferation of fibroblasts causes the deposition of collagen and other connective tissue in the alveoli, causing fibrosis and lung volume loss (see Fig. 36-1) (Fulmer, 1994). All of the factors in PF are not well understood. The mechanism and severity of PF may vary according to the type of cancer therapy and individual client variables. Radiation therapy, certain chemotherapeutic agents, and bone marrow transplant are potential causes of PF in oncology clients.

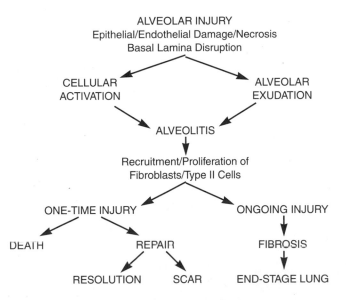

Figure 36–1 The pathogenesis of interstitial lung disease.

Source: Reprinted with permission from Fulmer JD: Interstitial lung disease. *In* Stein JH (ed): Internal Medicine. St. Louis, MO: Mosby Year Book, 1994, pp. 1681–1691.

Radiation therapy

The lungs are one of the most radiation-sensitive structures in the body and will almost invariably be damaged to some extent by radiation. The amount of damage to the lung tissue depends on the dose of radiation delivered, the volume of the irradiated lung tissue, the client's pre-existing pulmonary function, and concurrent chemotherapeutic agents (Jakacki, Schramm, Donahue, Haas, and Allen, 1995; Kimsey, Mendenhall, Ewald, Coons, and Layon, 1994; Mah et al., 1994; McDonald et al., 1995). While the overall incidence of lung disease resulting from radiation therapy is not known, with refined techniques for treatment planning and dose delivery, the incidence of clinically significant disease appears to be greatly decreased (Fulmer, 1994).

Radiation Pneumonitis—Acute Phase

Radiation pneumonitis results from the injurious effects of radiation therapy on lung tissue. The acute phase of radiation pneumonitis occurs 1 to 3 months following radiation therapy. Vascular damage, edema, and mononuclear cell infiltration of lung tissue are present, along with clinical symptoms of low-grade fever, congestion, and a sensation of fullness in the chest. More severe symptoms would include dyspnea, pleuritic chest pain, and a nonproductive cough (Anscher et al., 1994; McDonald et al., 1995). Dyspnea experienced by clients may be disproportional to the amount of lung irradiated, which may be caused by a generalized lymphocyte-mediated hypersensitivity reaction (Morgan and Breit, 1995; Roberts et al., 1993). The acute symptoms of radiation pneumonitis may be treated with corticosteroids over 2 to 3 weeks. However, while the client's symptoms may greatly improve, corticosteroids do not prevent the progression of interstitial fibrosis (McDonald et al., 1995).

Radiation Pneumonitis—Subacute Phase

The acute phase is followed by a subacute phase, which generally occurs 2 to 9 months following treatment. During this phase, the alveolar walls are infiltrated with cytokines, macrophages, and fibroblasts; the alveolar walls thicken; and the interstitium becomes edematous. Clients may appear asymptomatic during this seemingly latent period (Anscher et al., 1994; McDonald et al., 1995).

Radiation Pneumonitis—Chronic Phase

The late or chronic phase of radiation pneumonitis is characterized by alveolar fibrosis and capillary sclerosis, which result from the replacement of alveolar and endothelial cells with connective tissue; irreparable tissue damage ensues (Fulmer, 1994; McDonald et al., 1995). This phase can occur months or years following radiation treatment. The development of late radiation lung injury may be related to the effects of radiation on both the vascular and lung tissues of an individual. The most common symptoms experienced by clients in this phase are a nonproductive cough and dyspnea on exertion, although many patients may be asymptomatic. The severity of symptoms varies according to the amount of pulmonary damage that has occurred. If less than 50% of one lung is fibrosed, symptoms are generally minimal. If the volume of fibrosis is greater than this limit, the client may experience dyspnea and develop right-sided heart failure (McDonald et al., 1995).

Pediatrics

Large radiation doses affect the compliance and lung growth of children. Restrictive changes occurred in the lungs of children treated with 11 to 14 Gy to the whole lung. Lung irradiation in children less than 3 years old resulted in increased chronic toxicity (Benoist, Lemerle, Jeun, Scheinmann, and Paupe, 1982; Miller et al. 1986).

Chemotherapy

The increasing survival of clients who received chemotherapeutic agents has resulted in growing reports of pulmonary toxicity from various drugs. Chronic pneumonitis with subsequent lung fibrosis is the most common clinical presentation associated with chemotherapy (Santamauro, Stover, Jules-Elysee, and Maurer, 1994). The pulmonary effects may be identified days to many years following treatment. In general, chemotherapeutic agents cause toxicity by damaging endothelial cells and pneumocytes (Fischer, Tish Knobf, and Durivage, 1993), causing interstitial pneumonitis and eventual fibrosis (McDonald et al., 1995).

Bleomycin

Bleomycin is perhaps the most well-known cytotoxic agent with the potential for causing pulmonary fibrosis. The reported incidence in the literature of bleomycin-induced pulmonary toxicity varies from 5 to 50% (Fischer et al., 1993; Moore and Ruccione, 1992; Waid-Jones and Coursin, 1991). The incidence increases greatly with cumulative doses over 450 U (Moore and Ruccione, 1992; Waid-Jones and Coursin, 1991). Genetically impaired bleomycin metabolism may cause increased drug accumulation in lung tissue (Martin, 1991; McDonald et al., 1995; Waid-Jones and Coursin, 1991). Ferrous iron and oxygen combine with bleomycin to form its active complex. This active complex causes the generation of oxygen-free radicals in the lung tissue, causing progressive pulmonary damage and fibrosis (Martin, 1991; McDonald et al., 1995; Waid-Jones and Coursin, 1991).

In addition to the cumulative dose, other risk factors for pulmonary toxicity exist. Renal insufficiency can result in decreased bleomycin excretion. This is an important consideration for clients receiving regimens combining bleomycin and cisplatin. Bleomycin and cyclophosphamide is another combination associated with an increased risk of pulmonary toxicity. Smoking, age greater than 70 years, underlying pulmonary disease, and previous chest irradiation have been identified as risk factors for pulmonary toxicity in clients treated with bleomycin (Moore and Ruccione, 1992; Waid-Jones and Coursin, 1991). Bleomycin given concurrently with radiation therapy can produce severe lung toxicity. Bleomycin 500 U without radiation can be fatal in 1 to 2% of clients. However, as little as 30 U of bleomycin can be fatal when given with radiation therapy (McDonald et al., 1995). Because of the development of toxic oxygen-derived free radicals, high levels of oxygen in the lung (hyperoxia) have been associated with increased incidence of pulmonary toxicity. This is especially significant for clients undergoing general anesthesia. Clients who have received bleomycin and then undergone general anesthesia have been reported to develop acute respiratory distress syndrome 3 to 10 days after surgery, which can be rapidly fatal (Waid-Jones and Coursin, 1991).

Carmustine

Carmustine (BCNU) can produce pulmonary fibrosis in 20 to 30% of clients (Patterson, Wiemann, Lee, and Byron, 1993). Pulmonary fibrosis has been reported to occur as late as 17 years following treatment. This may be due to persistent, undetected pneumonitis that progresses to fibrosis or subclinical disease that progresses to fibrosis following exposure to another stimulus (O'Driscoll, Kalra, Gattamaneni, and Woodcock, 1995). Total dose of carmustine and client age at treatment (see "Pediatrics") are two significant factors in the development of PF. Total cumulative doses of more than 1500 mg/m2 have been associated with PF in 50% of clients (Ginsberg and Comis, 1982). Other reported factors in the development of carmustine-induced PF are cigarette smoking, pre-existing pulmonary disease, prior chest irradiation, and administration of other chemotherapeutic agents that produce pulmonary toxicities (Weiss, Poster, and Penta, 1981).

Other Chemotherapeutic Drugs

Various other chemotherapeutic agents have been associated with the development of PF. Like carmustine, busulfan-induced PF may appear years after treatment (Fischer et al., 1993; Snyder, 1986), and delayed onset of PF symptoms may occur with cyclophosphamide as well (McDonald et al., 1995; Patterson et al., 1993; Santamauro et al., 1994). Mitomycin can occasionally produce severe pneumonitis and fibrosis. The risk factors for mitomycin-associated PF are anesthesia, radiation therapy, vinblastine, and cyclophosphamide (Fischer et al., 1993; McDonald et al., 1995). PF developing after treatment with chlorambucil and lomustine appears to be dose-related. Doxorubicin and dactinomycin alone do not cause PF, but they can potentiate the development of radiation pneumonitis and fibrosis. Table 36-1 lists cytotoxic agents that, when combined with radiation therapy, produce pulmonary toxicity that is more severe than when either modality is used separately. Synergistic effects may also be seen with chemotherapy combinations (see Table 36-2). Methotrexate can produce pulmonary symptoms (i.e., hypersensitivity pneumonitis), but the development of PF is rare (Fischer et al., 1993; Santamauro et al., 1994).

Table 36–1
Chemotherapeutic Agents
That May Potentiate Pulmonary Toxicity
When Combined with Radiation Therapy

Bleomycin
Cyclophosphamide
Dactinomycin
Doxorubicin
Mitomycin
Nitrosureas
Paclitaxel
Vincristine

Source: Data from Choy and Safran, 1995; Fischer, Tish Knobf, and Durivage, 1993; McDonald, Rubin, Phillips, and Marks, 1995; Moore and Ruccione, 1992; Schweitzer, Juillard, Bajada, and Parker, 1995.

Table 36–2
Chemotherapy Combinations That
Potentiate Pulmonary Toxicity

Bleomycin–cisplatin
Bleomycin–cyclophosphamide
Bleomycin–doxorubicin
Bleomycin–vincristine
Mitomycin–cyclophosphamide
Mitomycin–vinca alkaloids
Nitrosureas–cyclophosphamide

Source: Data from Fischer, Tisch Knobf, and Durivage, 1993; Mah et al., 1994; McDonald, Rubin, Phillips, and Marks, 1995; Waid-Jones and Coursin, 1991.

Pediatrics

Developing lung tissue in children treated with carmustine may be especially prone to toxic effects. O'Driscoll et al. (1995) found a 100% incidence of PF in childhood survivors of brain tumors who were treated with carmustine. Of this group 47% eventually died from PF. Age less than 6 years at the time of treatment was closely correlated with increased mortality, while clients treated after the onset of puberty demonstrated the least pulmonary toxicity. Severe pulmonary toxicity was noted in infants who received vincristine, doxorubicin, and dactinomycin (Morgan, Baum, Breslow, Takashima, and D'Angio, 1988). Cyclophosphamide given to children during periods of rapid body growth can retard lung growth and cause decreased lung volumes (Santamauro et al., 1994). Bleomycin, mitomycin, and methotrexate have also been identified as causing late pulmonary toxicities in children (Greene and Fergusson, 1982). Periodic pulmonary function tests and respiratory assessments are necessary for children who have received radiation or chemotherapy that could adversely affect lung tissue (Maul-Mellott and Adams, 1987).

Bone marrow transplant

Bone marrow transplant (BMT) is a third cancer treatment modality that places clients at risk for PF through several mechanisms. Clients undergoing BMT receive high-dose chemotherapy, often with agents (cyclophosphamide, busulfan) known to produce pulmonary toxicity. Total body irradiation (TBI) can also cause pulmonary damage and fibrosis. The incidence of PF following TBI is decreasing, however, probably due to the use of fractionated, lower-dose TBI instead of single-dose TBI (Hartsell, Czyzewski, Ghalie, and Kaizer, 1995). High-dose chemotherapy and TBI produce pulmonary inflammation and interstitial pneumonitis (IP), which usually occurs 100 days or more post-transplant. BMT clients experience drastically compromised immune systems, making these clients susceptible to interstitial pneumonitis from infectious sources as well. Infectious IP may develop acutely post-transplant, but it more commonly develops months to several years following BMT. The causative agents may be viral (cytomegalovirus or varicella zoster), bacterial (pneumocystis carinii), or idiopathic (Anscher, Peters, Reisenbichler, Petros, and Jirtle, 1993; Hartsell et al., 1995). IP may also be a result of chronic graft vs. host disease (LeBlond et al., 1994).

The incidence of IP following BMT ranges from 20 to 50% (LeBlond et al., 1994). As with radiation therapy and chemotherapy described above, the inflammatory processes of IP produce progressive lung damage and eventual fibrosis, which may be fatal in some patients. These restrictive changes will usually stabilize within 1 to 3 years post-BMT (Corcoran-Buchsel, 1986); however, clients may experience significant activity restrictions because of dyspnea (Muscari Lin, Tierney, and Stadtmauer, 1993).

RISK PROFILE

Cancers: Large thoracic tumors requiring irradiation. Central nervous system malignancies requiring craniospinal irradiation (Jakacki et al., 1995). Pulmonary malignancies exhibiting lymphangitic spread. Alveolar malignancies.

Conditions: Cigarette smoking, elderly, pre-existing pulmonary disease, chronic pulmonary venous hypertension, pulmonary infection, previous thoracic irradiation, hyperoxia, impaired renal excretion, chronic aspiration.

Pediatrics: Age less than puberty for chemotherapy and radiation therapy (see specifics in text above).

Environment: Asbestos, silica dust, paraquat (herbicide).

Foods: None.

Drugs: See "Chemotherapy" above and Tables 36–1 and 36–2. Also, amiodarone, nitrofurantoin (Martin, 1991).

PROGNOSIS

The morbidity and mortality resulting from PF depend on numerous factors (see Table 36–3). Early PF is characterized by active alveolitis with minimal alveolar destruction and fibrosis. In advanced PF there is minimal alveolitis but widespread alveolar destruction and fibrosis (Fulmer, 1994). Because of the numerous factors involved in PF in the oncology client, overall survival is difficult to predict. In clients with idiopathic PF, Fulmer (1994) describes a 90% 5-year survival for young clients with minimal alveolitis and fibrosis. In contrast, clients with severe PF had a 5-year survival of less than 25%.

Table 36–3
**Factors Affecting Prognosis
in Oncology Clients with Pulmonary Fibrosis**

Pre-existing conditions (see Risk Profile)
Client age
Concurrent illness
Type and extent of malignancy
Extent of lung damage
Response to immunosuppressive therapy

Changes in pulmonary structure cause clients with PF to be susceptible to recurrent bacterial pneumonias. In severe cases, pulmonary hypertension and cor pulmonale can develop, which is associated with high morbidity and mortality (Fulmer, 1994; Syabbalo, 1991).

Little information is currently available that indicates why certain clients are more susceptible to toxic effects from cancer treatments. Rubin, Johnston, Williams, McDonald, and Finkelstein (1995) cite studies that suggest genetic susceptibility to the mechanisms that induce fibrosis. Models of drug- and radiation-induced lung toxicity, awareness of client risk factors, and improved detection techniques will improve client assessment and monitoring (Martin, 1991). As clinical oncology becomes more complex, more data will be needed on tumor and normal tissue response to individual and combination therapy (Mah et al., 1994).

TREATMENT

PF is an often progressive and sometimes fatal complication related to cancer therapy. Treatment objectives are to (1) suppress inflammation to prevent further lung tissue destruction and fibrosis and (2) palliate the symptoms and complications of PF (Fulmer, 1994). These objectives are complicated by the underlying malignancy and the fact that the development of PF may limit the efficacy of the treatment regimen as well as future treatment options (Haylock, 1987).

Surgery: Lung transplantation is accepted therapy for selected individuals who are unresponsive to medical therapy and considered cured of their primary malignancy. In most clients single-lung transplant is used (Fulmer, 1994; Santamauro et al., 1994). If surgery is required in clients treated with bleomycin or mitomycin, the FiO_2 during and after surgery should be kept as low as possible through continuous monitoring of oxygen saturation and periodic arterial blood gas (ABG) analysis (Waid-Jones and Coursin, 1991).

Pediatrics: When considering lung transplantation, one should know that the overall risk of secondary malignancies following cytotoxic therapy in children is 3 to 20% at 20 years (Santamauro et al., 1994).

Chemotherapy: See "Medications" below.

Radiation: Avoid single-dose total-body irradiation in persons undergoing BMT. Artificial pneumothorax has been used to decrease the lung volume irradiated in clients with large chest wall tumors (Christie, Spry, Lamb, and Sadler, 1993).

Medications

Corticosteroids are the mainstay of treating pulmonary inflammation. Typical therapy may be prednisone 1 mg/kg of ideal body weight for 6 to 8 weeks. The dose is gradually tapered to 15 to 20 mg daily until pulmonary function studies have been stable for 1 year; then the prednisone is slowly tapered off (Fulmer, 1994).

Clients may also be treated with agents such as cyclophosphamide, azathioprine, chlorambucil, methotrexate, colchicine, penicillamine, or cyclosporine. These agents have broad anti-inflammatory and/or antifibrotic properties, but their specific mechanisms of action are poorly understood. Except for corticosteriods, cyclophosphamide, and azathioprine, most reports of success with the above agents are anecdotal, and the cytotoxic agents and penicillamine can themselves directly injure lung tissue. The most success with pharmacotherapy was noted when clients were treated early in the disease process; however, despite some success PF eventually worsens in most cases (Hunninghake and Kalica, 1995).

Antibiotics may be necessary for superimposed pulmonary infections. Influenza and pneumococcal vaccines are strongly recommended (Fulmer, 1994).

Bronchodilators may be beneficial in clients with underlying obstructive pulmonary disease.

Diuretics and inotropics may be necessary in clients with cor pulmonale. Early detection of interstitial pneumonitis and prompt initiation of antimicrobial therapy may be beneficial in reducing the severity of interstitial pneumonitis following BMT (Lazarus, 1992).

Low-dose morphine (2.5 to 5.0 mg) may give relief for severe dyspnea in end-stage clients (Schmidt and Shell, 1994). An anxiolytic may also be given for anxiety accompanying dyspnea.

Procedures: Advanced PF and/or violent coughing may result in pneumothorax, necessitating chest tube placement, sometimes with pleurodesis (Fujiwara, 1993; Fulmer, 1994). Mechanical ventilation may be of limited benefit during acute exacerbation of symptoms. Chest x-rays, CT scans, and pulmonary function tests may be repeated at regular intervals to assess for progression of disease and response to treatment.

Other

Oxygen therapy may be required to improve client comfort and activity tolerance.

Fluid restriction and a low-sodium diet may be beneficial in persons with cor pulmonale.

Numerous therapies to suppress pulmonary inflammation and fibrosis are under investigation. Antioxidants show promise in inhibiting pulmonary injury. Niacin has been very effective in animal studies in preventing lung tissue injury from bleomycin, but no studies have yet been performed with humans. Since cytokines appear to play a role in initiating the inflammatory response, identifying and producing cytokine inhibitors may be one approach to therapy (Hunninghake and Kalica, 1995; Rubin et al., 1995). Transforming growth factor-beta, a growth factor present in lung tissue, strongly correlates with the development of PF in BMT clients following induction chemotherapy and with radiation pneumonitis and fibrosis in lung cancer clients (Anscher et al., 1994). This may be useful in detecting individuals at greater risk for PF and in suggesting a future role for growth factor inhibitors as well (Anscher et al., 1993).

ASSESSMENT CRITERIA: PULMONARY FIBROSIS

The assessment criteria for oncology clients with PF are listed in the table at the end of this section. In general, a client with early PF may state a history of gradually increasing dyspnea on exertion, possibly with a nonproductive cough. Clients may attribute their symptoms to the underlying malignancy or an expected aftermath of having received therapy. Lung auscultation may reveal diminished breath sounds and fine crackles, which may be diffusely spread throughout the lung fields, if the client has received chemotherapy, or localized to the area of radiation treatment.

Chest x-rays can show the presence of infiltrates and fibrotic changes, but high-resolution computerized tomography (CT) of the chest is more useful in determining the extent of pulmonary disease. The client's signs and symptoms may precede radiologic changes. Pulmonary function tests are useful in determining the amount of functional lung but do not indicate subclinical disease (Waid-Jones and Coursin, 1991). Ventilation/perfusion studies may indicate that the lung tissue is being ventilated but not adequately perfused because of capillary damage. DLCO (carbon monoxide diffusing capacity) may be the most sensitive test in measuring lung function by assessing the degree of alveolar capillary block (McDonald et al., 1995).

Lung biopsy is necessary to determine the cause of the pulmonary symptoms. Transbronchial lung biopsy is diagnostic in 37.5 to 50% of cases (Bensard, McIntyre, Waring, and Simon, 1993). Open lung biopsy is commonly done, although this requires thoracotomy and general anesthesia. Video thoracoscopic lung biopsy is a relatively new procedure that appears to obtain similar results to open lung biopsy with less mortality (Bensard et al., 1993). Bronchoalveolar lavage is an investigational procedure gaining acceptance that uses a flexible bronchoscope to obtain lung interstitium and fluid (Fulmer, 1994; Morgan and Breit, 1995).

Assessment criteria

Vital signs

Temperature	Normal; elevated if severe inflammation or infection.
Pulse	Tachycardia.
Respirations	Tachypnea.
Blood pressure	Normal; decreased with pulmonary hypertension.

History

Symptoms, conditions
Increasing dyspnea, especially with exertion.
Weight loss over several weeks.
Previous pulmonary infection or treatments known to cause PF.

Hallmark physical signs and symptoms
Nonproductive cough; rapid, shallow respirations; decreased thoracic expansion during inhalation/exhalation; crackles, diminished breath sounds.

Other physical signs and symptoms
Cyanosis (advanced disease).
Digital clubbing (advanced disease).
Use of accessory muscles of respiration (advanced disease).
Symptoms of right ventricular failure (advanced disease).

Psychosocial signs
Anxiety, restlessness.

Lab values

White blood cell (WBC) count	Elevated if infection is present.
Plasma-transforming growth factor-beta (experimental)	Elevated.

Diagnostic tests

Chest x-ray	Infiltrates; diffuse, mottled shadowing of lung fields (honeycomb lung). Enlarged pulmonary artery, right atrium, and ventricle in pulmonary hypertension.
Pulmonary function test	Normal airway resistance. Reduction in lung volume, forced vital capacity, and total lung capacity. Decreased DLCO (carbon monoxide diffusing capacity). Exercise-induced hypoxemia (early disease) or resting hypoxemia (advanced disease).
ABGs	PaO_2 may be normal at rest and decreased on exertion. $PaCO_2$ may be normal (owing to tachypnea) or may be increased in advanced disease.
CT scan of chest	Decreased lung volume; interstitial disease; pleural thickening; pneumothorax or pneumomediastinum.
Gallium lung scan	Can help distinguish treatment-induced inflammation from infectious processes (the latter will label heavily with gallium).

(continued)

ASSESSMENT CRITERIA: PULMONARY FIBROSIS *(continued)*

Lung biopsy	Inflammation, increased cellularity, and fibrosis.
Ventilation scan	May be normal owing to overexpansion of unaffected lung tissue.
Perfusion scan	Underperfusion if there is injury to microvasculature. Can show region of damage corresponding to irradiated area.
Cardiac catheterization with angiography (if pulmonary hypertension is suspected)	High pulmonary vascular resistance.
Other	Assess for contributing factors (see Risk Profile).

Source: Data from Bensard, McIntyre, Waring, and Simon, 1993; Fischer, Tish Knobf, and Durivage, 1993; Fujiwara, 1993; Fulmer, 1994; Howard, 1994; McDonald, Rubin, Phillips, and Marks, 1995; Morgan and Breit, 1995; Steuble, 1994; Waid-Jones and Coursin, 1991.

NURSING DIAGNOSIS

The nursing diagnosis will vary depending on the extent of PF and the degree of impairment experienced by the client. Possible diagnoses are as follows.

Activity intolerance related to dyspnea secondary to lung fibrosis.

Altered tissue perfusion related to hypoxia from decreased lung expansion secondary to lung fibrosis.

Anxiety related to dyspnea secondary to lung fibrosis.

Altered nutrition, less than body requirements, related to fatigue and dyspnea.

Risk for infection related to alteration in pulmonary structure and function and immunosuppressive therapy.

Risk for impaired skin integrity related to decreased mobility, corticosteroids, and decreased nutritional intake.

Decreased cardiac output related to pulmonary vascular resistance secondary to lung fibrosis.

Knowledge deficit related to the disease process and interventions.

NURSING INTERVENTIONS

Immediate nursing interventions

Assess temperature, pulse, respirations, and blood pressure.

Assess oxygen saturation, and determine need for supplemental oxygen.

Auscultate lung fields.

Place the client on bedrest in semi- or high-Fowler's position.

Assess for dehydration, edema, fluid overload.

Anticipated physician orders and interventions

Chest x-ray.
CT scan of chest.
Lung biopsy.
Corticosteroids.
Complete blood count (CBC), chemistry profile.
Chemotherapy and/or radiation therapy placed on hold.
Pulmonary function test with ABG analysis and DLCO.
Broad-spectrum antibiotic therapy.
Low-dose morphine, anxiolytic for severe anxiety and dyspnea.

Ongoing nursing assessment, monitoring, and interventions

Assess:
- Comfort and ease of breathing.
- Activity tolerance.
- Food and fluid intake q shift.
- Skin integrity.
- Lung sounds q2–4h; report increasing crackles and other adventitious lung sounds.
- For signs of hypoxia (restlessness, dyspnea, anxiety, cyanosis).
- For signs of pulmonary infection (elevated temperature, productive cough, crackles, coarse breath sounds).
- For signs of cor pulmonale (increased venous pressure, peripheral edema, distended neck veins, cyanosis, liver engorgement, systolic or diastolic murmur, prominent S_2 sound).

Measure:
- Oxygen saturation continuously until client no longer desaturates with activity; then titrate oxygen to maintain SaO_2 >92% at rest and with activity.
- Baseline PaO_2, and repeat as indicated by client condition.
- Intake and output (I and O) q8h until I = O.
- Weight qd.
- Dyspnea on 0 to 10 scale (0 = no dyspnea, 10 = severe dyspnea) q4h and with activity.
- Respiratory rate at rest q4h and with activity.

Send: CBC, chemistry profile.

Implement:
- Frequent rest periods following periods of activity.
- Calorie count for decreased nutritional intake.
- Small, frequent, high-calorie meals.
- Fluid and sodium restriction for cor pulmonale.
- Referrals to dietitian, social worker, physical therapist, occupational therapist, as indicated by assessment.

TEACHING/EDUCATION

Select items, based on client and significant others' assessed needs.

Discontinuation of chemotherapy/radiation therapy: *Rationale:* Radiation therapy and some chemotherapy drugs can cause your lung(s) to become inflamed, which can cause scars in your lungs (fibrosis). The type of cancer treatment you are getting may have to be changed to keep your lungs from being harmed.

Disease process of PF: *Rationale:* Radiation therapy, some chemotherapy drugs, and some lung infections can cause inflammation and scarring (fibrosis) of the lung tissue. Drugs can be given to treat the inflammation, prevent further lung damage, and improve some of your symptoms. However, the fibrosis in the lungs will not go away. Call your doctor or nurse if you are having more trouble breathing, if coughing becomes severe, or if you have pain in your chest.

Dyspnea: *Rationale:* Breathing oxygen through a tube or mask will help add more oxygen to your blood. This will help you feel less short of breath, make it easier for you to do certain activities, and make it easier for your heart to pump. You may find it easier to breathe when you sit forward with your hands or elbows on your knees, when you sit with your elbows placed on a pillow on a table, when you are lying in bed with your upper body raised on pillows. Practice slow, deep breathing, using your diaphragm: Place your hands on your stomach; you should feel your stomach rise and fall with each breath. Breathe out slowly through pursed lips. Breathe out for twice as long as you breathe in. This will help slow down your breathing and help your lungs take in more air (Foote, Sexton, and Pawlik, 1986). You may want to rate how hard it is for you to breathe on a 0 to 10 scale (0 = no problems with breathing, 10 = severe problems with breathing) to make it easier to tell your doctor or nurse how you are doing.

Rest and activity: *Rationale:* Plan what you are going to do according to how well you are feeling. Allow at least 90 minutes of complete rest between activities. You will know it is time to rest when you are taking more than ten breaths above your resting breathing rate. Do not plan activities within 1 hour of eating, since digesting food takes blood away from the muscles (Howard, 1994).

Anxiety: *Rationale:* Feeling short of breath may make you feel anxious and restless. The breathing exercises described above may help you feel more in control of your breathing. You may also want to learn exercises that will help you relax. You may try to imagine yourself in a peaceful place, or use television, reading, or music to distract yourself. It may take some practice to find activities that will work for you. Your nurse can tell you more about these activities. Your doctor may also prescribe some medicine to help you relax and feel more comfortable.

Corticosteroids: *Rationale:* Corticosteroids are medicines used in pulmonary fibrosis to "quiet down" the inflammation in the lung. This relieves some trouble with breathing and decreases further lung damage. There can be many side effects from this treatment, including a higher chance of infection (see "Preventing respiratory infection" below), high blood sugar, high blood pressure, mood changes, bleeding in the stomach or intestine, feeling hungry, bloating, facial swelling, easy bruising, and lower levels of potassium in your blood. You will be closely watched for any side effects.

Preventing respiratory infection: *Rationale:* The corticosteroids you are taking lower your body's ability to fight infection. Also, changes in your lung structure and the way it works make it easier for you to get an infection. You should have yearly flu and pneumococcal vaccines. Avoid people with coughs and colds; wash your hands often to get rid of germs you may have picked up on surfaces. Call your physician or nurse right away for a temperature over 100.5° F and/or a cough with yellow, green, or brown phlegm.

Tests and procedures: *Rationale:* A chest x-ray and CT scan of your chest will be done to check the type and amount of disease in your lungs. A small piece of lung tissue (lung biopsy) will also be taken to further decide what has caused your breathing trouble. This may be done through a small tube put down your airway into your lung or by going through the chest wall to get lung tissue. A pulmonary function test is a breathing test that will show how well your lung tissue is working. A blood sample will also be taken from a blood vessel in your wrist to see how well oxygen is getting from your lungs into your bloodstream. A probe may also be attached to your fingertip or earlobe to measure the oxygen in your bloodstream. Other tests may be done as well to get more information on your condition.

Pulmonary hypertension/cor pulmonale: *Rationale:* The fibrosis in your lungs can increase pressure in tiny lung blood vessels called capillaries. This can make it harder for your heart to pump blood to your lungs and, in time, may cause some degree of heart failure on the right side of your heart. You may need medicine to make it easier for your heart to work. You may be allowed less liquids and sodium (salt) so that your heart will have less fluid to pump. Report any of these symptoms to your doctor or nurse: more shortness of breath, swelling of ankles or legs, feeling faint, chest pain, or feeling that your heart is beating unevenly.

Nutritional requirements: *Rationale:* Weight loss can occur because of breathing trouble and feeling very tired, since your body also needs energy for eating and digestion. Eat small meals that are high in calories several times during the day. Your dietitian or nurse can help you with food choices and decide whether you will need extra nutrition from supplements.

EVALUATION/DESIRED OUTCOMES

1. The client is free from symptoms of respiratory infection.
2. Subjective relief of dyspnea is achieved; dyspnea rating < 3 on 0 to 10 scale.
3. Oxygen saturation > 92% with or without supplemental oxygen.
4. The client effectively demonstrates breathing techniques and positioning.
5. The client verbalizes strategies to control anxiety.
6. The client is able to organize and plan activities and rest periods. He or she has the resources available to assist with unmet needs.
7. Weight is stable; serum albumin > 3.5 g/dl. The client verbalizes the need for and content of high-calorie, frequent-small-meals diet.
8. Skin is without signs of breakdown.
9. The client is free from symptoms of cor pulmonale.
10. The client verbalizes purpose and potential side effects of medications.
11. The client verbalizes symptoms of worsening pulmonary disease requiring notification of physician or nurse.
12. The end-stage client has been referred to hospice and executed an advance directive, if desired.

DISCHARGE PLANNING

The oncology client with PF may need:

Supplemental oxygen and instruction in its use.
Intermittent caregiver to assist with activities of daily living (ADLs).
Assistance with meals, shopping, laundry, and housework.
Home nursing visits (if the client is homebound) to assess pulmonary status, review medications, and reinforce breathing and relaxation strategies.
Physical or occupational therapy for strengthening, conditioning, and modification of ADLs.
Hospice care for severe, end-stage pulmonary fibrosis.

FOLLOW-UP CARE

Anticipated care

Physician office visit within 1 week.
Chest x-ray every 2 to 3 months.
Pulmonary function test with ABGs and DLCO every 2 to 3 months.
Home nursing visit 1 to 2 times per week for 1 to 2 months.

Anticipated client/family questions and possible answers

Will the fibrosis in my lungs get better?

"The medication(s) you are taking will decrease the inflammation in your lungs and may improve some of your symptoms. However, fibrosis is 'scarring' of the lung tissue, so the changes in the lung will not disappear."

Will the fibrosis in my lungs get worse?

"The medication(s) you are taking should decrease the development of fibrosis. However, in time the lung fibrosis may get worse."

What can I do to help my family member/significant other with PF?

"Several effective ways to help him or her include:

Do not treat the person as an invalid because of his or her decreased activity tolerance;

Include the person in decision making;

Help the person establish a new routine at home;

Determine small tasks the person can accomplish; and

Plan activities or outings within the person's activity tolerance (Schmidt and Shell, 1994)."

What should I do if my breathing gets worse?

"Sit or lie quietly with your upper body upright. Put your oxygen back on if it was off. Practice your breathing exercises, and try to remain calm. Call your physician or the paramedics if your symptoms do not improve or become severe. If you have frequent problems with your breathing, you should have someone with you at all times."

What will happen with my cancer if I can't take radiation treatments?

"Since the radiation has damaged your lung, it is not advisable to continue with further lung radiation. Your oncologist can discuss with you whether other treatments (e.g., chemotherapy) are necessary and appropriate for you."

What will happen with my cancer if I can't take chemotherapy?

"Only certain chemotherapy drugs are known to cause lung damage. You may be able to have a different type of treatment (e.g., another chemotherapy regimen) that may not affect your lung tissue."

How can I increase my activity level?

"Remember to organize your day with short periods of activity followed by rest periods. You may gradually increase the amount of activity you do at one time, but continue to keep the same amount of time for rest periods."

Why is a nurse coming to my house?

"A nurse will come once or twice a week to listen to your heart and lungs, check your weight, talk to you about your medications, and see how well you are managing at home. He or she will also assess you for any other symptoms or side effects and answer your questions about your condition."

CHAPTER SUMMARY

PF is a complication of cancer treatment that can have a devastating effect on a person's quality of life. It is caused by pulmonary inflammation and tissue destruction, which in time results in lung fibrosis and restrictive lung disease. PF can compromise a person's ability to take part in meaningful activities, maintain employment, care for one's spouse or children, and maintain one's independence. Furthermore, it may prevent the client from receiving preferred cancer treatment or render the client unable to receive any cancer therapy at all.

PF is not preventable, but early detection may minimize its severity. Nursing care must focus on identifying clients at risk, teaching clients about the symptoms of PF they must report, and meticulous assessment for early pulmonary toxicity. Comprehensive, compassionate nursing interventions will help improve the client's ability to cope with PF. Research efforts will continue to focus on the mechanisms of PF, ways to interrupt the pathophysiologic processes, and identification of early indicators of the disease process.

TEST QUESTIONS

1. Early signs and symptoms of PF include:
   A. Productive cough, dyspnea at rest, fever
   B. Elevated $PaCO_2$, disorientation, fatigue
   C. Nonproductive cough, dyspnea with exertion, fine crackles
   D. Chest pain, course breath sounds, sore throat

1. Answer: C
The early signs and symptoms of PF are often mild in nature and may be attributed to other causes.

2. This cytotoxic drug is strongly associated with lung toxicity in children:
   A. Cisplatin
   B. Etoposide
   C. 5-Fluorouracil
   D. Carmustine

2. Answer: D
Carmustine has been associated with a high rate of lung fibrosis in children, especially in children under the age of 6.

3. The potential for radiation-induced pulmonary fibrosis is greatest in a client with:
   A. Large-volume lung irradiation
   B. Congestive heart failure
   C. Upper respiratory infection
   D. Lobectomy

3. Answer: A
Radiation damage to lung tissue depends on the volume of lung tissue irradiated, as well as the dose of radiation, pre-existing pulmonary function, and concurrent chemotherapeutic agents.

4. Pulmonary fibrosis results from damage to alveolar tissue and the:
   A. Bronchioles
   B. Gastrointestinal (GI) tract
   C. Alveolar capillary endothelium
   D. Central nervous system

4. Answer: C
Alveolar tissue and capillaries may become damaged; the capillary damage results in decreased alveolar perfusion, which may lead to further tissue damage.

5. A teaching strategy for a client with pulmonary fibrosis to reduce dyspnea-related anxiety would include:
   A. Light aerobic exercise
   B. Rapid, shallow breathing
   C. Lying flat in bed
   D. Slow deep breaths with exhalation through pursed lips

5. Answer: D
This breathing technique will help slow down breathing, increase the breathing capacity of the client's lungs, and help the client feel more in control of his or her breathing.

6. Concerns expressed by a client with pulmonary fibrosis may include:
   A. Difficulty in accomplishing daily activities
   B. Joy over increased cancer treatment options
   C. Increased need for complete dietary changes
   D. Dissatisfaction with alternating side effects of diarrhea and constipation

6. Answer: A
Increased difficulties with ADLs reflect a major realistic concern of a client with pulmonary fibrosis.

7. Teaching for a client beginning corticosteroid therapy would include:
   A. Signs and symptoms of respiratory infection
   B. Signs and symptoms of hypoglycemia
   C. Signs and symptoms of hypotension
   D. When improvement in fibrosed lung tissue can be expected

7. Answer: A
Corticosteroids can suppress the immune system, making the client prone to respiratory infection.

8. Client teaching to reduce the risk of pulmonary infection would include:
   A. The importance of weekly pneumococcal and influenza vaccines
   B. Avoiding persons with respiratory infections
   C. Increased bulk in the client's diet to rid the body of bacteria
   D. Decreasing systolic blood pressure to less than 90 mmHg

8. Answer: B
Avoidance of infected persons will decrease a client's potential to become infected from pathogens that are airborne or on surfaces.

9. Nursing assessment prior to administering bleomycin would include:
   A. Determining if the client is experiencing dyspnea on exertion
   B. Assessing for peripheral neuropathy
   C. Auscultating aortic valve for fine crackles
   D. History of diarrhea

9. Answer: A
Prior to each dose of bleomycin a client should be assessed for early signs of pulmonary toxicity, which would include dyspnea on exertion and fine crackles.

10. A client undergoing induction therapy for bone marrow transplant may be at risk for pulmonary fibrosis because of:
A. Liver damage
B. High-dose chemotherapy
C. Potential for hemorrhagic complications
D. Prolonged mucositis

10. Answer: B
High-dose chemotherapy, as well as total body irradiation and pulmonary infection, can cause inflammation and damage to lung tissue, which can lead to pulmonary fibrosis.

REFERENCES

Anscher MS, Murase T, Prescott DM, Marks LB, Reisenbichler H, Bentel GC, Spencer D, Sherouse G, Jirtle RL: Changes in plasma TGF beta levels during pulmonary radiotherapy as a predictor of the risk of developing radiation pneumonitis. Int J Radiat Oncol Biol Phys 30(3):671–676, 1994.

Anscher MS, Peters WP, Reisenbichler H, Petros WP, Jirtle RL: Transforming growth factor beta as a predictor of liver and lung fibrosis after autologous bone marrow transplantation for advanced breast cancer. New Engl J Med 328(22):1592–1598, 1993.

Benoist MR, Lemerle J, Jeun R, Scheinmann P, Paupe J: Effects on pulmonary function of whole lung irradiation for Wilm's tumor in children. Thorax 37(3):175–180, 1982.

Bensard DD, McIntyre RC, Waring BJ, Simon JS: Comparison of video thorascopic lung biopsy to open lung biopsy in the diagnosis of interstitial lung disease. Chest 103(3):765–770, 1993.

Choy H, Safran H: Preliminary analysis of a Phase II study of weekly paclitaxel and concurrent radiation therapy for locally advanced non-small cell lung cancer. Semin Oncol 22(Suppl 9):55–57, 1995.

Christie DRH, Spry NA, Lamb DS, Sadler HB: Artificial pneumothorax can be used to prevent lung toxicity in chest wall radiotherapy. Clin Oncol 5(4):257–259, 1993.

Corcoran-Buchsel P: Long-term complications of allogeneic bone marrow transplantation: Nursing implications. Oncol Nurs Forum 13(6):61–70, 1986.

Fischer DS, Tish Knobf M, Durivage HJ: The Cancer Chemotherapy Handbook, 4th ed. St. Louis, MO: Mosby, 1993.

Foote M, Sexton DL, Pawlik L: Dyspnea: A distressing sensation in lung cancer. Oncol Nurs Forum 13(5):25–31, 1986.

Fujiwara T: Pneumomediastinum in pulmonary fibrosis. Chest 104(1):44–46, 1993.

Fulmer JD: Interstitial lung disease. In Stein JH (ed): Internal Medicine. St. Louis, MO: Mosby Year Book, 1994, pp. 1681–1691.

Ginsberg SJ, Comis RL: The pulmonary toxicity of antineoplastic agents. Semin Oncol 9(1):34–51, 1982.

Greene PE, Fergusson JH: Nursing care in childhood cancer: Late effects of therapy. Am J Nurs 82:443–446, 1982.

Hartsell WF, Czyzewski EA, Ghalie R, Kaizer H: Pulmonary complications of bone marrow transplantation: A comparison of total body irradiation and cyclophosphamide to busulfan and cyclophosphamide. Int J Radiat Oncol Biol Phys 32(1):69–73, 1995.

Haylock PJ: Breathing difficulty: Changes in respiratory function. Semin Oncol Nurs 3(4):293–298, 1987.

Howard C: Respiratory disorders. *In* Swearingen PL (ed): Manual of Medical-Surgical Nursing Care: Nursing Interventions in Collaborative Management. St. Louis, MO: Mosby Year Book, 1994, pp. 1–42.

Hunninghake GW, Kalica AR: Approaches to the treatment of pulmonary fibrosis. Am J Respir Crit Care Med 151:915–918, 1995.

Jakacki RI, Schramm CM, Donahue BR, Haas F, Allen JC: Restrictive lung disease following treatment for malignant brain tumors: A potential late effect of craniospinal irradiation. J Clin Oncol 13(6):1478–1485, 1995.

Kimsey FC, Mendenhall NP, Ewald LM, Coons TS, Layon AJ: Is radiation treatment volume a predictor for acute or late effect on pulmonary function? Cancer 73(10):2549–2555, 1994.

Lazarus HM: Pharmacologic advances in bone marrow transplantation: Improvements in supportive care. Mediguide Oncol 12(2):1–6, 1992.

LeBlond V, Zouabi H, Sutton L, Guillon JM, Mayaud CM, Similowski T, Beigelman C, Autran B: Late CD8+ lymphocytic alveolitis after allogeneic bone marrow transplantation and chronic graft-versus-host disease. Am J Respir Crit Care Med 150(4):1056–1061, 1994.

Mah K, Keane TJ, Van Dyk J, Braban LE, Poon PY, Hao Y: Quantitative effect of combined chemotherapy and fractionated radiotherapy on the incidence of radiation-induced lung damage: A prospective clinical study. Int J Radiat Oncol Biol Phys 28(3):563–574, 1994.

Martin WJ: Pharmacologic and other chemical causes of interstitial lung disease. Chest 100(1):241–243, 1991.

Maul-Mellott SK, Adams JN: Childhood Cancer: A Nursing Overview. Boston: Jones and Bartlett, 1987.

McDonald S, Rubin P, Phillips TL, Marks LB: Injury to the lung from cancer therapy: Clinical syndromes, measurable endpoints, and potential scoring systems. Int J Radiat Oncol Biol Phys 31(5):1187–1203, 1995.

Miller RW, Fusner JE, Fink R, Murphy TM, Getson PR, Vogtova JA, Reaman GH: Pulmonary function abnormalities in long term survivors of childhood cancer. Med Pediatr Oncol 14:202–207, 1986.

Moore IM, Ruccione K: Late effects of cancer treatment. *In* Groenwald SL, Frogge MH, Goodman M, Yarbro CH (eds): Cancer Nursing: Principles and Practice. Boston: Jones and Bartlett, 1992, pp. 669–685.

Morgan E, Baum E, Breslow N, Takashima J, D'Angio G: Chemotherapy-related toxicity in infants treated according to the Second National Wilms' Tumor Study. Clin Oncol 6(1):51–55, 1988.

Morgan GW, Breit SN: Radiation and the lung: A reevaluation of the mechanisms mediating pulmonary injury. Int J Radiat Oncol Biol Phys 31(2):361–369, 1995.

Muscari Lin E, Tierney DK, Stadtmauer EA: Autologous bone marrow transplantation: A review of the principles and complications. Cancer Nurs 16(3):204–213, 1993.

O'Driscoll BR, Kalra S, Gattamaneni HR, Woodcock AA: Late carmustine lung fibrosis: Age at treatment may influence severity and survival. Chest 107(5):1355–1357, 1995.

Patterson DL, Wiemann MC, Lee TH, Byron WA: Carmustine toxicity presenting as a lobar infiltrate. Chest 104(1):315–317, 1993.

Roberts CM, Foulcher E, Zaunders JJ, Bryant DH, Freund J, Cairns D, Penny R, Morgan GW, Breit SN: Radiation pneumonitis: A possible lymphocyte-mediated hypersensitivity reaction. Ann Intern Med 119(10):696–700, 1993.

Rubin P, Johnston CJ, Williams JP, McDonald S, Finkelstein JN: A perpetual cascade of cytokines postirradiation leads to pulmonary fibrosis. Int J Radiat Oncol Biol Phys 33(1):99–109, 1995.

Santamauro JT, Stover DE, Jules-Elysee K, Maurer JR: Lung transplantation for chemotherapy-induced pulmonary fibrosis. Chest 105(1):310–312, 1994.

Schmidt SP, Shell JA: Lung cancer. *In* Otto SE (ed): Oncology Nursing. Louis, MO: Mosby Year Book, 1994, pp. 302–339.

Schweitzer VG, Juillard GJF, Bajada CL, Parker RG: Radiation recall dermatitis and pneumonitis in a patient treated with paclitaxel. Cancer 76:1069–1072, 1995.

Snyder CC: Oncology Nursing. Boston: Little, Brown, 1986.

Steuble BT: Cardiovascular disorders. *In* Swearingen PL (ed): Manual of Medical-Surgical Nursing Care: Nursing Interventions of Collaborative Management. St. Louis, MO: Mosby Year Book, 1994, pp. 43–111.

Syabbalo NC: How long do patients with cor pulmonale secondary to pulmonary fibrosis survive? Chest 99(1):263–264, 1991.

Thelan LA, Daire JK, Urden LD: Textbook of Critical Care Nursing: Diagnosis and Treatment. St. Louis, MO: CV Mosby, 1990.

Waid-Jones MI, Coursin DB: Perioperative considerations for persons treated with bleomycin. Chest 99(4):993–999, 1991.

Weiss RB. Poster DS, Penta JS: The nitrosureas and pulmonary toxicity. Cancer Treat Rev 8:111–125, 1981.

CHAPTER 37

SEIZURES

Catherine Ann Kernich, RN, MSN

CHAPTER OBJECTIVES

At the completion of this chapter, the reader will be able to:

Define the major classifications of seizures.

State the risk factors associated with the development of seizures in the oncology client.

Describe the immediate and ongoing nursing interventions for the client experiencing seizures.

Anticipate and prepare the client with seizures and his or her family for future care needs.

OVERVIEW

SEIZURE activity is a symptom of central nervous system (CNS) irritation resulting in excessive and abnormal neuronal discharges. Seizure activity may occur in individuals with primary or metastatic brain tumors, as a complication of therapies for CNS or systemic malignancies, or as a secondary effect of malignancy. A seizure may be an isolated event without any other associated neurologic symptoms, or it may occur with other symptoms suggestive of increased intracranial pressure (ICP) or encephalopathy. The new onset of seizures must be considered a medical emergency, the seizure treated appropriately, and the cause of the seizure investigated thoroughly and treated aggressively.

DESCRIPTION

Seizures are classified as partial or generalized. Proper classification of the seizure type will aid in diagnosing the cause of the seizure and will guide treatment. Partial seizures are caused by a focal area of abnormal electrical discharge within the brain. The clinical activity manifested by a partial seizure will vary according to the location of the seizure focus. Partial seizures are either associated with no loss of consciousness or with impaired consciousness, depending on the seizure focus and the spread of the electrical activity to other brain structures. The duration of partial seizures is usually 1 to 2 minutes. A simple partial seizure (SPS) is manifested by pure motor or pure sensory symptoms or autonomic symptoms without impaired consciousness. Complex partial seizures (CPSs) are usually associated with a combination of impaired consciousness, altered behavior, and motor or sensory symptoms. A CPS is often followed by a period of amnesia to the event and mild confusion.

Generalized seizures are caused by simultaneous involvement of both cerebral hemispheres, which leads to sudden loss of consciousness. The most common type of generalized seizure is the generalized tonic-clonic (GTC) seizure, formerly referred to as a grand mal. The tonic phase is characterized by muscle rigidity followed by the clonic phase of violent, rhythmic muscle contractions. The duration of the ictal phase of the GTC seizure is 2 to 5 minutes. It is usually followed by a post-ictal stupor, amnesia, and confusion. Transient focal weakness (Todd's paralysis) or sensory changes after a GTC seizure suggest a focal brain lesion. Prior to a CPS or a GTC seizure, the client may experience an aura. This subjective symptom of an impending seizure may include aphasia, circumoral numbness, dread, or an olfactory disturbance.

Seizures occurring in rapid succession without return to consciousness between events are called status epilepticus. Seizures without impaired consciousness that last more than 30 minutes are also considered status epilepticus. The most frequent causes of status epilepticus include noncompliance with anticonvulsant medications, trauma, metabolic disturbances, infections, and space-occupying lesions. Status epilepticus is a medical emergency because permanent brain damage and death can result from it. In fact, the mortality rate from GTC status epilepticus is between 3 and 20%.

Brain tumors

Seizures are one of the most frequent presenting signs of a brain tumor and occur in approximately 60 to 90% of clients with slow-growing tumors and 30% of clients with high-grade tumors. Seizures occur as a result of generalized increased ICP or by focal compression, invasion, or irritation of brain tissue. The type of seizure that the client with a brain tumor experiences is determined by the location of the tumor. In order of descending frequency, seizures are most common in frontal, parietal, and temporal lobe tumors (Jaeckle, Cohen, and Duffner, 1996.) Simple partial motor or GTC seizures are more common in tumors of the frontal lobe. Simple partial sensory seizures are produced by parietal lobe tumors. Temporal lobe tumors are likely to produce CPSs.

Approximately 17,000 adults in the United States are diagnosed with primary brain tumors each year (Posner, 1993.) Gliomas, including astrocytomas and glioblastoma multiforme, represent 40 to 60% of primary brain tumors. As more people with primary systemic cancers are being treated successfully, cerebral metastases represent approximately 30% of all brain tumors (Laws and Thapar, 1993.) In fact, an estimated one-quarter of individuals with cancer will develop a metastatic brain tumor, increasing the total number of individuals diagnosed with brain tumors to 150,000 per year (Posner, 1993; Snodgrass, 1994.) The lung is the most common primary site of cerebral metastasis (50%), followed by the breast (15%) and malignant melanoma (6%) (Laws and Thapar, 1993.) The incidence of brain metastases is highest in the 50- to 60-year-old population (Meehan, 1994.) Metastases to the brain are frequently multiple.

Reduction of the tumor load can decrease ICP and relieve compression on brain tissue, thereby assisting in the control of seizures. Surgical debulking of single tumors combined with focal radiation and adjunct chemotherapy can achieve these results. Multiple brain metastases or primary CNS lymphoma may require whole-brain irradiation with adjunct chemotherapy to reduce brain tissue compression. Stereotactic brain biopsy will diagnose the nature of the cerebral lesion. Craniotomy in itself increases the risk of seizure activity.

> **Pediatrics:** Seizures secondary to brain tumors are slightly less common in children because of their higher frequency of posterior fossa tumors (Jaeckle, et al., 1996).

The reader is referred to Chapter 26 for further information on brain tumors.

Metabolic encephalopathy

Metabolic conditions that disrupt water, pH and electrolyte balance, and energy metabolism can lead to metabolic encephalopathy, resulting in seizure activity. These include hyponatremia, hypocalcemia, hypomagnesemia, and renal or hepatic failure. The type of seizure that results from metabolic encephalopathy is usually GTC. Hypomagnesemia also disrupts neuronal excitability by influencing neurotransmitter function and ionic balance.

Neurotoxicity

Chemotherapeutic agents can cause neurotoxicity, leading to a broad spectrum of neurologic dysfunction, including seizures. The use of investigational drugs and protocols increases this risk. In addition, intrathecal chemotherapy can cause meningeal irritation leading to seizures.

CNS irradiation may cause neuronal cell damage and vasogenic edema, leading to necrosis of normal brain tissue. This radiation necrosis may not appear for months to years after treatment. The incidence varies according to client age, dose, and area irradiated. Acute cerebral irritation from CNS radiation and byproducts of tumor cell breakdown may lead to vasogenic edema, increased ICP, and seizures. CNS vascular changes are thought to be responsible for these abnormalities. Dexamethasone is frequently administered prophylactically during and immediately after cranial irradiation.

> **Pediatrics:** Children less than 3 years old and adults over 60 are at greatest risk for radiation necrosis (Meehan, 1994) as the radiation is more toxic to the developing brain and the brain that has already experienced volume loss.

RISK PROFILE

Cancers: Primary brain tumors, including gliomas and lymphomas; metastatic brain tumors, especially from cancers of the lung, breast, and from malignant melanoma; leptomeningeal carcinomatosis; acute lymphoblastic leukemia.

Conditions: Increased ICP; postoperative craniotomy; metabolic encephalopathy from hyponatremia, syndrome of inappropriate antidiuretic hormone (SIADH), hypocalcemia, hypomagnesemia, bone marrow transplant, or hepatic or renal failure; CNS infection.

Environment: History of whole-brain irradiation, intraventricular access devices, i.e., Ommaya reservoir.

Foods: None known.

Drugs: Noncompliance with anticonvulsant medications; chemotherapeutic agents, including cisplatin, cyclosporine, busulfan, and cytosine; intrathecal chemotherapy; immunosuppression resulting in CNS infection.

PROGNOSIS

Whether or not an individual who experiences seizure activity will develop epilepsy (i.e., experience two or more seizures) depends on the etiology of the seizure. If the precipitating factor was transient in nature and responsive to medical treatment, e.g., hyponatremia, the seizure is most likely an isolated event. Chronic therapy with anticonvulsant medications is not necessary. Seizures resulting from structural damage to brain tissue such as a brain tumor or radiation necrosis are more likely to recur and require long-term therapy with anticonvulsant medications. Seizures as a result of CNS infections may cause residual structural changes leading to epilepsy even after effective treatment of the infection.

TREATMENT

Surgery: Surgical biopsy or resection of cranial lesion.

Table 37–1
Common Anticonvulsant Medications

Medication	Dose	Therapeutic Range	Side Effects/Monitoring*
Phenytoin (Dilantin)	300–600 mg/day— may be given once/day.	10–20 μg/ml (40–79 μmol/L SI Units)	Agranulocytosis, ataxia, diplopia, nystagmus, gingival hyperplasia, hirsutism, lupus-like syndrome, rash. • CBC (complete blood count) with differential q 6 months.
Carbamazepine (Tegretol)	600–1200 mg/day in divided doses.	4–12 μg/ml (17–51 μmol/L SI Units)	Ataxia, aplastic anemia, diplopia, dizziness, drowsiness, hyponatremia, leukopenia, nystagmus. • CBC with diff weekly × 1 month, then q 3 months. • Liver studies q 3 months.
Valproic acid (Depakote, Depakene)	15–60 mg/kg/day in divided doses.	50–100 μg/ml (350–690 μmol/L SI Units)	Anorexia, ataxia, depression, drowsiness, leukopenia, liver toxicity, nausea, transient hair loss, tremor, vomiting. • Liver studies monthly × 6 months, then q 6 months. • CBC with diff q 3 months.
Phenobarbital	60–180 mg per day in divided doses.	*Adults:* 20–40 μg/ml (86–172 μmol/L SI Units) *Children and Infants:* 15–30 μg/ml (65–129 μmol/L SI Units)	Ataxia, decreased libido, depression, drowsiness, dulled sensorium, hyperactivity response in children, irritability, nystagmus. • CBC, SMA-12 q 6 months.
Clonazepam (Klonopin)	0.15–0.25 mg/kg/day in divided doses.	0.02–0.08 μg/ml, 15–60 ng/ml (48–190 μmol/L SI Units)	Ataxia, dizziness, drowsiness. • No specific recommendations.

* Authors differ as to monitoring requirements after initiation of anticonvulsant medications. Some recommend routine monitoring of drug levels, hematology, and hepatic enzymes. Others do not recommend routine monitoring and rely on clinical signs and symptoms to direct monitoring needs.

Chemotherapy

Administer nitrosoureas (BCNU, CCNU); procarbazine; IV or intrathecal methotrexate or cytosine arabinoside (adjunct therapy for treatment of a primary brain tumor that could cause seizure activity).

Decrease dosage or discontinue precipitant chemotherapeutic agent.

Radiation

Conventional fractionated limited-field radiation; interstitial radiotherapy (brachytherapy); stereotactic radiosurgery with gamma knife or linear accelerator (primary brain tumor).
Whole-brain radiation (metastases/CNS lymphoma).

> **Pediatrics:** Because of the developing brain, irradiation is deferred for as long as possible in the pediatric population.

Medications

Administration of IV anticonvulsant medications to stop seizure activity.
Administration of oral loading dose or maintenance of anticonvulsant medications to prevent further seizure activity (see Table 37–1).
Administration of high-dose corticosteroids in the event of increased ICP.
Administration of appropriate electrolytes to correct any abnormalities.
Antibiotics for suspected or documented CNS infections.

Procedures: ICP monitoring if increased ICP suspected with cerebral lesions or postoperative craniotomy.

Other

Seizure precautions.
Fluid restrictions for increased ICP.

ASSESSMENT CRITERIA: SEIZURES

Vital signs	
Respirations	Normal.
Pulse	Increased ictally.
Blood pressure	Increased ictally.
	Low blood pressure after prolonged status epilepticus.
Temperature	Fever with CNS infection or status epilepticus.
History	Description of seizure activity by reliable witness.
	Client report of aura and postictal symptoms.
	History of systemic malignancy.
Hallmark physical signs and symptoms	Alteration in consciousness or inappropriate behavior.
	Hyperreflexia.
	Normal neurologic exam interictally is common.
	Specific motor or sensory deficits.
Additional physical signs and symptoms	Altered language; headache; hemiparesis; nausea; papilledema; visual changes, including homonymous hemianopsia and diplopia; vomiting.

(continued)

ASSESSMENT CRITERIA: SEIZURES (continued)

Psychosocial signs	Memory deficits, personality changes.

Lab values

Anticonvulsant drug levels	Below established therapeutic levels.
Serum Na+	Low (<135 mEq/L, <135 mmol/L SI Units).
Serum Mg++	Low (<1.7 mg/dl, <1.5 mEq/L, <0.8 mmol/L SI Units).
Serum Ca+	Low (<8.5 mg/dl <2.3 mmol/L SI Units).
BUN, creatinine, and liver function studies	Abnormal.
White blood cell (WBC) count	Increased.
Cerebrospinal fluid (CSF) cultures*	Positive.
CSF protein*	Increased.
CSF cytology*	Positive.
CSF cell count*	Pleocytosis.

Diagnostic tests

Cranial CT scan with/ without contrast	Demonstrates contrast ring enhancement of tumor with associated edema and mass effect.
Cranial MRI with/without gadolinium	Demonstrates region of altered signal with surrounding edema and mass effect; most malignant tumors are enhanced with gadolinium.
EEG monitoring	Demonstrating seizure activity or interictal epileptiform spike-and-wave complexes.
Lumbar puncture after brain imaging	(CSF studies are performed only if no evidence of increased ICP exists.) See expected findings under Lab values above.

Other	ICP pressure monitoring.

* = lumbar puncture results.

NURSING DIAGNOSIS

The nursing diagnosis will vary, depending on the seizure type and etiology. Some of the common diagnoses and etiologies are described here.

Potential for ineffective airway clearance related to GTC seizure.

High risk for injury related to:

- Involuntary motor movements.
- Falls secondary to impaired consciousness during seizure activity.

Knowledge deficit related to:

- Seizure diagnosis.
- Use of anticonvulsant medications.
- Need for follow-up care.

Potential for alteration in tissue perfusion, cerebral, related to status epilepticus.

Table 37–2
Assessment and Documentation of Seizure Activity

Pre-ictal	Ictal	Post-ictal
Warning signs.	Sequence of progression of ictal signs.	Behavior.
Initial ictal signs.	Generalized or focal.	Weakness/paralysis.
	Type of motor activity and body parts involved.	Level of consciousness.
	Duration.	Orientation.
	Level of consciousness.	Vital signs.
	Incontinence.	Client description of aura and recall of event.
		Duration.
		Injury.

NURSING INTERVENTIONS

Immediate nursing interventions

Assess pre-ictal, ictal, and post-ictal phases (see Table 37–2).

Initiate seizure precautions; maintain patent airway with oral airway if it can be easily inserted into the client's mouth; turn client to a side-lying position; suction orally as needed; do not attempt to insert objects such as airways or tongue blades into the client's clamped mouth.

Protect the client's head and extremities from injury.

Remain with the client until seizure is complete.

Reorient as needed post-ictally.

Assess neurologic status q15min × 4, then q1h × 4.

Assess vital signs q15min × 4.

Electrocardiographic and blood pressure monitoring during IV phenytoin administration for detection of dysrhythmias or hypotension.

Monitor for respiratory depression if lorazepam or phenobarbital administered.

Anticipated physician orders and interventions

Oral loading dose of selected anticonvulsant medication.

Insertion of IV access.

IV lorazepam 0.1 mg/kg administered 2 mg/minute every 5 minutes until seizures are controlled or the maximum dose is reached for status.

IV phenytoin 15 to 20 mg/kg in normal saline (NS) at less than 50 mg/minute for status or as loading dose in initiation of phenytoin therapy.

IV phenobarbital 20 mg/kg administered at less than 100 mg/minute until seizures are controlled or the maximum dosage is reached for status.

Maintenance of anticonvulsant medications (see Table 37–1).

High-dose corticosteroids, especially dexamethasone, 4 to 20 mg four
times a day.

IV magnesium sulfate 500 mg (4mEq) in 50 to 100 ml of dextrose or
saline solution over 20 to 30 minutes for hypomagnesemia.

IV calcium gluconate 8 to 12 mg/kg administered over 6 to 8 hours for
hypocalcemia.

IV NS at 1.4 to 2.0 mEq/L/hour for hyponatremia.

IV phenytoin, lorazepam, and/or phenobarbital if seizure recurs within
30 minutes.

STAT anticonvulsant drug levels.

STAT electrolytes, calcium, and magnesium.

Discontinue any epileptogenic medications or treatments.

Ongoing nursing assessment, monitoring, and interventions

Assess: Neurological status q4h.

Measure: Vital signs q4h × 24, then q8h.

Send:
- Repeat anticonvulsant drug levels.
- Repeat serum electrolytes.

Implement:
- Seizure precautions, including suction equipment and an oral air-
way at bedside.
- Fluid restrictions as prescribed.

TEACHING/EDUCATION

Seizure precautions: *Rationale:* Equipment has been placed at your bedside
to help your breathing if you should have a seizure. To protect you from
injury until your seizures are under adequate control, you must stay on
bedrest or be with a nurse or family member while out of bed.

Anticonvulsant medications: *Rationale:* Medications have been prescribed
to prevent you from having another seizure. These medications may cause
side effects. The most common side effects are drowsiness and dizziness.
These usually wear off as your body adjusts to the new medications. Please
report any side effects to your nurse and doctor, as your dosage may need to
be adjusted. Your nurse can instruct you on your exact dosage at discharge.

EEG Testing: *Rationale:* An EEG measures the electrical activity within your
brain. Since a seizure is the result of abnormal electrical activity in the brain,
the EEG will help your doctor determine what type of seizure you had. This
will help your doctor in treating you. During the EEG, the technician will
place electrodes over your scalp and fix them in place with a special glue. The
technician may ask you to look at blinking lights or to breathe quickly and
deeply during the EEG to try to bring out a seizure to record. The procedure is

painless and safe and takes one to one and one-half hours to complete. Your nurse will help you wash the glue out of your hair after the procedure.

EVALUATION/DESIRED OUTCOMES

1. The client will have adequate seizure control at discharge.
2. The client and significant other will be able to state what to do if a seizure occurs.
3. The client and significant other will be able to state the name, dosage, and frequency of the prescribed anticonvulsant medications and their common side effects.
4. The client will have therapeutic anticonvulsant drug levels at discharge.
5. The client will have normal serum electrolytes at discharge.

DISCHARGE PLANNING

The seizure client may need:

Education of the client and significant other on care during a seizure.
Inpatient or outpatient rehabilitation for residual neurologic deficit occurring as a result of underlying disease process.
Referral to a support group, e.g., Epilepsy Foundation of America, 4351 Garden City Drive, Landover, MD 20785.

FOLLOW-UP CARE

Anticipated care

Ongoing outpatient care by a neurologist.
Outpatient laboratory testing for anticonvulsant drug levels.
Outpatient laboratory testing for serum electrolytes.

Anticipated client/family questions and possible answers

What do I do if a seizure occurs?
"If you experience an aura before a seizure, lie down on the floor to protect yourself from injury, and attempt to notify somebody in your immediate area that you feel a seizure coming on. After the seizure is over, notify your doctor that it occurred. He or she will instruct you as to whether or not to go to the emergency room."
"If you witness a seizure, loosen any tight clothing from around the person's neck to help ease breathing. Do not attempt to put something in the person's mouth to stop him or her 'from swallowing the tongue.' This really cannot happen and might actually interfere with breathing or cause injury. Hold the

person's head to one side to help drain secretions. Protect the person's head and arms and legs from injury, but do not restrain the person. Allow the person to sleep after a seizure. When the person wakes up, he or she may be confused and may need to be reoriented. You should notify the doctor that a seizure occurred."

What is the importance of drug levels?

"Periodic blood tests will be done to measure the amount of medication in your blood stream. Anticonvulsant medications require a certain level of medication in the blood in order to keep seizures under control. Your dosage will be adjusted according to the drug level, your body's tolerance of the medication, as well as the occurrence of any seizures. Drug levels are usually measured in the morning before you take your first dose of medication. Drug levels are commonly ordered 2 weeks after any change in dosage or with any signs or symptoms of drug toxicity.

CHAPTER SUMMARY

Seizures may represent a complication of a primary CNS tumor or of a systemic malignancy. The cause of the seizure activity will determine the type of seizure the client experiences as well as associated signs and symptoms. It will also direct diagnostic tests, nursing interventions, and medical management. Whatever the cause or type of seizure, the client and significant others will need psychological support and education to overcome the fear of recurrent seizures that often accompanies an initial event.

TEST QUESTIONS

1. The most common primary cancer to metastasize to the brain is:
   A. Bone
   B. Breast
   C. Kidney
   D. Lung

1. Answer: D
The lung is the most common primary cancer to metastasize to the brain, representing 50% of all brain metastases.

2. Which nursing intervention should be administered first to the client who is having a generalized tonic-clonic (GTC) seizure?
   A. Administer IV phenytoin as ordered.
   B. Establish effective airway.
   C. Protect client's extremities from injury.
   D. Obtain anticonvulsant drug levels.

2. Answer: B
The client who is having a GTC seizure may have increased secretions and is unable to clear the secretions during the seizure. Turning the client's head to one side during a seizure prevents aspiration and forces the tongue forward, preventing airway occlusion.

3. Seizures may occur as a result of all of the following electrolyte abnormalities *except:*
   A. Hypocalcemia
   B. Hyponatremia
   C. Hypokalemia
   D. Hypomagnesemia

3. Answer: C
Hypokalemia does not generally cause seizure activity.

4. The primary nursing diagnosis for the client during a GTC seizure is:
   A. Potential for ineffective airway clearance
   B. Knowledge deficit
   C. Memory, impaired
   D. Powerlessness

4. Answer: A
Potential for ineffective airway clearance is the primary nursing diagnosis during a GTC seizure. The risk of increased secretions and inability to clear these secretions leading to aspiration is high but potentially preventable.

5. Simple partial seizures (SPSs) are characterized by:
   A. Impaired consciousness
   B. Sensory or motor symptoms
   C. Post-ictal confusion
   D. Incontinence

5. Answer: B
Simple partial seizures do not involve any impairment of level of consciousness and are primarily characterized by pure motor or sensory symptoms.

6. The primary cause of radiation necrosis is:
   A. Toxic byproducts of tumor cell damage
   B. Increased ICP
   C. Metabolic encephalopathy
   D. CNS vascular changes

6. Answer: D
CNS vascular changes are thought to be the cause of radiation necrosis.

7. All of the following statements related to IV phenytoin administration are true *except:*
   A. EKG monitoring is essential to detect potential cardiac dysrhythmias.
   B. Phenytoin must be administered in normal saline solution.
   C. Phenytoin should be administered no faster than 50 mg/minute.
   D. Hypertension is a potential complication.

7. Answer: D
IV administration of phenytoin may cause hypotension.

8. Common side effects of carba-
   mazepine include all of the fol-
   lowing *except:*
   A. Hypernatremia
   B. Ataxia
   C. Aplastic anemia
   D. Nystagmus

8. Answer: A
   Carbamazepine may cause hyponatremia but not hypernatremia.

9. Status epilepticus is defined as:
   A. Any seizure that causes per-
      manent brain damage
   B. Seizures resistant to treat-
      ment with IV phenytoin
   C. Two or more seizures occur-
      ring in rapid succession
      without return to conscious-
      ness between them
   D. More than one seizure in a
      24-hour period

9. Answer: C
   Status epilepticus may cause permanent brain damage and may be
   resistant to phenytoin therapy, but
   these are not always true. Status
   epilepticus is two or more seizures
   in rapid succession without return
   of consciousness between the
   seizures.

10. Assessment criteria for the new
    onset of a seizure include all of
    the following *except:*
    A. Hypotension
    B. Personality changes
    C. Hyperreflexia
    D. History of headache

10. Answer: A
    The client's vital signs are usually
    normal between seizures. Hyperten-
    sion can occur ictally.

REFERENCES

Cooley ME, Davis L, Abrahm J: Cisplatin: A clinical review. Cancer Nurs 17(4):283–293, 1994.

Furlong TG, Gallucci BB: Pattern of occurrence and clinical presentation of neurological complications in bone marrow transplant patients. Cancer Nurs 17(1):27–36, 1994.

Jaeckle KA, Cohen ME, Duffner PK: Clinical presentation and therapy of nervous system
tumors. *In* Bradley WG, Daroff RB, Fenichel GM, Marsden CD (eds): Neurology in Clinical
Practice: The Neurological Disorders, 2nd ed. Boston: Butterworth-Heinemann, 1996, pp.
1131–1149.

Laws ER, Thapar K: Brain tumors. CA-A: Cancer Journal for Clinicians 43(5):263–271, 1993.

Meehan JL: Mobility and neurological function. *In* Gross J, Johnson BL (eds): Handbook of
Oncology Nursing, 2nd ed. Boston: Jones and Bartlett, 1994, pp. 490–495.

Newton HB: Primary brain tumors: Review of the etiology, diagnosis and treatment. Am Fam
Physician 49(4):787–797, 1994.

Posner JB: CA: Brain tumors. CA-A: Cancer Journal for Clinicians 43(5):261–262, 1993.

Snodgrass SM: Neurological aspects of cancer. *In* Weiner WJ, Goetz CG (eds): Neurology for
the Non-Neurologist, 3rd ed. Philadelphia: JB Lippincott, 1994, pp. 255–269.

CHAPTER 38

SEPSIS AND SEPTIC SHOCK

Phyllis G. Peterson, RN, MN, AOCN

CHAPTER OBJECTIVES

At the completion of this chapter, the reader will be able to:

Define septic shock.

List the factors that may predispose a client with cancer to the development of sepsis and septic shock.

Identify the signs and symptoms of sepsis in the oncology client.

Describe the nursing interventions that decrease the incidence of sepsis.

Describe and discuss nursing care of the oncology client with sepsis and/or septic shock.

OVERVIEW

INFECTION is a major cause of morbidity and mortality for the client with cancer. Infection, with its associated complications and processes, is responsible for at least 50% of deaths in clients with solid tumors (Ellerhorst-Ryan, 1993, p. 558). The process of infection is characterized by an inflammatory response to the presence of microorganisms in host tissue that is ordinarily sterile. Varying types of responses may be seen, depending on the immune competence of the host. The effectiveness of the response is a function of the status of the host and of the type and severity of the infection.

Sepsis occurs when the body can no longer restrict the response to injury to a single area. Clients with cancer are particularly at risk for infection because of impaired host defenses associated with malignant disease processes, as well as side effects and complications associated with cancer therapy.

DESCRIPTION

Immune response

The healthy client with an intact immune system is often able to mount an inflammatory response that will successfully overcome and neutralize the offending organisms. The inflammatory and immune responses serve to enhance the movement of nutrients and immune cells to the site of injury, thereby preventing the invasion and colonization of the host by foreign organisms (Secor, 1994). Because of the physiologic changes associated with malignant disease processes, as well as the complications of treatment, clients with cancer inevitably experience some degree of immune compromise over the course of their illness.

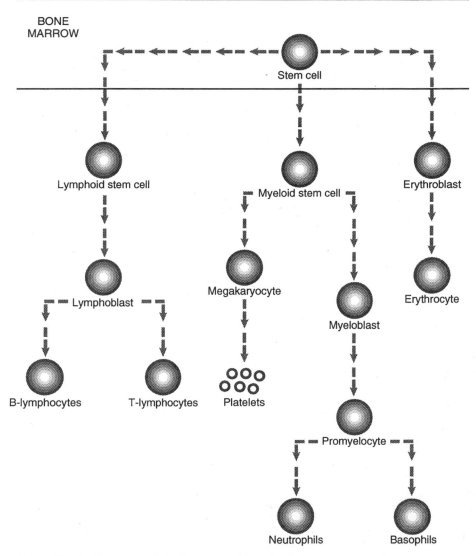

Figure 38–1 Illustration of the formation of blood cells from the stem cell in the bone marrow. Treatments or therapy that suppress the stem cells, or any of the blood cell precursors, can have adverse effects on the client's immune competence.

Leukocytes, or white blood cells (WBCs), are involved in both nonspecific and specific immune responses and are able to neutralize and destroy any substance that is recognized by the body as "foreign." Like all blood cells, leukocytes originate from stem cells that are formed and produced in the bone marrow (Fig. 38–1). Different types of leukocytes perform various specialized functions, which help to promote tissue healing and protect the body against injury from infectious organisms.

Neutrophils are phagocytic cells that are able to swallow up and destroy foreign particles. In response to substances that are released by damaged tissue, neutrophils travel to the site of injury to destroy the offending organisms. Lymphocytes serve to regulate and maintain the immune system by producing antibodies that facilitate the destruction of foreign proteins (Workman, Ellerhorst-Ryan, and Hargraave-Koertge, 1993).

Infection

When an organism or microbe is able to colonize and reproduce within a host, infection occurs. Disease results when the presence of the organism results in pathologic changes, inflammation, injury, or organ dysfunction in the host.

Causative Organisms

A wide variety of microorganisms may cause infection in the immunocompromised individual, ranging from toxin-producing pathogens to opportunistic organisms that normally pose very little threat to the healthy individual (Rubin and Ferraro, 1993). Changes in pharmacologic and medical therapeutics have changed the type of infections that may be found in the client with cancer. Bacteremia from gram-positive cocci now accounts for up to 60% of all septic episodes in persons with cancer. Morbidity and mortality rates tend to be lower for clients with gram-positive infections. The incidence of tuberculosis has shown a consistent increase nationwide over the last 8 years. Clients with lung cancer and lymphoproliferative disorders are most at risk for the development of this disease, which is often reactivation of an old infection (Koll and Brown, 1993).

The duration of immune compromise has been shown to have a direct effect on the type and severity of infections encountered by the client with cancer. Clients at greatest risk for a septic episode are those who have an absolute granulocyte count of < 100 mm³, and the risk increases exponentially with prolonged neutropenia.

A cancer diagnosis and prolonged treatment with immunosuppressive therapy will predispose the client to a variety of bacterial and opportunistic infections. During the first few days of severe neutropenia, bacteria tend to be the major causative organisms. These infections are often related to disruptions in skin and mucosal integrity related to chemotherapy and transmission of nosocomial infections via poor aseptic technique.

Respiratory tract infections are common. In many clients, damaged pulmonary tissue is rendered even more susceptible to secondary infections by opportunistic organisms such as *Aspergillus*. Ciliary function, local immune globulin production, and alveolar macrophage activity may be impaired because of the effects of cytotoxic therapy. Vomiting related to chemotherapy, with subsequent aspiration, is not uncommon.

Viruses are the most commonly occurring infection in the compromised host and may produce a variety of symptoms, including respiratory distress, changes in neurologic status, lesions in the skin and mucous membranes, and increased levels of immune compromise. Viruses are particularly problematic because a lifelong dormant infection may be reactivated by the onset of an immunosuppressed state. Fungal infections may be either a reactivation of a latent infection, which often attacks the lungs or nasal sinuses and then spreads to other areas, or a secondary infection either of the lungs or via an infected central line or catheter (Rubin and Ferraro, 1993). Candidiasis is the most common nosocomial fungal infection (Walsh, 1993).

Sepsis

The processes of infection, sepsis, and septic shock may be viewed as a continuum. In the presence of infection, the body mounts an inflammatory response that is characterized by two or more of the following conditions:

Temperature $< 36°$ C or $> 38°$ C $(< 96.8°$ F or $> 100.4°$ F)
Tachycardia
Tachypnea
WBC $> 12,000$ cells/mm^3 or $< 4,000$ mm^3 or $> 10\%$ immature forms
(bands)

Sepsis may be simply defined as a systemic response to infection (Ackerman, 1994). Substances in the microbial cell wall, usually an endotoxin, activate the clotting cascade and complement systems. This chain of chemical events further contributes to the capillary leak syndrome, vasodilation, and coagulopathies that are typically seen in septic clients. Endotoxin is a lipopolysaccharide component of the bacterial cell membrane of all gram-negative organisms, and is shed from the bacteria as they replicate or die (Secor, 1994). Endotoxin levels have been shown to be directly correlated with the severity of sepsis from gram-negative organisms.

During the early stages of sepsis, a high cardiac output is seen, with widespread vasodilation and normal or slightly elevated blood pressure readings. Cardiac ejection fraction is often decreased owing to circulating myocardial depressant factor, an enzyme that is thought to be released from the pancreas after a period of prolonged hypoperfusion (Kokiko, 1993). If the inflammatory response is allowed to continue uninterrupted, shunting and vasodilation increase. Capillary leak develops and may result in pronounced edema. Blood pressure begins to fall. Cardiac function is further depressed, and the falling blood pressure may not respond to fluid resuscitation, vaso-pressors, or inotropic agents (Weissner, Casey, and Zbilut, 1995).

Septic shock

If the body fails to initiate an adequate immune response or treatment fails, a state of vascular collapse ensues. Severe sepsis is associated with multior-gan dysfunction, hypoperfusion, and hypotension. Septic shock is defined as sepsis with a systolic blood pressure of < 90 mmHg or a reduction of > 40 mmHg from the baseline in spite of attempts at fluid resuscitation. Laborato-ry studies may reveal a hyperglycemia that requires administration of insulin and is associated with a poor prognosis (Wiessner, Casey, and Zbilut, 1995). The complete blood count (CBC) may demonstrate either leukopenia or leukocytosis. Thrombocytopenia is seen in most persons with severe sepsis. Initially, arterial blood gases will show mild hypoxemia with respiratory alkalosis, followed by respiratory acidosis with progression of the shock state (Kokiko, 1993). Because of hypoperfusion of vital organs, changes in mental status, oliguria, and lactic acidosis are often present (Ackerman, 1994).

Organ dysfunction and multisystem organ failure may be sequelae of septic shock. Hypoperfusion and systemic oxygen debt have been identified as factors that contribute to organ failure and subsequent mortality.

RISK PROFILE

All of the risk factors cited below are greater risks when occurring in the very young or elderly client, because of decreased production of T-lympho-cytes and limited inflammatory response.

Cancers: Acute leukemia; lymphoma; Hodgkin's disease; chronic leukemia; multiple myeloma; gastric, esophagus, colon, ovary, lung, and skin cancer; and melanoma.

Pediatrics: Acute and chronic leukemia.

Conditions: An absolute neutrophil count of 100 mm³, prolonged neutrope-nia, intensive and prolonged chemotherapy regimens, radiation therapy, gas-tric, small bowel and large bowel surgery, breaks in the integrity of the skin or mucous membranes, presence of foreign bodies such as venous ports and catheters, malnutrition, collagen vascular disease, diabetes, cardiac, or renal disease (Lee and Pizzo, 1993).

Environment: Exposure to contaminated water, animals, or air; treatment in a large teaching hospital (Ackerman, 1994).

Foods: Uncooked foods that are high in water content, i.e., tomatoes, lettuce, and raw fruits or vegetables. Uncooked shellfish, meats, and unpasteurized dairy products, and any food that is kept warm or held at room temperature for prolonged periods.

Drugs: Busulfan, chloramphenicol, cimetidine, cyclosporine, cytarabine, dactinomycin, daunorubicin, dexamethasone, doxorubicin, fludarabine, ganciclovir, hydroxyurea, indomethacin, isoniazid (INH), lomustine, mechlorethamine, melphalan, prednisolone, propranolol, Taxol (Tenenbaum, 1994), docetaxel (Taxotepe).

PROGNOSIS

Recovery from sepsis depends on the nature of the infectious organism(s), the degree and duration of neutropenia and immunocompromise, and the timely initiation of appropriate treatment. Mortality rates have remained essentially unchanged over the last several years, but this may be caused at least in part by the increased numbers of immunocompromised clients, increased use of invasive procedures, and increased placement of the very young and the very old in the intensive care unit (ICU) (Ackerman, 1994). In clients with cancer, the mortality rate for septic shock is approximately 75%. In clients with more than one organism, the mortality rate is greater than 90% (Truett, 1991). In clients with a fungal organism, even if treatment is successful, there is a 50% chance that the infection will recur if they undergo another period of immunosuppression.

TREATMENT

Survival from a septic episode depends on prompt initiation of broad-spectrum therapy, even before the causative organism has been identified.

Surgery: May be required in order to remove a medical appliance or device that is a focus of infection. Other indications include debridement of infected wounds and drainage of abscesses.

Chemotherapy: Not indicated.

Radiation: Used to shrink fungating lesions that act as a source of infection (Hilderley, 1993).

Medications

When it is feasible, decrease or cease using immunosuppressive agents such as corticosteroids.

Initiate therapy with broad-spectrum antibiotics, such as carbapenem, at the first sign of infection. Combination therapy may be given with a beta-lactam and an aminoglycoside. Combination therapy with two antimicrobials may decrease the chance that the client will develop resistance to the drugs.

Antifungals and antiviral agents and antipseudomonal penicillin may be indicated for prophylaxis in clients with severe immunocompromise. These drugs may also be needed for the neutropenic client with persistent fever who is already receiving treatment with broad-spectrum antibiotic therapy (Lee and Pizzo, 1993).

Vasoactive and inotropic drugs are given to correct hypotension that is unresponsive to fluid resuscitation and to maintain cardiac output and oxygen delivery.

Ibuprofen is useful in blocking arachidonic acid metabolism and stabilizes the cell membrane. Stabilization of the membrane of neutrophils decreases the release of sepsis mediators (Wiessner, Casey, and Zbilut, 1995).

Antipyretics serve to regulate temperature and help to lessen the detrimental effect of hypothermia on cardiac function.

Monoclonal antibodies against gram-negative endotoxins and against tumor necrosis factor-alpha have been developed and are under investigation (Brown, 1994; Opal et al., 1990).

Colony-stimulating factors (CSFs) may be administered to reduce the duration and severity of neutropenia.

Procedures

With the advent of fever or suspicious symptoms, obtain cultures of wounds, urine, sputum, and blood.

CT scans of the chest may be needed for the client with recurrent or persistent fever.

Assess venous catheter exit sites carefully for redness or tenderness, particularly along the subcutaneous tunnel of the catheter. Implanted catheters and medical devices may need to be removed in the event of persistent fever that does not respond to pharmacologic therapy.

Arterial line placement is required for continuous blood pressure monitoring and frequent blood sampling.

Pulmonary artery catheterization, although hazardous in the immunocompromised client, helps differentiate the type of shock (sepsis vs. other types) that is occurring and provides accurate evaluation of fluid resuscitation status.

Intubation and mechanical ventilation will be necessary for clients experiencing septic shock when (a) oxygenation cannot be maintained with increasingly high percentage of oxygen given with noninvasive oxygen delivery systems; and (b) respiratory muscle fatigue is indicated by rising CO_2 levels, or when arterial blood gas pH becomes acidemic in combination with decreased PaO_2 (Lee, Balk, and Bone, 1989).

Other

Nutritional support is indicated to prevent starvation, protect the gut, and maintain a positive nitrogen balance.

Prevent and correct fluid and electrolyte imbalances. Infuse crystalloid solutions to maintain optimal preload and urine output (Lawler, 1994). Initiate ventilatory support to maintain oxygenation, improve peripheral perfusion, and reduce the work of breathing (Rackow and Astiz, 1993).

ASSESSMENT CRITERIA: SEPSIS AND SEPTIC SHOCK

	Sepsis	Septic Shock
Vital signs		
Temperature	<36° C or >38° C (<96.8° F or >100.4° F)	<36° C or >38° C (<96.8° F or >100.4° F)
Pulse	Tachycardia	Tachycardia
Respirations	Tachypnea	Tachypnea
Blood pressure	Slightly above or below baseline.	Persistent hypotension that is unresponsive to fluid resuscitation.
History		
Symptoms, conditions	Increased cardiac output, warm, flushed skin, changes in behavior or mental status, intellectual impairment, hypoxia.	Decreased cardiac ejection fraction, pulmonary hypertension, anasarca, oliguria, coagulopathies.
Hallmark physical signs and symptoms	Weakness, malaise, temperature >38.0° C (100.4° F), confusion, restlessness, rigors.	Bilateral rales, persistent hypotension that is poorly responsive or refractory to treatment, oliguria or anuria, cyanosis, mental status changes, acute respiratory distress syndrome.
Psychosocial signs	Confusion, delirium, restlessness, agitation, and decreases in levels of consciousness (may be among the first symptoms of sepsis).	
Diagnostic tests	Cultures of blood and body fluids; x-rays of chest, abdomen; ultrasounds; gallium scans; CAT scans, MRI.	
Lab values		
Creatinine	Elevated	Elevated
Blood urea nitrogen (BUN)	Elevated	Elevated
Magnesium, serum	Decreased	Decreased
Calcium, serum	Decreased	Decreased
Potassium, serum	Elevated	Elevated

ASSESSMENT CRITERIA: SEPSIS AND SEPTIC SHOCK (continued)

	Sepsis	Septic Shock
Thyroid hormones	Suppressed	Suppressed
Growth hormone, serum	Elevated	Elevated
Cortisol, serum	Elevated	Elevated
Liver functions, serum	Elevated	Elevated
Glucose, serum	Elevated	Decreased (especially in terminal stages)

Source: Data from Ackerman MH: The systemic inflammatory response, sepsis, and multiple organ dysfunction: New definitions for an old problem. Crit Care Nurs North Am 6(2):243–250, 1994; and Lawler DA: Hormonal response in sepsis. Crit Care Nurs North Am 6(2):265–274, 1994.

NURSING DIAGNOSIS

The nursing diagnosis may vary, depending on the nature of the organism(s) that initiated the septic process, the client's previous state of health, and the complications engendered by the septic process. Possible diagnoses are as follows.

Alterations in tissue perfusion related to vasodilation secondary to release of cytokines.

Fluid volume deficit related to:
- Increased capillary permeability secondary to the inflammatory process.
- Venous pooling secondary to activation of the complement system.

Impaired gas exchange related to:
- Increased oxygen consumption secondary to hypermetabolic state.
- Circulatory abnormalities.

Altered nutrition, less than body requirements, related to:
- Increased metabolic requirements.
- Inadequate oral intake of nutrients.

Ineffective thermoregulation related to:
- Effects of circulating endotoxins associated with the septic process.
- Hypermetabolic state.

(Potential for) altered thought processes related to:
- Hypoperfusion of cerebral vessels.
- Sensory deprivation associated with hospital environment.

NURSING INTERVENTIONS

Immediate nursing interventions

Establish IV access, and obtain volumetric infusion pump.

Initiate aggressive fluid resuscitation to restore or maintain blood pressure to baseline.

Send STAT serum chemistry levels.

Submit cultures of blood and body fluids, suspicious drainage from wounds or lesions.

Obtain SaO$_2$ readings, and initiate oxygen therapy if indicated.

Assess intake and output (I and O).

Prepare for placement of long-term catheter or venous access device.

Prepare for possible intubation and ventilatory support.

Prepare for placement of enteral feeding tube.

Although hazardous in an immunocompromised client, anticipate possible placement of a pulmonary artery catheter.

Anticipated physician orders and interventions

Blood cultures from central line and peripheral site.

Broad-spectrum IV antibiotic therapy. First dose STAT.

STAT CBC with differential, disseminated intravascular coagulation (DIC) panel (prothrombin time/partial prothromboplastin time [PT/PTT], d-dimer, fibrinogen, fibrin degradation products), serum chemistry panel, SaO$_2$ readings.

Indwelling urinary catheter.

Vital signs q1h.

I and O q1h.

Central line insertion tray to bedside.

Intubation tray to bedside.

Bolus with 0.9% NaCl or lactated Ringer's solution IV; then infuse at 150 to 500 ml/hour.

Colloid (albumin, hetastarch) infusion may be used to prevent pulmonary edema secondary to fluid resuscitation in clients known to be hypoalbuminemic or to have increased capillary permeability (Parillo, 1990; Rackow, Falk, and Fein, 1983).

Begin dopamine infusion when hypotension continues after fluid resuscitation. Titrate to maintain mean arterial pressure (MAP) > 60 mmHg, while keeping the dose < 20 µcg/kg/minute. Add dobutamine and/or norepinephrine (levophed) if unable to maintain MAP > 60 mmHg at < 20 µcg/kg/minute dopamine.

Obtain blood cultures once every 24 hours for temperature > 38.5° C (> 101.3° F).

Ongoing nursing assessment, monitoring, and interventions

Assess:

- Vital signs q1h and PRN.
- For changes in vital signs indicative of worsening sepsis (falling blood pressure, drop in pulse rate, alterations in level of consciousness, decreased urine output).
- IV sites for redness, edema, and pain with each client contact.

- Catheter sites for redness, drainage, or tenderness.
- Wounds for drainage for odor, redness, and tenderness.
- Perirectal area for pain, redness, or induration.
- Oral mucosa for lesions.
- Skin for rashes or lesions.
- Skin color and turgor.
- For chills, rigors, or subjective complaints of pain or malaise.
- CBC for leukocytosis or leukopenia.
- Urine for adequacy of output color, foul odor, mucus, and pus.
- Lymphocyte counts, electrolytes, and serum protein for adequacy of nutritional status.
- Level of consciousness.

Measure:
- Vital signs q15 to 30 minutes during vasoactive drip titration or q1h when stable and PRN.
- I and O q1h.
- SaO$_2$ if/while mechanically ventilated, continuously until 4 to 8 hours after extubation.
- Daily weights.

Send: Blood and culture specimens every 24 hours for fever spikes.

Implement:
- Protective isolation if client is neutropenic.
- Measures to maintain and preserve integrity of protective barriers such as skin and mucous membranes.

TEACHING/EDUCATION

Because clients with cancer are at extremely high risk for infection and experience high rates of mortality and morbidity, infection should be prevented or detected in the early stages whenever possible. Effective teaching can help clients achieve a feeling of control over their own health and wellness, and prevent potentially lethal complications.

Protective isolation: *Rationale:* During the time your white blood cell count is low you are at risk for severe infections. In order to help you avoid the problem, we ask that your visitors be restricted to immediate family and children over the age of 12. No one who visits you should have a cold, flu, or history of recent respiratory viruses or recent vaccinations, and all visitors and staff must wash their hands before coming in contact with you. When out of your room, you will need to wear a face mask to protect you from the risk of an airborne infection such as a cold or flu.

Signs and symptoms of infection: *Rationale:* Chemotherapy drugs and your cancer can make you more at risk for serious problems for infections that ordinarily would not cause you to be ill. Early signs of infection that you may see are fever, chills, weakness, persistent aches and pains that have no obvious cause, and nausea, vomiting, and diarrhea.

Hygiene: *Rationale:* When your white blood cell count is low, germs that live on your skin can become a source of infection for you and cause you to be seriously ill. Bathe every day with a good antibacterial soap and be sure to wash your hands with soap and water every time you use the bathroom.

Oral care: *Rationale:* You may at times develop a sore mouth because of side effects of your chemotherapy or radiation. It is important to keep your mouth clean in order to avoid infection. Use a soft toothbrush or sponge toothettes, and a mild toothpaste or baking soda to cleanse your mouth after every meal and at bedtime. Do not use mouthwashes that contain alcohol, and do not use lemon-glycerin swabs.

Respiratory care: *Rationale:* The treatments and drugs you have received and your cancer place you at risk for respiratory infections. Avoid people who have coughs, sore throats, colds, or flu. Drink plenty of water. During periods when you are unable to be active, take plenty of deep breaths, and use the incentive spirometer to exercise your lungs and help you get rid of mucus and phlegm.

Medications: *Rationale:* You are receiving antibiotics to treat your infection. The doctor will send you home on an oral antibiotic to make certain that the infection is completely gone. Be sure to take all of the antibiotics that were ordered for you in the way they were prescribed, because the infection may return if it is inadequately treated.

Dietary restrictions: *Rationale:* When your white blood cell count is low, you are at risk for infection from germs found in food that will not cause you a problem when you have a normal white blood cell count. Do not eat raw shellfish or uncooked foods until you have your doctor's approval. Avoid foods that have been kept warm for a long period of time or at room temperature. Wash all fruits and vegetables thoroughly before eating them.

When to seek medical care: *Rationale:* Because your illness and treatment have put you at significant risk for infection, it is important that you look for signs and symptoms that may indicate you need to seek medical help. Call your doctor if you have fever greater than or equal to 38.5° C (100.3° F), chills, nausea, weakness, fatigue, diarrhea, or painful urination. Examine your body daily for rashes, sores, or painful or tender areas. Notify your doctor if you have a cough, shortness of breath, or purulent or rusty sputum.

EVALUATION/DESIRED OUTCOMES

1. The client will become and remain free of infection as evidenced by:
   Afebrile status.
   Chest clear to auscultation.

Blood and body cultures negative for bacterial, fungal, or viral organisms.

Normal patterns of elimination.

Intact skin and mucous membranes.

2. The client will demonstrate pertinent measures for prevention of infection.

3. Oral intake adequate for the nutritional needs of client.

4. The client is able to return to baseline level of activity (McNally and Stair, 1991).

DISCHARGE PLANNING

The neutropenic client may need:

Home health care referral for continuing IV antibiotic therapy, wound care, blood draws, training of self and significant others in medication administration, and environmental home assessment.

Placement in short-term intermediate care facility for IV antibiotic therapy and/or wound care.

FOLLOW-UP CARE

Anticipated care

Follow-up visit to health care provider within 1 week.

Outpatient lab studies for CBC and cell differential.

Home health care visits to assist with therapeutic regimen, evaluate status of infection, and provide client and family education.

Anticipated client/family questions and possible answers

What caused my infection?

"Your low white blood cell count left you at risk for infection from germs in your daily environment that ordinarily would not cause you to become ill."

When can I stop taking special precautions?

"We take frequent samples of your blood to evaluate your ability to fight infection. When the special white blood cell, called a neutrophil, rises to a level of 1000 or more, you can return to your normal lifestyle."

Isn't it safer for me to stay in the hospital until I get better?

"Germs that are found in the hospital environment are often stronger and harder to treat, even with IV antibiotics. The germs in your home are germs that your body is accustomed to, and they are less likely to cause you to become ill. As long as you don't have fever, chills, or other symptoms of infection and have someone to offer you help if necessary, it is usually safer for you to be at home."

CHAPTER SUMMARY

Sepsis is the thirteenth leading cause of death in the United States. Approximately 400,000 people develop sepsis each year, with a mortality rate of 20 to 50%. In the oncology population, septic episodes have a mortality rate as high as 90% because of altered immune status and compromised inflammatory response.

   Rates of infection can be decreased with strict adherence to aseptic technique and protective measures. Survival rates for the oncology client are improved if sepsis is detected and treated while still in the early stages. Because of immunocompromise, early signs and symptoms of sepsis in the oncology client are often subtle. Nurses must assess carefully for slight temperature elevations and changes in vital signs, localized areas of redness and tenderness on the body, and changes in level of consciousness and behavior. Prompt initiation of antibiotic therapy and fluid replacement can be lifesaving for the client with cancer.

TEST QUESTIONS

1. Which of the following is an early symptom of sepsis?
   A. Cold, clammy skin
   B. Confusion
   C. Hypoglycemia
   D. Decreased urine output

1. Answer: B
Immunocompromised clients are unable to mount a normal immune response. Changes in level of consciousness may be the only symptom of sepsis in the early stages, particularly in the elderly client.

2. Factors that predispose a client with cancer to bacterial infections include all of the following *except:*
   A. Disruptions in the mucosal lining
   B. Therapy with colony-stimulating factor
   C. Leukocytosis
   D. Skin lesions

2. Answer: B
Colony-stimulating factor is given to stimulate the production of neutrophils by the bone marrow, thereby augmenting the client's immune status.

3. Diseases that may adversely impact the client's immune status include:
   A. Diabetes
   B. Arthritis
   C. Hypertension
   D. Scleroderma

3. Answer: A
The diabetic client has impaired vasculature and neutrophil function.

4. The purpose of the inflammatory response is to:
   A. Prevent colonization of the host by foreign organisms
   B. Stimulate the release of cytokines
   C. Decrease the growth of bacteria within the host
   D. Facilitate movement of immune cells to the site of injury

4. Answer: D
The inflammatory response promotes the movement of nutrients and immune cells to the site of tissue injury.

5. Which client is at greatest risk for a septic episode?
   A. An acute leukemic
   B. A client with chronic leukemia who has a WBC count of 15,000
   C. A client with gastric cancer
   D. A client with an absolute neutrophil count of 94

5. Answer: D
Clients with severe neutropenia are at greatest risk for sepsis.

6. A severely neutropenic client is complaining of rectal tenderness. The *most appropriate* nursing intervention is to:
   A. Help the client maintain meticulous personal hygiene, especially in the perineal area.
   B. Notify the physician of the assessment finding.
   C. Give the client a diet that is high in fiber in order to avoid constipation.
   D. Administer a stool softener.

6. Answer: B
The symptom described is suggestive of rectal abscess, which can cause significant morbidity and mortality in the neutropenic client. The physician must be notified immediately so that antibiotic therapy can be initiated.

7. In advanced sepsis, laboratory studies are most likely to reflect:
   A. Decreased BUN
   B. Increased platelet count
   C. Respiratory acidosis
   D. Respiratory alkalosis

7. Answer: C
Respiratory acidosis is the result of alveolar hypoventilation, which results in carbon dioxide retention.

8. A neutropenic client has become febrile for the first time, with chills, malaise, and a temperature of 38.9° C (102° F). The nurse must make it a priority to:
   A. Obtain a prescription for treatment with broad-spectrum antibiotics
   B. Administer a scheduled dose of aspirin
   C. Initiate IV hydration to compensate for insensible fluid loss
   D. Submit cultures of the skin and oral mucosa

8. Answer: A
The neutropenic client requires immediate treatment with broad-spectrum antibiotic therapy with the first sign of infection. Cultures of blood, urine, and sputum are collected in order to help identify the causative organism(s).

9. A client is about to be discharged home with a neutrophil count of 400. Client education should include which of the following?
   A. Eat plenty of fresh fruits and vegetables.
   B. Take your temperature once a day and report any readings above 40° C (above 104° F) to your physician.
   C. Avoid people with contagious illnesses and respiratory infections.
   D. Use only moisturizing soaps in order to avoid damaging your skin.

9. Answer: C
In order to decrease the risk of infection, clients with neutropenia should be instructed to avoid individuals with contagious illnesses.

10. The client with sepsis requires nutritional support in order to:
    A. Maintain a negative nitrogen balance
    B. Increase protein starvation
    C. Protect the integrity of the microvessels of the brain
    D. Restore immune function

10. Answer: D
Adequate nutrition and nitrogen balance are required in order to support and restore immune function.

REFERENCES

Ackerman MH: The systemic inflammatory response, sepsis, and multiple organ dysfunction: New definitions for an old problem. Crit Care Nurs Clin North Am 6(2):243–250, 1994.

Ackerman MH, Evans NJ, Ecklund MM: Systemic inflammatory response syndrome, sepsis, and nutritional support. Crit Care Nurs Clin North Am 6(2):321–340, 1994.

Brown KK: Septic shock. Am J Nurs 94(10):21–22, 1994.

Dietz KA, Flaherty AM: Oncologic emergencies. *In:* Groenwald SL, Frogge MH, Goodman M (eds): Cancer Nursing: Principles and Practice. Boston: Jones and Bartlett, 1993, pp. 800–837.

Ellerhorst-Ryan JM: Infection. *In:* Groenwald SL, Frogge MH, Goodman M (eds): Cancer Nursing: Principles and Practice. Boston: Jones and Bartlett, 1993, p. 558.

Hilderley LJ: Radiotherapy. *In:* Groenwald SL, Frogge MH, Goodman M (eds): Cancer Nursing: Principles and Practice. Boston: Jones and Bartlett, 1993, p. 236.

Kokiko J: Septic shock: A review and update for the emergency department clinician. J Emergency Nurs 19(2):102–108, 1993.

Koll BS, Brown AE: Changing patterns of infections in the immunocompromised patient with cancer. Hematol/Oncol Clin North Am 7(4):753–767, 1993.

Lawler DA: Hormonal response in sepsis. Crit Care Nurs North Am 6(2):265–274, 1994.

Lee JW, Pizzo PA: Management of the cancer patient with fever and prolonged neutropenia. Hematol/Oncol Clin North Am 7(5):937–955, 1993.

Lee RM, Balk RA, Bone RC: Ventilatory support in the management of septic patients. Crit Care Clin 5:157–175, 1989.

McNally JC, Stair J: Potential for infection. *In:* McNally JC, Somerville ET, Miaskowski C, Rostad M (eds): Guidelines for Oncology Nursing Practice. Philadelphia: WB Saunders Co, 1991, pp. 191–202.

Opal SM, Cross AS, Kelly NM, Sadoff JC, Bodmer MW, Palardy JE, Victor GH: Efficacy of a monoclonal antibody directed against tumor necrosis factor in protecting neutropenic rats from lethal infection with *Pseudomonas aeruginosa.* J Infect Dis 161:1148–1152, 1990.

Parillo JE: Septic shock in humans: Advances in the understanding of pathogenesis, cardiovascular dysfunction and therapy. Ann Intern Med 113:227–242, 1990.

Rackow EC, Astiz ME: Mechanisms and management of septic shock. Crit Care Clin 9(2):219–237, 1993.

Rackow EC, Falk JL, Fein IA: Fluid resuscitation in circulatory shock: A comparison of the cardiorespiratory effects of albumin, hetastarch and saline solutions in patients with hypovolemic and septic shock. Crit Care Med 11:839–850, 1983.

Rubin RH, Ferraro MJ: Understanding and diagnosing infectious complications in the immunocompromised host: Current issues and trends. Hematol/Oncol Clin North Am 7(4):795–811, 1993.

Secor VH: The inflammatory/immune response in critical illness: Role of the systemic inflammatory response syndrome. Crit Care Clin North Am 6(2):251–264, 1994.

Tenenbaum L: Cancer Chemotherapy and Biotherapy: A Reference Guide. Philadelphia: WB Saunders Co, 1994.

Truett L: The septic syndrome: An oncologic treatment challenge. Cancer Nurs 14(4):175–180, 1991.

Walsh T: Management of the immunocompromised patient with evidence of an invasive mycosis. Hematol/Oncol Clin North Am 7(5):1003–1021, 1993.

Wiessner WH, Casey LC, Zbilut JP: Treatment of sepsis and septic shock: A review. Heart Lung 24(5):380–393, 1995.

Workman ML, Ellerhorst-Ryan J, Hartgraave-Koertge V: Nursing Care of the Immunocompromised Client. Philadelphia: WB Saunders Co, 1993.

CHAPTER 39

SPINAL CORD COMPRESSION

Denise Ann Forster, MSN, CRRN, CETN, LSW, CANP

CHAPTER OBJECTIVES

At the completion of this chapter, the reader will be able to:

Define spinal cord compression (SCC).

Identify types of cancers placing clients at highest risk for SCC.

Discuss symptoms heralding the onset of SCC.

Describe assessment parameters for the client at risk for or who has developed SCC.

Delineate nursing interventions for the client with SCC.

Educate the client and family regarding future care needs and health-promoting behaviors.

OVERVIEW

SCC is a potentially disabling oncologic emergency that requires swift recognition and intervention. The incidence of SCC is reported to be 5% in all clients with a malignant disease (Peterson, 1993). This condition is most commonly associated with cancers of the lung, breast, prostate, and kidney and with lymphoma, myeloma, and sarcoma (Held and Peahota, 1993). The spinal cord is compressed or injured as a direct or indirect result of a malignancy invading the intramedullary, intradural, extradural, or extravertebral space (Dyck, 1991).

DESCRIPTION

SCC is one of the complications that can arise as a part of the cancer disease process and that can result in a partial or total loss of various sensory and motor functions within the body. Regardless of the type of cancer or point of invasion, the mechanism of injury to the spinal cord remains the same. The cord becomes compressed through direct tumor involvement, metastases from a primary tumor site, or by vertebral collapse (due to a lytic process) either by directly impinging on the spinal cord or indirectly as a result of the impingement of bony fragments within the cord. "The pathophysiological response to SCC includes edema of the spinal cord, diminished blood supply at the cord and mechanical distortion of the neural tissue leading to paresis and paralysis" (Dyck, 1991).

Primary central nervous system (CNS) tumors account for only 1 to 3% of all cases. SCC can occur at any location on the spine, though it is most commonly found in the thoracic region (65% occurrence rate), followed by the cervical and lumbar sacral regions, which each have a 15% occurrence rate (Peterson, 1993).

The nature of the SCC symptomatology will depend on which segment of the spinal cord is affected. A neurologic exam will reveal sensory and motor functional level based on sensation and movement. In addition to the level of function, the diagnosis may be further classified as complete or incomplete. A complete injury is one in which there is no sparing of motor ability or sensation below the level of injury. Incomplete refers to an injury in which motor ability or sensation is spared to varying degrees.

It is imperative to recognize and treat SCC before additional damage occurs. It is also important to realize that subtle changes in motor ability and sensation can indicate a SCC and that bowel and bladder dysfunction or paralysis are actually late signs of SCC. Pain is considered the hallmark of SCC, presenting at a rate of up to 96% (Dyck, 1991). It should be noted, however, that it is possible to have asymptomatic SCC.

RISK PROFILE

Cancers: Of the lung, breast, prostate, kidney, and thyroid; myeloma, melanoma, sarcoma, lymphoma, leukemia, Hodgkin's, neuroblastoma, chordoma, neurofibroma, meningioma, glioma; dermoid, epidermoid, and gastrointestinal cancers.

Pediatrics: Wilm's tumor (rare).

Conditions: Cancer treatment leading to lytic lesions of the vertebrae.

Environment: None.

Foods: None.

Drugs: None.

PROGNOSIS

SCC is fatal only if it occurs in the cervical region of the spinal cord (C4 and above) and if it results in respiratory paralysis that is uncompensated for with mechanical ventilation. Prognosis as it relates to SCC is usually discussed in terms of survival and functional outcomes. Most sources agree that the primary prognostic factor related to functional outcomes is detection and intervention within 24 hours of SCC. This makes client and family education critical for those at risk for developing this oncologic emergency.

Tumor type is also a prognostic factor for functional outcome and survival. Thirty-two percent (32%) of clients with breast cancer and SCC experience a survival time greater than 6 months (median 4 months; range 0 to 56 months). The rates of survival for lung cancer after SCC onset is greater than 12 months in 9% of cases (Bach et al., 1990). In Eeles, O'Brien, Horwich, and Brada's (1991) review of 20 clients with SCC related to non-Hodgkin's lymphoma, the median survival was 8 months following the SCC. In this study, the pretreatment ambulant nonsensory impaired clients with SCC had survival rates of 104 months compared to the clients experiencing paresis or paralysis prior to treatment who survived only 6 months following treatment. Tumor histology and cord compression level were not found to be prognostic factors for survival.

A primary malignant spinal cord injury (SCI) lesion, even when it was treated aggressively with surgery and radiation, shows a median rate of survival as 1 year (Raney, 1991). Murray (1985) reported that clients with incomplete injuries, lymphomas, or solid tumors had lower survival rates and lower functional status at 1 year than those clients with primary CNS tumors or SCI related to radiation myelitis. Location of the lesion can also be a prognostic factor of functional outcome. Clients with a SCC occurring within the mid to lower thoracic levels may see less recovery due to poor collateral blood supply in this region as compared to the rest of the spine (Ratanatharathorn and Powers, 1991). Tumors located in the anterior of the vertebrae are more difficult to resect. Compressive lesions that do not infiltrate into the cord tissue have more favorable outcomes (Ratanatharathorn and Powers, 1991). No definite correlation between size, number or extent of metastases, and resultant disability has been established (Baldwin, 1993). Vertebral collapse along with an extradural tumor generally leads to a poorer prognosis (Dyck, 1991).

TREATMENT

Surgery

May or may not be palliative.

Laminectomy for spinal decompression.

Indications:
- Unknown primary.
- Spinal instability.
- Tumors that are radiation resistant.
- Previously irradiated spine.
- Intractable pain.
- Progressive neurologic regression due to deformity.

Spinal fusion (including instrumentation) to stabilize the spine by correcting deformities or replacing lytic or removed structures.

Bone grafts may be done in the absence of vertebrae body involvement.

Chemotherapy: The type of chemotherapy agent will depend on the type of primary tumor. Generally, chemotherapy is used as an adjuvant therapy.

Radiation

May or may not be palliative.

Parts are treated with a direct field to include the involved vertebral or paravertebral areas (two above and two below).

Note: Neurologic deterioration may occur as a result of progressive SCC or secondary to edema in the cord that is caused by radiation therapy.

Medications

Corticosteroids to decrease spinal cord edema administered when high suspicion of SCC occurs or immediately after diagnosis: methylprednisolone sodium succinate (Solu-Medrol) or dexamethasone.

Analgesics for pain control.

Enoxeparin (low molecular weight heparin) subcutaneously twice a day to decrease risk of deep vein thrombosis in clients with paralysis/paresis.

Rectal suppositories (bisacodyl and glycerin) for bowel routine for clients with neurogenic bowel.

Procedures: Possible halo vest application.

Other: Antiembolism stockings and sequential compression devices (the latter while the client is on bedrest).

Generally speaking, radiation therapy, surgery, and high doses of steroids are the treatment modalities of choice for SCC, either alone or in combination.

ASSESSMENT CRITERIA: SPINAL CORD COMPRESSION

	T7 and Below	T6 and Above (Secondary to Spinal Shock)
Vital signs		
Temperature	Normal range	Below 37° C (98.6° F).
Pulse	Normal range	50–60 beats per minute.
Respirations	Normal range	Increased if respiratory ability is compromised.
Blood pressure	Normal range	70–100/50–60 mmHg.
History		
Pain		May have sudden onset; may be unilateral or bilateral, severe, dull, or aching. *Local*—at or near tumor; aggravating factor is supine position. *Radicular*—caused by nerve root compression; aggravating factor: performing Valsalva maneuver.

(continued)

	Medullary—referred pain; is poorly localized, burning, or shooting pain.
Motor deficits	Weakness, tiredness, heaviness, stiffness in extremities. Ataxia. Loss of coordination/gait changes. Paralysis.
Sensory deficits	Decreased sensation (i.e., to pain, temperature). Hyperesthesias/dysethesias. Paresthesias. Numbness or tingling in the extremities. Bladder—dribbling, retention. Bowel—constipation, loss of urge to defecate, incontinence of stool. Sexual dysfunction.

Hallmark physical signs and symptoms	Pain, weakness, paresthesia, sensation loss, bowel and bladder dysfunction, numbness, decreased coordination and mobility, paralysis.

Additional physical signs and symptoms	Bradycardia, hypotension, hypothermia, respiratory compromise.

Psychosocial signs	Anxiety, denial, powerlessness.

Lab values	None.

Diagnostic tests

Magnetic resonance imaging (MRI)	Able to reveal extent of SCC, type of injury (soft tissue or bony injuries), and condition of soft tissues over the spinal cord, ligaments, intervertebral discs. Images entire spine.
Computerized axial tomography (CAT) scan	Able to reveal neural canal impingement, posterior element injuries, concomitant soft tissue injuries; unable to demonstrate anterior vertebrae body compression.
Myelography	Able to reveal area of SCC, cerebrospinal fluid flow, outline of the spinal cord and nerve roots, and presence of meningeal carcinomatosis with a cerebrospinal fluid (CSF) specimen.
Tomography	Able to reveal bony injury via longitudinal cross sections of the vertebral column.
Standard radiographs	Able to reveal bony injury.
American Spinal Injury Association (ASIA) scale	Comprehensive neurologic functional tool used to assess:
Motor function	International five-point scale for grading muscle strength.
Sensory function	Dermatomes.
Reflex activity	Deep tendon reflexes (if present) are a good sign. Depressed or not present below injury level in clients with recently developed SCC. Bulbocavernosus. Anal wink.

NURSING DIAGNOSIS

The nursing diagnosis will vary, depending on the extent and level of the SCI, which will manifest itself according to the level of injury. Only lesions of C3 and above are potentially life-threatening owing to paralysis and/or paresis of the respiratory musculature. Pain is usually the hallmark of this condition.

Impaired gas exchange related to inability to sustain spontaneous ventilation secondary to C4 injury or above.

Potential/actual impaired physical mobility related to paresthesia or paralysis from spinal cord injury secondary to SCC.

Risk for injury related to deep vein thrombosis, pulmonary emboli, falls, and dermal injuries secondary to loss of sensory perception.

Total incontinence related to neurogenic bowel and bladder secondary to spinal cord injury from SCC.

Pain (acute) related to SCC.

Risk for infection (urinary tract) related to neurogenic bladder with subsequent use of indwelling catheter, intermittent catheterization, urinary retention, or backflow from external collecting device.

Potential for self-care deficit related to spinal cord injury and activities of daily living will be variably affected, depending on the level of injury.

Sensory perceptual alterations (kinesthetic, tactile) related to SCC.

Risk of impaired skin integrity related to paresthesis and/or paralysis from SCC.

Risk for caregiver role strain related to need for assistance with activities of daily living.

Potential for autonomic dysreflexia related to upper motor neuron spinal cord lesion (T6 and above) once spinal shock has subsided (about 10 weeks).

Alteration in tissue perfusion related to SCC.

Knowledge deficit related to care needs following spinal cord injury and symptoms of SCC.

Potential for ineffective individual coping related to SCC.

NURSING INTERVENTIONS

Immediate nursing interventions

Institute appropriate immobilization: Maintain bedrest until spine is assessed to be stable, logroll only.

Assess respiration (quality and rate), pulse, and blood pressure q4–8h.
- Place suction equipment at bedside.
- Maintain patient airway, and provide oxygen with ambu-bag as necessary (C4 and above).

Assess client's neurologic status:
- Sensory perception (pinprick and temperature).

- Movement in lower extremities and upper extremities.
- Deep tendon reflexes while maintaining bedrest.

Assess for bladder dysfunction: If the client has not voided in 6 to 8 hours, consider straight catheterization of the client and/or insertion of an indwelling catheter.

Assess for pain: location and quality.

Provide call system that the client is able to use if hand function is impaired.

Assess for ataxia.

Provide support and allow the client maximum control over daily activities.

Anticipated physician orders and interventions

STAT MRI or x-ray of the spine.

Initiation of low molecular weight heparin therapy (Enoxeparin).

Application of sequential compression devices or antiembolism stockings.

Placement on ventilator (C4 and above).

Administration of medication:

- Analgesic for pain control.
- Administer corticosteroids to decrease spinal cord edema administered when high suspicion of SCC occurs or immediately after diagnosis: Methylprednisolone sodium succinate (Solu-Medrol) 30 mg/kg IV over 15 minutes within 8 hours of SCI, then 5.4 mg/kg IV every hour for 23 hours. Dexamethasone 10 mg IV initially followed by 4 mg q6h or dexamethasone 100 mg IV initially followed by 24 mg q6h.

Prepare for treatment:

- Surgery.
- Radiation.
- Combination.

Routine pre- and postoperative care.

Ongoing nursing assessment, monitoring, and interventions

Assess:

- Neurologic status q8h and PRN.
- Respiratory status (rate and depth) q8h PRN.
- Bladder functioning (hesitancy, urgency, retention, and abdominal discomfort from bladder spasms).
- Bowel functioning qd.
- Skin integrity for impaired circulation and breakdown.
- Lower extremities for deep vein thrombosis.
- Pathologic fractures.
- Quantity and quality of pain.

- Client's/family's ability to cope.
- For signs and symptoms of infection qd.

Measure:
- Vital signs q4h–q8h.
- Fluid intake and output q8h.

Send:
- Urine analysis culture and sensitivity if client develops neurogenic bladder.
- Doppler ultrasound of the legs to detect deep vein thrombosis.

Implement:
- Range-of-motion program.
- Turn schedule for clients with impaired mobility.
- Bowel routine using bisacodyl and glycerin suppositories along with digital stimulation and disimpaction if necessary, every other day.
- Bladder management program for clients with neurogenic bladder, including an intermittent catheter program or insertion of an indwelling catheter if necessary.
- Use of cervical collar or brace.
- Anti-foot-drop devices.
- Daily progressive mobility schedule as tolerated and indicated.
- Referral for rehabilitation: nursing (enterostomal therapy nurse), occupational therapy, and physical therapy.
- Encourage a balanced diet with sufficient fiber.
- Encourage use of incentive spirometry.
- Educate about spinal cord injury and changes in sexual functioning.

TEACHING/EDUCATION

Antiembolism stockings/sequential compression devices: *Rationale:* We are going to put these on both of your legs so that you won't develop blood clots in your legs while you are on bedrest.

Turning: *Rationale:* We are turning you so you don't get any bedsores or pressure ulcers. Also, it is important for your lungs and circulation to change position frequently.

Bedrest: *Rationale:* It is necessary for you to be flat in bed until all the tests are done, to make sure we don't allow any further damage to your spine.

Logrolling: *Rationale:* We need to keep your spine in a straight line so it is not injured while you are being turned.

Diagnostics: *Rationale:* These tests are being done to see if there are any problems with your spinal cord that could be causing the symptoms you are experiencing. These tests will help us to determine what the best course of treatment will be for you.

Indwelling urinary catheter placement or intermittent catheterization: *Rationale:* Your bladder is storing/leaking urine because there is injury to the nerves that help you control urination. Making sure your bladder is emptied on a regular basis will mean that it is less likely you will leak urine or get a bladder infection, and this precaution could prevent problems with your kidneys.

Bowel routine: *Rationale:* The nerves that help to control your bowels have been injured. Because of this, we need to insert suppositories in your rectum to help you have a bowel movement. This will help to prevent constipation or stool leakage during the day.

Symptoms and signs of SCC: *Rationale:* You need to tell us if your symptoms are changing in any way. This is important so that we can make changes in your treatment as soon as possible and prevent as many complications as possible.

EVALUATION/DESIRED OUTCOMES

1. SCC will be diagnosed and treatment initiated within 24 hours.
2. The client and his or her family will know to suspect SCC and present for follow-up immediately if symptoms are detected.
3. Baseline neurologic functioning will be maintained or restored following treatment.
4. Pain will be well controlled with analgesics or other interventions.
5. There are no signs of infection (surgical wound, bladder, or respiratory).
6. The client is free of radiation therapy complications.
7. The client experiences regular bowel movements and good bowel motility with or without bowel routine and use of suppositories.
8. Bladder program is established immediately in clients with neurogenic bladder, and the client is free of problems of distention, overflow, and stressed or mixed incontinence.
9. The client is free of stages I to IV pressure ulcers.
10. The client and/or the family is able to describe key elements of skin care program (i.e., turning while in bed, weight shifts when sitting).
11. The client and/or family is able to describe triggers, symptoms, and interventions for autonomic dysreflexia if SCI is at the level of T6 or above.
12. The client remains free of a deep vein thrombosis or pulmonary emboli.
13. The client is given as much control over environment and activity as possible; verbalizes understanding of condition and treatments.
14. The client is not unnecessarily fearful and remains communicative.
15. The lungs remain clear to auscultation and infection-free.

DISCHARGE PLANNING

The client with residual neurologic deficits may need:

Wheelchair, cushion, transfer board, and instructions for family on transfer techniques.

Enoxeparin, needles, and instructions on administration.

Hospital bed.

Respiratory management program and equipment.

Bladder management program and equipment.

Bowel management program and medication.

Follow-up care in an SCI clinic.

Pain control.

Home evaluation for accessability.

Ramps and other adaptive devices for the home or work.

Handicap display card for car.

FOLLOW-UP CARE

Anticipated care

Physician visit within 2 weeks (oncologist, surgeon).

Spinal cord injury team follow-up within 2 to 3 weeks.

Follow-up with home health nurse for monitoring of effective bowel and bladder, mobility, and skin care programs.

Administration of Enoxeparin at home and use of antiembolism stockings.

Resolution of spinal shock resulting in new onset of:

- Spasticity (often mistaken for returned functioning).
- Increase in sensory function (pain, temperature).
- Susceptibility to autonomic dysreflexia if SCC is at the level of T6 or above.

Anticipated client/family questions and possible answers

Could my SCI happen again or get worse?

"Yes, you can experience this complication again."

"Yes, depending on the location and type of cancer you have, this can affect a different part of the spinal cord in a different way, resulting in an increase in the effects of this complication you are experiencing. It is extremely important for you to know what the signs of an SCC are and seek medical attention immediately. Your physician will monitor your progress, using medical tests. By seeking medical attention quickly, you will give yourself the best opportunity to avoid more serious problems."

Will I be able to move and feel as I did before ever again?

"It is possible that your functioning may return to what it was before, or it may only partially return. It is recommended, however, that you focus on the abilities you have today and on staying as healthy as possible."

What must I do to take care of my skin daily?

"A spinal cord injury results in interrupted nerve pathways, including nerves to your skin. Having an SCI makes you more susceptible to developing pressure sores where your ability to touch or feel is either decreased or absent. Checking your skin daily, using a mirror for places you can't see directly, will help you to find problems before they become worse. Keeping your skin healthy will help you to avoid complications and possible hospitalizations."

What are weight shifts, and why do I need to do them?

"Performing a weight shift means lifting your body off of the surface of your wheelchair cushion every 15 to 20 minutes to allow the blood to return to the skin tissue on your buttocks on which you have been sitting. Without blood for prolonged periods of time, skin cells can die, resulting in a pressure ulcer (*note:* you also need to turn every 2 to 3 hours when in bed for the same reason). If you notice a red area anywhere on your skin that does not go away after a few hours, you should avoid pressure on that area until the color returns to normal."

Why can't I urinate or move my bowels as I used to?

"The nerve pathways that control your bladder and bowels have been interrupted because of your spinal cord injury. There are many ways to help you empty your bladder and move your bowels. Your health care team will help you decide a way that will best meet your needs and will teach you and your family how to carry this out when you are at home."

What should I do if I have the same symptoms again?

"Call your physician or come to the hospital immediately."

Why do I need therapy?

"Because of your spinal cord injury, you may need therapy to help you learn to be as independent with your daily activities as possible."

CHAPTER SUMMARY

Early detection and prompt treatment are critical in determining functional outcomes and future quality of life in the client with SCC. Nurses play a significant role with regard to teaching warning signs to clients who are at risk for developing SCC and reinforcing the need to avoid delays in seeking medical attention. Once an SCC occurs, the client must be appropriately immobilized until treatment goals are achieved. Providing and teaching proper bowel, bladder, and skin care is essential in assisting the spinal-cord-injured cancer client to prevent serious and life-threatening complications. Formal rehabilitation may be advisable to improve quality of life and enhance independent functioning. Follow-up care and thorough discharge planning will assist the client and his or her family in facing not only cancer but disability as well.

TEST QUESTIONS

1. The most common presenting symptom of SCC is:
   A. Numbness or tingling
   B. Weakness
   C. Urinary retention
   D. Pain

1. Answer: D
Pain is usually the first indicator that SCC is occurring and is often ignored or assigned to more benign causes.

2. SCC most often affects which part of the spine?
   A. Cervical
   B. Thoracic
   C. Sacral
   D. Lumbar

2. Answer: B
Seventy percent of all SCC injuries occur in the thoracic region.

3. Radiation therapy, teletherapy, is the only treatment for SCC.
   A. True
   B. False

3. Answer: B
Radiation therapy may be used alone or in conjunction with various surgical procedures and/or medications such as corticosteroids.

4. Which clients have the best prognosis for ambulation following treatment for SCC?
   A. Those who are discovered within the first 72 hours after onset of spinal cord compression
   B. Those who are ambulatory at the time of the SCC event
   C. Those who have an SCC at the lumbar level
   D. Those who are treated with adjuvant brachytherapy

4. Answer: B
For the best prognosis for ambulation, immediate detection is essential. Prognosis for survival is related to the nature of the neoplasm.

5. What is the estimated incidence of SCC due to cancer?
   A. 1%
   B. 5%
   C. 15%
   D. 25%

5. Answer: B
The estimated incidence of SCC secondary to cancer is 5%.

6. Laminectomy and spinal fusion are recommended for clients with vertebral collapse.
   A. True
   B. False

6. Answer: A
A laminectomy is performed to decompress the spinal cord. A spinal fusion may also be necessary if there has been vertebral collapse.

7. A complete lower motor neuron spinal lesion can result in a:
   A. Flaccid anal sphincter
   B. Spastic anal sphincter
   C. Pleural effusion
   D. Hemorrhagic cystitis

7. Answer: A
Most SCC will occur in the lower spinal area. The result is a flaccid anal sphincter. The client may complain of stool or flatus incontinence. This can be managed by performance of a regularly scheduled bowel routine.

8. SCC pain is typically:
   A. Nonexistent
   B. Worsened by a decreased atmospheric barometric pressure
   C. Increased by lying down
   D. Psychosomatic in nature

8. Answer: C
Pain, a hallmark sign of SCC, can be local, radicular, or medullary in nature. It can be constant, aggravated by movement, or increased by lying down.

9. Early recognition and treatment of metastatic spinal cord compression is essential because it:
   A. Increases survival rates
   B. Improves quality of life
   C. Increases nutritional protein stores
   D. Increases the chances of generalized muscular spasticity

9. Answer: B
Timely detection and treatment of SCC may not result in prolonged survival, but it may result in more positive functional outcomes and a higher quality of life.

10. What symptoms of SCC are most indicative of advanced compression?
    A. Severe pain
    B. Numbness and tingling
    C. Weakness
    D. Bowel and bladder incontinence

10. Answer: D
Incontinence due to SCC is an advanced sign and indicates that the autonomic nervous system has become impaired.

REFERENCES

Bach F, Larsen B, Rohde K, Borgensen SE, Gjerris F, Boge-Rasmussen T, Agerlin N, Rasmusson B, Stjernholm P, Sorensen PS: Metastatic cord compression. Acta Neurochir 107:37–43, 1990.

Baldwin PD: Epidural spinal cord compression secondary to metastatic disease: A review of the literature. Cancer Nurs 6(16):441–446, 1993.

Dyck S: Surgical instrumentation as a palliative treatment for spinal cord compression. Oncol Nurs Forum 18(3):515–521, 1991.

Eeles RA, O'Brien P, Horwich A, Brada M: Non-Hodgkin's lymphoma presenting with extradural spinal cord compression: Functional outcome and survival. Brit J Cancer 63(1):126–129, 1991.

Held JL: Identifying spinal cord compression. Nursing 24(5):28, 1994.

Held JL, Peahota A: Nursing care of the patient with spinal cord compression. Oncol Nurs Forum 20(10):1507–1516, 1993.

Murray P: Functional outcome and survival in spinal cord injury secondary to neoplasia. Cancer 55:197–201, 1985.

Peterson R: A nursing intervention for early detection of spinal cord compressions in patients with cancer. Cancer Nus 16(2):113–116, 1993.

Raney DJ: Malignant spinal cord tumors: A review and case presentation. J Neurosci Nurs 23(1):44–49, 1991.

Ratanatharathorn V, Powers W: Epidural spinal cord compression from metastatic tumor: Diagnosis and guidelines for management. Cancer Treat Rev 18:55–71, 1991.

Van Veldhuizen PJ, Stephens RL: Education of neoplastic spinal cord compressions. Kansas Med 94(5):130–132, 1993.

Zejdlik C: Management of spinal cord injury, 2nd ed. Boston: Jones and Bartlett, 1992.

CHAPTER 40

SUICIDAL IDEATION

Rosanne M. Radziewicz, MSN, RN, CS

CHAPTER OBJECTIVES

At the completion of this chapter, the reader will be able to:

Distinguish suicidal ideation, suicidal gestures, and suicide attempts.

Describe five risk factors of suicide for the client with cancer.

Identify four criteria for major depression among clients with medical illness.

Identify immediate nursing interventions for the client with cancer who

    1. Expresses hopelessness and despair.

    2. Expresses suicidal ideation.

    3. Makes a suicidal gesture or attempt.

Anticipate and prepare the client with suicidal ideation for discharge and future care needs.

OVERVIEW

THE diagnosis and treatment of cancer is often associated with psychological morbidity. Many clients with cancer meet the criteria of a psychiatric diagnosis, including moderate-to-severe depression, anxiety, and adjustment disorder (Fincannon, 1995; Ibbotson, Maguire, Selby, Priestman, and Wallace, 1994). Clients may become vulnerable to suicide when the diagnosis of cancer, its treatment, and a coexisting depression clouds the value, meaning, and quality of life. Although depression is relatively common, suicide in clients with cancer is rare. Perrone (1993) reports that adolescents with cancer tend to fight rather than succumb to death by suicide. Fox, Stanek, Boyd, and Flannery (1982) discovered that <0.2% suicides were diagnosed with cancer. The low frequency of suicides is thought to be due to under-reporting and inconsistency in classifying suicides with the oncology population (Allebeck and Bolund, 1991; Saunders and Valente, 1988). Compared to persons in the general population who attempt suicide, clients with cancer who do so experience nearly a twofold increase in mortality (Allebeck and

Bolund, 1991; Fox et al., 1982; Louhivuori and Hakama, 1979). Suicide may be seen as the only way out of unendurable pain, unmanageable symptoms, or depression. It is the responsibility of the healthcare professional to assess a client's suicidal ideation, reasonably evaluate suicidal risk, and respond in a safe and therapeutic manner to the client's suffering to alay further despair. Breitbart (1990) suggests that the therapeutic goal for clients with terminal illness is not precautions against suicide at all costs. Instead, the primary goals of treatment should be directed toward management of symptoms and pain, determining the need for treatment of depression, and relieving symptom distress. Providing the client with facts and options facilitates clear and informed decisions regarding care.

DESCRIPTION

Suicidal behavior

Suicidal behavior includes ideation, gestures, and intentional attempts to self-inflict death. Self-destructive behaviors such as smoking or overdrinking are considered risk behaviors, but these will not be addressed here.

Suicidal Ideation

Thoughts of harming oneself are known as suicidal ideation. Commonly, any person diagnosed with advanced cancer or depression, or who is seriously ill for any reason, may think about wanting to die. Many clients who express thoughts of ending their lives do not intend to commit suicide but are rather expressing feelings of powerlessness, frustration, and pain. Suicide is a choice that allows some sense of control in the midst of helplessness.

Suicidal ideation can be communicated verbally, behaviorally, or in writing if a client is unable to speak. Overt messages of suicidal ideation include "I'm going to kill myself" or "I'm a burden to my family and I'd be better off dead." More subtle messages can suggest suicidal ideation, such as a client's refusing further treatment or preparing a will. Because cancer is often seen as a terminal illness, preparing for death may be regarded by others as understandable or suggestive of the client's adjustment to his or her disease. Yet care must be used not to overlook a treatment for depression that could improve the client's outlook. If suicidal ideation or end-focused behaviors are untimely given the disease prognosis, then assessment of suicidal risk is indicated.

Suicidal Gestures

Suicidal gestures, also known as *parasuicide,* are specific actions that result in manipulation of the environment (McLaughlin, 1993). Suicidal gestures include self-destructive behaviors that may or may not be life-threatening, including minor wrist cutting or taking overdoses of benzodiazepines. It is suggested that gestures are an attempt to get relief from hopelessness or an attempt to retaliate against someone who hurt them (Roy, 1989). In the oncology client, a suicidal gesture may be a sign that the client is adjusting poorly to treatment or that pain control measures are no longer adequate. Often seen by healthcare providers as "attention seeking" or "game playing," all suicidal gestures must be considered a cry for help and treated seriously.

Suicide Attempt

Suicide is defined as an act to voluntarily end one's own life in response to an intolerable situation in which all alternatives are seen as hopeless. Suicide attempts are life-threatening, demonstrate poor coping with extreme life situations, and are challenges for the healthcare system. Suicide attempts that are usually fatal include overdoses of analgesics or other lethal drugs, hanging (strangulation), drowning, shooting, stabbing, carbon monoxide poisoning, or jumping from high places (Hatton and Valente, 1984; Saunders and Valente, 1988).

Rational suicide

The concept of rational suicide is described as a form of "justifiable suicide," or "autoeuthenasia." Rational suicide implies that a decision to end one's life is made free of depression, with a clear recognition of the causes of distress and of the consequences associated with suicide, and after all options to improve life have been explored (Saunders and Valente, 1988). Cancer is often seen by society as a terminal illness. For the client with cancer, rational suicide may be viewed as an option to regain control and maintain dignity. Engelhardt (1986) suggests that "very few competent individuals in our society appear actually to find suicide to be a rational alternative" (p. 106). Therefore, consultation with an ethics committee and assistance from mental health colleagues are important resources in resolving disputes that arise among healthcare professionals, clients, and their families about rational suicide.

Assisted suicide

Suicide is traditionally understood as the act of taking one's own life. Assisted suicide is defined by the American Nurses Association (ANA) as "making the means of suicide (e.g., providing pills or a weapon) available to a patient with knowledge of the patient's intention . . . [without] acting as the direct agent of death" (ANA, 1994, p. 1). Requests for assistance with suicide can be related to a number of factors, including fear of isolation, fear of loss of control, unrelieved pain, depression, concern for family coping, and hopelessness. The role of the nurse related to these difficult issues has been defined in the ANA Code for Nurses with Interpretive Statements, which states that "respect extends to all who require the services of the nurse for the promotion of health, the prevention of illness, the restoration of health, the alleviation of

Table 40–1
Vulnerability Factors That Increase Suicide Risk in Clients with Cancer

Vulnerability Factor	Significance
Advanced stage of disease	May be associated with multiple, poorly controlled symptoms (e.g., pain, nausea and vomiting, insomnia, depression).
Depression or hopelessness	Hopelessness is the key variable.
	Clients frequently have advanced disease and progressively impaired physical function.
	The client may feel alone, isolated, and abandoned.
Pain	Pain often is controlled inadequately.
	The meaning of pain to the client may be an agonizing death.
	Uncontrolled pain affects the family's ability to provide the client with emotional support.
Delirium	Loss of impulse control—the client more likely to act on suicidal thoughts.
Loss of control; feelings of helplessness	The most important factor relating to suicide risk.
	Associated with symptoms or deficits caused by cancer or treatment (e.g., loss of mobility, impaired bowel and bladder function, inability to eat and talk).
	Associated with some clients' need to maintain control over all aspects of their lives, including death.
Pre-existing psychopathology, major affective disorders, bipolar disorder, major depressive episode	Suicide is always of major concern with depressed clients. If depressive symptoms are severe or if suicide assessment shows risk of lethality, there is a reason for extreme concern. Manic depressive clients in the depressed phase are usually highly suicidal.
Schizophrenia	A high suicide risk exists if the client is experiencing hallucinations and delusions that are of a harmful nature.
Organic mental disorders (delirium)	Suicide may be a risk if the client is severely depressed, is impulsive, confused, delusional or hallucinating, or is using alcohol or drugs.
Substance use disorders	The combination of depression and impulsivity may account for the high incidence of suicide in clients who abuse substances.
Personality disorders (e.g., histrionic, antisocial, borderline)	Impulsive, demanding, and manipulative behavior coupled with depression may indicate suicidal risk.
Prior suicide attempts	Learned behavior from a family member can contribute to using suicide as a method of escape. The best indicator of suicide risk is a previous attempt.
Exhaustion	Multidimensional in the context of advanced multisymptomatic disease; includes physical, spiritual, emotional, and financial exhaustion, family exhaustion, and exhaustion of community and healthcare resources.

Source: Data from Barile L: The client who is suicidal. *In* Lego S (ed): The American Handbook of Psychiatric Nursing. Philadelphia: JB Lippincott, 1984, p. 339; Breitbart WS: Suicide. *In* Holland JC, Rowland J (eds): Handbook of Psychooncology. New York: Oxford University Press, 1990, pp. 291–300.

suffering, and the provision of supportive care of the dying. The nurse does not act deliberately to terminate the life of any person" (ANA, 1985, p. 3). Several states have proposed some form of physician-assisted legislation. Healthcare professionals in oncology often care for clients with terminal illness and are likely to face issues related to assisted suicide. Many difficult moral, legal, and ethical questions surround this controversial issue.

Withholding, withdrawing, and refusal of treatment

The discussion of withholding treatments or refusing treatment that might result in an earlier death are also common in clients with terminal cancer. The registered nurse participates in end-of-life decisions and actions. "Honoring the refusal of treatments that a patient does not desire, that are disproportionately burdensome to the patient, or that will not benefit the patient is ethically and legally permissible. Within this context, withholding or withdrawing life-sustaining therapies or risking the hastening of death through treatments aimed at alleviating suffering and/or controlling symptoms are ethically acceptable and do not constitute assisted suicide" (ANA, 1994, p. 2).

RISK PROFILE

Suicide is thought to be biopsychosocial in nature. Risk factors for suicide can be biologic (e.g., heredity, organicity, central serotonin system deficiency), psychologic (e.g., depression, high emotional distress), and social (e.g., lack of support, exhausted resources) in origin (Roy, 1989). The client with cancer may be particularly at risk for suicide because of symptom distress, psychologic morbidity, and social stresses associated with chronic illness and repeated hospitalization.

Cancers: Strong evidence exists that it is not the cancer diagnosis per se but rather the progression of cancer, level of physical and social impairment, and frequent losses associated with suffering that are important causes of depression and despair. Advanced cancer and rapidly progressing cancers, such as lung and gastrointestinal cancer are strongly linked with high suicide rates (Allebeck and Bolund, 1991; Hietanen and Lonnqvist, 1991). Cancer of the breast and genitals is found in a significant number of women with cancer who commit suicide (Allebeck and Bolund, 1991). Evidence shows an increase of suicide risk within the first 2 years of cancer diagnosis. Suicidal ideation can increase shortly after diagnosis, with exacerbations of the disease, and with treatment failure (Allebeck and Bolund, 1991; Hietanen and Lonnqvist, 1991). Because of the small sample sizes of many studies, it is not advised to base risk on type of cancer or length of time from diagnosis alone. Each individual's response to the disease may differ, based on other conditions.

Conditions: Previous history of suicide attempt(s); pre-existing psychopathology, particularly disorders of mood (see Table 40–1); expressed wish of being dead; family history of suicide; associated medical conditions (refer to Table 40–2); substance abuse; poorly controlled pain; psychological and spiritual distress; recent loss of a significant relationship; and hospital admittance. Table 40–3 summarizes data concerning suicide and its relationship to risk factors.

Demographics: Male gender (men tend to commit suicide sooner after diagnosis than women), Caucasian race (more likely than African American or Hispanic), increasing age (in men, rates rise with age above 45; in women

Table 40–2
Medical Causes of Depressive Symptoms

Endocrine Disorders
  Acromegaly
  Addison's disease
  Cushing's disease
  Diabetes mellitus
  Hyper/hypoadrenalism
  Hypoaldosteronism
  Hyper/hypoparathyroidism
  Hypopituitarism
  Hyper/hypothyroidism
  Insulinoma
  Pheochromocytoma
  Premenstrual syndrome

Nutrition Deficiency States
  Pellagra
  Pernicious anemia
  Wernicke's encephalopathy

Tumors
  Central nervous system
  Metastatic disease: breast, gastrointestinal,
    lung, pancreas, prostate

Infections
  Encephalitis
  Epstein-Barr virus
  Hepatitis
  Human immunodeficiency syndrome (HIV)
  Meningitis
  Mononucleosis
  Neurosyphilis
  Pneumonia
  Postinfluenza
  Tuberculosis

Others
  Alcoholism
  Electrolyte abnormalities: hypokalemia,
    hyponatremia
  Heavy metal poisoning
  Hypertension
  Postpartum disorders
  Rheumatoid arthritis
  Systemic lupus erythematosus
  Uremia

Neurologic
  Cerebral trauma
  Cerebrovascular disease
  Dementia
  Epilepsy: temporal lobe focus
  Huntington's chorea
  Hydrocephalus
  Multiple sclerosis
  Myasthenia gravis
  Narcolepsy
  Parkinson's disease
  Pick's disease
  Postconcussion
  Progressive supra nuclear palsy
  Stroke
  Subarachnoid hemorrhage
  Wilson's disease

Source: Data from Wise and Rundell, 1994; Jenike, 1984; Valente, 1993.

Table 40–3
Summarized Data of Suicide Mortality Related to Mental Health Risk Factor

Risk Factor	Suicide Mortality Rate
Previous suicide attempt	13–35% within first 2 years of previous attempt
Treated for primary depression	15–20% +
Diagnosis of schizophrenia	10%
Diagnosis of alcoholism, drug addiction	15%

Source: Data from Roy A: Suicide. *In* Kaplan HI, Sadoek BJ (eds): Comprehensive Textbook of Psychiatry/V, vol. 2, 5th ed. Baltimore: Williams and Wilkins, 1989, pp. 1414–1427.

the peak risk is about age 55, then the rate declines), unmarried status (widowed, divorced, living alone), social isolation, homosexual (gay men and lesbians have 3 to 5 times more suicide attempts than comparison groups of heterosexuals).

Social: Poor social support or family instability, being unemployed or retired, history of parental loss during childhood, history of child or sexual abuse.

Pediatrics: Family history of substance abuse and mood disorder, disciplinary crisis, disruption of a significant relationship.

Drugs: See Table 40–4 for drugs that may cause depressive symptoms.

PROGNOSIS

Suicide is considered a preventable cause of death, because most causes of suicide are treatable and the majority of suicidal persons communicate their self-destructive intentions to others, including healthcare providers (Valente, Saunders, and Grant, 1994). With any disease, there are clients whose suffering is so intense, resources so limited, disease so chronic, and who are treatment resistant, that suicide may be perceived as inevitable.

Psychiatric morbidity, particularly in the case of depression in clients with cancer, has been shown to increase based on distress from pain (Spiegel, Sands, and Koopman, 1994); specific symptoms; and, to a lesser degree, immobility over time (Kurtz, Kurtz, Given, and Given, 1995). Therefore, one may conclude that the prognosis for suicide is improved if the client's (1) needs are met through perceived support, (2) comfort and symptoms of treatment and disease are managed, and (3) depression is treated. It is not possible to predict with certainty if someone will harm himself or herself. There is conflicting evidence in the literature about clients at risk for suicide. It is necessary to examine the risk factors for suicide so that an informed statement concerning the actual risk can be documented. Health-

Table 40–4
Drugs That Contribute to Depressive Symptomatology

Analgesics/Anti-inflammatory
Ibuprofen
Indomethacin*
Baclofen
Cocaine
Opiates* (morphine, codeine)
Pentazocine
Phenacetin
Phenylbutazone

Anticonvulsants
Carbamazepine
Ethosuximide
Phenobarbital*
Phenytoin*
Primidone*

Antihistamines
Antihypertensive agents*
Clonidine
Guanethidine
Hydralazine
Hydrochlorothiazide
Methyldopa*
Propranolol
Reserpine
Spironolactone

Antimicrobials
Ampicillin
Cycloserine
Dapsone
Griseofulvin
Isoniazid
Metronidazole
Nalidixic acid
Nitrofurantoin
Procaine penicillin
Streptomycin
Sulfonamide
Tetracycline

Antineoplastics
Arathioprine
6-Azouridine
L-Asparaginase
Bleomycin
Cisplatin
Cyclophosphamide
Doxorubicin
Mithramycin
Procarbazine
Vinblastine
Vincristine

Antiparkinsonian Agents
Amantadine
Bromocriptine
Levodopa*
Hormones
ACTH*
Corticosteroids*
Estrogens/Oral contraceptives

Immunosuppressive Agents or Miscellaneous
Amphetamine withdrawal*
Caffeine
Cimetidine
Digitalis
Halothane
Inderal*
Metochlorpromide
Methysergide
Methrizamide
Phenylephrine

Immunotherapeutic Agents
Alpha interferon
Interleukin 2

Neuroleptics
Fluphenazine*
Haloperidol
Prochlorperazine

Sedatives/Tranquilizers
Barbiturates
Chloral hydrate
Diazepam*
Ethanol
Flurazepam*
Major tranquilizers
Minor tranquilizers
Triazolam*
Alprazolam

Stimulants
Amphetamine* (abuse)
Diethylpropion
Fenfluramine (abuse)
Methylphenidate
Ifosfamide

---

* Drug with a high incidence of depressive side effects.

Source: Data from Valente, 1993; Smith et al., 1994; Valente, Saunders, and Cohen, 1994.

care providers must rapidly assess clients who are at high risk for suicide and call for consultation when further help is indicated.

TREATMENT

The treatment of clients who exhibit suicidal ideation or gestures or who attempt suicide is primarily aimed at protecting the individual from harm. It is important in the case of clients who exhibit depressive symptoms to consider all possible medical (organic) and psychologic causes. Many organic disorders are often preceded by mental status changes, including depressed mood, before physical symptoms are noted. Treatment may entail reducing or removing any organic causes for the changed behavior (e.g., adjusting pain management therapy). Table 40–5 identifies the criteria for major depression among clients with medical illness.

Chemotherapy: Reconsider chemotherapeutic agents that may contribute to depressive effects. Promote the client's comfort with use of psychotropic drugs, and continue chemotherapy despite its side effects, if it is considered vital to treatment of the disease.

Radiation: Palliatively treat central nervous system (CNS) tumors, brain metastases.

Medications: Consult with the physician to taper medications that may con-

---

Table 40–5
Symptoms of Medical Illness (Cancer) and Major Depression

Criteria for Major Depressive Episode (DSM–IV) (American Psychiatric Association, 1994)
- A. Depressed mood or loss of interest or pleasure for 2 weeks.
- B. The presence of at least five of the following symptoms for at least 2 weeks:
  1. Significant unplanned weight loss or gain, or daily change in appetite.
  2. Insomnia (especially with early-morning awakening) or hypersomnia.
  3. Psychomotor agitation or retardation (observable by others) daily.
  4. Fatigue or loss of energy nearly daily.
  5. Feelings of worthlessness, excessive or inappropriate guilt, which may be delusional.
  6. Diminished ability to think or concentrate; complaints of indecisiveness.
  7. Recurrent thoughts about death (not just fear of dying); recurrent suicidal ideation with or without a specific plan; or a suicide attempt.

Criteria for Major Depression among Medically Ill/Hospitalized Clients (Massie, 1992)
Sad mood or mood incongruent with disease outlook.
Feelings of helplessness and hopelessness.
Feelings of guilt, of being a burden on others, worthlessness.
Loss of interest or pleasure.
Poor concentration.
Suicidal thoughts or plans.
Delusional thoughts.

tribute to depression (see Table 40–4); replace thyroid hormone for head and neck cancer clients with thyroid damage from irradiation; replace electrolytes to manage deficiencies related to treatment; medicate with antipsychotics (e.g., haloperidol, thiothixene, loxapine) for agitation related to delirium; initiate antidepressant medications if not contraindicated by medical status and if client is amenable to treatment. *(Note: Avoid tricyclic antidepressants in chronic suicidal clients because of the risk of cardiotoxicity in overdose.)*

Procedures: Neurologic workup (e.g., CT scan of head, lumbar puncture) may be indicated.

Other: Psychotherapy or supportive individual counseling to improve self-esteem, develop problem-solving skills, and reduce depression by counteracting cognitive distortions; social skills training or family counseling to enhance social support; electroconvulsive therapy for severe cases of major depression (contraindicated with increased intracranial pressure or with cerebral pathology such as space-occupying lesions).

ASSESSMENT CRITERIA: SUICIDAL IDEATION

The word "suicide" generally has a negative connotation and may be confusing to someone who does not have command of the English language. Using euphemisms such as "hurting yourself" or "ending it all" when assessing suicidality may be more acceptable and better understood.

Criteria	Risk Factors for Suicide	High Lethal Risk Factors for Suicide
History	Previous suicide attempts, previous psychiatric history (particularly disorders of mood), history of significant other's attempting or completing suicide, chemical dependence, recent significant loss (real or perceived).	Previous lethal suicide attempts (particularly if more than two previous attempts), previous admission(s) for suicidal ideation or attempts (lethal or nonlethal).
Hallmark physical signs and symptoms	Mood lifting following depressive period, giving away prized possessions, death-focused discussion, suicidal plan identified, available means to inflict self-injury.	Expresses wish to die and intent to commit suicide; asks questions about lethality of medications, etc.; discusses specific plan that is particularly lethal and has the means to harm self.

(continued)

ASSESSMENT CRITERIA: SUICIDAL IDEATION (continued)

Additional physical signs and symptoms	Depressive symptomatology, including weight changes (usually decreased), poorly controlled physical and/or emotional pain, sleep pattern disturbances (e.g., disturbances more frequent than usual, early-morning awakening, trouble falling asleep), somatic complaints.	Presence of psychosis with delusional thinking and command hallucinations.
Psychosocial signs	Ambivalence about living or dying, anhedonia, flat affect, guilt, helplessness, hopelessness, lack of eye contact, low self-esteem, social isolation.	Low frustration tolerance, thoughts highly focused on suicide or death, feelings of worthlessness.

Lab values

Possible biologic factors include:

CSF (cerebrospinal fluid) serotonin metabolite 5-hydroxyindoleacetic acid (5-HIAA)	Possibly decreased.
CSF norepinephrine metabolite-methoxy-4-hydroxyphenylglycol (MHPG)	Possibly increased.
Platelet monoamine oxidase (MAO)	Possibly low.
Platelet serotonin	Possibly low.
Platelet serotonin-2 receptor responsivity	Possibly high.

Possible other abnormal laboratory findings	Blunted plasma thyroid-stimulating hormone (TSH) response to infusion of thyrotropin-releasing hormone (TRH), altered urinary catecholamine ratios; nonsuppression of plasma cortisol after administration of dexamethasone.
Diagnostic tests	Depressive screening tools such as the Beck Depression Inventory (Beck, 1979), Hamilton Depression Rating Scale (Massie, 1992), or Hospital Anxiety and Depression Scale (Razavi, Delvaux, Farvacques, and Robaye, 1990) may be used as these are sensitive to clients with medical illness.

NURSING DIAGNOSIS

The first nursing diagnosis noted below is proper to suicidal behavior. Subsequent nursing diagnoses may be initiated as appropriate to client needs.

Risk for violence, self-directed, related to anxiety, fear, pain, dysfunctional grieving, identified risk of suicide, altered mental status.

Ineffective individual coping related to feelings of powerlessness, hopelessness.

Self-esteem disturbance related to feeling unworthy, lack of self-value, withdrawal.

Altered health maintenance related to depression, lethargy, lack of interest (anhedonia).

(Potential for) altered family process related to coping with client and/or family distress.

Self-care deficit, bathing/hygiene, feeding, dressing/grooming, related to inability to make decisions, feelings of helplessness and hopelessness associated with depression.

Knowledge deficit related to symptoms of depressive and suicidal behavior, pain management, responses to loss, treatment plan, need for support system, adaptive coping strategies to manage depression and/or illness.

NURSING INTERVENTIONS

Immediate nursing interventions

Interventions are designed to accomplish four tasks: (1) establish rapport with the client, (2) reduce distress by treating symptoms such as pain, depression, sexual concerns, etc., (3) identify level of suicide risk, and (4) protect the client from self-harm.

When a client begins to express despair, hopelessness, or death wishes, the first task is to listen to feelings, express concern, and establish a therapeutic relationship with the client. By listening, the healthcare professional gives "permission" to the client to further discuss issues and evaluate options. In the therapeutic relationship with the client, the healthcare professional can monitor periods of distress when quality of life is diminished and can anticipate periods of increased despair. Proactive interventions to reduce symptom distress can provide hope to the client and the family. Figure 40–1 presents an algorithm for managing suicidal clients in inpatient settings.

Suicidal Ideation

Respond nonjudgmentally to learn more about what the client is feeling.
Avoid discouraging further disclosure by using false assurances, encouraging treatment without listening to the client's concerns, or only

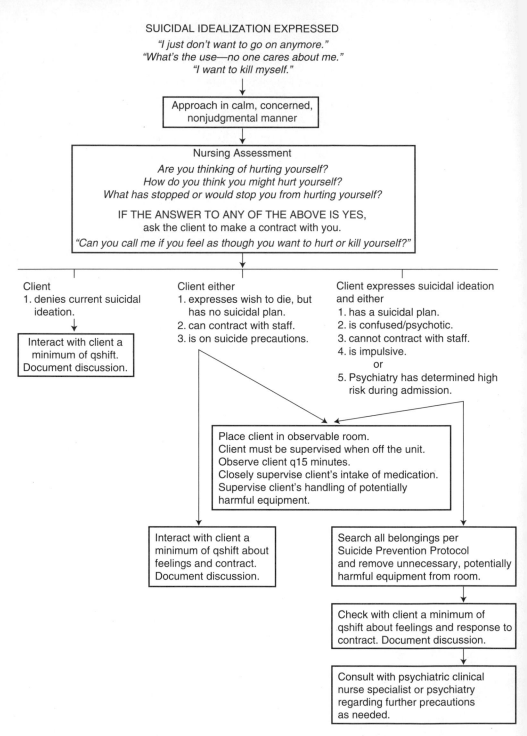

Figure 40–1 Algorithm for management of suicidal ideation in the hospitalized client with cancer.

focusing on positive aspects of the client's situation without hearing his or her distress signals.

Assess for and treat symptom distress (e.g., pain, nausea, fear).

Assess for suicidal ideation and behavioral control, according to the following criteria, by posing questions such as these suggested.

1. Presence of ideation of taking one's life.
   "What would you do if it got worse? Have you ever thought about hurting yourself?"
2. The client's perceived ability to control suicidal thoughts.
   "How likely are you to act on your thoughts?"
3. Possible methods of self-harm and/or a specific plan.
   "Do you have a plan? What specifically would you do to hurt yourself? Do you have the means?"
4. The client's perceived reasons that prevent acting on suicidal thoughts.
   "What has stopped or would stop you from hurting yourself?"
5. The client's ability to establish *no-harm contract* with staff. If the client is an outpatient, assess his or her ability to agree to call an appropriate resource if he or she is unable to control thoughts.
   "Can you call [identified resource] if you feel as if you would act on your thoughts?"
6. The client's ability to make goals for discharge and for the future.

Provide supportive interventions, reassurance, and emotional support frequently.

Provide further *suicide precautions,* based on the client's response (see Fig. 40–1):

a. Place the client in a highly observable room.

b. Restrict client to a specific area (supervised off-unit activity only).

c. Visually observe the client q15min noting level of activity; impulsive or potentially dangerous behavior; threats of harm to self, others, or property; safety of the environment.

d. Supervise and verify the client's intake of all medications (liquid medication may be used to ensure it is swallowed).

e. Supervise handling of potentially harmful equipment. In high-risk situations: search all personal belongings for sharp items and contraband; remove unnecessary harmful equipment from the room (e.g., plastic bags, phone cord, identification band with metal clasp, nursing call bell) while ensuring a communication system is in place if a nurse is needed.

Provide support to family who may be aware of the client's distress.

Consult with mental health colleagues regarding interdisciplinary intervention.

Consult with ethics committee for decision-making support as appropriate; document suicide risk assessment and interventions.

Suicidal Gesture or Attempt

In cases when the client attempts suicide in a care setting, in addition to all of the above implement the following:

Immediately remove client from the situation to a safe location.

Administer life support as needed.

Supervise the client's handling of potentially harmful items that cannot be removed (e.g., electric cord on necessary equipment).

Assign a sitter to continuously observe client within one arm's length at all times until he or she is further evaluated by psychiatry.

Medicate the client as prescribed to reduce the agitation or anxiety.

Impose restraints, if needed, to maintain client safety.

Notify the family/significant others regarding any change in the client's condition.

Document suicidal behavior, interventions, and outcome.

Anticipated physician orders and interventions

Psychiatric consultation for diagnostic evaluation and recommendations.

Suicide precautions.

Restraints (document duration, type of restraint, and rationale).

Document client behavior, interventions to promote safety, and client response.

Toxicology screen if behavior has immediate onset.

Medication to reduce agitation of delirium (e.g., haloperidol, thiothixene, lorazepam).

Medication to cautiously reduce anxiety (e.g., lorazepam, alprazolam), if needed.

Symptom management:

- Decrease/discontinue medications that may contribute to depression, disorientation, or further symptomatology (refer to Tables 40–2 and 40–4).
- Administer antidepressant medication (titrate to therapeutic effect and continue minimum of 4 months to prevent relapse).
- Adjust analgesic dosage to optimize pain relief.

Ongoing nursing assessment, monitoring, and interventions

Assess:

- Presence of suicidal ideation and ability to contract q8h and PRN.
- Level of social support.
- Presence of depression, cognitive impairment, symptom distress, and pain.

- Accuracy of the client's understanding of facts related to his or her condition.
- The client's consideration of alternative options and consequences of actions.

Implement:
- Suicide precautions appropriate to the client's behavior and verbalizations or as prescribed.
- Interventions for pain relief (see Chapter 33) and symptom control.
- Provision of information about condition, alternatives, and support; consideration of other reality-based and hope-inspiring strategies.

TEACHING/EDUCATION

Understanding cancer and its treatment: *Rationale:* Knowing about your cancer and how it can be treated may help you and your family make good choices for your health and future.

Ways to treat symptoms of your condition and treatment to provide hope: *Rationale:* Pain and other side effects of treatment can make you feel more depressed. Sometimes, as with any medical illness, you may have to try a few treatments before finding the best one. It is important not to become hopeless if the first treatment does not work. Call your doctor or nurse right away if you feel worse.

What depression feels like, how long it lasts, and ways to treat it: *Rationale:* Depression is not just "feeling blue," "down in the dumps," or feeling sad after a loss. Depression is an illness like high blood pressure or diabetes ("sugar") that day after day affects the way you eat, sleep, and think about yourself and the way you think about things. It can change how you "hear" what others tell you and can keep you from feeling hope. Depression is *not* a weakness; it is *not* your fault. It is an illness that can be helped with treatment. Treatment most often includes counseling and medication. As with other illnesses, the longer you have the depression before you get help, the harder it can be to treat. Most people who are treated for depression feel better and do what they used to in a few weeks. Chances are that treatment for depression will help you.

Warning signs of worsening mood and suicide: *Rationale:* Thoughts of death, of suicide, or wanting to end it all are often a part of depression. If you (your family member) has these thoughts, tell someone you trust now. Ask them to help you find professional help right away. Other signs of worsening mood include loss of interest in things you used to enjoy, including sex; feeling sad, blue, or down in the dumps; feeling slowed down or restless (unable to sit still); feeling unworthy or guilty; changes in appetite or weight loss or gain; problems with paying attention, thinking, remembering, or making choices; trouble sleeping or sleeping too much; loss of energy or feeling tired all the time; aches and pains; feeling hopeless or as if nothing will get better; feeling nervous or worried.

Suicide prevention resources: *Rationale:* The following are ideas of places and persons you can call for help if you should feel like hurting yourself at home. If you can't get hold of someone right away, try another place.

> A 24-hour community prevention hotline, your local health department, community mental health center, hospital, or clinic. They can help you or tell you where else you can go for help.
> Your family physician or other healthcare provider.

If your loved one talks strangely about hurting himself or herself or someone else or acts in a harmful way, either take your loved one to the emergency room or notify the police.

EVALUATION/DESIRED OUTCOMES

1. The client identifies no intent to act on suicidal ideation within the shift *or* will call for assistance if unable to control intensity of suicidal thoughts (ability to establish no-harm contract).
2. The client recognizes, expresses, and accepts own feelings of sadness, fear, and/or hopelessness as depression subsides.
3. The client identifies alternative self-care coping strategies in managing feelings and symptoms related to cancer and treatment throughout treatment period.
4. The client clearly understands the disease and treatment choices in order to make decisions based on facts as depression subsides or mental status clears.
5. The client identifies ways to manage symptoms at home and when to seek further intervention.
6. The client and family identify signs and symptoms of depression and warning signs of suicide.
7. The client and family identify resources that would be helpful should suicidal ideation or risk behavior occur.
8. The family identifies individual feelings and support available in response to verbalizations from the client about his or her personal distress.

DISCHARGE PLANNING

The suicidal client may need:

Follow-up appointment with outpatient psychiatric/mental health center for management of depression and suicidality.
Contact names and telephone numbers of resources for symptom control and crisis support.

Weapons safeguarded or removed from home if the original or recent suicide plan involved use of weapons.

Medications managed on a contracted basis in clinic (e.g., daily visit to obtain opiates) if suicidal plan involves overdosing.

Ongoing support for needs, including affirmation of healthy responses to stress, self-esteem, and control over one's life.

FOLLOW-UP CARE

Anticipated care

Physician office visit within the week for symptom management and discussion of further treatment options; other blood studies as appropriate to assess abnormalities.

Hospice/home health nursing visit once or twice a week for terminally ill clients.

Anticipated client/family questions and possible answers

I can't understand why someone would want to hurt themselves!

"Suicide is usually caused by many things that have added up over time. There are usually many reasons someone tries to take his or her life. Dealing with cancer and not being able to do things as before can make it harder to think a healthy future lies ahead. The effect of stress on the brain might also cause someone to feel like hurting himself or herself. After they have tried to fix things, some people get to a point where it seems too hard to go on living. They don't know where to turn for help or how to get away from the pain of living. Hurting themselves may seem like the only thing they *can* do. Most likely they don't think about how this will affect their family or others in their lives."

What can I do to help my loved one so they won't hurt themselves?

"It is normal to think about dying once in a while. If your loved one talks about wanting to hurt himself or herself, there is reason to ask for help. *Do not ignore remarks about suicide.* The most important thing anyone can do for their loved one who is depressed is to help him (or her) get help from someone specially trained to handle this problem. If your loved one is acting harmfully or talks about hurting himself (or herself), you need to consult with your doctor or take your loved one to the hospital for treatment. They may need to be hospitalized until they feel better, or get a different treatment if they are not feeling better. You might also help by checking whether or not your loved one is taking the medication correctly. Talk with the mental health specialist about ways to make your home more safe."

I didn't know he (or she) was going to do this. I feel terrible that I missed something!

"Sometimes, persons who want to hurt themselves do not tell someone they love. They may act the way they usually do. Others may give signs or talk about their feelings a lot. It is not uncommon for families to be surprised. Remember, you did not cause your loved one to hurt himself (or herself). No one can make another person commit suicide. No person can always stop another person from committing suicide either."

What do I do now that he (or she) tried to hurt himself (herself), or killed himself (herself)?
"When suicide has touched your life, your feelings about the event can be powerful. You may feel anger, guilt, love, confusion, self-blame, and self-pity. Suicide can cause chaos for those who knew the person. Everyone who cares about this person is hurt in some way. Children can be deeply hurt. I would suggest talking with someone you trust who can give you (your family) support through this difficult time. There are support groups for persons who love someone who has hurt himself or herself. It may help to know that many survivors, when they are ready, get through their grief and feel better."

CHAPTER SUMMARY

Suicide occurs at a significantly higher rate in clients with cancer, particularly those who have risk factors associated with this lethal choice. Because suicide has its origins in a biopsychosocial realm, risk factors must be assessed on several levels. Skill is needed to recognize the need for additional assessment of suicide risk in clients who present with risk factors or behaviors indicating a change in mood or outlook. Several simple questions will elicit information from the client that may provide relief for the client as well as an approach for maintaining safety on the part of inpatient and outpatient caregivers. In the case of treatable disease, all efforts must be aimed at identifying the causes of suicidal ideation, if possible, and working with the client to reduce those that can be managed. Ensuring that clients with terminal illness have all the facts related to their disease and treatment options provides them with choices. In addressing the emergency that is suicide with the client and family, nurses fulfill their duty to protect and preserve life, avoid doing harm, and create a relationship of trust and loyalty with their clients.

TEST QUESTIONS

1. Which of the following is *not* a risk factor for suicide?
   A. Expressed wishes of being dead
   B. Race/ethnicity
   C. Giving away prized possessions
   D. Expressed worries and fears

1. Answer: D
Worries and fears alone do not correlate with suicide. A client who is unable to problem-solve, has poor experience with crises, and has a low frustration tolerance is at risk.

2. Which of the following is the first nursing intervention for a client who expresses thoughts about hurting himself or herself?
   A. Offer options for symptom management.
   B. Implement suicide precautions.
   C. Assess intensity and immediacy of action.
   D. Enhance social support.

2. Answer: C
It is important not to "discount" suicidal expression by attempting to ameliorate possible risk factors before a full assessment is done. Asking a client about suicide does not result in suicide. Questioning the client's feelings of despair may open the discussion further and provide some relief for the client.

3. The primary nursing diagnosis for clients with active suicidal ideation is:
   A. Self-esteem disturbance
   B. Risk for violence: self-directed
   C. Altered family processes
   D. Sleep pattern disturbance

3. Answer: B
Although all the diagnoses noted under Nursing Diagnosis may be applicable to depression (a primary risk factor for suicide), the first priority when a client is actively suicidal is to protect him or her from harm.

4. Which chemotherapeutic drug may cause depressive side effects?
   A. Cisplatin
   B. Etoposide
   C. Methotrexate
   D. Taxol

4. Answer: A
Refer to Table 40–4.

5. An oncology client asks you about the lethality of taking more levorphanol than is prescribed for pain management at home. What would be the most appropriate response from the nurse?
   A. "Are you expecting to have more pain at home?"
   B. "We're only giving you a limited supply, so don't use it all at once."
   C. "What do you think your children will think of you if you take all those pills?"
   D. "Have you had thoughts of wanting to die?"

5. Answer: D
Two issues emerge from the scenario: the client appears concerned about pain, and there is a link drawn to the possibility of death. Further assessment before drawing a conclusion is indicated. A nurse may question the client about his or her pain further to clarify the issue. It would then be appropriate to question the client's ability to cope with the disease and its treatment.

6. Which attitude is appropriate on the part of the nursing staff?
   A. Suicide is an understandable choice for clients with cancer.
   B. Depression is an expected reaction for a client with cancer.
   C. Clients with cancer are more at risk for suicidal deaths than the general population.
   D. A client's lack of follow-through with treatment is evidence of noncompliance.

6. Answer: C
Attitudes affect the approach nurses have with clients. Clients with cancer are at higher risk for suicide owing to their chronic illness and its side effects. Although depression and suicide may be understandable in a client with terminal illness, it is important to assist the client in distinguishing correctable problems from those that cannot be relieved.

7. Which of the following criteria may indicate major depression for a client with cancer?
   A. Poor appetite and weight loss
   B. Loss of interest/pleasure in usual activities
   C. Feeling like a failure and worthless
   D. Loss of energy, fatigue

7. Answer: C
Clients with cancer often present with symptoms that can also be associated with depression, such as poor appetite, insomnia, weight loss, fatigue, and lack of concentration. One symptom that is definitely indicative of depression is self-reproach. Others include suicidal ideation, feeling punished, and feeling inappropriate or excessive guilt.

8. Mrs. X is admitted confused to the oncology unit following her last treatment for breast cancer. The report from the emergency room indicates that she was found by her son in her car in the garage. The car was running, and the garage door was closed. She did not expect his visit that day. He remarked that she had made vague statements about death the previous week. This is an example of:
   A. Suicidal ideation
   B. Suicidal gesture
   C. Suicide attempt
   D. Depression

8. Answer: C
This is an example of a suicide attempt. Mrs. X expressed some thoughts about death that may or may not have indicated a wish to control the process, but she did use lethal means and was clearly not expecting rescue. We are also led to believe that her disease was terminal, a factor increasing her risk of suicide. Assessment of her risk factors during her treatment for cancer might have prevented this suicide attempt.

9. In planning for the discharge of a newly diagnosed colon cancer client who has demonstrated suicidal behavior, the nurse should consider all of the following *except:*
   A. Hospice care
   B. Family involvement in a plan to remove weapons, etc., which the client may use to harm self
   C. Follow-up with mental health specialist
   D. Discussion of suicide hotline resources for immediate access

9. Answer: A
The suicidal client may need monitoring for signs of worsening mood or acting on harmful impulses. Ways to accomplish this include setting up a follow-up schedule, removing potential weapons, and considering medications that would best treat the underlying psychiatric disorder without posing a risk for harm. Hospice care is inappropriate for a newly diagnosed suicidal client.

10. What medication is inappropriate to give an agitated client with delirium who is threatening to harm himself or herself?
    A. Haloperidol
    B. Thiothixene
    C. Lorazepam
    D. Morphine

10. Answer: D
Agitated behavior that accompanies delirium best responds to treatment with antipsychotic agents or benzodiazepines. Haloperidol 5 mg intramuscularly every 30 minutes to 1 hour for one to four doses and thiothixene can be used for rapid control of behavior. Morphine can contribute to delirium.

REFERENCES

Allebeck P, Bolund C: Suicides and suicide attempts in cancer patients. Psychol Med 21:979–984, 1991.

American Nurses Association: Code for nurses with interpretive statements. Washington, DC: Author, 1985.

American Nurses Association: Position statement on assisted suicide. Washington, DC: Author, 1994.

American Psychiatric Association: Diagnostic and Statistical Manual of Mental Disorders, 4th ed. Washington, DC: Author, 1994.

Barile L: The client who is suicidal. *In* Lego S (ed): The American Handbook of Psychiatric Nursing. Philadelphia: JB Lippincott, 1984, p. 399.

Beck A: Cognitive therapy and emotional disorders. New York: New American Library, 1979.

Breitbart WS: Suicide. *In* Holland JC, Rowland J (eds): Handbook of Psychooncology. New York: Oxford University Press, 1990, pp. 291–300.

Breitbart WS: Cancer pain and suicide. *In* Foley KM, Bonica JJ, Ventafridda V (eds): Advances in Pain Research and Therapy. New York: Raven Press, 1990.

Engelhardt HT: Suicide in the cancer patient. Cancer 37(2):105–109, 1986.

Fincannon JL: Analysis of psychiatric referrals and interventions in an oncology population. Oncol Nurs Forum 22(1):87–92, 1995.

Fox BH, Stanek III EJ, Boyd SC, Flannery JT: Suicide rates among cancer patients in Connecticut. J Chronic Dis 35:89–100, 1982.

Hatton CL, Valente SM: Suicide, 2nd ed. New York: Appleton Century Crofts, 1984, pp. 34–148.

Hietanen P, Lonnqvist J: Cancer and suicide. Ann Oncol 2:19–23, 1991.

Ibbotson T, Maguire P, Selby P, Priestman T, Wallace L: Screening for anxiety and depression in cancer patients: The effects of disease and treatment. Eur J Cancer 30A(1):37–40, 1994.

Jenike MA: Depressed in the E.R. Emerg Med 16:102–120, 1984.

Kurtz ME, Kurtz JC, Given CW, Given B: Relationship of caregiver reactions and depression to cancer patients' symptoms, functional states and depression—a longitudinal view. Social Sci Med 40(6):837–846, 1995.

Louhivuori KA, Hakama M: Risk of suicide among cancer patients. Am J Epidemiol 109:59–65, 1979.

Massie MJ: Depression. In Holland JC, Rowland JH (eds): Handbook of Psychooncology. Oxford: Oxford University Press, 1992, pp. 283–290.

McLaughlin C: Suicidal behavior. Br J Nurs 2(22):1103–1105, 1993.

Perrone J: Adolescents with cancer: Are they at risk for suicide? Pediatr Nurs 19(1):22–25, 32–33, 1993.

Razavi D, Delvaux N, Farvacques C, Robaye E: Screening for adjustment disorders and major depressive disorders in cancer in-patients. Br J Psychiatry 156:79–83, 1990.

Roy A: Suicide. In Kaplan HI, Sadock BJ (eds): Comprehensive Textbook of Psychiatry/V: vol. 2, 5th ed. Baltimore: Williams and Wilkins, 1989, pp. 1414–1427.

Saunders JM, Valente SM: Cancer and suicide. Oncol Nurs Forum 15(5):575–581, 1988.

Smith MJ, Mouawad R, Vuillemin E, Benhammouda A, Soubrane C, Khayat D: Psychological side effects induced by interleukin-2/Alpha interferon treatment. Psycho-Oncol 3:289–298, 1994.

Spiegel D, Sands S, Koopman C: Pain and depression in patients with cancer. Cancer 74:2570–2578, 1994.

Valente SM: Evaluating suicide risk in the medically ill patient. Nurse Pract 18(9):41–50, 1993.

Valente SM, Saunders JM, Cohen MZ: Evaluating depression among patients with cancer. Cancer Pract 2(1):65–71, 1994.

Valente SM, Saunders JM, Grant M: Oncology nurses' knowledge and misconceptions about suicide. Cancer Pract 2(3):209–216, 1994.

Wise MG, Rundell JR: Concise guide to consultation psychiatry, 2nd ed. Washington, DC: American Psychiatric Press, 1994, p. 59.

CHAPTER 41

SUPERIOR VENA CAVA SYNDROME

Molly Loney, RN, MSN, OCN

CHAPTER OBJECTIVES

At the completion of this chapter, the reader will be able to:

Define superior vena cava syndrome (SVCS).

Differentiate between acute-onset and insidious-onset SVCS.

Identify the risk factors associated with SVCS in the pediatric and in the adult client with cancer.

Describe priority nursing interventions for managing the cancer client with SVCS for future care needs.

OVERVIEW

SVCS is an obstruction of the blood flow returning to the heart from the head, neck, upper thorax, and upper extremities. Because the vena cava is located in the confines of the mediastinum, any compression or obstruction can lead to venous congestion, reduced cardiac output, edema of surrounding structures, and hypoxia (Morse, Heery, and Flynn, 1985). The syndrome is a frequent initial presentation or complication of cancer. It has been estimated that 80 to 85% of all adult cases are due to cancer, with lung cancer causing 75% and lymphoma causing 10 to 15% of the malignant cases. Only 15% of adults with SVCS experience benign causes, such as thrombosis (Sculier and Feld, 1985).

DESCRIPTION

Anatomy

The superior vena cava (SVC) is a thin-walled blood vessel that carries venous drainage from the head, neck, upper extremities, and upper thorax to the heart. It is located in the right anterior mediastinum behind the sternum and is surrounded by lymph nodes that provide drainage from the right thoracic cavity and lower part of the left thorax. The SVC is in close proximity to other vital structures in the mediastinum, such as the vertebrae, trachea, esophagus, right bronchus, aorta, and pulmonary artery. The distal 2 cm of the vessel is within the pericardial sac. Because the SVC has a low pressure (less than 5 mmHg) and is confined within the mediastinum, it can be easily compressed by any adjacent fluid accumulation, disease process, or thrombosis (Abner, 1993).

Mechanisms of SVCS

Four mechanisms can cause compression that results in SVCS: (1) occlusion by an extrinsic mass; (2) occlusion by a mass invading the vessel wall; (3) occlusion by a thrombus around a central venous catheter; and (4) occlusion by a thrombus within the SVC (Miaskowski, 1991). Any compression of the SVC decreases venous return and increases venous congestion. Venous pressure rises, leading to third-spacing of fluid into adjacent tissue. Fluid accumulation only adds to the vena caval compression and may cause compression of other vital structures in the mediastinum, as well as pleural or pericardial effusion. Edema in the face, neck, upper thorax, and upper extremities is common. If the obstruction of venous blood flow is severe, cardiac filling and cardiac output decrease, with the risk of decreased cerebral perfusion and hypoxia. These sequelae are often accompanied by laryngeal and cerebral edema, which further place the client at risk for acute respiratory, cardiovascular, and neurologic distress.

The onset of SVCS can occur acutely or insidiously, with symptoms so subtle that the client and family have difficulty describing specific complaints. If the onset is gradual, collateral circulation has time to develop and compensate for the SVC's obstructed blood flow. The azygos vein is the only major vessel entering the SVC, carrying blood return from the posterior upper torso. It can play a critical role in providing for alternate routes for venous return with SVC obstruction. If the obstruction is located along the azygos vein, collateral circulation pathways can develop, and a pattern of large dilated veins will be visible on the client's upper chest. If the obstruction is located below the azygos vein, development of collateral circulation is unpredictable and more complex. At this point, venous pressure is higher, and the blood flow is circuitous through the inferior vena cava and its branches in the femoral and iliac veins. Turbulence of blood flow can impede collateral circulation and prevent compensation for the SVC compression (Morse et al., 1985).

In children, SVC obstruction is often accompanied by tracheal compression and acute respiratory distress. The trachea and right mainstem bronchus are less rigid than in adults, placing these structures at high risk for compression. Also, the intraluminal diameter of a child's trachea is small. Any tracheal edema can cause airway obstruction and a potentially fatal medical emergency (Lange, D'Angio, Ross, O'Neill, and Packer, 1993).

Whether acute or insidious in onset, SVCS can present as a frightening progression of symptoms that can be life-threatening if not recognized and treated.

RISK PROFILE

All the risk factors are greater when occurring in an elderly client with pre-existing coronary artery disease, hypertension, or heart failure.

Cancers: Lung (most commonly right-sided small cell or squamous cell tumors), lymphoma (most commonly non-Hodgkins' disease with right-sided perihilar lymph node involvement), thyoma, germ cell, and Kaposi's sarcoma.

Pediatrics: Lymphoma (more commonly non-Hodgkins' than Hodgkins' disease), neuroblastoma, and germ cell.

Conditions: Mediastinal metastases from the breast, esophagus, or testes or from colorectal cancers; thyroid goiter, tubercle bacillus mediastinitis, syphilitic aneurysm, mediastinal fibrosis (most commonly from histoplasmosis), sarcoidosis, and thrombosis. Thrombosis arises most commonly from central venous catheter or pacemaker lead placement; may also occur in clients with LeVeen shunt or a pulmonary artery catheter, or in those experiencing infection, volume depletion, liver disease, venous stasis, or leukocytosis.

Pediatrics: Cardiovascular surgery for congenital heart disease, placement of ventroatrial shunt for hydrocephalus, and thrombosis (most commonly from central venous catheter placement).

Environment: Previous radiation therapy to the mediastinum with mediastinal fibrosis (rare).

Food: None.

Drugs: None.

PROGNOSIS

Although SVCS can be accompanied by distressing symptoms, it rarely presents itself as a critical emergency. Death from the obstruction alone has not been described in the medical literature. Mortality comes from concurrent disease such as cancer in the mediastinum, which causes laryngeal edema, cerebral edema and hypoxia, and tracheal obstruction.

The prognosis depends on how rapidly obstruction develops, the degree of vena caval blockage, and the adequacy of collateral circulation. If venous return can be maintained to prevent hypoxia and ventricular strain, tissue damage and heart failure can be prevented even with acute onset. With the development of alternate circulation pathways, some causes of SVCS have resolved in time without treatment (Yahalom, 1993).

The overall prognosis also depends on the histologic diagnosis and prognosis of the underlying disease or causative mechanism. Benign causes can easily be treated and have a favorable prognosis. Malignant causes represent initial signs of an aggressive cancer, its recurrence, or metastatic spread. Median survival is 6 to 9 months following treatment of SVCS in clients with cancer, and only 1 to 2% of these clients live longer than 1 year (Robinson and Jackson, 1994).

> **Pediatrics:** Ninety percent of the cases of SVCS in children are iatrogenic and carry a favorable prognosis. With treatment, malignant causes of obstruction can result in long-term, disease-free survival (Yellin et al., 1992).

TREATMENT

The goals of treatment are first directed at preventing life-threatening symptom progression when the onset of SVCS is sudden and symptoms are severe. Priority is given to maintaining the airway and cardiac output, while stabilizing the client's hemodynamic status.

If the client is free of respiratory or cardiovascular distress, treatment focuses on symptom relief as well as on correcting the syndrome's underlying cause (Adelstein and Lichtin, 1995). In order to target specific causes of the SVC obstruction, treatment should be preceded by a thorough diagnostic workup, with histologic assays of suspected sites of malignancy.

Surgery

Thyroidectomy if goiter is retrosternal.

Aortic aneurysm resection or repair.

Percutaneous transluminal angioplasty with insertion of an expandable wire stent or balloon for vena caval stenosis that is resistant to noninvasive treatment.

Removal of central venous catheter if syndrome is caused by thrombosis that fails to resolve with anticoagulant or thrombolytic therapy.

Bypass grafting (using autologous graft from the saphenous vein or dacron prosthesis) of the SVC when the syndrome has a benign cause and persists for 6 months or more following conventional treatment (Doty, Doty, and Jones, 1990).

Chemotherapy: The treatment of choice for the syndrome when caused by small cell undifferentiated lung cancer, lymphoma, or disseminated cancer. Initial treatment for large mediastinal tumor (to shrink the mass, allowing for follow-up radiation therapy to a smaller field) (Morse et al., 1985). Combinations may be used, depending on the histology of the underlying cancer, i.e., cytoxan, methotrexate, and nitrogen mustard (Chernecky and Ramsey, 1984); cytoxan with oncovin, doxorubicin, methotrexate, and/or etoposide; cisplatin, procarbazine, and lomustin; or cisplatin and etoposide (Miaskowski, 1991).

> **Pediatrics:** Usual combination of cytoxan, oncovin, an anthracycline and steroids for lymphoma (Lange et al., 1993).

Radiation

First-line treatment for acute-onset syndrome with respiratory distress and when vital structures are compressed or invaded (i.e., trachea, esophagus, vocal cords, and pericardium).

Indicated when syndrome is caused by non-small cell lung cancer.

The total dose depends on tumor histology, radiologic sensitivity, symptom relief, tumor size, and client condition. The usual recommendation for adults is two to four high-dose fractions of 300 to 400 cGy, followed by conventional fractions of 150 to 200 cGy over 3 to 6 weeks (with total radiation dose reaching 3000 to 5000 cGy) (Yahalom, 1993). Subjective relief can be seen within 72 hours after treatment begins, and objective relief within 7 days (Ahmann, 1984).

Medications

Diuretics may be used to reduce edema associated with SVCS. *Caution:* Diuretics may further reduce venous return and cause dehydration and thrombosis.

Steroids to reduce edema associated with a large mediastinal tumor, risk of cerebral edema, or radiation therapy side effects (indicated if SVCS symptoms progress shortly after radiation therapy is started).

Bronchodilators, vasopressors, and antidysrythmics to stabilize the client during acute respiratory or cardiovascular distress.

Avoid central nervous system (CNS) depressants.

IV heparin drip to prevent or resolve thrombosis. The recommended starting dose is 150 to 300 U/kg/hour with titration as indicated to maintain the client's partial thromboplastin time (PTT) to $1\frac{1}{2}$ to 2 times the control value.

Heparin may also be instilled directly into the clotted catheter. *Caution:* Heparin may increase the risk of cerebral hemorrhage in clients with a high venous pressure.

Pediatrics: Systemic heparinization includes a bolus dose of 100 U/kg IV push followed by an IV drip at 25 U/kg/hour with titration according to the child's PTT.

Urokinase for identified thrombosis that fails to respond to heparin alone. The usual dose is 5000 IU instilled into an occluded central venous catheter. After 30 minutes, the residual is aspirated. If the occlusion continues, the process is repeated (Yahalom, 1993).

Prednisone 10 mg/m² orally four times per day to prevent or treat postirradiation tracheal edema (Lange et al., 1993).

Ketoconazole may be used to prevent SVCS recurrence when caused by histoplasmosis. *Caution:* Ketoconazole may increase the potency of corticosteroids.

Antianxiety medications, like Valium or Ativan, may be used to reduce respiratory strain from the client's anxiety-related hyperventilation.

Procedures: Not indicated.

Other: Supportive care with bedrest, elevation of head of bed, fluid and salt restrictions, and oxygen therapy.

ASSESSMENT CRITERIA: SUPERIOR VENA CAVA SYNDROME

The severity and range of symptoms in SVCS depend on how rapidly the obstruction develops, the obstruction's location and extension into mediastinal structures, and the availability of collateral circulation (Dietz and Flaherty, 1993). Hallmark symptoms include dyspnea, cough, facial edema and erythema, vein distention in the neck and thorax, and upper extremity edema (Morse et al., 1985).

Symptoms can arise suddenly in acute form or insidiously. Because the course of SVC obstruction is so variable, identifying a baseline assessment for each client is vital in monitoring for progression of the syndrome. Early recognition can prevent symptom progression to life-threatening airway obstruction, congestive heart failure, and cerebral hypoxia.

	Acute Onset	**Insidious Onset**	**Symptoms of Progression**
Vital signs			
Temperature	Elevated*	Baseline	Slightly elevated
Pulse	Tachycardic and bounding	Normal	Tachycardic and weak*
Respirations	Tachypneic*	Normal to tachypneic	Tachypneic*

* Symptoms common in children with SVCS.

	Acute Onset	Insidious Onset	Symptoms of Progression
Blood pressure	Increased initially, then hypotensive* and orthostatic	Normal, higher in arms than legs	Hypotensive*
CVP	Elevated	Slightly elevated	Elevated and climbing (above 12 mmHg)

History

	Acute Onset	Insidious Onset	Symptoms of Progression
Respiratory	Sudden and severe dyspnea,* shortness of breath, and stridor*	Dyspnea on exertion (DOE),* mild SOB, and dry cough	Progressive DOE*, SOB, and cough*
Cardiovascular	—	Epistaxis	—
Skin	Complaints of neck, facial edema and arm fullness, C/O ear fullness	C/O Stoke's sign (tight collar) or rings feeling tight	Progressive C/O of facial edema and arm swelling
Neurologic	C/O mood changes, headache,* lethargy,* and visual changes*	—	Progressive mood changes, Horner's syndrome (ptosis unilaterally with constricted pupil and anhidrosis from pressure on cervical sympathetic nerve)
Nutrition	Dysphagia	Weight gain in 1–2 weeks	Progressive dysphagia
Miscellaneous	Chest pain*	Pain at site of goiter or thrombosis, hoarseness*	Chest* or flank* pain (from pleural effusion), vocal cord paralysis

Hallmark physical signs and symptoms	Cyanosis,* sudden face and neck edema	Dilated superficial veins on thorax (on abdomen and groin if obstruction is azygous vein), erythema of face, neck, thorax	Cyanosis,* progressive edema of upper body.

Other physical signs and symptoms

	Acute Onset	Insidious Onset	Symptoms of Progression
Respiratory	Laryngospasm and sternal retractions on inspiration	Nail-bed cyanosis	Labored breathing (can lead to acute respiratory distress)
Cardiovascular	Gross neck and thorax vein distention	Veins in the hands do not collapse when raised over the head, hard to find vein for veni-puncture, frequent IV infiltration on the right side	Progressive neck and thorax vein distention (can lead to congestive heart failure)

(continued)

ASSESSMENT CRITERIA: SUPERIOR VENA CAVA SYNDROME *(continued)*

	Acute Onset	Insidious Onset	Symptoms of Progression
Skin (upper body)	Erythema of face and neck	Client "looks better," with fewer visible age lines and wrinkles, absence of pedal edema. Presence of early-morning periorbital, conjunctival and facial edema.	_____
Neurologic system	Changes in orientation* and level of consciousness (LOC)	_____	Progressive changes in LOC (can lead to stupor and coma)
Nutrition	_____	_____	Progressive weight gain
Psychosocial	Anxiety,* premonition of doom	Apprehension*	Apprehension*, irritability
Other	_____	Enlarged, nontender, and firm lymph nodes*	Enlarged, nontender, and firm lymph nodes*

Laboratory tests	None.
Diagnostic procedures	See Table 41–1.

* Symptoms common in children with SVCS.

NURSING DIAGNOSIS

The nursing diagnosis will vary, depending on the cause(s), speed of onset, and location of SVC obstruction. Common nursing diagnoses include:

(Potential for) ineffective breathing pattern related to airway obstruction secondary to laryngeal and/or tracheal edema.

(Potential for) decreased cardiac output related to ventricular strain secondary to decreased venous return to hypoxia.

(Potential for) decreased cerebral perfusion related to decreased venous return and cerebral edema.

(Potential for) fluid volume excess related to decreased SVC return and venous congestion in the upper thorax.

(Potential for) altered tissue perfusion related to thrombosis formation secondary to sluggish venous circulation.

(Potential for) altered skin integrity related to upper body venous congestion secondary to SVC obstruction.

(Potential for) altered communication related to vocal cord paralysis secondary to laryngeal edema.

Table 41–1
Diagnostic Tests for Superior Vena Cava Syndrome

Diagnostic Test	Risk	Findings
Chest x-ray	None	Mediastinal widening, right hilar mass, lymphadenopathy, pleural effusion, cardiomegaly.
Chest computerized tomography (CT)	Iodinated contrast can cause thrombosis	Mediastinal widening and mass with anatomical detail, tracheal compression, lymphadenopathy.
Magnetic resonance imaging (MRI)	None	Multidimensional image of vena cava and source of obstruction.
Venography	Iodinated contrast can cause thrombosis	Source of obstruction, pattern of collateral circulation.
Radionuclide scan of vena cava or angiography	Minimal with nonthrombogenic contrast	Source of obstruction, inferior vena cava involvement, pattern of collateral circulation.
Sputum cytology	None	Histologic diagnosis of cancer as SVCS cause.
Bronchoscopy	Bronchospasm and laryngeal	Histologic diagnosis of cancer as SVCS cause (if sputum is negative).
Biopsy (lymph node, bone marrow)	Minimal local bleeding	Histologic diagnosis of cancer as SVCS cause (if bronchoscopy is negative).
Ultrasound-guided transthoracic needle aspiration biopsy	Minimal with local bleeding	Histologic diagnosis of cancer, pattern of collateral circulation in and around mass (to minimize penetration during procedure).
Mediastinoscopy or thoractomy	High with anesthetic and bleeding complications	Histologic diagnosis of cancer when noninvasive tests are negative.

Source: Data from Abner, 1993; Belcher, 1992; Perez et al., 1978.

(Potential for) anxiety related to respiratory distress secondary to laryngeal and/or tracheal edema.

(Potential for) altered body image related to physical signs of venous congestion in head, neck, and upper thorax secondary to SVC obstruction.

Knowledge deficit related to unfamiliarity with sequelae, cause, and treatment of SVCS.

NURSING INTERVENTIONS

Immediate nursing interventions

Assess pulse, respirations, blood pressure, and central venous pressure (CVP) q15min until stable or acute respiratory and cardiovascular distress resolve.

Establish and maintain patent airway by elevating head of bed to a 45- to 90-degree angle at all times.

Monitor q15min for progressive symptoms leading to airway obstruction, increased intracranial pressure, and/or ventricular strain, until acute distress resolves.

Maintain blood flow by minimizing further constriction. Take blood pressure in lower extremities. Keep legs flat or below heart level.

Place suction equipment and oral airway at bedside.

Instruct the client to avoid any activity that may increase intrathoracic and intracranial pressure (i.e., bending, sneezing, or straining).

Measure intake and output (I and O) q2h.

Offer calm and simple explanations of treatment and supportive care being implemented to decrease symptoms.

Anticipated physician orders and interventions

Oxygen for cyanosis and respiratory distress.

Arterial blood gases (ABGs) to monitor for hypoxia, carbon dioxide retention, and respiratory acidosis.

STAT chest x-ray or computed tomography (CT) scan of the chest.

Complete blood count (CBC), platelets, prothrombin (PT), and PTT if thrombosis is suspected.

Thyroid function studies if goiter is present.

ECG if in acute cardiovascular distress.

Antidysrythmic medication administered for ECG changes.

Venous access to keep open IV (femoral vein or central venous catheter is preferable).

Administration of steroids.

Administration of diuretics, with fluid restriction and low-sodium diet.

Heparin by continuous IV infusion or urokinase IV push if thrombosis risk or occlusion is present.

Ketoconazole administration if client has histoplasmosis.

Radiation therapy initiated if cause of acute distress is suspected malignancy.

Ongoing nursing assessment, monitoring, and interventions

Assess:
- For progressive symptoms q4h and PRN:
  1. Respiratory pattern for airway obstruction (increased respirations with stridor, hyperventilation, increased rales/rhonchi, severe dyspnea).
  2. Tissue perfusion for hypoxia and bleeding (cyanosis, decreased peripheral pulses, hypotension, cool skin, occult bleeding from orifices/IV site).
  3. Mental status for increased intracranial pressure (severe

headache, visual changes, confusion, disorientation, lethargy to stupor or coma).
- For response to:
  1. Steroids (mood swings, weak involuntary muscles, glycosuria, insomnia).
  2. Diuretics (dehydration, hypovolemic shock, or thrombosis).
  3. Anticoagulant or thrombolytic therapy (bleeding or thrombosis).
  4. IV fluids (further venous congestion, ventricular strain, or infiltration at IV site).
  5. Radiation therapy (laryngospasm and stridor from laryngeal edema).
- For signs of compression to adjacent vital structures (larynx, trachea, lungs from pleural effusion, heart from pericardial effusion).
- For dysphagia, nausea, vomiting, or decreased gag reflex.
- For vocal cord paralysis.

Measure:
- Blood pressure, pulse, and respirations q1h × 4, then q4h if stable.
- I and O q2h × 24 hours, then q4h.
- Weight qd.
- CVP q4h × 24 hours if central venous catheter present.

Send:
- Repeat CBC, platelets, PT, and PTT q8h when the client is on anticoagulant or thrombolytic therapy.
- Repeat ABGs if on oxygen.
- Sputum for cytology.

Implement:
- Supportive care.
- Space activities of daily living (ADL) with frequent rest periods.
- Assist with ADL as needed.
- Avoid use of CNS depressants.
- Minimize/avoid added trauma to upper body (use pillows to support edematous arms, blood samples from pedal vein).
- Administer mild analgesic or sedative PRN as ordered.
- Offer small, frequent meals or liquids, with antiemetics PRN, as ordered.
- Assist in finding alternate methods of communicating if vocal cord paralysis is present.
- Encourage the client and family to express concerns and fears.
- Minimize noise and stress in client's room.
- Administer chemotherapy as ordered (avoid upper extremity IV site).

TEACHING/EDUCATION

Select items to include in client and family teaching, based on the client's pathophysiology.

Elevating the head: *Rationale:* Keeping your head up all the time will keep the backed-up blood in your upper body from making you uncomfortable and will make breathing easier.

Minimizing further venous constriction: *Rationale:* To keep your blood in your upper body from slowing down, it's important to prevent any pressure from tight clothes, rings, or blood pressure cuffs. Keeping your legs flat will keep you from getting as swollen in your head, neck, and arms.

Safety precautions: *Rationale:* Because we are watching very closely how you are breathing right now, we want to keep emergency equipment handy just in case you need help getting rid of the phlegm in your throat or help in breathing.

Antipressure activities: *Rationale:* It is very important to make sure you don't cough or sneeze, bend over, or strain when trying to have a bowel movement. Any of these simple activities can increase the pressure in your chest and head, making you more uncomfortable. Let us know if you feel as though you need to cough or sneeze, so that we can talk with your doctor. He or she may order some medicine to relieve those feelings.

Oxygen and ABGs: *Rationale:* Keeping this mask on will help you breathe a lot easier and will give you extra oxygen while we help decrease your neck swelling. The blood samples tell us if you're getting enough oxygen.

Symptoms of SVCS: *Rationale:* You and your family will need to watch for any signs of swelling in your face, neck, chest, and arms. Sometimes breathing gets harder with the swelling and you feel winded or like you can't quite catch your breath. You might have a cough, cloudy thinking, headache, blurred vision, and feel irritable or nervous for no reason. If you notice any of these signs, call your doctor right away so he or she can start treatment to help you feel better.

Diagnostic tests: *Rationale:* Your doctor needs to find out exactly what is making you have so much swelling and trouble breathing. Having an x-ray or scan of your upper body will help to find out whether anything is pressing on your superior vena cava and blocking the blood flow.

Dietary and fluid restrictions: *Rationale:* To keep the swelling from getting worse, you'll need to limit how much you drink and how much salt is in your diet for a few days.

Anticoagulant and thrombolytic therapy: *Rationale:* The medicine you're taking will keep your blood from clotting and blocking your circulation. Sometimes the medicine can cause side effects. Call your doctor if you feel dizzy or notice bleeding (in your phlegm, urine, bowel movement, or having menses) or bruising. It's important to be extra careful to keep from falling or bumping yourself.

Radiation therapy: *Rationale:* Your doctor has decided that the best way to decrease your swelling is to give you concentrated x-ray beams to shrink the disease that is pressing on your superior vena cava. Information should include frequency, what to expect from radiation therapy mapping and daily therapy, and possible side effects. Usually radiation therapy helps you feel a lot better in 2 or 3 days.

Surgical treatment: *Rationale:* In order to help you feel better and decrease the swelling in your upper body, a surgeon will be talking to you about having a procedure done in the operating room:

1. *Thyroidectomy.* By carefully removing your swollen thyroid gland, the pressure will be taken off your superior vena cava. Your blood can circulate normally again.
2. *Biopsy.* In order to take a sample of your lung/lymph nodes to study under the microscope, a biopsy of your main bronchus/mediastinum (over your middle chest bone) needs to be done. This will involve a specially trained doctor giving you a numbing medicine and inserting a tube in your airway/needle into your chest/ lymph nodes to get a specimen. The specimen can be studied to learn what kind of disease is causing your symptoms.
3. *Angioplasty.* In order to open up your blocked superior vena cava, the doctor will place a small tube/balloon into the blood vessel. This will let your blood go through the space that is blocked and decrease your symptoms.
4. *Graft.* In order to help your blood circulate around the place where it is blocked, a small piece of a dacron tube will be attached to your superior vena cava. Once it's stitched in place, it will work as part of your vena cava to keep blood going through your body. Your swelling and other symptoms should disappear.

Chemotherapy administration: *Rationale:* Your doctor has decided that the best way to decrease your swelling is to give you strong medicine that will shrink the mass that's pressing on your superior vena cava, and causing its blood flow to backup. Information should include administration expectations, possible side effects, frequency, and ways to minimize side effects. Usually chemotherapy can help you feel less swelling in 3 to 7 days.

Supportive care: *Rationale:* With the swelling in your face and upper body, it's normal to feel nervous and wonder if the symptoms will go away. Sometimes it helps to talk with someone about your concerns. If talking would help you, we have a member of our health team who is available.

EVALUATION/DESIRED OUTCOMES

1. CVP within normal limits (less than 5 mmHg).
2. Absence of airway obstruction, ventricular strain, and increased intracranial pressure.

3. Pulse, respirations, and blood pressure return to baseline within 3 to 7 days.
4. Subjective symptom relief within 72 hours, with decreased physical findings of SVC obstruction in 7 days.
5. Lungs are clear to auscultation within 72 hours.
6. Central venous catheter and SVC are free of additional thrombi after starting anticoagulant or thrombolytic therapy.
7. Dysphagia, nausea, and vomiting subside within 72 hours.
8. Absence of bleeding from high venous pressure or anticoagulant/thrombolytic therapy.
9. Treatment plans, supportive care, and follow-up needs are acknowledged by the client and family prior to discharge.
10. The client and family verbalize concerns regarding SVCS and its underlying cause(s) prior to discharge.

DISCHARGE PLANNING

The client with superior vena cava syndrome may need:

Short-term anticoagulant therapy and symptom management education.
Weekly home nursing visits for monitoring treatment side effects and medication compliance.
Oxygen therapy at home for advanced malignancy causing SVCS that doesn't respond to treatment.
Hospice follow-up for terminal phase of malignancy causing SVCS.

FOLLOW-UP CARE

Anticipated care

Office visit within 1 week of discharge.
Outpatient lab testing of CBC, platelets, PT, and PTT within 1 week of discharge.
Scheduled radiation therapy or chemotherapy as indicated by diagnostic workup.
Home health nursing visit once per week × 2 to 4 weeks for clients discharged on anticoagulant therapy.

Anticipated client/family questions and possible answers

Will this problem with obstruction of my superior vena cava happen again?
"It is possible that the disease causing the obstruction will return. It is very important for you to know the early signs of the obstruction and what to do if they occur."

"The surgery you had in the hospital will prevent the superior vena cava from becoming blocked again. The stent tubing/balloon/graft will let your blood flow freely."

"The radiation therapy/chemotherapy you are receiving will, it is hoped, shrink the mass that blocked your blood flow. Your doctor will order periodic x-rays or scans to check on your progress, besides asking you how you're feeling."

Why will a nurse be coming to my home?

"The nurse will visit to see how you are feeling and if the symptoms are continuing to disappear. She will also check on how you are tolerating your treatment and medications."

What should I do if the symptoms come back again?

"If you notice any of the symptoms of your superior vena cava being obstructed again, call your doctor right away. The sooner treatment can be started, the better you will feel and the less serious your obstruction will be."

CHAPTER SUMMARY

SVCS is an obstructive complication of lung cancer, lymphoma, and benign causes such as central venous catheter thrombosis. Its progression to airway obstruction, increased intracranial pressure, and congestive heart failure makes it a frightening and potentially fatal emergency. Although its onset can be sudden and acute, most cases develop gradually. Because initial symptoms can be subtle, close monitoring of clients at risk for the syndrome is needed. Early detection and treatment can prevent an acute emergency, as well as maintain the client's physical, mental, and psychosocial well-being.

TEST QUESTIONS

1. SVCS is primarily a disorder involving:
   A. Venous congestion
   B. Hypovolemia
   C. Pulmonary edema
   D. Atrial-ventricular node failure

1. Answer: A
SVCS results from blockage and congestion of venous blood flow returning to the heart from the upper body.

2. Mechanisms that can cause compression in SVCS include:
   A. Congestive heart failure
   B. Extrinsic or invasive mass
   C. Hepatomegaly
   D. Cerebral edema

2. Answer: B
Causative mechanisms include extrinsic or invasive mass; occlusion by a thrombosis, either in a central venous catheter or surrounding it; or thrombosis in the superior vena cava.

3. The client with SVCS has difficulty compensating with acute-onset symptoms because:
   A. Anxiety increases hypoxia
   B. Venous pressure is low
   C. Cardiac output increases
   D. Collateral circulation hasn't developed

3. Answer: D
Acute-onset SVCS has severe symptoms because collateral circulation hasn't had time to develop, as in insidious-onset SVCS.

4. Children with SVCS have a high risk for accompanying:
   A. Pleural effusion
   B. Congestive heart failure
   C. Tracheal compression
   D. Aspiration pneumonia

4. Answer: C
Children have vulnerable trachea, which can be easily compressed by the same disease process causing the SVCS. Children's tracheas are less rigid, with a smaller intraluminal diameter than adults.

5. Risk factors for developing SVCS include:
   A. Kaposi's sarcoma, sickle cell disease, and recent myocardial infarction
   B. Radiation mediastinitis, lymphoma, and central venous catheter placement
   C. Lower extremity thrombosis, pneumonitis, and malnutrition
   D. Coronary artery disease, hepatitis, and thyroid goiter

5. Answer: B
Risk factors for SVCS include Kaposi's sarcoma, radiation mediastinitis, lymphoma, central venous catheter placement, infection, elderly coronary artery disease, and thyroid goiter.

6. Common symptoms of SVCS in the adult and child include:
   A. Shortness of breath, dyspnea, and facial edema
   B. Tachypnea, dyspnea, and dry cough
   C. Horner's syndrome, anxiety, and neck vein distention
   D. Lymphadenopathy, plethora, and ear fullness

6. Answer: B
Common SVCS symptoms include dyspnea, facial edema, tachypnea, dry cough, anxiety, and lymphadenopathy.

7. The *primary* nursing diagnosis of clients with SVCS is:
   A. Fluid volume excess
   B. Decreased cerebral perfusion
   C. Altered skin integrity
   D. Ineffective breathing

7. Answer: A
Although each of these nursing diagnoses are involved, the primary diagnosis is fluid volume excess.

8. Priority nursing interventions for responding to acute-onset SVCS focus on:
   A. Maintaining venous return from lower extremities
   B. Maintaining patency of the airway
   C. Preventing dehydration
   D. Correcting electrolyte imbalance

8. Answer: B
Because of the high risk of airway obstruction and hypoxia from acute-onset SVCS, maintaining patency of the airway is the top nursing priority.

9. Important safety precautions to highlight in teaching the client with SVCS include:
   A. Elevating the head and feet
   B. Calling for assistance when getting out of bed
   C. Avoiding straining when trying to pass stool
   D. Refusing any invasive diagnostic tests

9. Answer: C
Safety precautions for preventing further complications from SVCS include elevating the head to maintain the airway and prevent venous congestion in the head and neck; keeping lower extremities flat; avoiding venous constrictions; and avoiding activities that might increase thoracic or intracranial pressure.

10. The overall prognosis of clients with SVCS depends on whether the:
    A. Cause is disease-related or iatrogenic
    B. The client is male or female
    C. Systemic circulation is adequate
    D. Diagnostic workup includes invasive tests

10. Answer: A
Overall prognosis of clients with SVCS is influenced by the underlying cause of the condition (worse if disease-related vs. iatrogenic), client's age, speed of onset, degree of obstruction of venous return, adequacy of collateral circulation around the superior vena cava, and ability to obtain a tissue sample with diagnostic tests.

REFERENCES

Abner A: Approach to the patient who presents with superior vena cava obstruction. Chest 103(Suppl 4):394S–397S, 1993.

Adelstein DJ, Lichtin AE: Oncologic toxicities and emergencies. *In* Sivak ED, Higgins TL, Seiver A (eds): The High Risk Patient: Management of the Critically Ill. Baltimore: Williams and Wilkins, 1995. pp. 866–869.

Ahmann FR: A reassessment of the clinical implications of the superior vena cava syndrome. J Clin Oncol 2(8):961–969, 1984.

Allegretta GJ, Weisman SJ, Altman AJ: Oncologic emergencies I: Metabolic and space-occupying consequences of cancer and cancer treatment. Pediatr Clin North Am 32(3):601–611, 1985.

Baker GL, Barnes HJ: Superior vena cava syndrome: Etiology, diagnosis, and treatment. Am J Crit Care 1(1):54–60, 1992.

Belcher AE: Cancer Nursing. St. Louis, MO: CV Mosby, 1992.

Chernecky CC, Krech RL, Berger BJ: Laboratory Tests and Diagnostic Procedures. Philadelphia: WB Saunders Co, 1993.

Chernecky CC, Ramsey R: Clinical Nursing Care of the Client with Cancer. Norwalk, CT: Appleton Century Crofts, 1984.

Christianson D: Caring for a patient who has an implanted venous port. Am J Nurs 94(11):40–44, 1994.

Davenport D, Ferree C, Blake D, Raben M: Radiation therapy in the treatment of superior vena caval obstruction. Cancer 42(6):2600–2603, 1978.

Dietz KA, Flaherty AM: Oncologic emergencies. *In* Groenwald SL, Frogge FL, Goodman M, Yarbro CH (eds): Cancer Nursing: Principles and Practice. Boston: Jones and Bartlett, 1993, pp. 651–653.

Doty DB, Doty JR, Jones KW: Bypass of superior vena cava: Fifteen years' experience with spiral vein graft for obstruction of superior vena cava caused by benign disease. J Thorac Cardiovasc Surg 99(5):889–895, 1990.

Escalante CP: Causes and management of superior vena cava syndrome. Oncology 7(6):61–68, 1993.

Francis CM, Phil D, Starkey IR, Errington ML, Gillespie IN: Venous stenting as treatment for pacemaker-induced superior vena cava syndrome. Am Heart J 129(4):836–837, 1995.

Jones LA: Superior vena cava syndrome: An oncologic complication. Semin Oncol Nurs 3(3):211–215, 1987.

Lange B, D'Angio G, Ross AJ III, O'Neill JA Jr, Packer RJ: Oncologic emergencies. *In* Pizzo PA, Poplack DG (eds): Principles and Practice of Pediatric Oncology. Philadelphia: JB Lippincott, 1993, pp. 951–972.

Miaskowski C: Oncologic emergencies. *In* Baird S, McCorkle R, Grant M (eds): Cancer Nursing. Philadelphia: WB Saunders Co, 1991, pp. 885–886.

Morse LK, Heery ML, Flynn KT: Early detection to avert the crisis of superior vena cava syndrome. Cancer Nurs 8(4):228–232, 1985.

Perez CA, Presant CA, Van Amburg AL III: Management of superior vena cava syndrome. Semin Oncol 5(2):123–134, 1978.

Robinson L, Jackson J: New approach to superior vena cava obstruction. Br Med J 308(6945):1697–1699, 1994.

Schweid L, Etheredge C, Werner-McCullough M: Will you recognize these oncological crises? RN 57(9):23–28, 1994.

Sculier JP, Feld R: Superior vena cava obstruction syndrome: Recommendations for management. Cancer Treat Rev 12(3):209–218, 1985.

Thelan LA, Davie JK, Urden LD, Lough ME: Critical Care Nursing: Diagnosis and Management. St. Louis, MO: CV Mosby, 1994.

Urban T, Lebeau B, Chastang C, Leclerc P, Botto MJ, Suavaget J: Superior vena cava syndrome in small-cell lung cancer. Arch Intern Med 153(3):384–387, 1993.

Yahalom J: Oncologic emergencies. *In* Devita VT Jr, Hellman S, Rosenberg SA (eds): Cancer: Principles and Practice of Oncology. Philadelphia: JB Lippincott, 1993, pp. 2111–2118.

Yellin A, Mandel M, Rechavi G, Neuman Y, Ramot B, Lieberman Y: Superior vena cava syndrome associated with lymphoma. Am J Dis Child 146(9):1060–1063, 1992.

CHAPTER 42

SYNDROME OF INAPPROPRIATE ANTIDIURETIC HORMONE SECRETION

Jan L. Hawthorne Maxson, MSN, RN, AOCN

CHAPTER OBJECTIVES

At the completion of this chapter, the reader will be able to:

Define the syndrome of inappropriate antidiuretic hormone secretion (SIADH).

Identify clients at risk for developing SIADH.

Describe nursing care as it relates to oncology clients with SIADH.

List interventions that involve clients and their families in the management of SIADH.

OVERVIEW

SIADH is a disorder characterized by the continued secretion and resulting elevated blood levels of antidiuretic hormone (ADH). Clients suffering from SIADH will exhibit signs and symptoms of fluid retention, an inability to excrete dilute urine, and dilutional hyponatremia. SIADH is a paraneoplastic disease, the most common underlying cause being a malignancy. Nurses caring for oncology clients who are at risk for or who have developed SIADH need to understand the pathophysiology involved, the clinical manifestation of the disorder, and the available treatment options.

DESCRIPTION

Normal physiology of ADH

To fully understand SIADH, one must have an understanding of how the body regulates water and the role of ADH (see Table 42–1).

The body is constantly regulating water by either conserving or excreting

Table 42–1
Feedback Mechanism Regulating the Release of Antidiuretic Hormone (ADH)

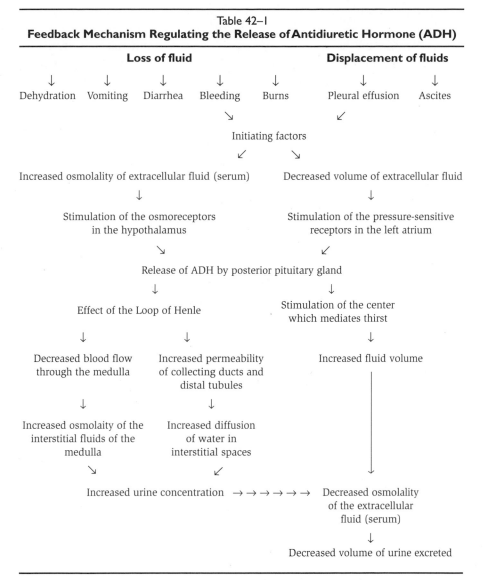

Source: From Yasko JM: Guidelines for Cancer Care: Symptom Management. Reston, VA: Reston Publishing, 1983.

it. Normally, ADH is released from the posterior pituitary gland in response to either increases in plasma osmolality or decreases in plasma volume. The release of ADH causes more water to be reabsorbed in the distal renal tubules and collecting ducts and leads to the production of urine in smaller amounts and in a more concentrated form. The resulting effect is plasma osmolality that is lowered by the dilutional effect of additional water to the plasma volume.

The mechanisms by which the brain regulates the secretion of ADH are twofold. A feedback loop of osmoreceptors in the hypothalamus and pressoreceptors in the left atrium and carotid sinus monitor plasma osmolality and plasma volume. When plasma osmolality increases or plasma volume decreases, these receptors send impulses to the hypothalamus and posterior pituitary to increase ADH secretion. When plasma osmolality decreases or the plasma volume increases, the reverse occurs, and ADH is inhibited, resulting in the urine volume becoming larger and more dilute. The overall result is that the plasma osmolality is held constant within a range of 286 to 294 mOsm/kg of water. Urine osmolality usually reflects that of the plasma.

Pathophysiology of SIADH

In SIADH, there is either an excess of ADH as a result of the ectopic production of the hormone, or the normal osmolar response to the osmoreceptors malfunctions. SIADH may also occur as a result of the direct effect on the renal system by external factors, such as chemotherapy or analgesics that mimic the action of ADH. The resulting pathophysiologic state is water intoxication, a state in which plasma water follows an osmotic gradient and moves intracellularly, resulting in intracellular edema. When excessive amounts of water are retained, plasma osmolality drops, and dilutional hyponatremia occurs. The normal homeostatic mechanisms to control ADH levels fail due to the ectopic production of ADH, and hyponatremia develops in the presence of urine that is not maximally dilute. If sodium-containing solutions are administered, the expansion of the intravascular space results in prompt natriuresis; the sodium is thereby lost, and the syndrome remains uncorrected. As urinary excretion of sodium increases, hyponatremia worsens, and urinary osmolality becomes inappropriately higher than plasma osmolality (see Table 42–2).

Multiple factors are known to stimulate ADH release. Besides changes in extracellular volume (i.e., hypovolemic states due to fluid or blood loss) and increased serum osmolality, stress is known to enhance ADH secretion. As a

Table 42–2
Laboratory Values in SIADH

	Value
Serum sodium	< 130 mEq/L (< 130 mmol/L SI Units)
Plasma osmolality	< 280 mOsm/kg
Urine osmolality	> 330 mOsm/kg
Urine sodium	> 20 mEq/L (> 20 mmol/L SI Units)

Source: Data from Dietz KA, Flaherty AM: Oncologic emergencies. *In* Groenwald SL, Frogge MH, Goodman M, Yarbro CH (eds): Cancer Nursing: Principles and Practice, 2nd ed. Boston: Jones and Bartlett, 1992, pp. 660–662.

portion of the body's stress response, mechanisms to conserve water are necessary in the event of hemorrhage or sweating. This phenomenon may explain why pain, surgery, and trauma also cause increased ADH secretion.

Various pharmacologic agents stimulate the release of ADH or potentiate the action of ADH on the renal tubules (see Table 42–3).

Table 42–3
Mechanisms Causing SIADH

Cause	Possible Mechanism
Pulmonary disorders	
Aspergillosis, tuberculosis, lung abscesses, viral pneumonia, or bacterial pneumonia.	Synthesis and secretion of ADH by benign pulmonary tissue.
CNS disorders and medical conditions	
Encephalitis, brain tumors, brain abscesses, cranial trauma (i.e., subarachnoid hemorrhage, skull fracture, cerebrovascular accident, subdural hematoma), and conditions as simple as experiencing pain or high stress levels.	Stimulation of the hypothalamic and posterior pituitary systems.
Malignancies	
Lung carcinomas (small cell or oat cell carcinoma), duodenal and pancreatic carcinoma, thymoma, Hodgkin's lymphoma, non-Hodgkin's lymphoma, and uterine carcinoma.	These neoplasms are capable of producing and secreting ADH identical to that made by the posterior pituitary. Malignant lung cancer cells also have the capacity to store and resecrete the hormone. Thoracic or mediastinal tumors can cause a rise in intrathoracic pressure, resulting in decreased venous return to the heart (decreased preload) and decreased cardiac output. The pressure receptors and the osmoreceptors are stimulated by these changes, and ADH is released, beginning the cycle of SIADH.
Drugs	
Narcotics, barbiturates, anesthetics, thiazide diuretics, and tricyclic antidepressants. Antineoplastic agents cyclophosphamide (Cytoxan) and vincristine (Oncovin).	Stimulation of ADH release.
Chlorpropamide (Diabinese), clofibrate (Atromid-S), and carbamazepine (Tegretol).	Stimulation of ADH release *or* potentiation of the action of ADH on the renal tubules.
Cisplatin	Unknown mechanism, possibly any of the above mechanisms.

Source: Adapted from Chernecky CC, Ramsey PW. Critical Nursing Care of the Client with Cancer. Norwalk, CT: Appleton-Century-Crofts, 1984.

There are three categories of disease-related causes of SIADH (see Table 42–3). These diseases or medical conditions include pulmonary disorders, central nervous system (CNS) disorders, and malignancies. Malignant tumors capable of the ectopic production of ADH are the most common cause of the syndrome. Lung carcinomas (small cell or oat cell carcinoma) account for the highest incidence of SIADH in clients with malignancies. In fact, SIADH is often the presenting symptom in clients with small cell lung cancer.

RISK PROFILE

Cancers: Lung (small cell or oat cell), duodenal, pancreatic, brain, esophagus, colon, ovary, laryngeal, leukemia (acute and chronic), mesothelioma, reticulum-cell sarcoma, prostate, bronchus, nasopharynx, thymoma, Hodgkin's lymphoma, non-Hodgkin's lymphoma, lymphosarcoma, and uterine.

Conditions: Aspergillosis, tuberculosis, lung abscesses, viral pneumonia, bacterial pneumonia, meningitis, encephalitis, brain tumors, brain abscesses, cranial trauma (i.e., subarachnoid hemorrhage, skull fractures, cerebrovascular accident, subdural hematoma), congestive heart failure, renal failure, liver disease with ascites, diabetic ketoacidosis, head injury, Addison's disease, hypothyroidism, pain, and stress.

Environment: None.

Foods: None.

Drugs: Vincristine, cisplatin, cyclophosphamide, thiazide diuretics, carbamazepine, oxytocin, acetaminophen, clofibrate, chlorpropamide, morphine, nicotine, ethanol, narcotics, barbiturates, general anesthesia, and tricyclic antidepressants.

PROGNOSIS

The overall prognosis for the client with SIADH depends on the underlying cause of the syndrome. SIADH usually will resolve as the primary condition regresses, but can persist despite control of the condition. SIADH may recur and suggest progression of the underlying disease, but recurrence is sometimes seen with stable disease during the maintenance phase of therapy. Neurologic impairment due to water intoxication is usually reversible and does not require long-term rehabilitation. Frequent assessment of the client and monitoring of the serum sodium level is needed in the initial period following SIADH.

TREATMENT

The management of SIADH depends on the severity of the hyponatremia, the client's clinical condition, and the underlying cause of the syndrome. When

SIADH is caused by a malignancy, it can only be controlled permanently by effective antitumor therapy. If tumor control cannot be reached, the client and his or her family must be taught how to manage chronic SIADH. Management of symptoms will increase the quality of life for the client. The client must be able to understand the rationale for and taught to report weight gain, weakness, lethargy, nausea, confusion, and possible drug side effects. The mainstay to control SIADH is to restrict fluids to 1 liter/day and to maintain the fluid restriction.

Surgery: Not indicated.

Chemotherapy: Primary treatment would be the appropriate combination chemotherapy regimen for the underlying oncologic condition causing SIADH. No other intervention will effectively suppress tumor production of ADH. Small cell lung cancer is often treated with vincristine, cyclophosphamide, and cisplatin, all agents which themselves have been associated with SIADH.

Radiation: Primary or adjuvant treatment for the underlying oncologic condition causing SIADH, as appropriate.

Medications

Any medications that can induce SIADH (see Table 42–3) must be withheld and substitutions made.

Medications used to treat SIADH assert their affects by blocking the action of ADH at the renal tubule. In the past, lithium carbonate was used. Currently, demeclocycline (a tetracycline derivative) has been used in doses of 800 mg to 1000 mg qd by mouth (Lowitz, 1985). It has been shown that lower doses than these appear to be ineffective. Many clients have been able to safely liberalize their fluid intake while taking this agent. Clients frequently develop azotemia or diabetes insipidus while taking demeclocycline. Both conditions are reversible when the drug is discontinued. Renal function should be carefully monitored while on this agent. If renal impairment exists, even the usual doses may lead to excessive systemic accumulation of the drug and possible liver toxicity.

Procedures: Not indicated.

Other

Clients who are comatose or present with serum sodium concentrations of less than 110 mEq/L require aggressive treatment with hypertonic saline (see Chapter 25).

Furosemide can be used to prevent fluid overload. Once the client's condition stabilizes, a fluid restriction of 1 liter/day and demeclocycline may be instituted.

ASSESSMENT CRITERIA: SYNDROME OF INAPPROPRIATE ANTIDIURETIC HORMONE SECRETION

The initial symptoms of SIADH are vague and easily attributed to the side effects of the treatment or the tumor itself. The severity of symptoms also depends on the serum sodium level and the length of time in which the syndrome develops. Clients who have developed SIADH over a long period of time may exhibit a lower severity of symptoms than those in whom the condition developed quickly. With this in mind, it is essential that the nurse identify and consistently assess those clients who may be at risk for developing SIADH. Common assessment data can be found in the table below.

	Serum Sodium <130 mEq/L <130 mmol/L SI Units	Serum Sodium <110 mEq/L < 110 mmol/L SI Units
Vital signs		
Temperature	At or below baseline	Same
Pulse	Rapid	Same
Respirations	Tachypneic, dyspnea on exertion (DOE)	Same
Blood pressure	Increased	Same
History	Be alert to clients with predisposing conditions—see Table 42–3.	
Hallmark physical signs and symptoms	Feeling tired, sleepy.	Weakness, lethargy, nausea and vomiting, anorexia.
Additional physical signs and symptoms	Normovolemia Edema is rarely seen.	Hypervolemia Weight gain, seizures, coma.
Psychosocial signs	Irritability, mental confusion.	Personality changes.
Lab values		
Osmolality, serum	Decreased <280 mOsm/Kg	Same
Osmolality, urine	Increased >330 mOsm/Kg	Increased >500 mOsm/Kg
Sodium, urine	Increased >20 mEq/L (>20 mmol/L SI Units)	Same
BUN, blood	Normal	Decreased
Creatinine, serum	Normal	Decreased
Potassium, serum	Normal	Decreased (probably dilutional)
Calcium, serum	Normal	Decreased (probably dilutional)

ASSESSMENT CRITERIA: SYNDROME OF INAPPROPRIATE ANTIDIURETIC HORMONE SECRETION *(continued)*

Diagnostic tests

Water-Load Test

Note: May only be used when serum sodium concentration >125 mEq/L and client is asymptomatic.	Comparison of the osmolality of timed urine and serum samples after administering a large quantity of water. <500 ml urine output 4 hours after water ingestion. Urine osmolality ≥180 mOsm/kg 5 hours after water ingestion. Urine osmolality >serum osmolality.	Test is contraindicated with serum sodium levels <125 mEq/L or <125 mmol/L SI Units.

Other	None

NURSING DIAGNOSIS

The nursing diagnosis will vary, depending on the cause(s) of SIADH. Some of the common diagnoses and etiologies are as follows.

(Potential for) altered cardiac output related to electrolyte imbalances and resulting dysrhythmias.

Acute confusion related to electrolyte imbalances, as evidenced by confusion, lethargy, coma.

Fluid volume excess related to serum hyponatremia and hypoosmolality of plasma, producing water intoxication.

Risk for injury related to electrolyte imbalances and resulting confusion and need for a protective environment.

Knowledge deficit related to unfamiliarity with sequelae and treatment of SIADH.

Effective management of therapeutic regimen for the treatment of SIADH.

NURSING INTERVENTIONS

Immediate nursing interventions

Assess pulse, respirations, blood pressure q4h × 48 hours.

Maintain an accurate measurement of intake and output (I and O). Calculate the I/O ratio for fluid balance q8h and q24h. Insert an indwelling urinary catheter, if necessary.

Initiate seizure precautions. Place suction equipment and an oral airway at the bedside.

Assess level of consciousness q4h, and record any changes in awareness, orientation, and/or behavior.

Auscultate breath sounds q8h.

Send STAT serum electrolyte panel.

Send STAT samples for urine osmolality and serum osmolality.

Obtain urine specific gravity q4–8h × 48 hours.

Obtain a baseline weight.

Establish IV access, and obtain volumetric infusion pump.

Assess skin color, temperature, and moisture.

Anticipated physician orders and interventions

Assess lab data when available, and compare them to baseline and normal values.

Assess results of water-load test. (*Note:* This test should not be performed unless client's serum sodium level is 125 mEq/L or more.)

Decrease/discontinue chemotherapy and other medications that may stimulate ADH release.

Maintain fluid restriction at 800 to 1000 ml fluid/24 hours.

Administer hypertonic saline (3% NaCl) with potassium chloride at a rate of 1 liter per every 6 to 8 hours to restore serum sodium.

Administer furosemide (initial dose of 40 to 80 mg IV) with additional doses administered as needed to produce hypotonic diuresis.

Demeclocycline (after condition stabilizes) as prescribed.

Ongoing nursing assessment, monitoring, and interventions

Assess:
- Those clients who are at risk for recurrence, because the initial symptoms are usually vague and attributed to other causes.
- Mental status and level of consciousness q4h and PRN.
- For anorexia, nausea, and vomiting, and medicate with antiemetics PRN as prescribed.
- For sudden weight gain.
- The I/O ratio for fluid balance q8h and q24h.
- For signs of fluid overload and congestive heart failure (CHF) q8h (rales, tachypnea, dyspnea, S_3, tachycardia, jugular vein distention [JVD], peripheral edema, bounding pulses).
- Breath sounds q8h, and record any changes.
- For clients undergoing the water-load test, observe for and report nausea, abdominal fullness, fatigue, desire to defecate, shortness of breath, chest pain.

Measure:
- Pulse, respirations, and blood pressure q4h.

- I and O q8h and q24h.
- Weight qd.

Send:
- Repeat urine electrolytes and urine osmolality in 24 hours and PRN.
- Repeat serum creatinine and BUN in 24 hours and PRN.
- Repeat serum electrolytes and serum osmolality in 24 hours and PRN.

Implement:
- Fluid restriction as prescribed.
- Seizure precautions.
- Water-load test, if serum sodium level exceeds 125 mEq/L and client is asymptomatic.

TEACHING/EDUCATION

Select items based on client's pathophysiology:

Discontinuation of chemotherapy: *Rationale:* Certain chemotherapy drugs may produce or aggravate SIADH. Some of your drugs may make it difficult for your body to rid itself of water. Your doctor may need to change the chemotherapy drugs you are receiving.

Blood and urine samples: *Rationale:* Blood and urine samples will be taken over the next few days. They are needed to measure the amount of salt and water in your body.

IV line placement: *Rationale:* The IV line allows us to easily take blood samples and to give you necessary treatments with fluids and medications.

Urinary catheter placement: *Rationale:* Accurate urine measurement is very important for people with low salt levels. The catheter allows us to collect all of your urine for exact measurements. We may also give you medicine that will make your kidneys produce more urine. The catheter prevents you from having to get up frequently to go to the bathroom.

Fluid restriction: *Rationale:* It is important to limit how much fluid you drink to keep the fluid from building up in your body while your kidneys aren't able to rid the body of extra fluid.

Signs and symptoms of hyponatremia: *Rationale:* You and your family need to be alert for the signs of a low salt level, because early treatment helps you to feel better and could prevent a medical emergency. Signs could include any of the following: feeling tired or weak, mental confusion, feeling sleepy, losing your appetite, nausea, vomiting, weight gain, seizures, coma.

EVALUATION/DESIRED OUTCOMES

Resolution of SIADH will be manifest by the following:

1. Serum and extracellular osmolality return to normal levels.
2. Serum sodium returns to normal levels.
3. Urine osmolality and specific gravity return to normal levels.
4. Serum potassium returns to normal levels.
5. Lungs are clear to auscultation, and the client is free of any respiratory difficulty.
6. Diuresis has been achieved.
7. The client is producing 30 to 50 ml of urine each hour.
8. Nausea, vomiting, and anorexia have subsided.
9. The client's mental status has returned to baseline.
10. The client can tolerate continuation of prescribed chemotherapy.
11. Fluid restriction requirements are understood by the client and caregiver prior to discharge.

DISCHARGE PLANNING

The client with SIADH may need:

Instruction on I and O measurement and documentation.
Instruction on the requirements for fluid restriction maintenance, if continued restrictions are necessary.
Instruction on the signs and symptoms of SIADH.
Guidelines for when it would be necessary to contact the physician for medical intervention.

FOLLOW-UP CARE

Anticipated care

Physician office visit within 1 week.
Outpatient lab testing for serum electrolytes within 1 week.
Other blood work as needed (serum osmolality, K^+, BUN/creatinine, etc.).
Continuation of fluid restrictions as needed.
Home care nursing visit once per week × 2 weeks for clients discharged to home needing continued short-term assessment.

Anticipated client/family questions and possible answers

Will this problem with low salt/sodium in my blood happen again?
"It is possible that this may happen again. That's why it is very important for you to know the signs of a low salt level and to know when to call your doctor or nurse, if you notice them."

Will I be able to continue my chemotherapy?

"You will be able to continue the therapy for the cancer once your lab values are back to normal and when your body can tolerate the effects of the chemotherapy drugs again."

Why will a nurse be coming to my home?

"A nurse will be coming to see if the low salt problems are happening again. The nurse will listen to your lungs, weigh you, check the fluid intake/output records you are keeping, check your legs for swelling, check your blood pressure, heart and breathing rate; ask you about any nausea, vomiting, or poor appetite; and talk with you to see how alert you are. All of these checks help the nurse determine if the problem with low salt in your blood is developing again."

Why do I have to limit my fluids?

"The low salt level in your blood is caused by your body's retaining too much fluid. As a result, the salt level in your blood becomes lower because the salt is diluted in too much fluid. By limiting the amount of fluids you drink, you begin to reduce the amount of fluid that can be retained in your body. So, if there is less fluid in your body, the salt level will not be as diluted and will return to a normal level, and your body will be back in balance again."

CHAPTER SUMMARY

SIADH is a paraneoplastic disease, the most common underlying cause being a malignancy. The primary clinical manifestations of the syndrome are caused by water intoxication. The severity of the symptoms depends on the degree of the abnormality of the serum sodium level, as well as on the rapidity with which the syndrome develops. The insidious onset of SIADH can delay early diagnosis, which makes it imperative that the nurse be aware of those clients at risk and their predisposing factors. Involving clients and their caregivers is crucial in the effective management of SIADH, since compliance with fluid restrictions, monitoring signs and symptoms, and reporting changes is necessary to reverse the syndrome. SIADH is an easily treated condition when the physician, nurse, client, and caregivers all cooperate with one another.

TEST QUESTIONS

1. Which chemotherapeutic agents may induce SIADH?
   A. Doxorubicin
   B. Mitomycin
   C. Taxol
   D. Vincristine

1. Answer: D
Vincristine and cyclophosphamide are known to stimulate the release of ADH from the posterior pituitary gland. Cisplatin has also been linked with SIADH.

2. Which type of cancer accounts for the highest incidence of SIADH in clients with malignancies?
   A. Acute lymphocytic leukemia
   B. Lung cancer (small cell or oat cell)
   C. Uterine cancer
   D. Non-Hodgkin's lymphoma

2. Answer: B
Many medical conditions are associated with SIADH, but malignant tumors capable of the ectopic production of ADH are the most common cause of the syndrome. Lung carcinomas (small cell or oat cell carcinomas) account for the highest incidence of SIADH in clients with malignancies.

3. When SIADH is developing, which of the following signs and symptoms occur?
   A. Weight loss, mouth sores
   B. Alopecia, anemia, hyperkalemia
   C. Mental confusion, weakness, nausea and vomiting
   D. Abdominal pain, diarrhea

3. Answer: C
The inappropriate secretion of ADH causes the client to retain fluid. The primary clinical manifestations of the syndrome are due to the resulting water intoxication from the retained fluid.

4. One cause of SIADH in clients who do not have cancer includes:
   A. Cranial trauma
   B. Cerebrovascular accident
   C. Septic shock
   D. Cardiomyopathy

4. Answer: A
Hyponatremia and SIADH are common features associated with cranial trauma. It is believed that the stimulation of the hypothalamic and posterior pituitary systems is the mechanism associated with CNS disorders and SIADH.

5. Appropriate treatment for SIADH includes:
   A. Restricting fluid intake to 1000 ml per day
   B. Utilizing effective stress-management techniques
   C. Treating bacterial pneumonia with the appropriate antibiotics
   D. All of the above

5. Answer: D
Stress, pain, and bacterial pneumonia can all be associated with the development of SIADH. The treatment of these primary disorders can either prevent or control SIADH. Limiting fluid intake reduces the amount of fluid that can be retained.

635 Chapter 42 • **Syndrome of Inappropriate Antidiuretic Hormone Secretion**

6. Which of the following is the primary treatment for SIADH?
   A. Radiation therapy
   B. Appropriate chemotherapy regimen for the underlying malignancy
   C. Restricting fluid intake to 1000 ml per day
   D. Increasing fluid intake while the client is receiving chemotherapy

6. Answer: B
Only the appropriate chemotherapy regimen for the underlying malignancy will effectively suppress tumor production of ADH.

7. What would be the primary nursing intervention for the nursing diagnosis of fluid volume excess in a client with SIADH?
   A. Measurement of I and O
   B. Assess level of consciousness
   C. Obtain weight three times a day (TID)
   D. 12-lead electrocardiogram now

7. Answer: A
Measurement of intake/output is of primary importance in monitoring for fluid retention. Weight should be obtained daily. Changes in mental status and level of consciousness are indications of hyponatremia.

8. What intervention would you expect the physician to prescribe for a client with SIADH?
   A. Administer hypertonic normal saline.
   B. Administer 1000 mg acetaminophen TID.
   C. Maintain fluid restriction equal to 4000 ml qd.
   D. Increase vincristine chemotherapy.

8. Answer: A
The administration of hypertonic saline raises the serum sodium level.

9. To obtain a water-load test, the client's serum sodium level must be _____ or more.
   A. 120 mEq/L (120 mmol/L)
   B. 125 mEq/L (125 mmol/L)
   C. 130 mEq/L (130 mmol/L)
   D. 135 mEq/L (135 mmol/L)

9. Answer: B
To perform a water-load test, the client must be asymptomatic and have a serum sodium that exceeds 125 mEq/L (125 mmol/L).

10. ADH is secreted from which part of the body?
    A. Posterior pituitary gland
    B. Adrenal glands
    C. Cerebral cortex
    D. Renal tubules

10. Answer: A
    ADH is secreted from the posterior pituitary gland in response to either increases in plasma osmolality or decreases in plasma volume.

REFERENCES

Batcheller J: Disorders of antidiuretic hormone secretion. AACN Clin Issues Crit Care Nurs 3(2):370–378, 1992.

Batcheller J: Syndrome of inappropriate antidiuretic hormone secretion. Crit Care Nurs Clin North Am 6(4):687–692, 1994.

Beitel-Wardrop J: Restoring the balance: Identification and management of syndrome of inappropriate antidiuretic hormone in critical care. CACCN 5(3):20–25, 1994.

Boh DM, Van Son A: The water load test. Am J Nurs 82(1):112–123, 1982.

Bryce J: SIADH: Recognizing and treating syndrome of inappropriate antidiuretic hormone secretion. Nursing 24(4):33, 1994.

Chernecky CC, Ramsey PW: Critical Nursing Care of the Client with Cancer. Norwalk, CT: Appleton Century Crofts, 1984.

Dietz KA, Flaherty AM: Oncologic emergencies. In Groenwald SL, Frogge MH, Goodman M, Yarbro CH (eds): Cancer Nursing: Principles and Practice, 2nd ed. Boston: Jones and Bartlett, 1992, pp. 660–662.

Escuro R, Adelstein D, Carter S: Syndrome of inappropriate secretion of antidiuretic hormone after infusional vincristine. Cleveland Clin J Med 59(6):643–644, 1992.

Fuhrman T, Runyan T, Reilley T: SIADH following minor surgery. Can J Anaesthesia 39(1):97–98, 1992.

Lindaman C: SIADH: Is your patient at risk? Nursing 22(6):60–63, 1992.

Lowitz BB: Paraneoplastic syndromes. In Haskell CM (ed): Cancer Treatment, 2nd ed. Philadelphia: WB Saunders Co, 1985, pp. 905–906.

Miaskowski C: Oncologic emergencies. In Baird SB, McCorkle R, Grant M (eds): Cancer Nursing: A Comprehensive Textbook. Philadelphia: WB Saunders Co, 1991, p. 880.

Mizobuchi M, Kunishige M, Kubo K, Komatsu M, Bando H, Saito S: Syndrome of inappropriate secretion of ADH (SIADH) due to small cell lung cancer with extremely high plasma vasopressin level. Int Med 33(8):501–504, 1994.

Moore JM: Metabolic Emergencies. In Johnson BL, Gross J (eds): Handbook of Oncology Nursing. New York: Wiley, 1985, pp. 476–482.

Otto C, Richter W: Syndrome of inappropriate antidiuretic hormone secretion induced by different drugs. Ann Pharmacother 28(10):1199–2000, 1994.

Rohaly-Davis J: Hematologic emergencies in the intensive care unit. Crit Care Nurs Q 18(4):35–43, 1995.

Wachsberg R, Kurtz A: Use of furosemide in patients with syndrome of inappropriate antidiuretic hormone secretion. Radiology 182(3):898, 1992.

Yasko JM: Guidelines for Cancer Care: Symptom Management. Reston, VA: Reston Publishing, 1983.

CHAPTER 43

TUMOR LYSIS SYNDROME

Jeanene (Gigi) Robison, MSN, RN, OCN

CHAPTER OBJECTIVES

At the completion of this chapter, the reader will be able to:

Describe the pathophysiology of tumor lysis syndrome (TLS).

State the risk factors associated with TLS in the oncology client.

Differentiate the manifestations of TLS that are related to hyperuricemia, hyperkalemia, hyperphosphatemia, or hypocalcemia.

Describe measures to prevent and manage the metabolic complications of TLS.

Anticipate and prepare the client with TLS for future care needs.

OVERVIEW

TLS is a potentially fatal metabolic condition that occurs in some clients with cancer. This syndrome most commonly occurs in clients who have a large tumor cell burden (i.e., leukemia, lymphoma, tumor with multiple metastases) that is rapidly proliferating and very sensitive to the cytotoxic effects of therapy. TLS has occurred much less often in clients with metastatic solid tumors and has rarely occurred spontaneously in clients newly diagnosed with cancer. It primarily results when a large volume of tumor cells are rapidly destroyed by cytotoxic therapy (i.e., chemotherapy, corticosteroids, biologic response modifiers, or radiation). The intracellular contents (potassium, uric acid, phosphorus, and nucleic acids) are released from the tumor cells when they are destroyed, and these contents are emptied systemically into the extracellular circulation (Tsokos, Balow, Spiegel, and Magrath, 1981). TLS usually manifests within the first 24 to 48 hours after the initiation of a specific cancer therapy and may persist for 5 to 7 days post-therapy (Cohen, Balow, Magrath, Poplack, and Ziegler, 1980). The large-volume cell kill is advantageous in the treatment of the disease. However, TLS may be a severe or fatal sequela of effective therapy. It can create life-threatening metabolic abnormalities, including hyperkalemia, hyperuricemia, hyperphosphatemia, hypocalcemia, and metabolic acidosis. Death may be the result of acute renal failure or cardiopulmonary arrest due to dysrhythmias (Malik, Abubakar, Alam, and Khan, 1994).

DESCRIPTION

TLS is characterized by the development of acute hyperuricemia, hyperkalemia, hyperphosphatemia, and hypocalcemia, with or without acute renal failure. These alterations may occur individually or in combination, and may occur despite prophylactic measures (Hande and Garrow, 1993; Malik et al., 1994). These metabolic abnormalities occur when the kidneys are unable to process and excrete the large amounts of intracellular products and metabolites that are released when tumor cells are destroyed. The adequacy of renal function and the amount of tumor burden affect the magnitude of these metabolic abnormalities. This section will describe the pathophysiologic process for each of these metabolic abnormalities.

Hyperuricemia

Several factors may contribute to hyperuricemia in the client with cancer. First, high growth fractions, bulkiness of tumor, and sensitivity to chemotherapy are tumor-related factors that increase uric acid production. Before the client begins chemotherapy treatments, the uric acid levels may be elevated. The client's body increases renal excretion to compensate for a moderate elevation of uric acid (Stucky, 1993). Second, the degree of elevation in the leukocyte count and the degree of spleen, liver, and lymph node enlargement are factors that affect both serum uric acid levels and uric acid excretion in the client with leukemia or lymphoma. Uric acid excretion is highest in clients with acute lymphoblastic leukemia, and it is increased in clients with acute nonlymphoblastic leukemia (Pocheldy, 1973). Third, uric acid metabolism is altered in clients with leukemia and lymphoma, due to an increased formation or destruction of white blood cells. Increased nucleic acid metabolism results, which causes an increased output of nucleoprotein and metabolites and increased uric acid formation (Stucky, 1993; Pocheldy, 1973). Finally, hyperuricemia may result from tumor cell destruction, primarily occurring after cytotoxic therapy, and also rarely occurring spontaneously (Sklarin and Markham, 1995; Jasek and Day, 1994). Since cancer cells undergo periods of rapid growth and development, they contain higher levels of nucleic acids than do normal cells. When the cancer cells are destroyed, the nucleic acids are converted into uric acid by the liver (Lawrence, 1994; Cunningham, 1982). Because of its relative insolubility, even very small increases in the serum uric acid may lead to precipitation of uric acid crystals in the highly concentrated and acidified urine of the distal tubules and collecting ducts in the kidneys and in the ureters. This may result in obstructed urine flow, decreased glomerular filtration rate, and increased hydrostatic pressure. Continued precipitation can result in a decreased capacity and number of nephrons to clear the urates. This may ultimately lead to acute renal failure (Drakos, Bar-Ziv, and Catane, 1994; Lawrence, 1994; Stucky, 1993; Tsokos et al., 1981).

Hyperkalemia

High serum potassium levels may be due to a number of factors. Hyperkalemia may result from the release of potassium from a massive volume of lysed tumor cells. This would have a significant impact on the body's intravascular and interstitial fluids, since the potassium content of intracellular fluids is 150 mEq/L and that of intravascular and interstitial fluids is only 5 mEq/L (Cassmeyer, 1983). In addition, the rapid lysis of tumor cells may cause uric acid nephropathy, and a concomitant decreased urinary excretion of potassium may result.

Hyperkalemia has neuromuscular, cardiac, and gastrointestinal (GI) effects. Potassium excess causes nerve and muscle irritability, since the cell membrane potential is decreased (partially depolarized) and the cell becomes more excitable. The client may complain of muscle twitching, muscle cramps, and paresthesias (such as tingling and burning). Hyperkalemia also increases GI peristaltic movement, which results in hyperactive bowel sounds and diarrhea. Even small changes in serum potassium can cause life-threatening changes, especially in cardiac muscles. When serum potassium levels are 7.5 to 8.0 mEq/L (7.5 to 8.0 mmol/L SI Units) or greater, cardiac electrical conduction is delayed. ECG changes can occur, including tall T waves, flat P waves, and wide QRS complexes. These ECG changes are due to slowed repolarization and delayed conduction of impulses, primarily at the atrioventricular node. Severe hyperkalemia soon leads to muscle weakness and flaccid paralysis, since an overstimulation of muscles produces an accumulation of lactic acid. The heart will eventually stop, as the cardiac cycle is halted in diastole (Drakos et al., 1994; Hawthorne, Schneider, and Workman, 1992; Soltis, 1983).

Hyperphosphatemia, hypocalcemia, and hypomagnesemia

High serum phosphorus levels also result when a large number of tumor cells are lysed. Hypocalcemia and renal failure are two clinical problems related to hyperphosphatemia. Hypocalcemia occurs due to the inverse relationship between dissolved calcium and phosphorus. In TLS, high levels of serum inorganic phosphate binds with free ionized calcium, calcium phosphate salts form, and the serum calcium level is lowered. When the calcium phosphate salts precipitate in the kidneys, renal insufficiency or failure occurs (Dietz and Flaherty, 1993; Methany, 1987).

Hypocalcemia has a significant effect on a person's body, since free ionized calcium is needed for nerve functions and for smooth, skeletal, and cardiac muscle function. When serum calcium levels are low, depolarization of the cell membranes occur, and the nervous system and muscle tissue is more excitable. The client may experience tetany, convulsions, diarrhea, dysrhythmias, or cardiac arrest (Dietz and Flaherty, 1993; Hawthorne et al., 1992).

Magnesium is closely interrelated with calcium metabolically. Low calcium levels increase magnesium absorption and decrease serum magnesium levels. Low serum magnesium levels lead to increased neuromuscular irritability. Hypomagnesemia may be occurring in a client with hypocalcemia who is unresponsive to the therapy administered to correct the low calcium levels. Hypomagnesemia needs to be treated with oral or parental magnesium in order to minimize the neuromuscular irritability related to hypocalcemia (Soltis, 1983).

Metabolic acidosis

Metabolic acidosis, which is characterized by the primary loss of HCO_3 from the extracellular fluid, may develop due to hyperuricemia, acute renal failure, or lactic acidosis (Malik et al, 1994). It is identified from arterial blood gas analysis when the pH is low and the HCO_3 and $PaCO_2$ levels are decreased (Guzzetta, 1981).

Complications of tumor lysis syndrome

Two major complications may cause mortality in clients with TLS. The first complication is acute renal failure, which may result from hyperuricemia and hyperphosphatemia. The second complication is cardiopulmonary arrest, which may result from hyperkalemia or hypocalcemia.

RISK PROFILE

All the risk factors below are greater when occurring in an elderly client.

Cancers

Hematopoietic tumors that are highly proliferative and sensitive to cytotoxic treatment: TLS most commonly occurs in clients with acute lymphoblastic leukemia, acute myelogenous leukemia, high-grade lymphomas (i.e., Burkitt's lymphoma), or non-Hodgkin's lymphoma.

Other hematopoietic tumors: TLS may also occur in clients with chronic myelogenous leukemia in blastic transformation, chronic lymphocytic leukemia, or prolymphocytic leukemia.

Large tumor burden: TLS may occur in clients with hematologic malignancies, Burkitt's lymphoma with extensive abdominal masses, extensive lymph node involvement, multiple metastases, or significant ascites secondary to cancer (Drakos et al., 1994). Elevated lactate dehydrogenase (LDH) levels may also indicate a large tumor burden (Haskell, 1985; Cohen et al., 1980).

Solid tumors: TLS occurs much less often in clients with solid tumors, and it occurs in clients with rapidly progressive disease, large tumor burdens, and liver metastasis. TLS has been reported in clients with small cell lung cancer, medulloblastoma, metastatic breast cancer, rapidly growing ovarian cancer, hepatoblastoma, metastatic melanoma, metastatic GI adenocarcinoma, soft tissue sarcoma, Merkel carcinoma, metastatic or locally advanced squamous cell carcinoma of the vulva, and seminoma.

Spontaneous occurrence in clients with cancer: Rarely, TLS has occurred in clients before cancer therapy has been initiated (Jasek and Day, 1994), and it has recurred spontaneously after cytotoxic treatment (Sklarin and Markham, 1995).

Pediatric tumors: TLS also occurs in pediatric clients with hematopoietic malignancies (acute lymphocytic leukemia, acute myelogenous leukemia, lymphomas), nonhematopoietic malignancies (i.e., stage IVS neuroblastoma, rhabdomyosarcoma), and large tumor burdens.

Conditions

Dehydration

Pretreatment metabolic disturbances: Clients are at higher risk when they have (1) elevated serum potassium levels due to compromised renal function, acidosis resulting from sepsis, dehydration, adrenal insufficiency as steroids are tapered, or certain medications (i.e., indomethacin, potassium supplements, and potassium-sparing diuretics); and/or (2) low calcium levels due to hypomagnesemia, acute pancreatitis, vitamin D deficiency, diarrhea, multiple blood transfusions, or anorexia (Drakos et al., 1994; Dietz and Flaherty, 1993).

Pretreatment renal insufficiency: Clients are at higher risk when their serum creatinine level is greater than 1.6 mg/dl. Oliguric clients are at a significantly higher risk of developing renal failure than nonoliguric clients (Hande and Garrow, 1993; Silverman and Distelhorst, 1989).

High white blood cell count, lymphadenopathy, splenomegaly, and elevated LDH (LDH greater than 1500 IU/L): Clients are at higher risk when these conditions exist in combination with large tumor burdens (Dietz and Flaherty, 1993; Hande and Garrow, 1993; Haskell, 1985).

Environment: None.

Food: None.

Drugs

Aggressive doses of chemotherapy, such as induction therapy for leukemia or lymphoma.

Agents that have potent myelosuppressive activity, such as the antitumor antibiotic agents or Fludarabine.

Other cytotoxic agents, such as corticosteroids, tamoxifen, intrathecal methotrexate, alpha interferon, tumor necrosis factor-alpha, monoclonal antibody R24, adoptive chemoimmunotherapy.

Drugs that potentiate metabolic abnormalities:
- Potassium supplements, potassium-sparing diuretics, and indomethacin potentiate hyperkalemia.
- Phosphates, furosemide, mithramycin, gallium nitrate, and anticonvulsants potentiate hyperphosphatemia and hypocalcemia.
- Thiazide diuretics potentiate hyperuricemia. (Dietz and Flaherty, 1993)

PROGNOSIS

The overall mortality rates for clients with cancer who develop TLS are not known. The occurrence and resolution depend on:

The tumor's sensitivity to the cytotoxic effects of therapy.
The volume of tumor cell burden.
The early identification of clients at high risk for developing TLS.
The early initiation of preventive measures (i.e., hydration fluids, allopurinol).

Authors have described the morbidity and mortality of many clients who have developed TLS. In several case studies, the TLS resolved after treatment, although a few clients died from other causes (Drakos et al., 1994; Gold, Malamud, LaRosa, and Osband, 1993; Shamseddine, Khalil, and Wehbeh, 1993; Dirix et al., 1991; Loosveld, Schouten, Gaillard, and Blijham, 1991; Simmons and Somberg, 1991). In other case studies, the clients died from complications that developed after TLS evolved, even though they received appropriate treatment (Sklarin and Markham, 1995; Jasek and Day, 1994; Malik, Abubakar, Alam, and Khan, 1994; Cannon, Spilove, Rhodes, Garfinkel, and Pezzimenti, 1993). When clients exhibit clinically significant manifestations of TLS, authors agree that these clients are often admitted to the intensive care unit (Lawrence, 1994) and that mortality is high (Malik et al., 1994).

One classic study described the morbidity and mortality of 37 clients with Burkitt's lymphoma (Cohen et al., 1980). Six clients died within 1 month of induction therapy. Five deaths were related to complications of the therapy and disease, and only one death was attributed to complications related to TLS. This client, with a uric acid level of 16.0 mg/dl, died primarily because of intractable renal failure. All the other clients survived remission induction therapy and the associated metabolic complications.

Another study (Hande and Garrow, 1993) described the morbidity and mortality of 102 clients receiving combination chemotherapy for non-Hodgkin's lymphoma (intermediate to high-grade histology). The authors determined the frequency of laboratory TLS (LTLS) and clinical TLS (CTLS). Clients were considered to have LTLS if two of the following metabolic changes occurred within 4 days of treatment: a 25% increase in the serum phosphate, potassium, uric acid, or blood urea nitrogen (BUN) concentrations, or a 25% decline in the serum calcium concentration. CTLS was defined as LTLS plus one of the following: a serum potassium level greater than 6 mmol/L (6 mEq/L), a creatinine level greater than 221 μmol/L (2.5 mg/dl), or a calcium level less than 1.5 mmol/L (6 mg/dl), the development of a life-threatening dysrhythmia, or sudden death. The results of this study were that LTLS occurred in 42% of clients and that CTLS occurred in 6% of clients. Therefore, clinically significant TLS is a rare occurrence in clients with lymphoma when they are receiving allopurinol, but TLS can occur in clients with all types of non-Hodgkin's lymphoma.

TREATMENT

Surgery: Debulking surgery for bulky abdominal disease may be indicated, if the disease can be resected adequately.

Chemotherapy: Not indicated.

Radiation: Indicated for clients with cancer that infiltrates the kidney (e.g., lymphoma, leukemia). Radiation therapy to the kidney before the client receives chemotherapy should reduce the tumor burden (Dietz and Flaherty, 1993).

Medications: See Table 43–1.

Table 43–1
Medications and Fluids to Prevent and Manage the Metabolic Complications of Tumor Lysis Syndrome

Goal of Treatment	Medications and Fluids	Rationale
Prevent/manage hyperuricemia	Initiate allopurinol administration. Reduce dosage 3–4 days into chemotherapy. Reduce/discontinue dosage if hyperuricemia is controlled.	Allopurinol inhibits uric acid synthesis.
Force diuresis to maintain urine flow at 150 to 200 ml/hour	Determine that the client is well hydrated (at least 3000 ml/m²/day) the day before treatment is initiated, the day(s) of treatment, and for at least 48 hours after treatment. Administer parenteral fluids if oral fluids are not tolerated or if oral intake is not sufficient.	Diuresis dilutes excess electrolytes and increases their excretion.
Maintain fluid balance	Administer nonthiazide diuretics (i.e., loop diuretics, such as furosemide, or osmotic diuretics, such as mannitol) if urine output falls below fluid intake. Initiate low-dose dopamine and nonthiazide diuretics in clients with pre-existing evidence of fluid retention (i.e., marked edema or ascites) or oliguria.	Diuretics increase urine flow.

(continued)

Table 43–1 (continued)

Goal of Treatment	Medications and Fluids	Rationale
Manage hyperkalemia	Discontinue IV administration of potassium-containing fluids. Initiate furosemide. Administer one or two of the following drugs, based on the client's condition: cation-exchange resins, such as oral kayexalate or a kayexalate retention enema; IV fluids containing glucose and insulin; or calcium gluconate.	Decrease the body's intake of potassium, and increase the body's loss of potassium. Hypertonic glucose solution facilitates movement of potassium from extracellular space to intracellular space. Insulin is required to prevent hyperglycemia, secondary to administration of hypertonic glucose.
Manage hyperphosphatemia	Initiate phosphate-binding antacids. Initiate hypertonic glucose and insulin infusion.	Increase the body's loss of phosphates. Hypertonic glucose solution facilitates movement of phosphorus from extracellular space to intracellular space.
Manage hypocalcemia	Administer calcium gluconate IV for severe ECG changes.*	Calcium gluconate increases cardiac muscle tone and the force of systolic contractions.
Urinary alkalinization (urine pH > 7)	Administer sodium bicarbonate IV solution.** Discontinue when serum uric acid level is normal (< 10 mg/dl). Administer acetazolamide 250–500 mg IV daily, if the above measure is ineffective.	Prevent uric acid crystal formation and correct metabolic acidosis.

* Controversy surrounds the administration of calcium supplements to correct hypocalcemia. Some authors recommend the administration of oral or parenteral calcium supplements to correct symptomatic hypocalcemia (Malik et al., 1994; Hawthorne et al., 1992; Silverman and Distelhorst, 1989). Other authors state that these treatment measures are contraindicated because they may cause further formation of the calcium-phosphate salts, which may promote greater deposits in the soft tissues (Stucky, 1993; Nace and Nace, 1985). Therefore, measures for treating hypocalcemia must be individualized and used cautiously.

** Another treatment controversy regards the use of sodium bicarbonate infusions. Several authors acknowledge the benefit of using sodium bicarbonate infusions for urinary alkalinization (Malik et al., 1994; Stucky, 1993; Simmons and Somberg, 1991); others recommend limiting its use until the serum uric acid level has normalized (Dietz and Flaherty, 1993); and others do not recommend its use (Jasek and Day, 1994; Hande and Garrow, 1993). This treatment controversy has evolved because an alkaline pH, although it increases the solubility of uric acid, increases the risk for calcium phosphate precipitation in the renal tubules. Also, alkalosis may predispose the patient to neuromuscular irritability by further lowering the calcium level. Therefore, therapeutic measures for preventing renal complications must be individualized and used cautiously (Stucky, 1993).

Table 43–1 *(continued)*

Goal of Treatment	Medications and Fluids	Rationale
Treat cancer	Initiate cytotoxic therapy within 24–48 hours of admission. Postpone cytotoxic therapy until metabolic abnormalities are controlled, adequate urine output is achieved, or dialysis has begun.	Early treatment slows tumor cell growth. Cytotoxic therapy is often the cause of the tumor lysis syndrome.

Table 43–2
**Suggested Criteria for Hemodialysis Therapy
in Clients with Tumor Lysis Syndrome**

Clients who do not respond to other treatment measures to correct metabolic abnormalities.

Clients who have the following serum blood values:
Potassium ≥6 mEq/L (6 mmol/L SI Units)
Uric acid > 10 mg/dl (590 µmol/L SI Units)
Creatinine ≥10 mg/dl (880 µmol/L SI Units)
Phosphorus > 10 mg/dl (3.2 mmol/L SI Units) or rapidly rising phosphorus level

Clients with the following conditions:
Fluid volume overload
Symptomatic hypocalcemia
Severe renal insufficiency

Procedures

Leukopheresis may be employed when the white blood cell count is extraordinarily elevated (e.g., 100,000/mm^3) to reduce both the tumor burden and the risk of TLS (Dietz and Flaherty, 1993).

Hemodialysis is recommended for clients with TLS who meet the suggested criteria (see Table 43–2).

ASSESSMENT CRITERIA: TUMOR LYSIS SYNDROME

Vital signs

Temperature	Normal
Pulse	Slow, weak, irregular with severe hyperkalemia (rare).
Respirations	Rapid, shallow if client experiencing shortness of breath or rales secondary to fluid overload.
Blood pressure	Elevated with renal insufficiency/failure. Decreased with severe hyperkalemia or hypocalcemia.

(continued)

ASSESSMENT CRITERIA: TUMOR LYSIS SYNDROME (continued)

History

Symptoms, conditions	See Risk Profile, especially "Conditions."
Weight pattern	Stable, or increasing owing to renal insufficiency.

Hallmark physical signs and symptoms

Early signs: diarrhea, lethargy, muscle cramps, nausea, paresthesias, vomiting, weakness.

Additional physical signs and symptoms

Hyperuricemia
1. GI effects: nausea, vomiting, anorexia, diarrhea.
2. Renal effects: flank pain, hematuria, cloudy urine, crystalluria, urine pH <7, decreased or absent urine output, weight gain, hypertension, edema.
3. Miscellaneous: pain and swelling at joints, lethargy.

Additional physical signs and symptoms

Hyperkalemia
1. Cardiac effects: cardiac arrest.
2. Neuromuscular effects: nerve and muscle irritability (twitching), muscle cramps or spasms, paresthesias, muscle weakness.
3. GI effects: nausea, diarrhea, intestinal colic.

Hyperphosphatemia
1. Renal effects: decreased or absent urine output, edema, hypertension, weight gain.
2. Metabolic effect: hypocalcemia, which may be accompanied by neurologic and cardiac signs and symptoms.

Hypocalcemia
1. Cardiac effects: cardiac arrest.
2. Neurologic symptoms: muscle cramping and twitching, tetany, grimacing, carpopedal spasm, laryngospasm, convulsions, seizures, paresthesias, confusion, loss of recent memory, delirium, lethargy.

Psychosocial signs

Apprehension, confusion, delirium.

Lab values

Uric acid, serum	High (>8.0 mg/ dl; or >475 μmol/L SI Units)
Potassium, serum	High (>5.5 mEq/L; or >5.5 mmol/L SI Units)
Phosphorus, serum	High (>7.0 mg/dl; or 2.26 mmol/L SI Units)
Calcium, serum	Low (≤7.0 mg/dl; or 1.75 mmol/L SI Units)
Blood urea nitrogen (BUN), serum	High (>50 mg/dl; ≥17.85 mmol/L SI Units)
Creatinine, serum	High (>1.6 mg/dl; or 140.8 μmol/L SI Units)
LDH, serum	High (>1500 IU/L)
Arterial blood gas (pH, HCO_3, $PaCO_2$)	Low in metabolic acidosis

ASSESSMENT CRITERIA: TUMOR LYSIS SYNDROME *(continued)*

Diagnostic tests	
Chvostek's sign	Positive sign (facial muscle twitch) with hypocalcemia.
Trousseau's sign	Positive sign (hand moves into a position of palmer flexion, which is carpopedal spasm, after occlusion of arterial blood flow in the arm) with hypocalcemia.
ECG	*Hyperkalemia:* 1. ECG changes: peaked and narrow T waves, shortening of Q-T interval, widened QRS complex with decreased amplitude, sine wave (blending of QRS into T wave), loss of P wave. 2. Dysrhythmias: ventricular tachycardia, ventricular fibrillation, asystole. *Hypocalcemia:* 1. ECG changes: prolongation of Q-T interval and S-T segment, lowering and inversion of T wave, slowed ventricular repolarization. 2. Dysrhythmias: ventricular dysrhythmias, 2:1 heart block.
Deep tendon reflexes	Hyperactive reflexes related to hyperkalemia and hypocalcemia.
Other	Assess content and rate of IV fluids.

NURSING DIAGNOSIS

The nursing diagnosis will vary, depending on the metabolic and clinical manifestations of TLS. Some of the common diagnoses are as follows.

Tissue perfusion, altered (renal), related to uric acid crystal and calcium phosphate salt formation in the kidneys.

Urinary elimination, altered, related to uric acid nephropathy and acute renal failure.

Fluid volume excess related to vigorous hydration and/or to renal insufficiency.

Decreased cardiac output related to dysrhythmias associated with hyperkalemia or hypocalcemia.

Injury, risk for, related to seizures and convulsions associated with hypocalcemia.

Sensory alterations (tactile) due to paresthesias associated with hyperkalemia or hypocalcemia.

Confusion related to hypocalcemia.

Knowledge deficit related to:
- High risk for developing TLS.
- Management of the metabolic and clinical manifestations of TLS.

NURSING INTERVENTIONS

Immediate nursing interventions

Assess pulse, respirations, blood pressure, and mental status.
Auscultate lung sounds and assess presence of cough.
Measure strict intake and output (I and O).
Monitor urine color, appearance, and pH.
Establish/maintain patent IV access. Obtain volumetric infusion pump.

Anticipated physician orders and interventions

IV hydration fluid rate at 3000 ml/m^2/day or greater.
Initiate allopurinol at a dose of 600 to 900 mg/day (or 500 mg/m^2/day).
  Reduce dosage to 300 to 450 mg/day (or 200 mg/m^2/day) 3 to 4 days
  into chemotherapy.
Reduce/discontinue dosage if hyperuricemia is controlled. Reduce
  dosage of allopurinol for pediatric clients.
Serum electrolytes, BUN, creatinine, uric acid, phosphorus, calcium, and
  magnesium STAT and q6h.
Arterial blood gas for clients with respiratory distress, hyperuricemia, or
  acute renal failure.
Decrease/discontinue chemotherapy and other medications that may
  contribute to the metabolic abnormalities associated with TLS.
IV nonthiazide diuretic (e.g., furosemide, mannitol) administration if
  urine output < 100 ml/hour.
Indwelling urinary catheter placement, if the client has altered mental
  status or if there is evidence of urinary retention.
Nasogastric tube placement for the administration of allopurinol
  and/or phosphate-binding agents, if the client is unable to tolerate
  oral medications.
Topical cream and antipruritic medication administration for rashes associated with allopurinol.

Emergency measure initiation for cardiac, respiratory, or renal failure
Cardiopulmonary resuscitation. Admit to intensive care unit.
Mechanical ventilation.
Pulmonary artery catheter.
Hemodialysis, if client meets suggested criteria (see Table 43–2).

Hyperuricemia
Administer IV solution of sodium bicarbonate (100mEq/L initially; adjust
  as needed).
Discontinue infusion when serum uric acid level is < 10 mg/dl.
Administer acetazolamide 250 to 500 mg IV daily, if IV solution of sodi-
  um bicarbonate is not effective in lowering the uric acid level.

Hyperkalemia

Administer oral kayexalate, 15 to 30 g with 50 ml of 20% sorbitol, two to four times daily for serum potassium levels less than 7 mEq/L.

Administer kayexalate retention enema, 50 g in 200 ml of 20% sorbitol, if the client is unable to tolerate oral medications. The best effect is achieved if the enema is retained for 30 to 60 minutes. Indicated for clients with serum potassium levels less than 7 mEq/L.

Administer hypertonic glucose IV infusion (usually 250 ml of 10 to 20% glucose solution) and insulin (10 to 20 units of regular) for oliguric clients, or for clients with serum potassium levels of 6.5 to 7.5 mEq/L.

Administer sodium bicarbonate 50 mEq as IV bolus, or 50 to 150 mEq added to 1 liter D5W or D10W as an IV infusion for clients with potassium levels greater than 7 mEq/L, metabolic acidosis, or significant ECG changes.

Administer 1 to 3 amps of 10% calcium gluconate over 3 to 5 minutes IVP (intravenous pyelogram), with continuous ECG monitoring, for clients with serum potassium levels greater than 7 mEq/L, or significant ECG changes.

Obtain a 12- lead ECG, if serum potassium level is greater than 6 mEq/L, or if serum calcium level is less than 8 mg/dl.

Maintain cardiac monitoring, if the client is at a high risk of developing TLS or if severe ECG changes occur.

Notify the physician immediately for changes in pulse and blood pressure.

Discontinue administration of IV fluids containing potassium.

Discontinue medications that promote potassium retention (e.g., potassium-sparing diuretics).

Restrict dietary intake of potassium.

Hyperphosphatemia

Administer phosphate-binding antacids, such as Amphogel, Basaljel, or Neutraphos.

Administer hypertonic glucose and insulin infusion for severe hyperphosphatemia.

Administer stool softeners or laxatives, if constipation occurs because of the phosphate-binding antacids.

Discontinue medications containing phosphates.

Restrict dietary intake of phosphates, especially soft drinks.

Hypocalcemia

Administer 1 to 3 amps of 10% calcium gluconate over 3 to 5 minutes IVP, with continuous ECG monitoring for significant ECG changes caused by of hypocalcemia.

Hypomagnesemia

Administer oral or parenteral magnesium for serum magnesium levels less than 1.5 mEq/L, with concurrent hypocalcemia or hyperkalemia.

Ongoing nursing assessment, monitoring, and interventions

Assess:

- For renal effects (e.g., urine output < 100 ml/hour, cloudy urine, pH < 7, hematuria, flank pain), and notify the physician immediately if any of these occur.
- For peripheral, periorbital, scrotal, and presacral edema, and medicate with diuretics as ordered.
- For respiratory changes by auscultating lung sounds and assessing presence of cough q8h, and assessing respiratory rate and depth q4h.
- •: For distended neck veins, by having client lie in bed with head of bed elevated 30 to 60 degrees.
- For nausea and vomiting, and medicate with antiemetics as ordered.
- For diarrhea, and medicate with antidiarrheals as ordered.
- For neuromuscular signs and symptoms, such as lethargy; twitching; muscle cramps, spasms, or weakness; tetany; numbness, tingling; grimacing; carpotunnel spasm; laryngospasm; or seizures, convulsions.
- For mental status changes, such as confusion, delirium, or loss of recent memory q8h.
- For positive Trousseau's sign or Chvostek's sign q8h.
- For pain and swelling at joints.
- For clients at risk for fluid overload (e.g., elderly clients, clients who have a history of cardiac problems).

Measure:

- Pulse and blood pressure q4h and PRN, depending on the client's condition.
- Respiratory rate q8h.
- Strict I and O: q2h if client is exhibiting signs/symptoms of TLS; q4h if client is at high risk for developing TLS.
- Determine that urine output is at least 3000 ml/day.
- Weight qd.

Send:

- Serum electrolytes, BUN, creatinine, uric acid, calcium, phosphorus, magnesium q6–12h, until the client's blood chemistries and physical condition are stable.
- Urine analysis (to monitor crystals, pH, and blood in urine) q12h, until client's blood chemistries and physical condition are stable.

Implement:

- Seizure precautions, until serum calcium > 7.0 mg/dl.
- Potassium and/or phosphate intake restriction, as prescribed.
- Low-fiber diet, if diarrhea occurs.

TEACHING/EDUCATION

Select items, based on the client's pathophysiology.

TLS: *Rationale:* This is a syndrome that may occur when a person has large amounts of tumor cells and when they receive treatment to kill these cells. The tumor cells break open or "lyse" when they die. Then the cells release their contents, which include potassium, uric acid, and phosphorus. Too much of these substances can cause serious or fatal problems in a person, including: (1) the kidneys may have trouble getting rid of water and waste from the body, (2) the muscles and nerves may be more excitable, and (3) the heart may not work as well, or may stop. Also, too much phosphorus can lead to a lack of calcium, which can lead to more problems.

Risk factors for developing tumor lysis syndrome: *Rationale:* It is important to know if you are at risk for developing tumor lysis syndrome, so that you can watch for the signs and symptoms. Also, you can take measures to prevent this syndrome from occurring, such as increasing your fluid intake or taking allopurinol as ordered. Persons with fast-growing tumors, such as leukemia or lymphoma, are at risk. Persons who have a large amount of tumor, such as tumor that has spread to several places in the body or tumor in many lymph nodes, are also at risk.

Signs and symptoms of tumor lysis syndrome: *Rationale:* You, and those close to you, need to watch for signs of tumor lysis syndrome, because early treatment helps you feel better and live a better quality of life. Tell us if you notice any of these signs:

Nausea, vomiting, lack of appetite, or watery stools.
Muscle cramps, spasms, twitching, or weakness.
Numbness or tingling.
Increased tiredness.
Side pain, cloudy urine, or blood in urine.
Weight gain or swelling.
Shortness of breath.
Pain and swelling at joints.

IV blood samples: *Rationale:* Several blood samples will be taken before you start your chemotherapy, during your treatment, and after it. These are needed to track the amount of potassium, uric acid, phosphorus, calcium, and other substances in your blood.

Decrease/discontinue chemotherapy, anticancer drugs, any other drugs that may be causing problems: *Rationale:* Some chemotherapy drugs, anticancer drugs, and other drugs may be affecting your body's balance of fluids, potassium, uric acid, phosphorus, calcium, and other substances. You may receive your anticancer treatment at a later time. Some of your drugs may be changed or alternated with other drugs.

IV line placement: *Rationale:* The IV line allows us to easily take blood samples and to give you the needed treatments with fluids and drugs.

Increasing fluids: *Rationale:* Drinking more fluids helps prevent tumor lysis syndrome from occurring. Also, more fluids are an important part of treatment if it does occur. You need to drink lots of fluids (8 to 10 glasses a day, or the amount that your doctor orders). Continue drinking fluids for 2 days after your last dose of chemotherapy. Tell your doctor or nurse if you are unable to drink fluids during or after your chemotherapy.

Strict measurement of I and O: *Rationale:* Accurate measurement of fluids taken in (i.e., drinks, soups, gelatin, ice cream, IV fluids) and of output (i.e., urine, stools, vomitus) is critical in persons with tumor lysis syndrome. You need to keep track of the fluids that you take in by mouth. Also, you need to save your urine in a container in the toilet, so that we can correctly measure your urine output. This measurement will tell us if your kidneys are working well.

Drugs to treat TLS: *Rationale:* You may be given several drugs to treat this syndrome. Allopurinol is a drug that you take by mouth to prevent uric acid buildup. You may be given other drugs to correct the potassium, phosphorus, or uric acid levels in your body.

Indwelling urinary catheter placement: *Rationale:* Accurate urine measurement is very important, especially for persons who are confused or who are retaining urine. The catheter prevents any urine from spilling before it is measured. We may give you drugs that will make your kidneys make more urine, so the catheter keeps you from having to get up often and go to the bathroom.

Stomach tube placement: *Rationale:* Placing a tube through the nose and into the stomach may be needed, if you are unable to swallow your drugs by mouth.

Seizure precautions: *Rationale:* Persons with low calcium levels are at risk for having seizures. To protect the person, the bed side rails need to be padded. Also, a padded tongue blade needs to be placed near the bed to prevent the tongue from closing off the person's breathing during a seizure. An oral airway may also be kept at the bedside.

Dietary changes: *Rationale:* Foods or drinks with potassium or phosphorus will be limited in your diet for a few days to bring your blood levels back to normal. Also, you may be placed on a low-fiber diet if you have diarrhea.

EVALUATION/DESIRED OUTCOMES

1. Serum potassium decreases to 5.5 mEq/L (5.5 mmol/L SI Units) or less within 48 hours.

2. Serum uric acid decreases to 8 mg/dl (476 µmol/L SI Units) or less within 48 hours.
3. Serum phosphorus decreases to 7 mg/dl (2.25 mmol/L SI Units) or less within 48 hours.
4. Serum calcium increases to 7 mg/dl (1.74 mmol/L SI Units) or more within 48 hours.
5. Pulse, blood pressure, and respiratory rate return to baseline within 72 hours.
6. Urinary output is maintained at 100 ml/hour or greater.
7. Urine pH is maintained at 7 or greater.
8. Indwelling urinary catheter is discontinued within 72 hours.
9. Nausea, vomiting, and diarrhea subside within 48 hours.
10. Nasogastric tube is discontinued within 48 hours.
11. Renal effects (i.e., flank pain, hematuria, cloudy urine, crystalluria, weight gain, edema) subside within 72 hours.
12. Cardiac effects (ECG changes, dysrhythmias) subside within 72 hours.
13. Neuromuscular effects (muscle cramps, spasms, twitching, or weakness; paresthesias; hyperactive reflexes; positive Chvostek's sign or Trousseau's sign) subside within 72 hours.
14. Lungs are clear to auscultation within 48 hours.
15. The client and/or caregiver verbalizes understanding of management of the metabolic and clinical manifestations of TLS.

DISCHARGE PLANNING

The client with tumor lysis syndrome may need:

Intermittent blood work drawn at home or at an outpatient facility.
Instruction of client and significant others to report signs and symptoms of TLS to physician or primary health care provider immediately.
Training in I and O measurement and documentation.

FOLLOW-UP CARE

Anticipated care

Physician office visit within 1 week.
Outpatient lab testing for serum electrolytes, uric acid, phosphorus, and calcium within the next week.
Other blood work, as appropriate (i.e., magnesium, BUN, creatinine, etc.).
Home health nursing visit once per week for 2 weeks.
Continuation of high fluid intake and dietary restrictions of potassium and phosphorus.

Anticipated client/family questions and possible answers

Can I develop tumor lysis syndrome again?

"It is possible that this syndrome could happen again. It is very important for you to know the signs of tumor lysis syndrome, and to know what to do when you recognize these signs."

"Tumor lysis syndrome could return in persons who receive more anticancer treatment for cancer in the blood or lymph system, for cancer that is fast-growing, or for cancer that has spread in the body. Also, it is more likely to return in persons who are dehydrated or who have imbalances in their blood work."

"Because of this, you must know the signs of tumor lysis syndrome and call your doctor or nurse if you notice them." (Refer to "Signs and symptoms of tumor lysis syndrome" in the Teaching/Education section.)

When can I continue my chemotherapy?

"When your lab values are back to normal and your body can tolerate the side effects of the drug again. This is usually within 1 or 2 weeks."

Why will a nurse be coming to my home?

"The nurse will come to see whether any problems caused by the tumor lysis syndrome are occurring again. The nurse will take blood samples from your vein; listen to your lungs with a stethoscope; weigh you; take your blood pressure, heart and breathing rate; ask about any recent nausea, vomiting, or diarrhea; ask about the amount and color of your urine; ask about any muscle cramps, spasms, or weakness; talk with you to see how alert you are; and ask you if you have any questions or concerns."

CHAPTER SUMMARY

TLS is a metabolic complication that primarily occurs in clients who have a fast-growing, large tumor cell burden that is very sensitive to the cytotoxic effects of anticancer therapy. More commonly, clients will exhibit laboratory manifestations, which include moderate elevations in serum potassium, uric acid, and phosphorus levels, and a decline in serum calcium levels. Because of the increasing use of preventive measures, such as hydration fluids and allopurinol, clinically significant manifestations of tumor lysis syndrome occur more infrequently. These manifestations include critical elevation in serum potassium (> 7 mEq/L, > 7 mmol/L SI Units), critical decrease in serum calcium (< 6.0 mg/dl, < 1.49 mmol/L SI Units), renal insufficiency or failure, life-threatening dysrhythmias, or sudden death. Clients who exhibit clinically significant manifestations of TLS are experiencing an acute oncologic emergency and have a worse prognosis than those who are exhibiting only laboratory manifestations of TLS. Treatment and nursing care are related to the presence of specific laboratory and clinical manifestations of TLS, the severity of the manifestations, and the rapidity of development of the problem. A definitive understanding of potassium, uric acid, phosphorus, and calcium homeostasis is essential to the underlying treatment and care.

TEST QUESTIONS

1. TLS results when massive amounts of tumor cells are lysed and release their intracellular contents, which include:
   A. Phosphorus, calcium, sodium, and potassium
   B. Potassium, uric acid, phosphorus, and nucleic acids
   C. Uric acid, nucleic acids, phosphorus, and magnesium
   D. Nucleic acids, potassium, albumin, and sodium

1. Answer: B
The intracellular contents released when massive amounts of tumor cells are lysed include potassium, uric acid, phosphorus, and nucleic acids. Serum calcium levels decrease because of the increase in serum phosphorus levels.

2. TLS is most likely to occur in clients with:
   A. Small cell lung cancer
   B. Metastatic breast cancer
   C. Acute leukemia
   D. Metastatic ovarian cancer, with ascites

2. Answer: C
TLS is most likely to develop in clients with hematologic tumors that are highly proliferative and sensitive to cytotoxic treatment, such as acute leukemia, high-grade lymphomas, and non-Hodgkin's lymphoma.

3. Clients are at higher risk for developing TLS when the following conditions exist before they receive their cytotoxic treatment:
   A. Dehydration, renal insufficiency, lymphadenopathy
   B. Hypervolemia, high white blood cell count, acidic urine
   C. Dehydration, alkaline urine, diarrhea
   D. Hypervolemia, cardiac dysrhythmias, splenomegaly

3. Answer: A
Dehydration, pretreatment metabolic disturbances, pretreatment renal insufficiency, high white blood cell count, splenomegaly, lymphadenopathy, and elevated LDH levels are conditions that place clients at higher risk for developing TLS.

4. The primary nursing diagnosis of clients with TLS is:
   A. Risk for injury related to convulsions
   B. Confusion related to hypocalcemia
   C. Excess fluid volume
   D. Alteration in tissue perfusion (renal)

4. Answer: D
TLS is a metabolic disorder that can lead to renal insufficiency or failure. Renal tissue perfusion is altered because of the development of uric acid crystals and calcium phosphate salts in the kidneys.

5. Early signs and symptoms of TLS include:
   A. Nausea, vomiting, muscle cramps, lethargy
   B. Diarrhea, decreased urine output, intestinal colic
   C. Nausea, vomiting, paresthesias, EKG changes
   D. Diarrhea, cloudy urine, muscle weakness

5. Answer: A
Early signs of TLS include nausea, vomiting, diarrhea, muscle cramps, paresthesias, lethargy, and weakness. Progressive, or late, signs, include renal effects, cardiac effects, and intestinal colic.

6. To prevent TLS from developing in high risk clients, treatment should include all of the following *except:*
   A. Increasing fluid intake to at least 3000 ml/m^2/day
   B. Decreasing the serum uric acid concentration
   C. Limiting the urinary flow rate to 30 ml/hour
   D. Increasing the solubility of uric acid in the urine

6. Answer: C
Methods to prevent TLS from developing include hydration fluids, allopurinol, and urinary alkalinization. A urinary flow rate of at least 100 ml/hour is the desired outcome.

7. The nurse needs to closely monitor the client for signs and symptoms of TLS from the onset, e.g., _____ hours after therapy is initiated, and continuing for _____ days.
   A. 1 to 2 hours; 5 to 7 days.
   B. 6 to 12 hours; 3 to 5 days.
   C. 12 to 24 hours; 7 to 10 days.
   D. 24 to 48 hours; 10 to 14 days.

7. Answer: A
Tumor lysis syndrome may begin 1 to 2 hours after cytotoxic therapy is initiated and may continue for 5 to 7 days.

8. Mr. Jones, a 48-year-old man who was recently diagnosed with Burkitt's lymphoma, is receiving his first chemotherapy treatment today. He has vomited all of his lunch. You have auscultated rales in his lungs. His vital signs are: T: 98.7° F, P: 84, R: 26, BP: 116/82. His urinary output was 150 ml in the last 2 hours. The first physician order that the nurse will anticipate and implement is:
   A. Insert urinary catheter STAT.
   B. Obtain serum electrolytes, uric acid, phosphorus, and calcium STAT.
   C. Insert nasogastric tube STAT.
   D. Administer thiazide diuretic STAT.

8. Answer: B
To determine if a client is developing tumor lysis syndrome, blood work needs to be drawn. This will monitor for the four hallmark signs of TLS: hyperkalemia, hyperuricemia, hyperphosphatemia, and hypocalcemia.

9. A client diagnosed with TLS would most likely be taught about:
   A. Seizure precautions
   B. High-calcium diet
   C. Fluid restriction
   D. Strict measurement of I and O

9. Answer: D
Accurate measurement of I and O in clients with TLS is critical in determining fluid balance, development of renal insufficiency, and need for diuretics.

10. An expected outcome for a client with TLS would be:
   A. Serum calcium level decreases to 9 mg/dl within 48 hours.
   B. Urinary output is maintained at 50 ml/hour or greater.
   C. Serum potassium level decreases to 5.5 mEq/L or less within 48 hours.
   D. Cardiac enzymes will be within normal limits within 24 hours.

10. Answer: C
Expected outcomes include: (1) serum potassium, uric acid, and phosphorus levels need to decrease to normal ranges, and serum calcium levels need to increase to the normal range; (2) urinary output needs to be maintained at 100 ml/hour; and (3) cardiac effects (ECG changes, dysrhythmias) need to subside within 72 hours.

REFERENCES

Cannon LM, Spilove L, Rhodes R, Garfinkel H, Pezzimenti J: Acute tumor lysis syndrome complicating fludarabine treatment of prolymphocytic leukemia. Conn Med 57(10):651–654, 1993.

Cassmeyer VL: Mechanisms for maintaining dynamic equilibrium. In Phipps WJ, Long BC, Woods NF (eds): Medical-Surgical Nursing: Concepts and Clinical Practice, 2nd ed. St. Louis, MO: CV Mosby, 1983, pp. 296–326.

Cohen LF, Balow JE, Magrath IT, Poplack DG, Ziegler JL: Acute tumor lysis syndrome: A review of 37 patients with Burkitt's lymphoma. Am J Med 68(4):486–491, 1980.

Cunningham SG: Fluid and electrolyte disturbances associated with cancer and its treatment. Nurs Clin North Am 17:579–593, 1982.

Dietz KA, Flaherty AM: Oncologic emergencies. In Groenwald SL, Goodman M, Frogge MH, Yarbro CH (eds): Cancer Nursing: Principles and Practice, 3rd ed. Boston: Jones and Bartlett, 1993, pp. 800–839.

Dirix LY, Prove A, Becquart D, Wouters E, Vermeulen P, Van Oosterom A: Tumor lysis syndrome in a patient with metastatic Merkel cell carcinoma. Cancer 67(8):2207–2210, 1991.

Drakos P, Bar-Ziv J, Catane R: Tumor lysis syndrome in nonhematologic malignancies: Report of a case and review of the literature. Am J Clin Oncol 17(6):502–505, 1994.

Gold JE, Malamud SC, LaRosa F, Osband ME: Adoptive chemoimmunotherapy using ex vivo activated memory T-cells and cyclophosphamide: Tumor lysis syndrome of a metastatic soft tissue sarcoma. Am J Hematol 44(1):42–47, 1993.

Guzzetta C: Cardiopulmonary arrest and resuscitation. In Kenner CV, Guzzetta CE, Dossey BM (eds): Critical Care Nursing: Body—Mind—Spirit. Boston: Little, Brown, 1981, pp. 329–392.

Hain RD, Rayner L, Weitzman S, Lorenzana A: Acute tumor lysis syndrome complicating treatment of stage IVS neuroblastoma in infants under six months old. Med Pediatr Oncol 23(2):136–139, 1994.

Hande KR, Garrow GC: Acute tumor lysis syndrome in patients with high grade non-Hodgkin's lymphoma. Am J Med 94(2):133–139, 1993.

Haskell CM (ed): Cancer Treatment, 2nd ed. Philadelphia: WB Saunders Co, 1985.

Hawthorne JL, Schneider SM, Workman ML: Common electrolyte imbalances associated with malignancy. AACN Clin Iss Crit Care Nurs 3(3):714–723, 1992.

Jasek AM, Day HJ: Acute spontaneous tumor lysis syndrome. Am J Hematol 47(2):129–131, 1994.

Lawrence J: Critical care issues in the patient with hematologic malignancy. Semin Oncol Nurs 10(3):198–207, 1994.

Loosveld OJ, Schouten HC, Gaillard CA, Blijham GH: Acute tumor lysis syndrome in a patient with acute lymphoblastic leukemia after a single dose of prednisone. Br J Haematol 77(1):122–123, 1991.

Malik IA, Abubakar S, Alam F, Khan A: Dexamethasone-induced tumor lysis syndrome in high-grade non-Hodgkin's lymphoma. South Med J 87(3):409–411, 1994.

Methany NM: Fluid and electrolyte balance: Nursing considerations. Philadelphia: JB Lippincott, 1987.

Nace CS, Nace GS: Acute tumor lysis syndrome: Pathophysiology and nursing management. Crit Care Nurs 5(3):26–34, 1985.

Patterson KL, Klopovich P: Metabolic emergencies in pediatric oncology: The acute tumor lysis syndrome. J Pediatr Oncol Nurs 4(3–4):19–24, 1988.

Pocheldy C: Hyperuricemia in leukemia and lymphoma. New York State J Med (May):1085–1091, 1973.

Shamseddine AI, Khalil AM, Wehbeh MH: Acute tumor lysis syndrome with squamous cell carcinoma of the vulva. Gynecol Oncol 51(2):258–260, 1993.

Silverman P, Distelhorst CW: Metabolic emergencies in clinical oncology. Semin Oncol 16(6):504–515, 1989.

Simmons ED, Somberg KH: Acute tumor lysis syndrome after intrathecal methotrexate administration. Cancer 67:2062–2065, 1991.

Sklarin NT, Markham M: Spontaneous recurrent tumor lysis syndrome in breast cancer. Am J Clin Oncol 18(1):71–73, 1995.

Soltis B: Fluid and electrolyte imbalance. *In* Phipps WJ, Long BC, Woods NF (eds): Medical-Surgical Nursing: Concepts and Clinical Practice, 2nd ed. St. Louis, MO: CV Mosby, 1983, pp. 327–357.

Stucky LA: Acute tumor lysis syndrome: Assessment and nursing implications. Oncol Nurs Forum 20(1):49–59, 1993.

Tsokos GC, Balow JE, Spiegel RJ, Magrath IT: Renal and metabolic complications of undifferentiated and lymphoblastic lymphomas. Medicine 60:218–228, 1981.

CHAPTER 44

TYPHLITIS IN PEDIATRICS

Gretchen A. Vaughn, RN, MSN

AND

Lisa M. Moles, RN, MSN

CHAPTER OBJECTIVES

At the completion of this chapter, the reader will be able to:

Describe the etiology and pathophysiology of typhlitis in children.

State the risk factors associated with typhlitis in children.

Identify the clinical signs and symptoms of typhlitis in children.

Describe the nursing care of children with typhlitis.

Discuss the client/family education and discharge preparations for children with typhlitis.

OVERVIEW

TYPHLITIS, derived from the Greek word "typhlon" (cecum), is a pathologic condition of the gastrointestinal (GI) tract associated with immunosuppression. More specifically, it is an inflammatory and/or necrotic process involving the cecum and/or the terminal ileum and appendix. The term typhlitis has been used synonymously with neutropenic enterocolitis, necrotizing enterocolitis, and ileocecal syndrome. Typhlitis was initially described at autopsy of children with leukemia (Wagner, Rosenberg, Fernbach, and Singleton, 1970). Typhlitis is now recognized to occur also in clients with other disorders, such as aplastic anemia, lymphoma, acquired immune deficiency syndrome (AIDS), and following organ or bone marrow transplantation (Sloas, Flynn, Kaste, and Patrick, 1993). The incidence of typhlitis in children with leukemia after chemotherapy ranges from 10 to 24% (Paulino, Kenney, Forman, and Medeiros, 1994). However, the incidence of typhlitis in other disorders remains unknown. The overall incidence of typhlitis can be expected to increase as a result of more aggressive chemotherapy regimens, advances in transplantation technology, and the increasing occurrence of AIDS in the population.

DESCRIPTION

Typhlitis is a condition of the intestines that may occur in children or adults who receive chemotherapy and then become neutropenic. Typhlitis only becomes evident during periods of neutropenia (Sloas et al., 1993), and the longer a client is neutropenic, the greater is the risk that typhlitis will develop. Reports of typhlitis have been more common in children than adults (Wade, Nava, and Douglass, 1992).

The etiology of typhlitis is complex and not entirely understood. It is believed to be an inflammatory and/or necrotizing process that primarily involves the cecum but may occur at other parts of the intestines (Katz, Wagner, Gresik, Mahoney, and Fernbach, 1990). Typhlitis has a predilection for the cecum for a variety of reasons. The cecum has decreased vascularity, decreased lymphatic drainage, and increased distensibility compared to other parts of the colon (Hiruki, Fernandes, Ramsey, and Rother, 1992). These factors promote the possibility of necrosis, infection, and swelling that are common in typhlitis.

In order for typhlitis to develop, the integrity of the mucosal wall of the intestines first becomes compromised either by leukemic infiltration, chemotherapy toxicity, or both. This alteration of the mucosal wall, or mucositis, can be present anywhere in the GI system. When clients are febrile and neutropenic following chemotherapy, they are given broad-spectrum antibi-

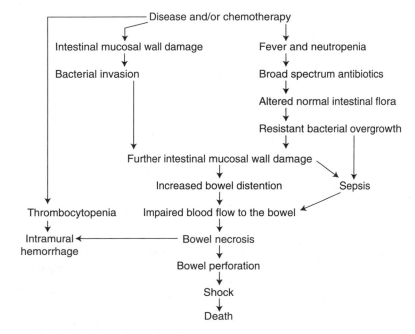

Figure 44–1 Pathophysiology of typhlitis.

otics. These antibiotics reduce the normal intestinal flora, which allows bacterial invasion and overgrowth of resistant bacteria. The infection in the bowel can be caused by gram-positive or gram-negative organisms and/or by fungi (Hiruki et al., 1992). These potent bacteria and/or fungi invade the bowel wall and cause more extensive damage. The bowel responds to the bacterial invasion by distending, which impairs the blood flow to the area. The ischemic area becomes weakened and necrotic, which puts the client at greater risk for intramural hemorrhage, continued necrosis, and perforation of the bowel. The blood flow to the intestines and entire GI tract may also be compromised if the client becomes septic and hemodynamically unstable (see Figure 44–1).

The clinical symptoms common in clients with typhlitis include abdominal pain (usually but not exclusively in the right lower quadrant), abdominal distention, recurrent fever up to 38.3 to 40° C (101 to 104° F), upper or lower GI bleeding, nausea, vomiting, and diarrhea. In a few cases, a right lower quadrant mass or respiratory distress have also been described. These symptoms must be carefully monitored and evaluated to rule out other abdominal processes such as appendicitis, intussusception, intramural hemorrhage, small bowel obstruction, segmental pseudomembranous colitis, and diverticulitis (Jones and Wall, 1992). A differentiating factor between typhlitis and appendicitis is that diarrhea and GI bleeding are much more frequent in typhlitis.

The clinical course of typhlitis often follows a pattern of mild/moderate complaints initially, with worsening symptoms over a period of several days. Some clients may stabilize with medical management for days to weeks until their absolute neutrophil count recovers. Other clients with confirmed typhlitis can have progressive symptoms, including the concurrent development of sepsis despite aggressive medical management. For some clients, surgical management may also become necessary.

Diagnostic tests that help to differentiate typhlitis from other conditions include plain abdominal films and ultrasounds. Computed tomography (CT) scans of the abdomen are indicated when the abdominal x-rays and ultrasounds are inconclusive (see Assessment Criteria). A barium enema is not usually part of the diagnostic workup because of the risk of perforation.

RISK PROFILE

Cancers: Hematologic malignancies account for the majority of cases of typhlitis. These include acute nonlymphocytic leukemia, acute lymphocytic leukemia, myelodysplastic syndrome, and lymphoblastic lymphoma. Typhlitis has also been described in children with solid tumors treated with aggressive chemotherapy regimens and in adults with multiple myeloma and metastatic breast cancer.

Conditions: Fever and neutropenia can be seen in clients with various conditions. Clients at risk for fever and neutropenia include those with AIDS, cyclic neutropenia, and aplastic anemia and in those who have had a bone marrow or solid tumor transplant.

Environment: None.

Foods: None.

Drugs: Clients who develop typhlitis usually have received a combination of chemotherapy agents. Common drugs include cytosine arabinoside, etoposide, daunorubicin, methotrexate, vincristine, and corticosteroids such as prednisone and dexamethasone.

PROGNOSIS

The prognosis for recovery from typhlitis has historically been grim. Many cases were found only on autopsy, including 10% of children in one series who had died from leukemia (Angel, Bhaskar, Wrenn, Lobe, and Kumar, 1992). Survival of typhlitis has ranged between 0 and 50% (Sloas et al., 1993). As early diagnosis and treatment become more common, the prognosis has been improving. The single most important factor in the recovery process is the increase to normal of the neutrophil count. In clients who have a prolonged period of neutropenia, the risk of a poor outcome from the typhlitis is increased.

TREATMENT

Surgery: The role of surgical intervention remains controversial. The client with neutropenia is considered a poor surgical candidate for a major abdominal procedure owing to the risks of peritonitis, sepsis, or impaired wound healing. It is unclear when the benefits outweigh the risks of surgery for the client with typhlitis. However, there is consensus for surgical intervention if transmural bowel necrosis or perforation is highly suspected or confirmed.

Chemotherapy: Not indicated.

Radiation: Not indicated.

Medications

    Prompt treatment with parenteral broad spectrum antibiotics is essential. Antibiotic therapy options may reflect the particular institution's standard regimen used for febrile neutropenic clients.

    Antifungal therapy is indicated in the presence of a fungal infection or after prolonged fevers that are unresponsive to other antibiotics.

    Colony-stimulating factors are used in the treatment of typhlitis to help the client recover from the neutropenia more quickly.

    Use pain medications as indicated. It is important to note that there are many concerns about the use of narcotics for pain management. Narcotics have the potential to cause a worsening abdominal distention or ileus; therefore, some would recommend that they be used sparingly.

The use of anticholinergic (particularly antidiarrheal) agents is contraindicated because these agents decrease the GI tract motility.

Vasopressors may be indicated to maintain blood pressure and perfusion for the client with sepsis.

Procedures

Placement of additional IV catheters to infuse IV fluids, antibiotics, total parenteral nutrition (TPN), blood products, and vasopressors.

Placement of a nasogastric (NG) tube is necessary for bowel decompression.

Other: IV fluids are given to maintain adequate hydration and electrolyte balance. Parenteral nutrition is used while the client is NPO (nothing by mouth) for bowel rest. Blood products are given during the period of myelosuppression that follows chemotherapy.

Typhlitis is a diverse process that varies in presentation and severity. Therefore, the treatment plan for each client may vary. The treatment may range from conservative medical management to surgical intervention. For all clients with typhlitis, however, a favorable outcome depends upon early recognition, diagnosis, and prompt medical interventions, including antibiotic administration, fluid, electrolyte, and blood product support. All of these treatment interventions are life-sustaining measures necessary until the client is no longer neutropenic and the typhlitis has resolved.

ASSESSMENT CRITERIA: TYPHLITIS IN PEDIATRICS

Vital signs	
Temperature	Fever up to 104° F; hypothermic if sepsis develops.
Pulse	Normal to tachycardic; thready and weak if sepsis develops.
Respirations	Normal; labored and shallow as abdominal distention worsens.
Blood pressure	Normal; hypotensive if sepsis develops or hypertensive if acute pain is uncontrolled.
History	
Symptoms, conditions	Chemotherapy administration up to 14 days (approximately) prior to onset of typhlitis.
Hallmark physical signs and symptoms	Neutropenia, fever, moderate-to-severe abdominal pain and distention, hypoactive-to-absent bowel sounds.
Additional physical signs and symptoms	Abdominal pain (localized to the right lower quadrant or diffuse, intermittent cramping or constant dull ache), diarrhea (watery and/or bloody), nausea, vomiting, mucositis, tympany, ileus, rebound tenderness.

ASSESSMENT CRITERIA: TYPHLITIS IN PEDIATRICS (continued)

Psychosocial signs	Irritability, anxiety.

Lab values	
Absolute neutrophil count (ANC)/mm³	Decreased, neutropenic.
Platelets	Decreased, thrombocytopenic.
Hemoglobin	Normal
Microorganisms	Common bacterial isolates include *Pseudomonas, Escherichia coli, Klebsiella,* and *Clostridium.* Common fungal isolates include *Candida, Aspergillus,* and *Cryptococcus.*
Other	Altered renal function tests due to diarrhea, dehydration, vomiting, ascites, and sepsis.

Diagnostic tests	
Abdominal radiograph (plain film)	May reveal a nonspecific bowel gas pattern in the right lower quadrant, a fluid-filled, distended cecum with dilated small bowel loops, and decreased-to-absent large bowel gas (Katz et al., 1990).
Abdominal ultrasound	Often demonstrates more clearly the thickened bowel wall and dilated loops of the bowel with a characteristic "thumb-printing" pattern that indicates edema or hemorrhage.
Abdominal CT scan	A sensitive test and can be used to rule out appendicitis and intussusception when the plain film and ultrasound are not conclusive.

NURSING DIAGNOSIS

The priority of the following nursing diagnoses may change, depending on the severity and presentation of the disease process.

(Potential risk for) infection related to:
- Low absolute neutrophil count (ANC).
- Positive blood or stool culture.
- Mucositis.
- Altered skin integrity.
- Postoperative complications.

(Potential for) fluid volume deficit related to:
- Fluid loss through vomiting, gastric suction, and diarrhea.
- Decreased oral intake secondary to NPO status for bowel rest.

(Potential for) altered nutrition, less than body requirements, related to:
- Nausea, vomiting, and diarrhea.
- Decreased oral intake secondary to NPO/bowel rest.
- Increased metabolic demands (i.e., fever, tissue healing).

Pain related to:
- Abdominal distention.
- Mucositis, esophagitis, gastritis.
- Intestinal obstruction.
- Surgical intervention.

(Potential for) knowledge deficit related to typhlitis disease process, treatment, and sequelae.

NURSING INTERVENTIONS

Immediate nursing interventions

Assess heart rate, blood pressure, respirations, and temperature q4h initially, then q1–2h if clinical status worsens.

Obtain blood cultures before first dose of antibiotics are given. Administer initial doses of antibiotics STAT.

Keep client NPO.

Maintain patent NG tube to low intermittent suction to promote abdominal decompression.

Closely monitor and record abdominal assessment q4h and PRN if clinical status worsens:
- Measure abdominal girth to detect changes in abdominal distention.
- Assess bowel sounds, color of abdomen, tympany, any palpable mass, tenseness, or pain.
- Assess for nausea, vomiting, diarrhea, GI bleeding.

Anticipated physician orders and interventions

Broad-spectrum antibiotics. Repeat blood cultures each 24 hours in presence of continued fever.

CBC with differential qd.

Transfuse client with packed red blood cells, platelets, and granulocytes to maintain hemostasis.

Serum electrolyte panel qd.

IV fluids/parenteral nutrition to maintain adequate hydration and electrolyte balance. Intake and output (I and O) q4–8h.

Colony-stimulating factors qd.

Pain medications as needed. (See Chapter 33 for further information on this aspect of care.)

Abdominal radiographs qd or as clinically indicated.

Vasopressors as indicated to maintain blood pressure and perfusion. (See Chapter 38 for further details of managing perfusion in the client with typhlitis who becomes septic and requires vasopressors.)

Ongoing nursing assessment, monitoring, and interventions

Assess:
- Abdomen for color, bowel sounds, tympany, palpable mass, tenseness, or pain q4h.
- For abdominal distention q4h.
- For GI bleeding.
- For nausea and vomiting.
- Respiratory status q4h.

Measure:
- Blood pressure, heart rate, respiratory rate, and temperature q4h, then q1–2h if clinical condition worsens.
- Amount of NG tube output/emesis/stool.
- NG tube output/emesis/stool for occult blood.
- Abdominal girth q4h.
- I and O q4–8h.
- Weight qd.

Send:
- Blood and stool for cultures.
- CBC with differential.
- Serum renal and liver function tests.

Implement:
- Antibiotic therapy.
- NPO for bowel rest.
- Gastric decompression with use of NG tube.
- Blood product support and colony-stimulating factors.
- Fluid and electrolyte replacement and nutritional support.
- Pain management therapy.

TEACHING/EDUCATION

IV antibiotics: *Rationale:* A fever is the most common sign of infection in a person who has a low neutrophil count. Infection can cause some of the damage in the bowel that is part of typhlitis. Until your body (your child's body) can fight off an infection with the white blood cells, intravenous antibiotics are used to keep the infection under control. If fevers continue after the antibiotics have been used for a few days, then more or different antibiotics are added to get the infection under control. It is better to give the antibiotics into the vein than by mouth because more of the drug is able to fight the infection.

IV blood samples for CBC: *Rationale:* There are three main types of cells in your (your child's) blood: platelets, red blood cells, and white blood cells. Platelets help to make a clot and prevent bleeding. Red blood cells carry hemoglobin, which is used to carry oxygen throughout the body. White blood cells, especially the neutrophils (which are also called granulocytes), are needed to defend against infection.

It is important to know what your (your child's) platelet count is because of the risk of bleeding in the bowels. When the platelet count is low, the doctors will order a platelet transfusion to help prevent bleeding. If you (your child) would need surgery, the platelet count also needs to be close to normal levels.

The hemoglobin in the blood carries oxygen through your (your child's) body. The walls of the bowels can become more damaged if there is not enough oxygen there. When the hemoglobin is low, the doctor will order a packed red blood cell transfusion to help the bowels have enough oxygen supplied to them.

The white blood cells (especially the neutrophils) are used to fight bacterial infections. They also help with healing in an area of infection. Infection can add to the damage that is in your (your child's) bowels. There are a couple of ways to help raise the neutrophil count. Medicines like G-CSF (granulocyte colony-stimulating factor) can be given to help the bone marrow make more granulocytes (or neutrophils). It may take days to weeks to see the neutrophil count rise while G-CSF is given. As the neutrophil count starts to recover, it may increase and decrease for the first several days. This is because the cells are not staying in the blood stream. They go to the areas of infection in the bowel and throughout the body to help heal the tissues.

Giving white blood cell transfusions can also help bring up the neutrophil count. But the increase only lasts for several hours because the cells are destroyed as they kill bacteria. That's why white blood cell transfusions need to be given once or twice a day to help keep the count up.

NG tube/NPO status: *Rationale:* Your (your child's) bowels are weakened from the side effects of the chemotherapy. When any food or liquids move through the bowels, there is pressure on the bowel walls. The pressure could cause the bowel to burst. Then the bacteria and germs that are usually kept inside the bowels would be spilled into the abdominal space. This could cause a serious infection. The nasogastric tube is needed to keep the fluid out of the bowels so the pressure in the bowel is able to stay low. This is also why you (your child) can't eat and drink. NPO is the hospital term that means "nothing by mouth."

Frequent measurement of abdominal girth, serial physical exams, and abdominal x-rays: *Rationale:* As the pressure inside your (your child's) bowel increases or decreases, it will cause the outside of the abdomen to change in size or appearance. The doctors need to tell when changes in pressure are happening so they can decide if the treatment needs to be changed. The measurement of the abdominal girth and the physical exams are simple ways to watch what is happening. The abdominal x-rays provide a more detailed description about what is happening inside the bowel.

Surgery consult: *Rationale:* It is helpful for the surgeons to know about you (your child) so they can be ready if you need surgery. It is hoped that your (or your child's) bowel will get better without an operation. The surgeons are able to help you decide if you (your child) should have surgery.

IV fluid administration: *Rationale:* Your (your child's) body needs certain amounts of water and other substances such as salt, potassium, and bicarbonate to function properly. During this time you (your child) are not allowed to eat or drink, the IV fluids are needed to provide these things to the body. If you (your child) are having vomiting or diarrhea, these substances are being lost from the body and need to be replaced.

TPN: *Rationale:* Your (your child's) body needs calories to survive and to provide energy. All of the cells need energy to be able to do their work. During this time you (your child) cannot have any food by mouth, it is very hard to provide enough calories by just using regular IV fluids. TPN (total parenteral nutrition) is a combination that includes sugar, water, vitamins, minerals, and fat. Using TPN is the best way to provide nourishment for you (your child) during the time that you (your child) can't eat or drink.

Pain management: *Rationale:* No one wants you (your child) to be in pain. It is important that your (your child's) pain level be watched and treated. Pain is a symptom that could show changes in your (your child's) condition. Changes in treatment are sometimes needed when your (your child's) condition changes. The doctors will check to see how much pain medicine is being used and how you (your child) feel about the current pain control plan. This will help the doctors know if the pain is getting better or worse and if the dosage of pain medicine needs to be adjusted.

EVALUATION/DESIRED OUTCOMES

1. The client will not experience intestinal perforation.
2. GI bleeding will diminish within 24 hours of the initiation of medical management.
3. The client will exhibit negative blood and stool cultures within 24 hours of starting antibiotics.
4. Nausea, vomiting, and diarrhea will diminish within 24 to 48 hours after NPO and NG tube placement.
5. Serum electrolyte panel will return to normal values within 72 hours of starting IV fluid support.
6. The client's pain will be controlled during hospitalization.
7. Abdominal film, ultrasound, and CT scan will not indicate progression of typhlitis within 72 hours of the initiation of medical management.
8. The client will be afebrile before discharge.
9. The complete blood count (CBC) with differential will return to normal values before discharge.

10. The client and/or family members will verbalize understanding of the tests, procedures, and interventions for the child with typhlitis during hospitalization.
11. Family members will demonstrate the appropriate skills for the child's care at home prior to discharge.

DISCHARGE PLANNING

The client with typhlitis may need:

Short-term enteral or parenteral nutrition if unable to take adequate food and fluids orally.

Family members to manage the enteral or parenteral intake.

Intermittent home nursing visits to assist with the nutrition regimen, and to obtain blood specimens that monitor the nutritional status and blood cell count recovery.

FOLLOW-UP CARE

Anticipated care

Physician office visit within 1 week.

Home nursing visit for outpatient lab testing of TPN labs (renal and liver function tests), and CBC one to two times per week until client is able to resume full oral diet and all blood cell counts have recovered.

Continued packed red blood cell and/or platelet transfusions as indicated either per home nursing visit, in outpatient clinic, or on short-stay unit.

Weekly weight assessment in physician's office.

Resumption of chemotherapy after bowel has healed and blood cell counts have recovered.

Anticipated client/family questions and possible answers

Will this problem with my (my child's) bowels happen again?

"It is possible that this problem will happen again. We will watch for it during the next time that your (your child's) neutrophil count is low after chemotherapy. It is helpful for you (your child) to know the signs of typhlitis and to report them promptly when they occur."

Why will a nurse be coming to my home?

"The nurse will come to take blood samples to see if a transfusion is needed. The nurse may also come to your home to give you (your child) the transfusion. Blood samples also are used to plan any changes in the TPN or other nutritional sources. The nurse will also check to see how well you (your child) can eat and drink."

When can chemotherapy be given again?

"Several things need to happen before more chemotherapy can be given. The blood cell counts need to be back to normal without transfusions. Blood cultures need to be negative, and the course of antibiotics must be finished. Also, we wait for the bowel to heal before chemotherapy is given. Generally it is safe to give the next cycle of chemotherapy a week or two after your (your child's) discharge from the hospital."

CHAPTER SUMMARY

Typhlitis is an intestinal complication that occurs in some children undergoing cancer therapy. It may be seen in children with leukemia, lymphoma, or other solid tumors that require aggressive chemotherapy. Despite varying diagnoses and chemotherapy regimens, children with typhlitis share common factors. They are profoundly neutropenic, develop fever, and require hospitalization for IV antibiotics. In spite of medical management, frequently the client's condition does not improve. They may have persistent neutropenia, fever, abdominal pain and distention, as well as other symptoms of typhlitis. This situation becomes an oncologic emergency because of the risk of bowel perforation and potential life-threatening peritonitis or sepsis in the client who has no neutrophils.

Careful assessment and timely nursing interventions contribute to improved outcomes for the clients with typhlitis. The care of these children is focused on monitoring for and preventing perforation, and providing supportive care until the child's neutrophil count recovers and the bowel tissue heals. Nurses play an integral role in the care of the child with typhlitis.

TEST QUESTIONS

1. The greatest risk for a client with typhlitis is:
   A. Infection
   B. Ileus
   C. Perforation
   D. Neutropenia

1. Answer: C
Perforation of the bowel can cause overwhelming peritonitis, contributing to sepsis and, potentially, to death.

2. Typhlitis is most often associated with which type of cancer in children?
   A. Hodgkin's lymphoma
   B. Osteogenic sarcoma
   C. Astrocytoma
   D. Acute nonlymphocytic leukemia

2. Answer: D
Typhlitis occurs most often in children with a hematologic malignancy such as acute nonlymphocytic leukemia; although less often it is seen in children with a variety of solid tumors following aggressive chemotherapy.

3. Typhlitis is usually treated by which of the following types of interventions?
   A. Chemotherapy
   B. Radiation
   C. Surgery
   D. Medications

3. Answer: D
Side effects from chemotherapy and radiation can both contribute to the development of typhlitis. Medications are the most common type of treatment intervention; surgery is reserved for cases of necrosis or perforation.

4. Diagnostic tests for the client suspected of having typhlitis include all of the following *except:*
   A. Abdominal ultrasound
   B. Barium enema
   C. Abdominal CT scan
   D. Abdominal x-ray

4. Answer: B
A barium enema is contraindicated in the client with suspected typhlitis because of the risk for intestinal perforation.

5. The pathophysiology of typhlitis is related to all of the following *except:*
   A. Broad-spectrum antibiotics use
   B. Decreased vascularity of the cecum
   C. Mucositis
   D. Leukocytosis

5. Answer: D
Broad-spectrum antibiotics promote the growth of resistant bacteria or fungus in the bowel; the risk for necrosis in the cecum is higher than for other sections of the bowel owing in part to the decreased vascularity; mucositis of the intestinal tract allows for bacterial invasion of the bowel wall.

6. What are possible clinical signs and symptoms associated with typhlitis?
   A. Hepatomegaly and alopecia
   B. Constipation and fever
   C. Afebrile and skin rash
   D. Abdominal pain and diarrhea

6. Answer: D
These are two of the most common clinical signs and symptoms of typhlitis.

7. Typhlitis most commonly occurs in the:
   A. Cecum
   B. Duodenum
   C. Stomach
   D. Jejunum

7. Answer: A
Typhlitis most commonly occurs in the cecum because of its decreased vascularity, decreased lymphatic drainage, and increased distensibility.

8. Which of the following factors does *not* put the client at risk for potential alteration in nutritional status?
   A. Nausea and vomiting
   B. Watery diarrhea
   C. Neutropenia
   D. Increased metabolic demands

8. Answer: C
Neutropenia alone does not put the client at risk for potential alteration in nutritional status.

9. An expected outcome for the client with typhlitis would be:
   A. CBC will return to normal within 24 hours.
   B. Pain will be managed during hospitalization.
   C. Cultures will be negative prior to starting antibiotics.
   D. The client will be afebrile within 48 hours after starting antibiotics.

9. Answer: B
Pain management is a very important expected outcome for the client with typhlitis.

10. Which one of the following types of medications is contraindicated for the client with typhlitis?
    A. Broad-spectrum antibiotics
    B. Colony-stimulating factors
    C. Antidiarrheal agents
    D. Pressors

10. Answer: C
The use of anticholinergic (particularly antidiarrheal) agents is contraindicated because they decrease the GI tract motility.

REFERENCES

Aitken TJ: Gastrointestinal manifestations in the child with cancer. J Pediatr Oncol Nurs 9(3):99–109, 1992.

Angel CA, Bhaskar NR, Wrenn E, Lobe TE, Kumar APM: Acute appendicitis in children with leukemia and other malignancies: Still a diagnostic dilemma. J Pediatr Surg 27(4):476–479, 1992.

Earnest D, Schneiderman D: Other diseases of the colon and rectum. In Sleisenger M, Fordtran J (eds): Gastrointestinal Disease: Pathophysiology, Diagnosis, Management, 4th ed. Philadelphia: WB Saunders Co, 1989, pp. 1592–1631.

Gavan DR, Hendry GMA: Colonic complication of acute lymphoblastic leukaemia. Br J Radiol 67(797):449–452, 1994.

Hiruki T, Fernandes B, Ramsay J, Rother I: Acute typhlitis in an immunocompromised host. Report of unusual case and review of the literature. Dig Dis Sci 37(8):1292–1296, 1992.

Jones B, Wall SD: Gastrointestinal disease in the immunocompromised host. Radiol Clin North Am 30(3):555–576, 1992.

Katz JA, Wagner ML, Gresik MV, Mahoney DH, Fernbach DJ: Typhlitis: An 18 year experience and postmortem review. Cancer 65:1041–1047, 1990.

Kunkel JM, Rosenthal D: Management of the ileocecal syndrome: Neutropenic enterocolitis. Dis Colon Rectum 29:196–199, 1986.

Panzarella C, Duncan J: Nursing management of physical care needs. In Foley GV, Fochtman D, Mooney KH (eds): Nursing Care of the Child with Cancer. Philadelphia: WB Saunders Co, 1983, pp. 347–348.

Paulino AFG, Kenney R, Forman EN, Medeiros LJ: Typhlitis in a patient with acute lymphoblastic leukemia prior to the administration of chemotherapy. Am J Pediatr Hematol Oncol 16(4):348–351, 1994.

Sloas MM, Flynn PM, Kaste SC, Patrick CC: Typhlitis in children with cancer: A 30 year experience. Clin Infect Dis 17(3):484–490, 1993.

Smith LH, VanGulick AJ: Management of neutropenic enterocolitis in the patient with cancer. Oncol Nurs Forum 19(9):1337–1344, 1992.

Wade DS, Nava HR, Douglass HO: Neutropenic enterocolitis: Clinical diagnosis and treatment. Cancer 69(1):17–23, 1992.

Wagner M, Rosenberg H, Fernbach D, Singleton E: Typhlitis: A complication of leukemia in childhood. Am J Roentgenol 109(2):341–350, 1970.

Index

Note: Pages in *italic* indicate illustrations; those followed by t refer to tables.